Michael T. Murray ND is a leading researcher, lecturer and writer in the field of natural medicine, and a member of the faculty of the Bastyr College, Seattle. He is a consultant to the natural food/supplement industry, and the co-author of *A Textbook of Natural Medicine*.

Joseph E. Pizzorno Jr ND is president and co-founder of the Bastyr College, and a prominent educator, lecturer and writer in natural medicine. He is the editor of two journals in the field, and the co-author of *A Textbook of Natural Medicine*.

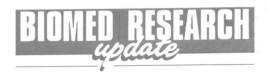

Study Reveals Potent Antioxidant Activity of OptiZinc®

Researchers at Creighton University, Omaha Nebraska, have found that OptiZinc®, a dietary zinc supplement, possesses antioxidant activity comparable to vitamins E,C and beta carotene, significantly more antioxidant activity than other forms of zinc tested.

The findings, announced April 10th at the Federation of American Societies for Experimental Biology (FASEB) conference in Atlanta, were presented by Dr. Debasis Bagchi, Assistant Professor at Creighton University of Pharmaceutical Sciences.

According to Dr. Bagehi, "OptiZinc could serve as a useful dietary supplement in helping to neutralise harmful free radicals caused by pollution, tobacco smoke, excess sunlight and other sources."

Vitamins E, C and Beta-carotene have gained in popularity over recent years primarily due to their antioxidant role in the human body. Antioxidants neutralise free radicals, which are highly reactive molecules that can cause significant cellular damage. Many scientists now believe that free radical damage can lead to cancer, heart disease, cataracts, arthritis and other chronic diseases, as well as premature aging.

The researchers compared the free radical scavenging effects of Optizinc with vitamins E, C and beta-carotene plus other forms of zinc such as zinc oxide, sulphate, citrate, gluconate and

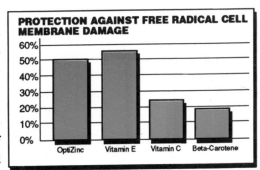

Chart 1. Percent Inhibition of TPA-induced LDH cell membrane leakage of various antioxidants in vitro

Continued over....

picolinate. According to Dr. Bagechi, OptiZinc was nearly as effective as vitamin E, more effective than vitamin C and Beta carotene, and four to six times more effective than other forms of Zinc tested.

Zinc, an essential trace mineral, is vital for cell growth and immune function but a growing body of research is showing that zinc plays an important role in the body's antioxidant system as well. A 1993 study at the University of California, Davis Department of Nutrition, showed that OptiZinc helped reduce excess levels of superoxide free radicals produced by white blood cells.

"OptiZinc's ability to neutralise free radicals is not its only health-promoting effect", states Bagchi. "It also helps detoxify cellular membranes by displacing toxic metabolites and heavy metals from biological tissues."

According to Bagchi, OptiZinc may serve as a new weapon in preventing certain chronic diseases, increasing longevity and promoting good health.

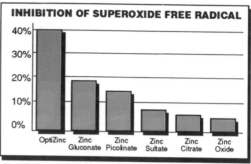

Chart 2. Percent Inhibition of superoxide free radical by various zinc supplements in vitro

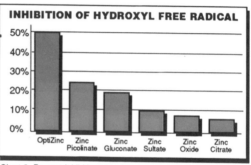

Chart 3. Percent Inhibition of hydroxyl free radical by various zinc supplements in vitro

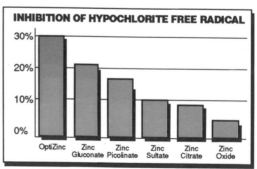

Chart 4. Percent Inhibition of hypochlorite free radical by various zinc supplements in vitro

AN ENCYCLOPAEDIA OF NATURAL MEDICINE

Michael T. Murray N.D.
Joseph E. Pizzorno N.D.

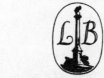

LITTLE, BROWN AND COMPANY
BOSTON NEW YORK TORONTO LONDON

A *Little, Brown* Book

© Joseph Pizzorno and Michael Murray, 1990.

First published in 1990 by
Macdonald Optima, a division of
Macdonald & Co. (Publishers) Ltd

Reprinted in 1992, 1993
Reprinted by Little, Brown and Company (UK) 1995
Reprinted 1996

British Library Cataloguing in Publication Data

Murray, Michael
    Encyclopaedia of natural medicine
    1. Medicine, Naturopathy
    I. Title   II. Pizzorno, Joseph
    615.5'35

ISBN 0 316 87779 4

Little, Brown and Company (UK)
Brettenham House
Lancaster Place
London WC2E 7EN

Typeset in Parlament by Leaper & Gard Ltd, Bristol

Printed and bound in Great Britain by
BPC Hazell Books Ltd
A member of
The British Printing Company Ltd

TO THE BEAUTY, TRUTH AND WISDOM OF NATUROPATHIC MEDICINE.

This book is dedicated both to naturopathic medicine and all the natural healing arts of the past and of the future, and to those physicians and healers who have bestowed the virtues of the 'healing power of nature' throughout history and those who will do so in the future.

Contents

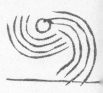

CONTENTS

Acknowledgments

Most of all I would like to acknowledge that inner voice that has guided me in my life, providing me with inspiration, strength and humility at the most appropriate times.

I have also been blessed by having wonderful parents whose support and faith have never waned. If every child was loved as much as I was it would truly be a wonderful world. Thank you Mom and Dad.

This work represents a great deal of things to me, including commitment and dedication. In addition to my parents, people who have truly inspired me include Terry Lemerond, Dr Ralph Weiss, Anthony Robbins, Dr Ed Madison, Dr Bill Mitchell, Phi Nu Sigma fraternity and the entire JBC community. A special thanks to all of those who have helped me 'live with passion'.

And finally, I am deeply honoured to have Dr Joe Pizzorno, not only as my co-author, but also as a valued friend.

Michael T. Murray, ND

Many people have helped me through my life – to be a better human being, to be a healer, to be an educator. Hopefully, this work will help to repay all the caring I have received.

In particular, I would like to thank my parents Joe and May Pizzorno for their love and support, May Ann Feller for humanising me, John Bastyr ND for inspiration, Jeff Bland PhD for helping me see how to bring science into natural medicine and Sheila Quinn for friendship and helping make John Bastyr College a reality.

Finally, and most important, my appreciation and love for my wonderful wife Lara and daughter Raven for their inexhaustible love and patience. They mean the world to me.

Joseph E. Pizzorno Jr ND

The publishers would like to thank Jennie Smith for the illustrations.

Preface

This book was written in an effort to update the public's knowledge on the use of 'natural' medicines in the maintenance of health and treatment of disease. It dispels a common myth about the use of natural remedies – that natural medicine is 'unscientific'. This book contains information based on firm scientific inquiry and represents countless hours of research. This is without question the most thoroughly researched and referenced book on the use of natural medicines ever written for the public.

The book must not be used in place of a physician or qualified healthcare practitioner. It is designed for use in conjunction with the services provided by physicians practising natural medicine. Readers are strongly urged to develop a good relationship with a physician knowledgeable in the art and science of natural and preventive medicine, such as a naturopathic physician. In all cases involving a physical or medical complaint, ailment or therapy, please consult a physician. Proper medical care and advice can significantly improve the quality and duration of your life.

With this in mind, it can be stated that the information in this book is meant to be used, not simply read. Commit yourself to following the guidelines of natural healthcare as outlined in this book and you will be rewarded immensely. Your reward will be a life full of health, vitality and vigour.

Michael T. Murray ND
Joseph E. Pizzorno, ND

PART ONE

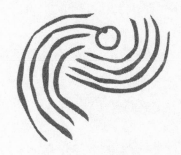

*Introduction
to
natural medicine*

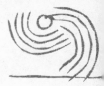

1

What is natural medicine?

The doctor of the future will give no medicine, but will interest his patient in the care of the human frame, in diet and in the cause and prevention of disease.

Thomas Edison

Introduction

A revolution is occurring in health care. Science and medicine now have in their possession the technology and understanding necessary to appreciate the value of 'natural' therapies. Edison's words above are truly prophetic. And at the forefront of this revolution is naturopathic medicine.

Although the term naturopathy was not used until the late 19th century, its philosophical roots can be traced back to Hippocrates. It is a system of health-oriented medicine which stresses maintenance of health and prevention of disease. It contrasts with the current disease-oriented system greatly. For example, physicians often tell patients 'Your blood pressure is a little elevated. We'll need to have you come in every few months to check on it' (meaning it's not bad enough for drugs yet); or 'Your Pap smear came back a class III. We'll need to repeat it in two months to see if it changes' (meaning hopefully it will get better on its own, but if it doesn't we'll do a cone biopsy, i.e. surgically remove the inner part of the cervix); or 'Sure, you're tired. You're getting older now, it's normal.'

Each of these is an example of an easily treatable condition which frequently progresses to significant disease because appropriate preventive measures are not employed; this is exactly what happens in our current health care (don't we mean disease-treatment?) system. The average westerner has an unhealthy, disease-promoting lifestyle, but the tools the typical medical doctor has (i.e. drugs and surgery) never address this underlying factor. Although effective when appropriately applied (such as surgery for appendicitis), drugs and surgery often have too many side effects to be used in the treatment of many early, common and/or recurring problems people have.

In contrast, the naturopathic physician is trained in finding the underlying cause rather than treating or suppressing the symptoms. Naturopathic doctors don't wait for disease to progress before they institute appropriate preventive measures. Remember, an ounce of prevention is worth a pound of cure. The examples given above (precancerous changes on the cervix, hypertension, symptoms attributed to 'old age') are easily preventable diseases in the making.

- Cervical cancer is the second most common malignancy found in women aged 15–34, but what the typical doctor doesn't know is that 67 per cent of patients with cervical cancer are deficient in one or more nutrients,[1] and as a group have a level of serum beta-carotene (critical for the prevention of cancer of cells like those in the cervix) only one-half that of normal women.[2]

- Over 90 per cent of people with high blood pressure have 'essential' or 'idiopathic' hypertension,[3] meaning the typical doctor does not know what is causing the elevation. The naturopathic doctor knows – it is virtually always due to dietary and lifestyle factors.[4]

- When properly diagnosed, elderly patients are often found to have easily treatable problems which are causing unnecessary debility, e.g. over half of those over 60 have been found to have hypochlorhydria (low levels of hydrochloric acid in the stomach) which leads to malnutrition,[5,6] and other problems such as osteoporosis.[7]

The more one studies the causes of the common health problems of our age, the more apparent it becomes that naturopathic medicine has much to offer. Thomas Edison's 'doctor of the future' is here today, and has been available since the turn of the century when the first naturopathic college was established.

History

Naturopathic medicine grew out of alternative healing systems of the 18th and 19th centuries, but traces its philosophical roots to the Hippocratic school of medicine (*circa* 400 BC). Over the centuries, natural medicine and techno-medicine (a term coined to refer to the currently dominant school of medicine) have alternatively diverged and converged, shaping each other, often in reaction.

Prehistoric people believed that disease was caused by magic or supernatural forces, such as devils or angry gods. Hippocrates, breaking with this superstitious belief, became the first naturalistic doctor in recorded history. Hippocratic practitioners assumed that everything in nature had a rational basis; therefore, the physician's role was to understand and follow the laws of the intelligible universe. They viewed disease as an effect and looked for its cause in natural phenomena – air, water, food, etc. They used the term *vis medicatrix naturae*, the healing power of nature, to denote the body's ability to heal itself.

Naturopathy, or 'nature cure', is both a way of life and a concept of healing employing various natural means of preventing and treating human disease. The earliest mechanisms of healing associated with the term naturopathy involved a combination of hygienics and hydrotherapy. The term itself was coined in 1895 by Dr John Scheel of New York City to describe his method of health care. But earlier forerunners of these concepts already existed in the history of natural healing, both in America and in the Austro-Germanic European core.

Benedict Lust (whose teachings and organisational energy initiated naturopathy in the US) began using the term 'naturopathy' in 1902 to name the eclectic compilation of doctrines of natural healing that he envisioned as the future scope of natural medicine, and to include the best of what is now known as nutritional therapy, natural diet, herbal medicine, homeopathy, spinal manipulation, exercise therapy, hydrotherapy, electrotherapy, stress reduction and nature cure. In one of the many journals and books he published, 'The principles, aim and program of the nature cure', he described naturopathy[8]:

> The natural system for curing disease is based on a return to nature in regulating the diet, breathing, exercising, bathing and the employment of various forces to eliminate the poisonous products in the system, and so raise the vitality of the patient to a proper standard of health.
>
> THE PROGRAM OF NATUROPATHIC CURE
>
> 1. ELIMINATION OF EVIL HABITS, or the weeds of life, such as over-eating, alcoholic drinks, drugs, the use of tea, coffee and cocoa that contain poisons, meat eating, improper hours of living, waste of vital forces, lowered vitality, sexual and social aberrations, worry, etc.
>
> 2. CORRECTIVE HABITS. Correct breathing, correct exercise, right mental attitude. Moderation in the pursuit of health and wealth.
>
> 3. NEW PRINCIPLES OF LIVING. Proper fasting, selection of food, hydropathy, light and air baths, mud baths, osteopathy, chiropractic and other forms of mechano-therapy, mineral salts obtained in organic form, electropathy, heliopathy, steam or Turkish baths, sitz baths, etc. . . .
>
> There is really but one healing force in existence and that is Nature herself, which means the inherent restorative power of the organism to overcome disease. Now the question is, can this power be appropriated and guided more readily by extrinsic or intrinsic methods? That is to say, is it more amenable to combat disease by irritating drugs, vaccines and serums employed by superstitious moderns, or by the bland intrinsic congenial forces of Natural Therapeutics, that are employed by this new school of medicine, that is Naturopathy, which is the only orthodox school of medicine? Are not these natural forces much more orthodox than the artificial resources of the druggist? The practical application of these natural agencies, duly suited to the individual case, are true signs that the art of healing has been elaborated by the aid of absolutely harmless, congenial treatments.

Naturopathic medicine grew and flourished in the United States in the early part of the 20th century until the mid-1930s, when several factors resulted in the opportunity for the medical profession to establish the foundation for its current virtual monopoly of health care: foundations supported by the chemical and drug industries began heavily subsidising medical schools; the medical profession finally stopped using their 'heroic' therapies (blood letting and mercury dosing) and were able to replace them with therapies that were more effective for treating symptoms and much less toxic; and the medical profession became much more politically astute and, using the tremendous technological advances in surgery promoted by the two world wars, were able to convince both the public and politicians of the apparent superiority of their system, resulting in the passing of legislation that severely restricted the viability of other health care systems.[9]

Philosophy

Vis medicatrix naturae – the healing power of nature. Fundamental to the practice of naturopathic medicine is a profound belief in the ability of the body to heal itself, given the proper opportunity. The strict corollary of this is, to quote Hippocrates, 'do no evil', i.e. very carefully avoid both practices which weaken the body's ability to heal itself and therapies which take over a function of the body. Needless to say, this philosophy has limits, and at times the body needs more than just supportive help. The goal of the naturopathic doctor in such situations is to use the least invasive intervention that will have the desired therapeutic effect. This philosophical approach necessitates a broad range of diagnostic and therapeutic skills and accounts for the eclectic interests of the naturopathic profession.

Since the days of Benedict Lust, naturopathic medicine has continued in its eclectic ways. Although the profession has evolved into a primary healthcare system providing services from natural childbirth and family practice through to preventive and therapeutic medicine, the principles are still the same – education of the patient in the laws of healthy living, support of the body's own healing abilities and the use of natural and non-toxic therapies. Key to the success of naturopathic treatments is the high level of involvement of patients in their own healing process.

Naturopathic medicine is 'vitalistic' in its approach, i.e. life is viewed as more than just the sum of biochemical processes, and the body is believed to have an innate intelligence that is always striving for health. Vitalism maintains that the symptoms accompanying disease are not directly caused by the morbific agent, e.g. bacteria; rather, they are the result of the organism's intrinsic response or reaction to the agent and the organism's attempt to defend and heal itself. Symptoms, then, are part of a constructive phenomenon that is the best 'choice' the organism can make, given the circumstances. In this construct, the role of the physician is to aid the body in its efforts, not to take over the functions of the body.

Health is viewed as more than just the absence of disease; it is considered to be a vital dynamic state which enables a person to thrive in, or adapt to, a wide range of environments and stresses. People who 'catch' every cold that comes by are not healthy when they are symptom free; they can be considered healthy only when they stop being overly susceptible to infection.

Health and disease can be looked at as points on a continuum, with death at one end and optimal function at the other. As the typical person goes through life, s/he drifts away from optimal function and moves relentlessly towards progressively greater dysfunction. Although such deterioration is endorsed by our society as the normal expectation of aging, it does not happen to animals in the wild, or to those few fortunate peoples who live in an optimal environment, i.e. no pollution, low stress, regular exercise and abundant natural, nutritious food. Death is indeed inevitable, but progressive disability is not.

Areas of therapy

Many naturopaths choose to specialise in specific areas of therapy while others choose to be eclectic. A wide variety of different types of therapy can be employed by the naturopathic physician in the treatment of an individual, including nutrition, botanical medicines, homeopathy, acupuncture, physiotherapy, counselling and lifestyle modification. These areas will be briefly described below.

Nutrition

Clinical nutrition, or the use of diet as a therapy, serves as the foundation of naturopathic medicine. There is an ever increasing body of knowledge that supports the use of wholefoods and nutritional supplements in the maintenance of health and treatment of disease. Many common conditions can be treated effectively by dietary measures, including acne, arthritis, asthma, atherosclerosis, depression, diabetes (type II), eczema, gout, hypertension, irritable bowel syndrome, premenstrual syndrome and ulcerative colitis.

Botanical medicine

Plants have been used as medicines since antiquity. With the advent of the pharmaceutical industry in this century, the popularity of herbal medicine declined (although 25 per cent of all prescription drugs contain ingredients isolated from plants). Currently there is a renaissance occurring in the appreciation of plants as medicinal agents. Technology now exists which allows for greater understanding of the manner in which herbs promote health and restore balance in disease. Naturopathic physicians are professionally trained herbalists and know both the historical uses of plants as well as modern pharmacological mechanisms.

Homeopathy

The term 'homeopathy' is derived from the Greek word *homeos*, meaning similar, and *pathos*, meaning disease. Homeopathy is a system of medicine that treats a disease with a dilute, potentised agent, or drug, that will produce the same symptoms as the disease when given to a healthy individual, the fundamental principle being that like cures like. This principle was actually first recognised by Hippocrates, who noticed that herbs given in low doses tended to cure the same symptoms they produced when given in toxic doses. Homeopathic medicines are derived from a variety of plant, mineral and chemical substances.

Acupuncture

Acupuncture is an ancient Chinese system of medicine involving the stimulation of certain specific points on the body to enhance the flow of vital energy (*chi*) along pathways called meridians. Acupuncture points can be stimulated by the insertion and withdrawing of needles, the application of heat (moxibustion), massage, laser, electrical means, or a combination of these methods. Traditional Chinese acupuncture implies a very specific acupuncture technique and knowledge of the oriental system of medicine including yin and yang, the five elements, acupuncture points and meridians, as well as a method of diagnosis and differentiation of syndromes quite different from that of western medicine.

Hydrotherapy

Hydrotherapy may be defined as the use of water in any of its forms (hot, cold, ice, steam, etc.) and methods of application (sitz bath, douche, spa and hot tubs, whirlpool, sauna, shower, immersion bath, pack, poultice, foot bath, fomentation, wrap, colonic irrigations, etc.) in the maintenance of health or treatment of disease. It is one of the ancient methods of treatment. Hydrotherapy has been used to treat disease and injury by many different cultures, including the Egyptians, Assyrians, Persians, Greeks, Hebrews, Hindus and Chinese.

Physical medicine

Physical medicine refers to the use of physical measures in the treatment of an individual. This includes the use of physiotherapy equipment such as ultrasound, diathermy and other electromagnetic techniques, therapeutic exercise, massage, joint mobilisation (manipulation) and immobilisation techniques, and hydrotherapy.

Counselling and lifestyle modification

Counselling and lifestyle modification techniques are essential to the naturopathic physician. A naturopath is a holistic-minded physician formally trained in the following counselling areas:
- interviewing and responding skills, active listening, assessing body language and other contact skills necessary for the therapeutic relationship;
- recognising and understanding prevalent psychological issues including developmental problems, abnormal behaviour, addictions, stress, sexuality, etc.;
- various treatment measures including hypnosis and guided imagery, counselling techniques, correcting underlying organic factors and family therapy.

Therapeutic approach

The therapeutic approach of the naturopathic doctor is basically two-fold: to help patients heal themselves (alas, most patients still come only when they are sick, too few while they are still healthy); and to use the opportunity to guide and educate the patient in developing a more healthy lifestyle.

A typical first visit to a naturopathic doctor takes one hour. The goal is to learn as much as possible about the patient, using thorough history taking, physical examination, laboratory tests, radiology and other standard diagnostic procedures. The patient's diet, environment, exercise, stress and other aspects of lifestyle are also evaluated. Once a good understanding of the patient's health and disease is established (making a diagnosis of a disease is only one part of this process), the doctor and patient work together to establish a treatment and health promoting programme.

Although every effort is made to treat the whole person, and just his/her disease, the limits of a short description like this necessitate the description of typical naturopathic therapies of those conditions previously described in a simplified, disease-oriented manner.

Cervical dysplasia

The typical treatment for the patient with cervical dysplasia, a precancerous condition of the cervix, would include:

- **Education** about factors that increase the risk of cervical cancer, such as smoking (risk = 3.0), multiple sex partners (risk = 3.4) and the use of oral contraceptives (risk = 3.6).[10]
- **Prevention**: her nutrition would be optimised (through diet and supplementation), particularly in regards to those nutrients known to be deficient (often a result of oral contraceptive use) in women with cervical dysplasia and whose deficiencies are known to promote cellular abnormalities – folic acid,[11] betacarotene,[4] vitamin C,[12] vitamin B6[13] and selenium.[4]
- **Treatment**: the vaginal depletion pack (a traditional mixture of botanical medicines placed against the cervix) would be used to promote sloughing of the abnormal cells.[14] For a woman with a class III Pap the process would usually involve about six visits for the vag packs, the taking of three or four nutritional supplements, and the modification of her diet and lifestyle.

The advantages of this approach are many: the causes of the cervical dysplasia have been identified and resolved, so the problem should not recur; no surgery is used, thus no scar tissue is formed; and the cost, particularly considering that many women with cervical dysplasia have recurrences when treated with standard surgery, is reasonable.

Essential hypertension

The patients with so-called idiopathic or essential hypertension can be very effectively treated, if they are willing to make the necessary lifestyle changes.

- **Diet**: numerous studies have shown that excessive dietary salt in conjunction with inadequate dietary potassium is a major contributor to hypertension[15,16,17]; that dietary deficiencies in calcium,[18,19] magnesium,[20,21] essential fatty acids[22,23] and vitamin C[24] all contribute to increased blood pressure; and that increased consumption of sugar,[25] caffeine[26] and alcohol[27] are all associated with hypertension.
- **Lifestyle**: smoking,[28] obesity,[29] stress[30] and a sedentary lifestyle are all known to contribute to the development of high blood pressure.
- **Environment**: exposure to heavy metals such as lead[31] and cadmium[32] increase blood pressure.

- **Botanical medicine**: many herbal medicines are used when necessary for the patient's safety, initially to lower his/her blood pressure rapidly until the slower, but more curative, dietary and lifestyle treatments can have their effects. Included are such age-old favourites as garlic (*Allium sativa*),[34] mistletoe (*Viscum album*),[34] hawthorn (*Crataegus monogyna*)[35] and others.[36]

The causes of high blood pressure are not unknown, they are unheeded!

Aging

Aging in our society is feared and its supposed treatment is highly commercialised. Considering the average person's lifestyle, the progressive disability of aging is not surprising. What is surprising is the willingness of some people simply to accept aging as unavoidable, and of others to expect to find miracles in bottles – be they drugs or vitamins. Unnecessary premature aging is preventable, but once again prevention is dependent on the willingness of the individual to adopt a healthy lifestyle and the ability and knowledge of their doctor to help them. The degenerative diseases typical of older people can often be treated, but are much more easily prevented – they are virtually all either caused by or accelerated by an unhealthy lifestyle. Instead of covering here specific diseases which are common in the elderly, such as atherosclerosis (the leading cause of death in the US), leucoplakia (a common precancerous condition) and diabetes (which affects 4 per cent of the US population), we will briefly discuss some of the most common lifestyle and health problems which underlie those diseases which cause most of the unnecessary death and disability of aging.

Hypochlorhydria, food allergy, nutritional deficiencies, intestinal toxaemia, the western diet, inappropriate farming techniques, stress, cigarette smoking, alcohol consumption, food additives, environmental pollution and a sedentary lifestyle are the primary causes of virtually all disease and disability in our society. Although each alone will not necessarily cause a specific disease in any given individual, cumulatively they seriously impair the ability of the body to function.

Let's consider how the typical westerner becomes progressively unhealthy.

- He eats foods which are deficient in minerals (such as zinc) since they are grown in synthetically fertilised soils.
- The low intake of zinc results in hypochlorhydria (the enzyme which produces hydrochloric acid in the stomach is carbonic anhydrase, a zinc-dependent metallo-enzyme) which leads to maldigestion and further nutritional deficiencies.
- The problem is further compounded by the development of food allergies, since he eats only relatively few different foods many times a day. (How often do you eat wheat?)
- Not only does he eat relatively few foods, but they are highly refined, resulting in the loss of important nutrients, and they are high in saturated fats and sugar, and low in important non-nutrients such as fibre, leading to further metabolic dysfunction.
- Now that the body's defences have been weakened, consider the constant exposure to various poisons – cigarette smoke, alcohol, inner city air, food additives, infectious bacteria, etc.

- He now starts getting sick.

At first he experiences minor inconveniences, such as frequent colds, coughs in the morning, and fatigue (momentarily relieved by caffeine consumption), but they progress. After a few years, he starts being bothered by a progressive sexual dysfunction as his prostate enlarges (due to a deficiency of zinc[37] and essential fatty acids[38]); he develops adult-onset diabetes (due directly to his western diet,[39] excessive sugar consumption, deficiencies in such nutrients as chromium[40,41] and biotin,[42] and many other controllable factors); and his blood pressure is elevated. Of course, he actually dies from lung cancer induced by his two-pack-a-day habit.

Lifestyle modification is crucial to the successful implementation of naturopathic techniques – health does not come from a doctor, pills or surgery, but rather from the patient's own efforts to take proper care of themselves. Unfortunately, our society expends considerable resources inducing disease-promoting habits. While it is relatively easy to tell a patient to stop smoking, get more exercise and reduce their stress, such lifestyle changes are difficult in the context of peer group pressure, habit and commercial pressure. The naturopathic doctor is specifically trained to assist the patient in making the needed changes. This involves many aspects: helping the patient acknowledge the need; setting realistic, progressive goals; establishing a support group of family and friends, or of others with similar problems; identifying the stimuli which reinforce the unhealthy behaviour; and giving the patient positive reinforcement for their gains.

Education

The education of the naturopathic physician is extensive, and incorporates much of the diversity that typifies the natural healthcare movement. The training programme is very similar to conventional medical education, with the primary differences being in the therapeutic sciences. To be eligible to enroll, prospective students must first successfully complete a conventional premedicine programme. The naturopathic curriculum then takes an additional four years to complete.

The first two years concentrate on the standard human biological sciences covering anatomy, physiology, biochemistry, pathology, microbiology, etc. The second two years are oriented towards the clinical sciences of diagnosis and treatment. Although the standard diagnostic techniques of physical, laboratory and radiological examination are taught, what makes the programme unique is its emphasis on preventive diagnosis, such as diet analysis, the early physical signs of nutritional deficiencies, and on natural therapies, such as nutrition, botanical medicines, homeopathy, acupuncture, natural childbirth, hydrotherapy, fasting, physical therapy, exercise therapy, counselling and lifestyle modification.

The future of naturopathic medicine

To the uninformed, naturopathic medicine, as well as the entire concept of natural medicine, appears to be a fad that will soon pass away. To the informed, it is clear that naturopathic medicine will be to the forefront of medical practice in the future.

One of the great fallacies promoted by the United States medical establishment is that there is no firm scientific evidence for the use of many natural therapies. This assumption is simply not true. During the 1970s and 1980s there has been an explosion of information in the scientific literature supporting the use of natural medicines. Science and medicine now have in their possession the technology and understanding necessary to appreciate many aspects of natural medicine. It is becoming increasingly common for medical organisations that in the past have spoken out strongly against naturopathic medicine now to endorse such naturopathic techniques as lifestyle modification, stress reduction, exercise, consuming a high fibre diet rich in wholefoods and other dietary measures, and many others.

This illustrates the shift that is occurring in medicine. What were once scoffed at are now becoming generally accepted as effective alternatives. In fact in most instances the naturopathic alternative offers significant benefit over standard medical practices. Undoubtedly in the future many of the concepts, philosophies and practices of naturopathy will be vindicated.

Many of the advances in medicine in the future will be naturopathic in philosophy. For example, through genetic engineering it is now feasible for many substances natural to the body to be produced in the laboratory. Although it must be emphasised that these substances should be reserved for end-stage disease and should in no way circumvent appropriate preventive measures, appropriate use of many of these substances could be considered naturopathic in essence. Examples of such substances are monoclonal antibodies directed against specific tumour antigens; various antiviral and immuno-enhancing substances natural to the body in the treatment of acquired immunodeficiency syndrome (AIDS) such as interferon, interleukin, thymosin, etc.; atrial natriuretic peptide in severe congestive heart failure; and human growth hormone in the treatment of growth hormone deficiency.

Certainly the future looks very bright for naturopathic medicine.

Summary

Naturopathic medicine makes sense. The basic approach of a naturopathic physician is: discover and eliminate the causes of disease; when treatment is necessary, use the most natural, non-toxic and least invasive therapy available; treat the whole person; teach the patient to develop a healthy diet and lifestyle; and trust in the *vis medicatrix naturae*, the healing power of nature.

Further information on naturopathic medicine

For non-professionals

Healthy and Wise, a free newsletter of articles on health issues published approximately quarterly by the John Bastyr College Clinic, 1408 NE 45th, Seattle, WA 98105, USA, tel. 206-632-0354.

The Naturopath, a monthly newspaper containing news and articles about natural health care, from 1920 N. Kilpatrick, Portland, OR 97217, USA, tel. 503-285-3807.

For professionals

Pizzorno, J.E. and Murray, M.T. *A Textbook of Natural Medicine*, John Bastyr College Publications, 1988; 144 NE 54th, Seattle, WA 98105, USA, tel. 206-523-9585; volume I $150, Volumes I+II $225, one year of updates $75.

PART TWO

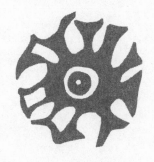

*Principles
of
health*

2

Basic principles of health

Introduction

Health is a term that is difficult to define; a definition somehow tends to place unnecessary boundaries on its meaning. The World Health Organisation defines health as 'a state of complete physical, mental, and social well being, not merely the absence of disease or infirmity'. This definition provides a positive range of health well beyond the absence of sickness.

The question of health or disease often comes down to individual responsibility. In this context, responsibility means choosing a healthy alternative over a less healthy one. If you want to be healthy, simply make healthy choices.

Many features of our health and lifestyle are based on habit and marketing hype. Not only do features of our parents' lifestyle usually become intricately woven into the fabric of our own lives but the time, energy and money spent on marketing bad health practices also has its effect – the mass media constantly bombards us with messages affecting health, diet and lifestyle.

The first step in achieving and maintaining health is taking personal responsibility. The second step is taking the appropriate action to achieve the results you desire. Achieving and maintaining health is usually quite easy if an individual follows the basic principles of health – positive mental attitude, a healthy diet and exercise. The importance of these three essential components of a healthy lifestyle are discussed below, along with additional suggestions for attaining optimum health.

Positive mental attitude

The most important factor in maintaining or attaining health is a consistent 'positive mental attitude'. More and more evidence is accumulating that what we think, feel and internally represent has a tremendous effect on the way our body functions. Our mind is so powerful, yet we only utilise a fraction of its capabilities. If only there was an 'owner's manual' that would allow each one of us to maximise our own mind. It is quite obvious this is what many people are looking for, as there is always a so-called self-help book near the top of the bestsellers list. Many of these books are extremely valuable reading and are capable of inducing change in people if they take action. There appears to be several basic themes in all of these types of books, but as for real substance they all are trying to help a person achieve 'self actualisation'.

Self-actualisation is a concept developed by Abraham Maslow, the founding father of humanistic psychology. His work and theories were the result of intense research on psychologically healthy people over a period of over 30 years. Maslow was really the first psychologist to study healthy people. He strongly believed the study of healthy people would create a firm foundation for the theories and values of a new psychotherapy.

Maslow discovered that healthy individuals are motivated toward self-actualisation, a process of 'ongoing actualisation of potentials, capacities, talents, as fulfilment of a mission (or call, fate, destiny, or vocation), as a full knowledge of, and acceptance of, the person's own intrinsic nature, as an increasing trend toward unity, integration, or synergy within the person'.

Maslow developed a five-step pyramid of human needs in which personality development progresses from one step to the next. The needs of the lower levels must be satisfied before the next level can be achieved. When needs are met, the individual moves toward well being – health.

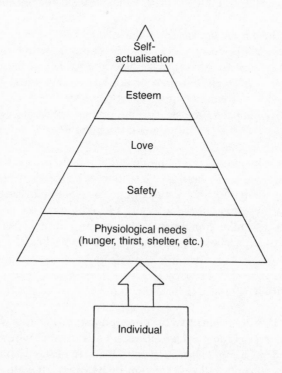

Figure 2.1 Maslow's hierarchy of needs.

The primary needs, which form the base of the pyramid, are basic survival or physiological needs – the satisfaction of hunger, thirst, sexuality and shelter. These are essential biological needs. The next step consists of needs for safety – security, order and stability. These feelings are essential in dealing with the world. If these needs are satisfied, the individual can progress to the next step – love. This level refers to the ability to love and be loved. The next step, self-esteem, requires approval, recognition and acceptance. These elements contribute strongly to high self-esteem and self-respect. The final step is self-actualisation – the utilisation of one's creative potential for self-fulfilment.

Maslow studied self-actualised people and noted they had striking similar characteristics. Here in an abbreviated form are some of Maslow's findings.

- Self-actualised people perceive reality more effectively than others and are more comfortable with it. They have an unusual ability to detect the spurious, the fake and the dishonest in personality. They judge experiences, people and things correctly and efficiently. They possess an ability to be objective about their own strengths, possibilities and limitations. This 'self-awareness' enables them clearly to define values, goals, desires and feelings. They are not frightened by uncertainty.

- Self-actualised people have an acceptance of self, others and nature. They can accept their own human shortcomings, without condemnation. They do not have an absolute lack of guilt, shame, sadness, anxiety, defensiveness, but they do not experience these feelings in unnecessary or unrealistic degrees. When they do feel guilty or regretful, they do something about it. Generally, they will feel bad about discrepancies between what is and what ought to be.

- Self-actualised people are relatively spontaneous in their behaviour, and far more spontaneous than that in their inner life, thoughts and impulses. They are unconventional in their impulses, thoughts and consciousness. They are rarely unconventional, but they seldom allow convention to keep them from doing anything they consider important or basic.

- Self-actualised people have a problem-solving orientation towards life instead of an orientation centred on self. They commonly have a mission in life, some problem outside themselves that enlists much of their energies. In general this mission is unselfish and is involved with the philosophical and the ethical.

- Self-actualised people have a quality of detachment and a need for privacy. It is often possible for them to remain above the battle, to be undisturbed by that which upsets others. The meaning of their life is self-decision, self-governing and being an active, responsible, self-disciplined, deciding person rather than a pawn or a person helplessly ruled by others.

- Self-actualised people have a wonderful capacity to appreciate again and again the basic pleasures of life such as nature, children, music and sexual experience. They approach these basic experiences with awe, pleasure, wonder and even ecstasy.

- Self-actualised people commonly have mystic or 'peak' experiences or times of intense emotions in which they transcend self. During a peak experience they experience feelings of limitless horizons, feelings of unlimited power and at the same time feelings of being more helpless than ever before; there is a loss of place and time, and feelings of great ecstasy, wonder and awe, and finally the experience ends with the conviction that something extremely important and valuable has happened so that the person is to some extent transformed and strengthened by the experience.

- Self-actualised people have deep feelings of identification, sympathy and affection for other people, in spite of occasional anger, impatience or disgust.
- Self-actualised people have deeper and more profound interpersonal relationships than most other adults, but not necessarily deeper than children. They are capable of more closeness, greater love, more perfect identification, more erasing of ego boundaries than other people would consider possible. One consequence is that self-actualised people have especially deep ties with rather few individuals and their circle of friends is small. They tend to be kind or at least patient to almost everyone, yet they do speak realistically and harshly of those whom they feel deserve it, especially the hypocritical, pretentious, pompous or the self-inflated individual.
- Self-actualised people are democratic in the deepest possible sense. They are friendly towards everyone regardless of class, education, political beliefs, race or colour. They believe it is possible to learn something from everyone. They are humble in the sense of being aware of how little they know in comparison with what could be known and what is known by others.
- Self-actualised people are strongly ethical and moral. However, their notions of right and wrong and of good and evil are often not conventional ones.
- Self-actualised people have a keen, unhostile sense of humour. They don't laugh at jokes that hurt other people or are aimed at others' inferiority. They can make fun of others in general, or of themselves, when they are foolish or try to be big when they are small. They are inclined towards thoughtful humour that elicits a smile, is intrinsic to the situation, and spontaneous.
- Self-actualised people are highly imaginative and creative. The creativeness of a self-actualised individual is not of special talent, such as Mozart, but is rather similar to the naive and universal creativeness of unspoiled children.

Self-actualisation doesn't happen all at once. It happens by degrees, subtle changes accumulating one by one. The first step is taking personal responsibility for your own positive mental state, your life, your current situation and your health. The next step is taking action to make the changes you desire.

This action may involve reading a book, going to a seminar, possibly seeking the aid of a professional counsellor. Or, it may simply be a matter of doing the things that you have been telling yourself to do for years, but before now you have been putting off. Take action! Make healthy choices in all aspects of your life, and you will be rewarded.

Diet

What is a healthy diet?

Quite simply, it is a diet which provides optimum levels of all known nutrients and low levels of food components which are detrimental to health, such as sugar, saturated fats, cholesterol, salt and additives. Dietary intake and energy expenditure must be adjusted to maintain appropriate weight for height (see Chapter 58, Obesity).

A healthy diet is rich in whole 'natural' and unprocessed foods. It is especially high in plant foods, such as fruits, vegetables, grains, beans, seeds and nuts, as these foods contain not only valuable nutrients but also dietary fibre which has remarkably healthy properties (see Chapter 4, Dietary fibre). A healthy diet must contain adequate, but not excessive, quantities of protein. A healthy diet also includes a least eight glasses of water per day.

The American Dietetic Association and American Diabetes Association, in conjunction with other committees, have developed a convenient tool for the rapid estimation of calories, protein, fat and carbohydrates called the exchange system. Originally designed for use in formulating dietary recommendations for diabetics, the exchange system is now used in the calculation and design of virtually all therapeutic diets. The exchange system presented below is a healthier version of the basic exchange system.

Foods are arranged in lists (exchange lists). Each item in a list can be exchanged for another item in the list. The diet is prescribed by allotting the number of exchanges allowed per list for one day. The exchange lists are as follows:

List 1 – milk
List 2 – vegetables
List 3 – fruits
List 4 – breads, cereals and starches
List 5 – dried beans and pulses
List 6 – meats
List 7 – fats

Using the exchange system

The exchange lists on pages 24 to 28 can be utilised to construct a healthy diet. According to most experts, the diet for a healthy person should have the following.
- At least 50 grams (2 oz) fibre.
- Carbohydrates should make up between 60 and 70 per cent of the total intake of calories.
- Fats should make up 20 to 30 per cent of total calories.
- Proteins should make up 10 to 15 per cent of total calories.

Of the carbohydrates ingested, 90 per cent should be complex carbohydrates and other naturally occurring sugars. Intake of refined carbohydrate and concentrated sugars (including honey, fruit juices, dried fruit, as well as sugar and white flour) should never account for more than 10 per cent of the total calorie intake. The intake of poly-unsaturated fats should be equal to or greater than the intake of saturated fats.

It is very easy to construct a diet which meets these recommendations using the exchange lists. In addition, the recommendations given below ensure a high intake of vital wholefoods rich in nutritional value, and highlight the importance of vegetables in the diet.

To determine how many calories you need per day multiply your ideal body weight in kilograms (2.2 pounds per kilogram) by the following calories, depending upon your activity level.

- Little physical activity   30 calories
- Light physical activity   35 calories
- Moderate physical activity   40 calories
- Heavy physical activity   45 calories

Using this calculation, a 70 kg (154 pound) man who has a moderate physical activity level would need 2,800 calories to maintain that weight. A 50 kg (110 pound) woman with a moderate activity level would require 2,000 calories. In order to lose 1 pound of fat by diet alone in one week an individual would need to have a negative calorie intake (burn more calories than eaten) of 500 calories per day or 3,500 calories per week.

For a diet of approximately 3,000 calories, the following recommendations can be made for exchange servings per day:

List 1 – milk, 1 serving
List 2 – vegetables, 20 servings
List 3 – fruits, 10 servings
List 4 – breads, cereals and starches, 16 servings
List 5 – beans, 4 servings
List 6 – meats, 4 servings
List 7 – fats, 10 servings

Such a recommendation would result in an intake of approximately 3,000 calories, of which 65 per cent are derived from complex carbohydrates and naturally occurring sugars, 20 per cent are derived from fat, and 15 per cent protein. (Remember: 1 gram of fat = 9 calories, 1 gram of protein = 4 calories and 1 gram of carbohydrate = 4 calories.) The dietary fibre intake with these recommendations would be approximately 124 grams, while the protein intake would be approximately 136 grams, well above the recommended daily allowance of protein intake for adults of 0.8 mg per kilogram (2.2 lb) body weight.

For a diet of 2,500 calories, the following recommendations can be made for exchange servings per day:

List 1 – milk, 1 serving
List 2 – vegetables, 18 servings
List 3 – fruits, 10 servings
List 4 – breads, cereals and starches, 12 servings
List 5 – beans, 2 servings
List 6 – meats, 4 servings
List 7 – fats, 8 servings

The dietary fibre intake with these recommendations would be approximately 96 grams, while the protein intake would be approximately 110 grams.

For a diet of 2,000 calories, the following recommendations can be made for exchange servings per day:

List 1 – milk, 1 serving
List 2 – vegetables, 12 servings

List 3 – fruits, 8 servings
List 4 – breads, cereals and starches, 9 servings
List 5 – beans, 2 servings
List 6 – meats, 4 servings,
List 7 – fats, 6 servings

The dietary fibre intake with these recommendations would be approximately 74 grams and the protein intake would be 92 grams.

For a diet of 1,500 calories, the following recommendations can be made for exchange servings per day:

List 1 – milk, 1 serving
List 2 – vegetables, 10 servings
List 3 – fruits, 6 servings
List 4 – breads, cereals and starches, 6 servings
List 5 – beans, 2 servings
List 6 – meats, 2 servings
List 7 – fats, 5 servings

The dietary fibre intake with these recommendations would be approximately 60 grams, the protein intake would be 68 grams.

For a diet of 1,200 calories, the following recommendations can be made for exchange servings per day:

List 1 – milk, 1 serving
List 2 – vegetables, 9 servings
List 3 – fruits, 4.5 servings
List 4 – breads, cereals and starches, 5 servings
List 5 – beans, 1 serving
List 6 – meats, 2 servings
List 7 – fats, 4 servings

The dietary fibre intake with these recommendations would be approximately 45 grams, the protein intake 57 grams.

For a diet of 1,000 calories, the following recommendations can be made for exchange servings per day:

List 1 – milk, 1 serving
List 2 – vegetables, 6 servings
List 3 – fruits, 4 servings
List 4 – breads, cereals and starches, 4 servings
List 5 – beans, 1 serving
List 6 – meats, 2 servings
List 7 – fats, 3 servings

The dietary fibre intake with these recommendations would be approximately 36 grams, the protein intake 49 grams.

Exchange lists

List 1 – milk

Non-fat milk	1 cup
Skim milk (omit 1 fat exchange)	1 cup
Low-fat yogurt (omit 1 fat exchange)	1 cup
Whole milk (omit 2 fat exchanges)	1 cup
Yogurt (omit 2 fat exchanges)	1 cup

Nutrient composition per serving

Protein	8 g
Fat	trace
Carbohydrate	12 g
Fibre	0
Calories	80

List 2 – vegetables

This list shows the kind of vegetables to use for one vegetable exchange: 1 exchange = ½ cup of raw or cooked vegetables. (Starchy vegetables are included in the bread exchange, list 4.)

Asparagus	Chicory	Onions
Aubergine/eggplant	Chinese cabbage	Radishes
Bean sprouts	Courgette/zucchini	Rhubarb
Broccoli	Cucumber	String beans
Brussels sprouts	Green pepper	Tomatoes
Cabbage	Greens	Tomato juice
Carrots	Lettuce	Turnips
Cauliflower	Mushrooms	Watercress
Celery		

Nutrient composition per serving

Protein	2 g
Fat	0
Carbohydrate	5 g
Fibre	2 g
Calories	25

List 3 – fruit

Apple	1 small	Nectarine	1 small
Apple juice	⅓ cup	Orange	1 small
Apricots, fresh	2 medium	Orange juice	½ cup
Apricots, dried	4 halves	Peach	1 medium
Banana	½ small	Pineapple	½ cup
Blackberries	½ cup	Pineapple juice	⅓ cup
Cherries	10 large	Plums	2 medium
Dates	2	Prunes	2 medium
Figs, fresh	1	Raisins	2 tbsp
Figs, dried	1	Raspberries	½ cup
Grapefruit	½	Strawberries	¾ cup
Grapefruit juice	½ cup	Tangerine	1 medium
Grapes	12		
Grape juice	¼ cup		
Melon			
Cantaloupe	¼ small		
Honeydew	⅛ medium		
Watermelon	1 cup		

Additional fruit exchanges

Honey	1 tbsp	1½	
Jams, preserves	1 tbsp	1½	equivalent
Syrup	1 tbsp	1½	fruit exchanges
Sugar	1 tbsp	1	

Nutrient composition per serving

Protein	0
Fat	0
Carbohydrate	10 g
Fibre	2 g
Calories	40

List 4 – breads, cereals and starches

Bread
White	1 slice
Whole wheat	1 slice
Rye or pumpernickel	1 slice
Plain roll	1
Hamburber bun	½

List 4 continued

Cereals

Bran flakes	½ cup
Other ready-to-eat unsweetened cereal	¾ cup
Puffed cereal (unfrosted)	1 cup
Cereal (cooked)	½ cup
Rice or barley (cooked)	½ cup
Pasta (cooked): spaghetti, noodles, macaroni	½ cup
Flour	2½ tbsp
Wheat germ	¼ cup

Starchy vegetables

Corn	⅓ cup
Corn on cob	1 small
Lima beans	½ cup
Parsnips	⅔ cup
Peas, green (canned or frozen)	½ cup
Potato	1 small
Potato (mashed)	½ cup
Pumpkin	¾ cup

Prepared foods

Biscuit, 2 in diameter (omit 1 fat exchange)	1
Crackers, round butter type (omit 1 fat exchange)	5
Potatoes, french fried, length 2 to 3½ in (omit 1 fat exchange)	8
Potato crisps/chips (omit 2 fat exchanges)	15

Nutrient composition per serving

Protein	2 g
Fat	0
Carbohydrate	15 g
Fibre	2
Calories	70

List 5 – dried beans and pulses

Any of the following beans, or any other dried beans and pulses, can be used as one bean exchange, where 1 exchange = ½ cup of cooked beans.

Chick peas	Lima beans
Kidney beans	Soy beans (omit 1 fat exchange)
Lentils	Split peas

List 5 continued

Nutrient composition per serving

Protein	7 g
Fat	0.5 g
Carbohydrate	15 g
Fibre	8 g
Calories	90

List 6 – meat

Bacon, beef, ham, lamb, pork and veal can fall into the low-fat, medium-fat or high-fat categories below, depending on the cut; 1 exchange = 1 oz in each case.

Low fat

Poultry

Chicken	1 oz
Pheasant	1 oz
Turkey	1 oz

Fish

Any fresh or frozen	1 oz
Clams, oysters, scallops, shrimps	5 or 1 oz
Tinned salmon, tuna, mackerel, crab	¼ cup
Tinned sardines (drained)	3
Cheese, low-fat	1 oz
Dried beans and peas	½ cup (omit 1 bread exchange)

Medium fat

For each exchange of medium-fat items omit ½ a fat exchange.

Offal (heart, kidney, liver, etc.)	1 oz
Cheese, medium-fat	1 oz
Egg	1
Peanut butter	2 tbsp

High fat

For each exchange of high-fat items omit 1 fat exchange.

Poultry

Duck	1 oz
Goose	1 oz
Cheese, high-fat (hard cheeses)	1 oz

List 6 continued

Nutrient composition per serving

Protein	7 g
Fat	3 g
Carbohydrate	0
Fibre	0
Calories	55

List 7 – fats

To plan a diet low in saturated fat, select only those exchanges in the left-hand column

Margarine*	1 tsp	Butter	1 tsp
Avocado (4 in diameter)†	⅛	Cream, light	2 tbsp
Oil: corn, cottonseed,		Cream, sour	2 tbsp
safflower, soy,		Cream, heavy	1 tbsp
sunflower, flaxseed	1 tsp	Cream cheese	1 tbsp
Oil, olive†	1 tsp	French dressing§	1 tbsp
Olives†	5 small	Lard	1 tbsp
Almonds†	10 whole	Mayonnaise§	1 tsp
Peanuts†	20 whole	Salad dressing,	2 tsp
Walnuts	6 small	mayonnaise type	2 tsp
Nuts, other†	6 small		

*Made with corn, cottonseed, safflower, soy, or sunflower oil only.
†Fat content is primarily monounsaturated.
§If made with corn, cottonseed, safflower, soy or sunflower oil, can be used on fat-modified diet.

Nutrient composition per serving

Protein	0
Fat	5 g
Carbohydrate	0
Fibre	0
Calories	45

Note: In these calculations:
1 gram of fat yields 9 calories
1 gram of protein yields 4 calories
1 gram of carbohydrate yields 4 calories
1 ounce = 28 or (more approximately) 25 grams

Exercise

The health benefits of regular exercise cannot be overstated. The immediate effect of exercise is stress on the body; however, with a regular exercise programme the body adapts. The body's response to this regular stress is that it becomes stronger, functions more efficiently and has greater endurance.

Physical benefits of exercise

The entire body benefits from regular exercise largely as a result of improved cardio-vascular and respiratory function. Simply stated, exercise enhances the transport of oxygen and nutrients into cells. At the same time, exercise enhances the transport of carbon dioxide and waste products from the tissues of the body to the bloodstream and ultimately to the organs that remove waste from the body.

Regular exercise is particularly important in reducing the risk of coronary artery disease. It does this by lowering cholesterol levels, improving blood and oxygen supply to the heart, increasing the functional capacity of the heart, reducing blood pressure, reducing obesity and exerting a favourable effect on blood clotting.

Psychological and social benefits of exercise

Regular exercise not only makes people look better, but also makes them feel better. Tensions, depressions, feelings of inadequacy and worries diminish greatly with regular exercise.

The value of an exercise programme in the treatment of depression cannot be overstated. Exercise alone has been demonstrated to have a tremendous impact on improving mood and the ability to handle stressful situations. In a study published in the *American Journal of Epidemiology* it was found that increased participation in exercise, sports and physical activities is strongly associated with decreased symptoms of depression (feelings that life is not worthwhile, low spirits, etc.), anxiety (restlessness, tension, etc.) and malaise (rundown feeling, insomnia, etc.).[1]

How to start an exercise programme

The first thing to do is to make sure you are fit enough to start an exercise programme. If you have been mostly inactive for a number of years or have a previously diagnosed illness, see your physician first.

If you are fit enough to begin, the next thing to do is select an activity that you feel you would enjoy. The best exercises are the kind that get your heart moving – walking briskly, jogging, bicycling, crosscountry skiing, swimming, aerobic dance and racquet sports are good examples.

Intensity of exercise

Exercise intensity is determined by measuring your heart rate (the number of times your heart beats per minute). Exercise physiologists recommend training at a level of between 70 per cent and 80 per cent of your maximal heart rate, and never exceeding 85 per cent of your maximal heart rate.

To determine your maximal heart rate simply subtract your age from 220. Then to determine your training range multiply this number by 70 percent and 80 per cent. For example, if you are 40 years old your maximal heart rate would be 180, your training range would be between 126 and 144, and you would never exceed a heart rate of 153 beats per minute.

A minimum of 15 to 20 minutes of exercising at your training heart rate at least three times a week is necessary to gain any significant benefit from exercise.

Supportive measures

A number of measures can support the basic essentials of health. Several of these will be briefly mentioned below.

Body work

Massage, spinal adjustment and manipulation, rolfing, and other types of body work are extremely valuable measures in attaining and maintaining health. The majority of the benefits derived from body work relate to improvements in circulation and nerve supply to the areas worked on.

Nutritional supplements

Vitamins and mineral supplements can provide valuable nutrition which may be lacking in our diet. The concept behind supplementing the diet in seemingly healthy people is that low levels of vitamins and minerals within our bodies may be preventing us from achieving optimum health. A high-potency multiple vitamin and mineral supplement is strongly recommended.

Herbal tonics

Herbal tonics are defined as agents which have strengthening effects and which tone up the entire body or specific organ structures or body functions. These herbs can help protect against the development of disease in a particularly weak organ or body system. For example, if your family has a history of heart disease it might be appropriate to take hawthorn berries (*Crataegus monogyna*), a botanical medicine and food with confirmed tonic effects on the heart. If stress is a particular problem, then utilise *Panax ginseng* as discussed in Chapter 10, Stress.

Summary

This chapter on the surface may appear to be quite elementary. However, the recommendations are often all that are needed to attain and regain health if an individual follows them. The reason so many people are unhealthy in western societies is directly related to the choices they make about their diet and lifestyle. For example, alcohol and smoking are very detrimental to our health, yet a large portion of our population smoke and drink. Choose health!

It is often difficult to 'sell' people on health. In order to be healthy it takes commitment. The reward is often difficult to see or feel. It is usually not until the body fails us in some manner that we realise that we haven't taken care of it. Ralph Waldo Emerson said 'The first wealth is health'.

The reward for most people maintaining a positive mental attitude, eating a healthy diet and exercising regularly is a life filled with very high levels of energy, joy, vitality and a tremendous passion for living.

3

Detoxification

This chapter identifies toxins in the body and natural ways to support the detoxification and elimination of these harmful compounds. Toxic substances are everywhere – in the air we breath, the food we eat and the water we drink. Even our bodies and the bacteria in the intestines produce toxic substances. It can be strongly said that the health of an individual is largely determined by the ability of the body to detoxify.

Types of toxic substances

Heavy metals

Included in this category are lead, mercury, cadmium, arsenic, nickel and aluminium. These metals tend to accumulate within the brain, kidneys and immune system, where they can severely disrupt normal function.[1-6] The typical person has more lead and other heavy metals in their body than is compatible with health. It is conservatively estimated that up to 25 per cent of the US population suffer from heavy metal poisoning to some extent. Hair mineral analysis is a good screening test for heavy metal toxicity.[1]

Most of the heavy metals in the body are a result of environmental contamination due to industry. For example, in the United States alone, lead from industrial sources and leaded petrol contribute more than 600,000 tons of lead to the atmosphere, to be inhaled or – after being deposited on food crops, in fresh water and soil – to be ingested.[1]

Common sources of heavy metals, in addition to industrial sources, include lead from the solder in tin cans, pesticide sprays and cooking utensils; cadmium and lead from cigarette smoke; mercury from dental fillings, contaminated fish and cosmetics; and aluminium from antacids and cookware.[1]

Early signs of heavy metal poisoning are vague, or associated with other problems. Early symptoms can include headache, fatigue, muscle pains, indigestion, tremors, constipation, anaemia, pallor, dizziness and poor coordination. The person with even

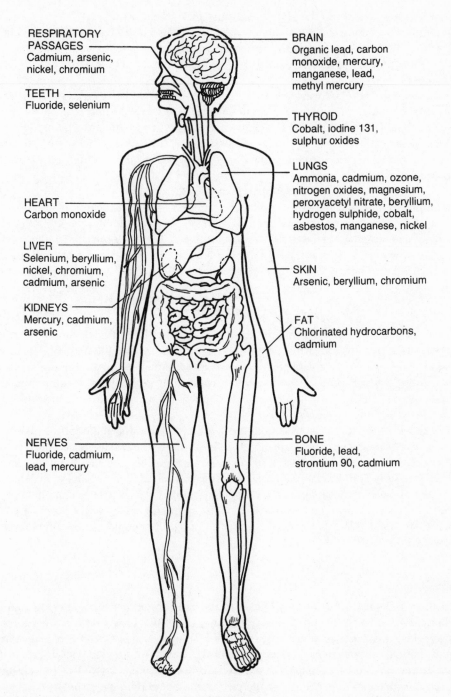

Figure 3.1 Main targets of major air pollutants

RESPIRATORY
PASSAGES
Cadmium, arsenic,
nickel, chromium

TEETH
Fluoride, selenium

HEART
Carbon monoxide

LIVER
Selenium, beryllium,
nickel, chromium,
cadmium, arsenic

KIDNEYS
Mercury, cadmium,
arsenic

NERVES
Fluoride, cadmium,
lead, mercury

BRAIN
Organic lead, carbon
monoxide, mercury,
manganese, lead,
methyl mercury

THYROID
Cobalt, iodine 131,
sulphur oxides

LUNGS
Ammonia, cadmium, ozone,
nitrogen oxides, magnesium,
peroxyacetyl nitrate, beryllium,
hydrogen sulphide, cobalt,
asbestos, manganese, nickel

SKIN
Arsenic, beryllium, chromium

FAT
Chlorinated hydrocarbons,
cadmium

BONE
Fluoride, lead,
strontium 90, cadmium

mild heavy-metal toxicity will experience impaired ability to think or concentrate. As toxicity increases, so do the severity of signs and symptoms.[1-6]

Numerous studies have demonstrated a strong relationship between childhood learning disabilities (and other disorders including criminal behaviour) and body stores of heavy metals, particularly lead.[7-12] (See Chapter 47, Hyperactivity and learning disorders.)

More and more information is accumulating that indicates chronic heavy metal toxicity is a major problem in our modern society. Every effort should be made to reduce heavy metal levels. This is particularly true in individuals who are exposed to high levels of heavy metals. Some professions with extremely high exposure include battery makers, petrol station attendants, printers, roofers, solderers, dentists and jewellers.[1]

Nutritional factors which combat heavy metal poisoning include a high potency multiple vitamin and mineral supplement; minerals such as calcium, magnesium, zinc, iron, copper and chromium; vitamin C and B-complex vitamins; sulphur-containing amino acids (methionine, cysteine and taurine) and high sulphur containing foods like garlic, beans, onions and eggs; and water-soluble fibres such as guar gum, oat bran, pectin and psyllium seed. [1,13]

Toxic chemicals, drugs, alcohol, solvents, formaldehyde, pesticides, herbicides and food additives

This category of toxins is primarily dealt with by the liver. It is staggering to contemplate the tremendous load placed on the liver as it detoxifies the incredible quantity of toxic chemicals it is constantly exposed to. Chapter 8, Liver support, discusses compounds which support the liver's detoxification mechanisms such as methionine, antioxidants, choline, and the botanicals dandelion root, milk thistle, artichoke leaves and curcuma root.

Exposure or toxicity to food additives, solvents (cleaning materials, formaldehyde, toluene, benzene, etc.), pesticides, herbicides and other toxic chemicals can give rise to a number of symptoms. Most common are psychological and neurological symptoms such as depression, headaches, mental confusion, mental illness, tingling in extremities, abnormal nerve reflexes and other signs of impaired nervous system function. The nervous system is extremely sensitive to these chemicals. Respiratory tract allergies and increased rates for many cancers are also noted in people chronically exposed to chemical toxins.[14-30]

Microbial compounds

Toxins produced by bacteria and yeast in the gut can be absorbed, causing significant disruption of body functions. Examples of these types of toxins include endotoxins, exotoxins, toxic amines, toxic derivatives of bile and various carcinogenic substances.[31] Gut-derived microbial toxins have been implicated in a wide variety of diseases including liver diseases, Crohn's disease, ulcerative colitis, thyroid disease, psoriasis, lupus erythematosis, pancreatitis, allergies, asthma and immune disorders.[31-8]

In addition to toxic substances being produced by microorganisms, antibodies formed against microbial antigens can cross-react with the body's own tissues, thereby causing autoimmunity. The list of autoimmune diseases which have been linked to cross-reacting antibodies includes rheumatoid arthritis, myasthenia gravis, diabetes and autoimmune thyroiditis.[39-41]

To reduce the absorption of toxic substances it is recommended that the diet be rich in fibre, particularly the water-soluble fibres, such as those found in vegetables, guar gum, pectin, oat bran and other vegetables. Fibre has an ability to bind to toxins within the gut and promote their excretion.

The immune system as well as the liver is responsible for dealing with the toxic substances that are absorbed from the gut.

Breakdown products of protein metabolism

The kidneys are largely responsible for the elimination of toxic waste products of protein breakdown (ammonia, urea, etc.). The kidneys can be supported in their important function by drinking adequate amounts of water and avoiding excessive protein intake.

The diagnosis of toxicity

A number of special laboratory techniques are useful in detecting toxins in the body. For heavy metals, the most reliable measure of chronic exposure is the hair mineral analysis. Reliable results of hair analysis are dependent upon:

- a properly collected, cleaned and prepared sample of hair; and
- the test being performed by experienced personnel using appropriate analytical methods in a qualified laboratory.

For determining exposure to the second category of toxins, i.e. toxic chemicals, a detailed medical history by an experienced physician in these matters is essential. When appropriate the laboratory analysis for this group of toxins can involve measuring blood and fatty tissue for suspected chemicals. It is also necessary to measure the effect that these chemicals have on the liver. The most sensitive test for measuring the effect these toxic chemicals have on the liver is the serum bile acid assay. Other tests for liver function (serum bilirubin and liver enzymes) are also important, but are less sensitive.

Physicians use a number of special laboratory techniques to determine the presence of microbial compounds, including tests for the presence of:

- abnormal microbial concentrations and disease-causing organisms (stool culture);
- microbial byproducts (urinary indican test); and
- endotoxins (microclot generation test).

The determination of the presence of high levels of breakdown products of protein metabolism and kidney function involves both blood and urine measurement of these compounds. Table 3.1 lists diseases which have been associated with various pollutants and Table 3.2 lists the clinical characteristics of some pollutants.

Table 3.1 Diseases which have been associated with various pollutants

Manifestation	Pollutant
Aging (premature)	Ozone, PAN*, other oxidants, radiation
Alopecia (loss of hair)	Lead, arsenic, radiation
Anaemia	Lead, molybdenum, vanadium
Asthma	
Allergic	Fungi, pollen; TDI†, cobalt, epoxy resins
Non-allergic	Respiratory pollutants
Ataxia	Manganese, mercury, lead
Bone disease	Strontium, fluorides
Brain involvement	Boron, carbon monoxide, lead, mercury, zinc
Bronchitis	Irritating gases
Cancer	
Abdomen	Nickel carbonate
Bones	Strontium
Gall bladder	Nitrosamines
Lungs	Asbestos, beryllium , nickel carbonate, benzo[a]pyrene
Nose, sinuses	Selenium, nickel carbonate, chromium, strontium
Skin	Arsenic
Testicles	Cadmium
Coronary heart disease	Carbon monoxide, cadmium, hydrogen sulphide
Cyanosis	Nitrites, carbon monoxides
Dental caries	Selenium
Dermatitis	Nickel, chromium, arsenic, formaldehyde, organophosphates
Emphysema	Most respiratory pollutants
Eye irritation	Ozone, PAN*, formaldehyde, nitrogen oxides, acrolein, ammonia
Fever	Manganese, zinc, boron, other metals
Fibrosis (scarring) of lungs	Quartz, silica, selenium, cobalt, iron
Gastroenteritis	Lead, mercury, fluorides, arsenic, zinc, selenium
Hypertension, arteriosclerosis	Cadmium, barium, organophosphates, carbon monoxide
Headaches	Lead, fluoride, carbon monoxide
Kidney disease	Lead, mercury, selenium, cadmium
Leukaemia	Atomic explosions, radionuclides
Liver disease	Molybdenum, selenium, chlorinated hydrocarbons
Melanosis (dark skin)	Arsenic
Mesothelioma	Asbestos
Mutagenic agents	Chlorinated hydrocarbons, lead, arsenic, cadmium, radionuclides, mercury
Myalgia (muscle weakness and pain)	Flourides, lead
Nasal irritation (septum)	Nickel, chromium, arsenic, selenium
Visual reduction	Ozone, selenium, fluoride

*PAN, 1–(2–pyridylazo)–2–napthol.
†TDI, toluene 2, 4–diisocyanate.

Table 3.2 Clinical characteristics of certain pollutants

Pollutant	Characteristic
Arsenic	Dark skin, loss of hair
Asbestos	Ferruginous bodies
Barium	Thyroid disease
Boron	Brain damage
Cadmium	Hypertension, emphysema, osteoporosis
Carbon monoxide	Carboxyhaemoglobin
Chromium*	Nasal irritation
Cobalt*	Thyroid disease, asthma
Fluoride	Skin (maculae), dental fluorosis
Iron*	Siderosis
Lead	Anaemia, gastrointestinal symptoms
Hydrogen sulphide	Rotten egg odour
Manganese*	Ataxia, tremor
Mercury	Tremor
Nickel carbonate	Nasal irritation
Nitrites	Cyanosis
Ozone	Eye irritation
Quartz	Silicosis
Selenium*	Odour of garlic, tooth decay
Tellurium	Garlic-like odour
Titanium	Yellow discoloration of skin
Vanadium	Respiratory symptoms
Zinc*	Fever

*Trace quantities of these elements are essential for life.

Detoxification by fasting

Fasting is often used as a detoxification method as it is one of the quickest ways to increase elimination of wastes and enhance the healing processes of the body. Fasting is defined as abstinence from all food and drink except water for a specific period of time, usually for a therapeutic or religious purpose. This process spares essential tissue (e.g. vital organs) while utilising non-essential tissue (e.g. fatty tissue and muscle) for fuel.

Although therapeutic fasting is probably one of the oldest known therapies, it has been largely ignored by the scientific community. The most recent development in the study and promotion of fasting has been the formation of the International Association of Professional Natural Hygienists (IAPNH).[42] This organisation comprises doctors specialising in therapeutic fasting as an integral part of total health care.

Research into fasting has been reported since 1880. Since then, medical journals have carried articles on the use of fasting in the treatment of obesity, chemical poisoning, arthritis, allergies, psoriasis, eczema, thrombophlebitis, leg ulcers, the irritable bowel syndrome, impaired or deranged appetite, bronchial asthma, depression, neurosis and schizophrenia.[43-56]

A most encouraging use of fasting was published in the *American Journal of Industrial Medicine* in 1984.[50] This study involved patients who had ingested rice oil contaminated with polychlorinated-biphenyls or PCBs. All patients reported improvement in symptoms, and some observed 'dramatic' relief, after undergoing seven to ten day fasts. This research supports past studies conducted by Inamura of PCB-poisoned patients and indicates the therapeutic effects of fasting. Caution must be used, however, when fasting after significant contamination with fat-soluble toxins like pesticides. The pesticide DDT has been shown to be mobilised during a fast and may reach blood levels toxic to the nervous system.[57] For this reason it is a good idea to include those guidelines given below under basic detoxification programme (page 39).

The short fast

The short fast (three to five days) is a good chance for the body to acquire optimal rest, both mental and physical. Longer fasts require strict medical supervision, but the short fast can usually be conducted at home rather than as an inpatient. Before starting an unsupervised fast, it is a very good idea to consult your physician.

Although a short fast can be started at any time, it is better to begin on a weekend during a time when you can be inactive. The more rest, the better results as energy can be directed towards healing, instead of other body functions.

Prepare for a fast on the day before eating is stopped by making the last meal one of only fresh fruits and vegetables (some authorities recommend a full day of raw food to start a fast). Only water – distilled or spring water is best – should be consumed while fasting. (Some authorities recommend fruit or vegetable juice, but this is actually an elimination diet rather than a fast.) The quantity of water should be dictated by thirst, but at least a few glasses every day. No coffee, juice, soft drinks, cigarettes, or anything else by mouth should be taken except water. Herbal teas can be quite supportive of a fast, but they should not be sweetened.

Exercise is not usually encouraged while fasting. It is a good idea to conserve energy and allow maximal healing. Short walks or light stretching are useful, but heavy workouts tax the system and inhibit repair and elimination.

Cleansing the skin with lukewarm water is encouraged, but extremes of temperature can be tiring. Deodorants, soaps, sprays, detergents, synthetic shampoos and exposure to other chemicals should be avoided. These only hinder elimination and add to the body's detoxification and elimination burden.

Sunlight is essential for healthy cells, but excessive exposure will strain the body's protective systems. At least 10–20 minutes of direct sun exposure per day is beneficial while fasting.

Rest is one of the most important aspects of a fast. A nap or two during the day is recommended. Less sleep will usually be required at night, since daily activity is lower.

Enemas are usually not necessary, but this will depend on an individual's health. If constipation is a usual problem, a longer prefast period of fresh fruits and vegetables will assist elimination.

Body temperature usually drops during a fast, as do blood pressure, pulse and respiratory rate – all measures of the slowing of the metabolic rate of the body. It is important, therefore, to stay warm.

Breaking a fast

In breaking a fast, as outlined in Table 3.3, an individual is encouraged to eat slowly, chew thoroughly, limit quantities and eat foods at room temperature. While breaking a fast, and in the days that follow, it can be very helpful to record carefully what is eaten and note any adverse effects. Many of today's health problems are due to food allergies and overeating.

Table 3.3 Breaking your fast

	Breakfast	Lunch	Dinner
Day 1	One of the following: melon, nectarine, pineapple	A different fruit from the breakfast list	8 oz of any fruit
Day 2	12 oz of one type of fresh fruit	14 oz of whole pears or citrus fruit	Raw vegetable salad with leafy greens, tomato, celery and cucumber, or 2 pears, 2 apples and avocado
Day 3	Resume healthy diet (raw fresh fruits, raw/steamed vegetables, whole grains, nuts, seed, and legumes)		

Basic detoxification programme

Detoxification does not have to be an unpleasant experience and does not have to be performed only while on a fast. Actually, the best approach is to detoxify gradually. The basic detoxification programme outlined below is suitable for a gradual long-term detoxification programme. The same recommendations are appropriate if an individual chooses to fast, as it is important to support the body against severe toxaemia as stored toxins are dumped into the bloodstream.

Lipotropic formulas or silymarin from *Silybum marianum* (see Chapter 8, Liver support) and vitamin C should always be used when detoxifying to help the liver remove toxic compounds from the blood effectively. A gel-forming fibre like psyllium seed, guar gum, pectin or oat bran should also be used to prevent reabsorption of toxic chemicals dumped in the intestinal tract by the bile. Goldenseal root (*Hydrastis canadensis*) effectively supports the lymphatic system during a detoxification programme.

- The diet should be as natural as possible, high in fruits and vegetables and low in animal products.
- At least 2 quarts of distilled or purified water should be drunk daily.

Supplements

- High-potency multiple vitamin and mineral formula.
- Lipotropic formula:
    Choline, 1 gram/day.
    L-methionine, 1 gram/day.
- Vitamin C, 1 gram three times per day.
- Fibre supplement, 1–2 tablespoons at night before retiring.

Botanical medicines

- The standard dose of *Silybum marianum* is based on its silymarin content, 70–210 mg of silymarin three times daily.
- *Hydrastis canadensis* (goldenseal):
    Dried root (or as tea), 1 to 2 g.
    Tincture (1:5), 4 to 6 ml (1 to 1.5 tsp).
    Fluid extract (1:1), 0.5 to 2.0 ml (1/4 to 1/2 tsp).
    Powdered solid extract (4:1), 250–500 mg.

Summary

Detoxification of harmful substances is a continual process in the body. The ability to detoxify and eliminate toxins largely determines an individual's health. A number of toxins (heavy metals, solvents, pesticides, microbial toxins, etc.) are known to cause significant health problems.

A rational approach to aiding the body's detoxification mechanisms can include the use of periodic short fasts (3–5 days) or longer medically supervised fasts. However, to support the body's detoxification processes truly, a long-term detoxification programme is recommended. This involves adopting a healthy diet and lifestyle as outlined in Chapter 2.

4

Dietary fibre

This chapter discusses the major diseases of western society and how they relate to one key component of the diet – dietary fibre (DF). The term 'western diet' is used throughout this chapter, as well as in many other parts of this book. It refers to the typical diet of western people; it is also referred to as 'foods of commerce'. It consists of a high intake of refined carbohydrates, saturated fats, processed foods and cholesterol, and an extremely low intake of DF. In one year, the average American consumes 100 lb of refined sugar, 55 lb of fats and oils, 300 cans of soda pop, 200 sticks of gum, 18 lb of sweets and candy, 5 lb of potato crisps, 7 lb of corn chips, popcorn and pretzels, 63 dozen doughnuts, 50 lb of cakes and biscuits and 20 gallons of ice cream.[1] This translates to an annual total population consumption of 100 billion oz of cola, and other equally startling figures. When we consider the $4 billion food manufacturers spend on advertising each year in the States, however, these numbers are not surprising.

The fibre hypothesis

The dietary fibre hypothesis, popularised by the work of Burkitt and Trowell, has two basic components:

- a diet rich in foods which contain plant cell walls (i.e. whole grains, legumes, fruits and vegetables) is protective against a wide variety of diseases, in particular those that are prevalent in western society; and
- a diet providing a low intake of plant cell walls is a causative factor in the aetiology of these diseases and provides conditions under which other aetiological factors are more active.[2-5]

Although well known, the work of Burkitt and Trowell is actually a continuation of the landmark work of Weston A. Price,[6] who brought attention to the 'foods of commerce' in the early part of the 20th century. Dr Price, a dentist, travelled the world observing changes in orthodontic parameters as various cultures discarded traditional dietary practices in favour of a more 'civilised' diet. He was able to follow individuals as well as cultures over periods of 20 to 40 years, and carefully documented the onset of degenerative diseases as their diets changed.

Burkitt formulated the following sequence of events, based on extensive studies examining the rate of diseases in various populations (epidemiological data) and his own observations of primitive cultures[2]:

- First stage – the primal diet of plant eaters contains large amounts of unprocessed starch staples; there are few examples of subsequently mentioned diseases.
- Second stage – commencing westernisation of diet, obesity and diabetes commonly appear in privileged groups.
- Third stage – with moderate westernisation of the diet, constipation, haemorrhoids, varicose veins and appendicitis become common.
- Fourth stage – finally, with full westernisation of the diet, ischaemic heart disease, diverticular disease, hiatal hernia and cancer become prominent.

Diseases highly associated with a low-fibre diet	
Metabolic	Obesity, gout, diabetes, kidney stones, gall stones
Cardiovascular	Hypertension, cerebrovascular disease, ischaemic heart disease, varicose veins, deep vein thrombosis, pulmonary embolism
Colonic	Constipation, appendicitis, diverticulitis, diverticulosis, haemorrhoids, colon cancer, irritable bowel syndrome, ulcerative colitis, Crohn's disease
Other	Dental caries, autoimmune disorders, pernicious anaemia, multiple sclerosis, thyrotoxicosis, dermatological conditions

Definition and composition of dietary fibre

Originally, the definition of dietary fibre was restricted to the sum of plant compounds that are not digestible by the secretions of the human digestive tract. This definition is vague, since it depends on an exact understanding of what exactly is not digestible. For our purposes the term 'dietary fibre' will be used to refer to the components of plant cell walls as well as the indigestible residues.

The composition of the plant cell wall varies according to the species of plant. Typically, the dry cell wall contains 35 per cent cellulose, 45 per cent non-cellulose polysaccharides, 17 per cent lignins, 3 per cent protein and 2 per cent ash.[3,7] It is important to recognise that dietary fibre is a complex of these constituents, and supplementation of a single component does not substitute for a diet rich in high-fibre foods. However, in some clinical conditions the use of specific components is a useful adjunct to a healthy diet. Table 4.1 summarises the classifications of dietary fibres.

Table 4.1 Classification of dietary fibre

Fibre class	Chemical structure	Sources	Physiological effect
Cellulose	Unbranched 1-4-beta-D-glucose polymer	Principle plant wall component Wheat brean	Increases faecal weight and size
Non-cellulose polysaccharides:			
Hemicellulose	Mixture of pentose and hexose molecules in branching chains	Plant cell walls Oat bran	Same as above Binds bile acids
Gums	Branched chain uronic acid containing polymers	Karaya, gum arabic	Laxative
Mucilages	Similar to hemicelluloses	Found in endosperm of plant seeds Guar, legumes, psyllium	Hydrocolloids that bind steroids and delay gastric emptying Heavy metal chelation
Pectins	Mixture of methylesterified galacturan, galactan and arabinose in varying proportions	Citrus rind, apple, onion skin	As above
Algal polysaccharides	Polymerised D-mannuronic and L-glucuronic acids	Algin, carrageenan	As above
Lignins	Non-carbohydrate polymeric phenylpropene	Woody part of plant: Wood (40–50%) Wheat (25%) Apple (25%) Cabbage (6%)	Antioxidants Anticarcinogenic

Cellulose

The best known component of the plant cell wall is cellulose. Wheat bran is an example of a fibre rich in cellulose. Cellulose is relatively insoluble in water, but it has an ability to bind water. This ability to bind water accounts for its effect of increasing faecal size and weight, thus promoting regular bowel movements. Although cellulose cannot be digested by humans, it is partially digested by the microflora (the bacteria) of the gut. This natural fermentation process, which occurs in the colon, results in the degradation of about 50 per cent of the cellulose, and is an important source of short chain fatty acids (SCFA).[3,4] SCFA have very important properties in the colon and are discussed below.

Table 4.2 Dietary fibre constituents of the food groups

Food group	Main dietary fibres
Fruit and vegetables	Cellulose, hemicellulose, lignin, pectic substances, cutin, waxes
Grains	Cellulose, hemicellulose, lignin, phenolic esters
Seeds and legumes	Cellulose, hemicellulose, pectic substances, guar gum
Seed husk of *Plantago ovata*	Mucilage
Food additives	Gum arabic, alginate, carrageenan, carboxymethylcellulose

Non-cellulose polysaccharides

The majority of polysaccharides in the plant cell wall are a non-cellulose type. They are water-soluble compounds which possess diverse properties. Included in this class are hemicelluloses, gums, mucilages, algal polysaccharides and pectin substances.[3,4,7]

Beneficial effects of dietary fibre

Decreased intestinal transit time
Delayed gastric emptying resulting in reduced after-meal elevations of blood
    sugar
Increased satiety
Increased pancreatic secretion
Increased stool weight
More advantageous intestinal microflora
Increased production of short chain fatty acids
Decreased serum lipids
More soluble bile

Hemicelluloses

Perhaps the most popular hemicellulose source is oat bran. Hemicelluloses contain a mixture of small sugar molecules (pentose and hexose) in branched-chain configurations of much smaller size than cellulose. The hemicelluloses are more important fibre components than cellulose fibres. As well as promoting regular bowel movements, these compounds exert many other effects. The hemicelluloses are also a much more important source of short chain fatty acids.[3,4,7]

Gums

Plant gums are a complex group of water-soluble gel-forming compounds. They are produced by the plant in response to injury, and are commercially produced by incising a plant or tree and collecting the fluid extract. Gums are used as emulsifiers, thickeners and stabilisers by the food industry and as laxatives in pharmaceuticals.[3,4,7] Examples of plant gums are karaya and gum arabic.

Mucilages

Structurally mucilages resemble the hemicelluloses, but they are not classed as such due to their unique location in the seed portion of the plant. They are generally found within the inner layer (endosperm) of the plant seeds, where they are responsible for retaining water to prevent the seed from drying.

Guar gum, found in most beans (legumes), is the most widely studied plant mucilage. Commercially, guar gum is isolated from the endosperm of *Cyamopsis tetragonolobus*, a plant cultivated in India for livestock feed. Guar gum is used commercially as a stabiliser, thickening and film-forming agent in the production of cheese, salad dressings, ice cream, soups, toothpaste, pharmaceutical jelly, lotion, skin cream and tablets. Guar gum is also used as a laxative.

Guar gum and other mucilages, including pectin and glucomannan, are perhaps the most potent cholesterol-lowering agents of the gel-forming fibres. Guar gum has been shown to reduce fasting and after-meal glucose and insulin levels in both healthy and diabetic subjects; and it has decreased body weight and hunger ratings when taken with meals by obese subjects.

Psyllium seed husk (*Plantago ovata*) is another example of a mucilage fibre. It is widely used as a bulking and laxative agent.[3,4] It possesses many of the same qualities as guar gum, except that it has a greater effect as a laxative.

Pectin and pectin-like substances

These compounds are found in all plant cell walls, as well as in the outer skin and rind of fruits and vegetables; for example, the rind of an orange contains 30 per cent pectin, apple peel 15 per cent and onion skins 12 per cent.

The gel-forming properties are well known to anyone who has made jelly or jam. These same gel-forming qualities are responsible for the cholesterol-lowering effects of pectins. Pectins lower cholesterol by binding the cholesterol and bile acids in the gut and promoting their excretion.

Algal polysaccharides

Included in this fibre category are compounds which are produced from seaweeds (algae) – alginic acid, agar and carrageenan. These compounds are used extensively by the food industry. Alginate has been shown to inhibit heavy metal uptake in the gut, as do other gel-forming fibres. Agar is used as a thickening agent and it has laxative activity.

Carrageenan is used in milk and chocolate products due to its ability to react with milk proteins. Unlike other plant polysaccharides, carrageenan appears to be detrimental to human health.[3,4] In rats, carrageenan has been shown to promote ulceration and damage of the intestines.[4] Other rat studies have shown carrageenan to produce colon cancer, birth defects and hepatomegaly (liver enlargement).[8]

Lignins

Lignins are plant products of low molecular weight and are typically composed of cinnamic acid, cinnamyl alcohol, propenylbenzene and allylbenzene precursor units. Many plant lignins show important properties, such as anticancer, antibacterial, anti-fungal and antiviral activity. Plant lignins are changed by the gut flora into entero-lactone and enterodiol, two compounds which are believed to be protective against cancer, particular breast cancer.[9]

Miscellaneous fibre-associated compounds

Phytic acid stores minerals such as calcium, phosphorus, magnesium and potassium in the plant. Dietary phytates adversely affect the uptake and utilisation of many minerals, including calcium, iron and zinc. The major sources of phytate in the diet are cereal grains. However, most of the phytate is destroyed by heat and phytase during the leavening of bread.[3,4,5] Consumption of raw grains or unleavened bread may result in mineral deficiency as a result of the phytates preventing mineral absorption.

Physiological effects of dietary fibre

It is beyond the scope of this chapter to detail all known effects of dietary fibre on humans. Instead, we will concentrate on the effects of greatest significance (stool weight, transit time, digestion, lipid metabolism, short chain fatty acids and colon flora) and a selection of diseases highly correlated with (the lack of) dietary fibre (colon diseases, obesity and diabetes).

Stool weight and transit time

Fibre has long been used in the treatment of constipation. Dietary fibre, particularly the water-insoluble fibres such as cellulose (e.g. wheat bran), increase stool weight as a result of their water-holding properties.[3-5] Transit time, the time taken for passage of material from the mouth to the anus, is greatly reduced on a high-fibre diet.

Cultures consuming a high-fibre diet (100–170 grams/day) usually have a transit time of 30 hours and a faecal weight of 500 grams. In contrast, Europeans and Americans who eat a typical low-fibre diet (20 grams/day) have a transit time of greater than 48 hours and a faecal weight of only 100 grams.[4,7] The increased intestinal transit time associated with the western diet allows prolonged exposure to various carcino-genic compounds within the intestines.[2-5,10,11]

Fibre should not only be thought of in the treatment of constipation, but also of diarrhoea due to the irritable bowel syndrome (see Chapter 51, Irritable bowel syndrome). When fibre is added to the diet of subjects with abnormally rapid transit times (less than 24 hours) it causes slowing of the transit time.[3,4] Dietary fibre acts to normalise bowel movements.

Dietary fibre's effect on transit time is apparently directly related to its effect on stool weight and size. A larger, bulkier stool passes through the colon more easily, requires less pressure to be produced during defaecation, and subsequently less straining.[2-5] This results in less stress on the colon wall and therefore avoids the ballooning effect which results in diverticula. It also prevents the formation of haemorrhoids and varicose veins.

Digestion

Although dietary fibre increases the rate of transit through the gastrointestinal tract, it slows gastric emptying. This results in food being released more gradually into the small intestine, and as a result blood glucose levels will rise more gradually.[2-5] Pancreatic enzyme secretion and activity also increase in response to fibre.[12]

A number of research studies have examined the effects of fibre on mineral absorption. Although the results have been somewhat contradictory, it now appears that large amounts of dietary fibre may result in impaired absorption and/or negative balance of some minerals. Fibre as a dietary component does not appear to interfere with the minerals in other foods; however, supplementary fibre, especially wheat bran, may result in mineral deficiencies.[3-5]

Lipid metabolism

The water-soluble gels and mucilaginous fibres like oat bran, guar gum and pectin are capable of lowering serum lipid (i.e. cholesterol and triglyceride) levels by greatly increasing their faecal excretion as well as preventing their manufacture in the liver. The water-insoluble fibres like wheat bran have much less effect in reducing serum lipid levels.[2-5]

Short chain fatty acids (SCFAs)

The fermentation of dietary fibre by the intestinal flora produces three main end products:
- short chain fatty acids;
- various gases; and
- energy.

The SCFAs – acetic, propionic and butyric acids – have many important physiological functions.

Proprionate and acetate are transported directly to the liver and utilised for energy production, while butyrate provides an important energy source for the cells that line the colon. In fact, butyrate is the preferred source for energy metabolism in the colon.[3] Butyrate production may also be responsible for the anticancer properties of dietary fibre.[3,13,14] Butyrate has been shown to possess impressive anticancer activity in animals and humans.[13,14]

Intestinal bacterial flora

Dietary fibre improves all aspects of colon function.[2-5] Of central importance is the role it plays in maintaining a suitable bacterial flora in the colon. A low-fibre intake is associated with both an overgrowth of endotoxin-producing bacteria (bad guys) and a lower percentage of lactobacillus (good guys) and other acid loving bacteria.[3] A diet high in dietary fibre promotes the growth of acid loving bacteria through the increased synthesis of short chain fatty acids, which reduce the colon pH.

Diseases associated with a lack of dietary fibre

Diseases of the colon

The evidence documenting the protective effect of dietary fibre on colon cancer is overwhelming. There is evidence for similar strong links with other common diseases of the colon – diverticulitis, diverticulosis, irritable bowel syndrome, ulcerative colitis and appendicitis.[2-5]

Obesity

A diet deficient in dietary fibre is an important causative factor in the development of obesity.[2-5] Dietary fibre plays a role in preventing obesity by:
* increasing the amount of necessary chewing, thus slowing the eating process;
* increasing faecal calorie loss;
* improving digestive hormone secretion;
* improving glucose tolerance; and
* inducing a state of satiety (feeling of sufficient food intake).

Diabetes mellitus

Population studies and clinical and experimental data show diabetes mellitus to be one of the diseases most clearly related to inadequate dietary fibre intake.[2-5] Clinical studies that have demonstrated the beneficial therapeutic effect of dietary fibre on diabetes have further substantiated this association. Fibre's prevention and improvement of diabetes is due to its effects on glucose and, subsequently, insulin levels.

A high-complex-carbohydrate, high-fibre diet reduces after-meal elevations in glucose levels (largely by delaying gastric emptying and thereby reducing insulin secretion) and increases tissue sensitivity to insulin.[3] Fermentation products of fibre, chiefly short chain fatty acids, also enhance liver glucose metabolism and may further contribute to the therapeutic effects of dietary fibre on diabetes.

Summary

A diet high in plant cell walls is associated with a decreased incidence (see page 42) of most of the degenerative diseases of western society. While this is largely due to increased levels of dietary fibre, such a diet is also high in other important nutrients, most of which are also deficient in the western diet.

It is clear from the scientific literature that the best source of dietary fibre is from wholefoods, although specific types of fibres have their use in the treatment of specific diseases. Further, even with a diet high in dietary fibre, when as little as 18 per cent of the total calories are in the form of refined carbohydrates, many of the beneficial effects of dietary fibre are greatly reduced.[3] There is no substitute for a healthy diet, i.e. a diet composed of foods as close to their original form as possible.

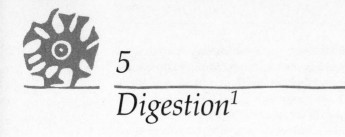

5
Digestion[1]

Most of the foods we eat are simply too large to be absorbed into our cells. The food molecules are therefore broken down by the process of digestion, the organs that collectively perform this function comprising the digestive system.

The digestive system extends from the mouth to the anus. It consists of the gastro-intestinal tract and its appendage organs, e.g. salivary glands, the liver and gallbladder, and the pancreas.

Digestion occurs as a result of both physical and chemical processes. The physical changes of food are brought about by grinding, crushing and mixing the food mass (chyme) with digestive juices during propulsion through the digestive tract. The digestive juices are responsible for the chemical breakdown of chyme. The active compounds in the digestive juices are primarily enzymes.[2]

Components of the digestive tract

Mouth and oesophagus

The mouth receives food and reduces it in size by chewing and mixing it with saliva. Saliva contains the enzyme salivary amylase (ptyalin) which breaks down starch molecules into smaller sugars. Chewing food thoroughly is the first aspect of good digestion.

The oesophagus then transports food and liquids from the oral cavity (the mouth) to the stomach.

Stomach

The stomach is primarily responsible for digestion of proteins and ionisation of minerals.

The stomach secretes gastric acid (hydrochloric acid) and various hormones and enzymes. Although much is said about hyperacidity (as often occurs with peptic ulcers), probably more significant health problems are caused by lack of gastric acid secretion. (Hypochlorhydria refers to deficient gastric acid secretion, while achlorhydria refers to a complete absence of gastric secretion.) There are many symptoms and signs that suggest impaired gastric acid secretion, and a number of specific diseases have been found to be associated with insufficient gastric acid output.[1,3–13]

Several studies have shown that the ability to secrete gastric acid decreases with age[14,15] – low stomach acidity has been found in over half of those over age 60. One

---

Low gastric acidity

Common symptoms of low gastric acidity

Bloating, belching, burning and flatulence immediately after meals
A sense of 'fullness' after eating
Indigestion, diarrhoea or constipation
Multiple food allergies
Nausea after taking supplements
Itching around the rectum

Common signs of low gastric acidity

Weak, peeling and cracked fingernails
Dilated blood vessels in the cheeks and nose (in non-alcoholics)
Acne
Iron deficiency
Chronic intestinal parasites or abnormal flora
Undigested food in stool
Chronic candida infections
Upper digestive tract gasiness

Diseases associated with low gastric acidity

Addison's disease	Lupus erythematosis
Asthma	Myasthenia gravis
Coeliac disease	Osteoporosis
Dermatitis herpetiformis	Pernicious anaemia
Diabetes mellitus	Psoriasis
Eczema	Rheumatoid arthritis
Gallbladder disease	Rosacea
Graves disease	Sjogren's syndrone
Chronic autoimmune disorders	Thyrotoxicosis
Hepatitis	Hyper- and hypothyroidism
Chronic hives	Vitiligo

---

study of the elderly found that their tissue nutrient levels could be saturated only through the use of injecting the nutrient directly into the body; oral supplementation was ineffective. The authors speculated this was due to defective digestive secretions and absorption.[16]

The best method of diagnosing a lack of gastric acid is a special procedure known as the Heidelberg gastric analysis.[1,17-21] This technique utilises an electronic capsule attached to a string. The capsule is swallowed and then kept in the stomach with the aid of the string. The capsule measures the pH of the stomach and sends a radio message to a receiver which then records the pH level. The response to a bicarbonate challenge is the true test of the functional ability of the stomach to secrete acid.[21] After the test, the capsule is pulled up from the stomach by the string attached to it.

Since not everyone can have detailed gastric acid analysis to determine the need for gastric acid supplementation, a practical method of determination is often used. If an individual is experiencing any signs and symptoms of gastric acid insufficiency, as listed in the box on page 51, or has any of the diseases listed in the box, the method outlined below on page 55 should be employed.

Small intestine

The small intestine participates in all aspects of digestion, absorption and transport of ingested materials. It secretes a variety of digestive and protective substances as well as receiving the secretions of the pancreas, liver and gallbladder.

The 21-foot-long (over 6 metres) small intestine is divided into three segments: the duodenum is the first 10 to 12 inches (25–30 cm); the jejunum is the middle portion and is about 8 feet long (2.4 metres); and the ileum is about 12 feet long (3.6 metres). Absorption of minerals occurs predominantly in the duodenum, absorption of water-soluble vitamins, carbohydrates and protein occurs primarily in the jejunum, and the ileum absorbs fat-soluble vitamins, fat, cholesterol and bile salts.

Diseases involving the small intestine often result in malabsorption syndromes characterised by multiple nutrient deficiencies. Examples of common causes of malabsorption include coeliac disease (gluten intolerance), food allergy or intolerance, intestinal infections and Crohn's disease.

The pancreas and its enzymes

The pancreas produces enzymatic secretions required for the digestion and absorption of food. Each day the pancreas secretes about 2½ pints (about 1½ litres) of pancreatic juice into the small intestine. Enzymes secreted include lipases which digest fat, proteases which digest proteins, and amylases which digest starch molecules.

- Lipases – the pancreatic lipases, along with bile, function in the digestion of fats. Deficiency of lipase results in malabsorption of fats and fat soluble vitamins.
- Amylases are enzymes which break down starch molecules into the smaller sugars. Amylase is secreted by the salivary glands as well as the pancreas.
- Proteases secreted by the pancreas (trypsin, chymotrypsin and carboxypeptidase) function in digestion by breaking down protein molecules into single amino acids.

Incomplete digestion of proteins creates a number of problems for the body including the development of allergies and formation of toxic substances produced during putrefaction (the breakdown of protein material by bacteria).

As well as being necessary for protein digestion, the proteases serve several other important functions. For example, the proteases, as well as other digestive secretions, are largely responsible for keeping the small intestine free from parasites (including bacteria, yeast, protozoa and intestinal worms).[22] A lack of proteases or other digestive secretions greatly increases an individual's risk of having an intestinal infection.

Liver and biliary system

The major functions of the liver include the metabolism of proteins, carbohydrates and fats; detoxifying hormones, toxins and drugs; and the synthesis of physiological substances. The liver also manufactures bile which is either secreted into the small intestine or stored in the gallbladder. Bile is extremely important in the digestion of fat and fat-soluble vitamins.[2]

Like pancreatic enzymes, bile also serves to keep the small intestine free from micro-organisms. Each day about 1½ (1 litre) of bile is secreted into the small intestine, with about 99 per cent reabsorption.

Large intestine (colon)

The large intestine is about 5 feet in length and functions in the absorption of water, electrolytes and, in limited amounts, some of the final products of digestion. The large intestine also provides temporary storage for waste products, which serve as a medium for bacteria.

The health of the colon is largely determined by the types of foods that are eaten. In particular, dietary fibre is of critical importance in maintaining the health of the colon (see Chapter 4, Dietary fibre).

Therapeutic uses of protein-digesting enzymes

Pancreatin

Pancreatin refers to preparations of pancreatic enzymes isolated from fresh hog pancreas.[23] Pancreatin is most often employed in the treatment of pancreatic insufficiency characterised by impaired digestion, malabsorption, nutrient deficiences and abdominal discomfort. Pancreatin is also used by physicians in the treatment of cystic fibrosis and inflammatory and autoimmune diseases like rheumatoid arthritis, scleroderma, athletic injuries, tendinitis, etc.

It is best to use a full-strength undiluted pancreatic extract (8–10X USP) with additional enzymes added (see bromelain below). Lower potency pancreatin products are often diluted with salt, lactose or galactose.

Bromelain

Bromelain, the protein-digesting enzyme found in pineapple, is useful as an aid to protein digestion. Bromelain is quite effective as a substitute for pancreatic enzymes in the treatment of pancreatic insufficiency, but best results are obtained if it is used in combination with pancreatin and ox ,bile.[24] Bromelain has also been shown in many studies to aid the body's response to inflammation and swelling.[25]

Papain

This a protein-digesting enzyme isolated from the unripe papaya fruit. It is often used alone and in formulas as a digestive aid. Papain has been shown to be able to digest wheat gluten and render it harmless in coeliac disease subjects[26,27]; taking a papain supplement (500–1,000 mg) with meals may allow some individuals to tolerate gluten.[28]

Other uses

The protein-digesting enzymes are also important in preventing tissue damage during inflammation and the formation of fibrin clots.[29] Proteolytic enzymes increase the breakdown of fibrin, a process known as fibrinolysis. Fibrin's role in the promotion of inflammation is to form a wall around the area of inflammation which results in the blockage of blood and lymph vessels, which in turn leads to swelling. Fibrin can also cause the development of blood clots which can become dislodged and produce strokes or heart attacks. Proteolytic enzymes are therefore often used therapeutically in the treatment of thrombophlebitis, a disease in which blood clots develop in veins, which become inflamed; the clots can then dislodge to cause strokes or heart attacks.[3]

The proteases are also essential in preventing the deposit of immune complexes in body tissues. This is extremely important in the treatment of an autoimmune disease like rheumatoid arthritis. Studies have shown proteolytic enzymes to be quite effective in immune complex disease and have been suggested to be of value in the treatment of AIDS.[30,31]

Indigestion

The term indigestion is often used to describe a feeling of gaseousness or fullness in the abdomen. It can also be used to describe heartburn. Indigestion can be attributed to a great many causes, including decreased secretion of digestive juices and enzymes. Digestion may be improved by using digestants, which by definition are compounds which aid in digestive function. Commonly used digestants include hydrochloric acid and pancreatic enzyme preparations.

Antacids are also used to relieve symptoms of indigestion; however detailed clinical studies have shown that neutralisation or suppression of gastric acid is of no therapeutic benefit.[32] The substantial amount of money spent on antacid products each year thus appears to be wasted.

A suitable alternative to the use of antacids in the treatment of indigestion is the use of herbal bitters. Bitters are believed to work by stimulating digestion as a result of activating the bitter-taste receptors on the tongue. Stimulation of bitter-taste receptors activates a number digestive processes including the secretion of digestive juices. Examples of commonly used bitters include gentian root (*Gentiana lutea*), goldenseal root (*Hydrastis canadensis*), wormwood (*Artemisia absinthium*), chamomile flowers (*Matricaria chamomilla*) and dandelion root (*Taraxacum officinale*).

Gentian is perhaps the most widely used bitter. Clinical studies have demonstrated that gentian-containing formulas are effective in relieving indigestion.[33,34] Administration of teas made of gentian and other bitters are most effective when they proceed a meal by 15 to 30 minutes.

The irritable bowel syndrome

A history of alternating constipation and diarrhoea may be indicative of the irritable bowel syndrome, a functional disorder of the large intestine. (A functional disorder means there is no evidence of accompanying structural defects of disease.)

Irritable bowel syndrome (described in detail in Chapter 51) is characterised by some combination of:
- Abdominal pain
- Altered bowel function, constipation or diarrhoea
- Hypersecretion of colonic mucus
- Dyspeptic symptoms (flatulence, nausea, anorexia)
- Varying degrees of anxiety or depression

Less acceptable synonyms include nervous indigestion, spastic colitis, mucous colitis and intestinal neurosis. If constipation alone is the problem please consult Chapter 29.

Aids to digestion

To improve digestion, digestive aids can be used. The most commonly used digestive aids are hydrochloric acid, pancreatin and enzyme preparations.

Hydrochloric acid

- Begin by taking one hydrochloric acid (HCl) capsule (10 grains) at your next large meal. At every meal of the same size after that take one more capsule. (One capsule at the next meal, two at the meal after that, three at the next meal and so on.)
- Continue to increase the dose until you reach seven capsules or when you feel a warmth in your stomach, whichever occurs first. A feeling of warmth in the stomach means that you have taken too many capsules for that meal, and you need to take one less capsule for that size meal. It is a good idea to try the large dose again at another meal to make sure that it was the HCl that caused the warmth and not something else.

- After you have found the largest dose that you can take at your large meals without feeling any warmth, maintain that dose at all meals of similar size. You will need to take less at smaller meals.
- When taking a number of capsules it is best to take the capsules throughout the meal.
- As your stomach begins to regain the ability to produce the amount of HCl needed to digest your food properly you will notice the warm feeling again and will have to cut down the dose level.

Other digestive aids

- Pancreatin: 4X USP, two to four tablets with meals; 8X USP, one to two tablets with meals.
- Bromelain: 250 to 500 mg with meals.
- Papain: 500 to 1,000 mg with meals.
- *Gentian lutea*: dried rhizome and roots, 1–2g, or as tea tincture (1:5), 4 to 6 ml (1 to 1½ tsp).

Summary

Proper digestion is a requirement for optimum health, and incomplete or disordered digestion can be a major contributor to the development of many diseases. The problem is not only that ingestion of foods and nutritional substances are of little benefit when breakdown and assimilation are inadequate, but also that incompletely digested food molecules can be inappropriately absorbed into the systemic circulation. This can lead to various diseases and the development of food allergies.

6

Immune support

The immune system is perhaps one of the most complex and fascinating systems of the human body. While the workings of other bodily systems (respiratory, cardiovascular, digestive, musculoskeletal, etc.) have been well known for some time, it has only been relatively recently that researchers, scientists and physicians have understood the basic structure and functions of our immune system. Immunology, the study of the immune system, is one of the most dynamic fields of study involving the human body.

The immune system is composed of the lymphatic vessels and organs (thymus, spleen, tonsils and adenoids and lymph nodes), white blood cells (lymphocytes, neutrophils, basophils, eosinophils, monocytes, etc.), specialised cells residing in various tissues (macrophages, mast cells, etc.) and specialised serum factors. The immune system's prime function are protecting the body against infection and the development of cancer.

The various components of the immune system will be described, followed by a discussion of nutrients and herbs important in enhancing the immune system.

The immune system

Thymus gland

The thymus is the major gland of our immune system. It is composed of two soft pinkish-grey lobes lying like a bib just below the thyroid gland and above the heart. The thymus is responsible for many functions of the immune system, including the production of T lymphocytes, a type of white blood cell responsible for cell mediated immunity. (Cell mediated immunity refers to immune mechanisms not controlled or mediated by antibodies.) Cell mediated immunity is extremely important in resistance to infection by mould-like bacteria, yeast (including *Candida albicans*), fungi, parasites and viruses (including *Herpes simplex* and Epstein-Barr). Cell mediated immunity is also critical in protecting against the development of cancer and allergies.

The thymus gland also releases several hormones such as thymosin, thymopoeitin and serum thymic factor with regulate many immune functions. Low levels of these hormones in the blood are associated with depressed immunity and an increased susceptibility to infection. Typically, thymic hormone levels will be very low in the elderly, individuals prone to infection, AIDS patients and when an individual is exposed to undue stress.[1]

Ensuring optimal thymus gland activity, thymic hormone levels and cell mediated immunity depends upon:

- prevention of thymic involution or shrinkage;
- use of nutrients that act as cofactors for the thymic hormones;
- stimulation of thymus gland activity.

Prevention of thymic involution The thymus gland shows maximum development immediately after birth. During the ageing process the thymus gland undergoes a process of shrinkage or involution. The reason for this involution is that the thymus gland is extremely susceptible to free radical and oxidative damage caused by stress, radiation, infection and chronic illness.

Antioxidants such as vitamin C, vitamin E, selenium, zinc and beta-carotene can prevent thymic involution and enhance cell mediated immune functions.[1-5] Individuals who are under stress, who have weak immune systems or who are exposed to high levels of pollutants may need to supplement their diets with these important nutrients to prevent thymic involution and to enhance cell mediated immunity.

Nutrients required for thymic hormone manufacture Many nutrients function as important cofactors in the manufacture, secretion and function of thymic hormones. Deficiencies of any one of these nutrients results in decreased thymic hormone action and impaired immune function.[1,2] Zinc, vitamin B6 and vitamin C are perhaps the most critical nutrients. Supplementation with these nutrients has been shown to increase thymic hormone function and cell mediated immunity.[1-5] Zinc is particularly effective in restoring depressed cell mediated immunity in the elderly, largely as a result of enhancing the production, secretion and activity of the thymic hormones.[1]

Stimulation of thymus gland activity Stimulation of thymus gland activity can best be done by using high quality thymus and botanical extracts. Studies have demonstrated that the administration of extracts of calf thymus tissue can significantly increase immune function, particularly in the elderly or debilitated.[6-9] The immune enhancing effects of an orally administered thymus extract have been demonstrated in a variety of viral infections including AIDS, upper respiratory tract infections in children and viral hepatitis.

Perhaps the most widely used herb for enhancement of the immune system is *Echinacea angustifolia*. Studies have shown that echinacea has profound immune enhancing effects, many of which may be mediated via the thymus gland.[1,10,11] Other herbs which positively effect the thymus gland include liquorice (*Glycyrrhiza glabra*) and European mistletoe (*Viscum album*).[12-15]

Lymph, lymphatic vessels and lymph nodes

Approximately one-sixth of the entire body consists of the space between cells. Collectively this space is referred to as the interstitium and the fluid contained within the space is referred to as the interstitial fluid. This fluid flows into the lymphatic vessels and becomes the lymph.

Lymphatic vessels usually run parallel to arteries and veins, draining waste products from tissues and transporting the lymph to lymph nodes which filter the lymph. The cells responsible for filtering the lymph are macrophages, large cells which engulf and destroy foreign particles including bacteria and cellular debris. The lymph nodes also contain B-lymphocytes, the white blood cells which are capable of initiating antibody production in response to the presence of viruses, bacteria, yeast and other organisms.

Lymphatic function can be improved by increasing the circulation of lymph through regular exercise and diaphragmatic breathing. Those herbs which stimulate macrophage activity may also improve lymph function. Included in this category are the herbs goldenseal (*Hydrastis canadensis*), echinacea (*Echinacea angustifolia*) and Korean ginseng (*Panax ginseng*).[1,10,11,16]

The spleen

The spleen is the largest mass of lymphatic tissue in the body. In addition to producing lymphocytes, engulfing and destroying bacteria and cellular debris, the spleen is responsible for destroying worn-out blood cells and platelets. The spleen also serves as a blood reservoir. During times of demand, such as haemorrhage, the spleen can release its stored blood and prevent shock.

Spleen tissue extracts may be of benefit in enhancing immune function, as many potent immune-system-enhancing compounds secreted by the spleen are small molecular weight peptides, e.g. tuftsin is composed of only four amino acids. Orally administered spleen extracts have been shown to possess some physiological action in increasing white blood cell counts in extreme deficiencies of both lymphocytes and neutrophils (see page 60), as well as being of some benefit in patients with malaria and typhoid fever.[17] Goldenseal (*Hydrastis canadensis*) may also improve spleen function through its ability to enhance the blood flow through this important organ, as well as increasing macrophage activity.[1,16,18]

The liver

Although not considered a lymphatic organ, the liver produces the majority of lymph in the body. In addition, the integrity of the lymphatic system is highly dependent on special types of macrophage (Kupffer cells) that exist in the liver. Kupffer cells are responsible for filtering bacteria, yeast (like *Candida albicans*) and toxic foreign compounds that are absorbed by the gastrointestinal tract. These cells, when functioning properly, are extremely effective in filtering the blood; healthy Kupffer cells have been shown to engulf and destroy a single bacteria in less than 1/100 second. Those factors which enhance Kupffer cell and macrophage activity are discussed below.

White blood cells

White blood cells fall into two major groups.

- The first group is the granular white blood cells. These cells develop in the bone marrow and are characterised by the presence of granules within the cytoplasm, and lobed nuclei. The three kinds of granular white blood cells are neutrophils, eosinophils and basophils.
- The non-granular white blood cells have no granules and their nuclei are spherical rather than lobed. The two kinds of non-granular white blood cells are the lymphocytes and the monocytes.

Virtually all known vitamins and minerals are essential for normal functioning of white blood cells.[1,2] Perhaps the most well known and important nutrients for the immune system are vitamins A, B6 and C, and the trace mineral zinc. As well as being necessary for the white blood cells, these important nutrients function in the manufacture, secretion and function of thymic hormones and other chemical compounds which are necessary for white blood cell function.[4,5]

Many herbs possess direct white blood cell enhancing effects, including goldenseal (*Hydrastis canadensis*), echinacea (*Echinacea angustifolia*), Korean ginseng (*Panax ginseng*), Siberian ginseng (*Eleutherococcus senticosus*) and liquorice (*Glycyrrhiza glabra*).[1,10,11]

Neutrophils These cells actively phagocytise – engulf and destroy – bacteria, tumour cells and dead particulate matter. Neutrophils are especially important in preventing bacterial infection.

Eosinophils and basophils These cells are involved in allergic conditions. They secrete histamine and other compounds which are designed to break down antigen-antibody complexes, but which also promote allergic mechanisms.

Lymphocytes There are several types of lymphocytes – T cells, B cells, natural killer cells, etc.

T cells stand for thymus-derived lymphocytes. These cells orchestrate many immune functions and are the major components of cell mediated immunity (discussed on page 57 under thymus). There are different types of T cells, including helper T cells, which help other white blood cells to function; suppressor T cells, which inhibit and control white blood cell functions; and cytotoxic T cells, which attack and destroy foreign tissue, cancer cells and virus infected cells.

B cells are responsible for producing antibodies – large protein molecules which bind to foreign molecules (antigens) on bacteria, viruses, other organisms and tumour cells. After the antibody binds to the antigen it sets up a sequence of events that ultimately destroys the infectious organism or tumour cell.

Natural killer cells or NK cells received their name because of their ability to destroy cells that have become cancerous or infected with viruses. They are the body's first line of defence against cancer development.

Monocytes Monocytes are the garbage collectors of the body. These large white blood cells are responsible for cleaning up cellular debris after an infection, and are also responsible for triggering many immune responses.

Macrophages   As stated earlier, the lymph is filtered by specialised cells known as macrophages. Macrophages are actually monocytes that have taken up residence in specific tissues like the liver, spleen and lymph nodes. These large cells phagocytise or engulf foreign particles including bacteria and cellular debris. Macrophages are essential in protecting against invasion by mircoorganisms as well as against damage to the lymphatic system.

Many herbs possess direct macrophage enhancing effects, including goldenseal (*Hydrastis canadensis*), echinacea (*Echinacea angustifolia*), Korean ginseng (*Panax ginseng*), Siberian ginseng (*Eleutherococcus senticosus*) and liquorice (*Glycyrrhiza glabra*).[1,10,11,16,19–21]

Mast cells   Mast cells are basophils which have taken up residence primarily along blood vessels. The mast cell, like the basophil, is responsible for releasing histamine and other compounds involved in allergic reactions.

Special chemical factors

There are a number of special chemical factors which enhance the immune system (interferon, interleukin II, complement, etc.). These compounds are produced by various white blood cells, e.g. interferon is produced primarily by T cells, interleukins are produced by macrophages and T cells, and complement fractions are manufactured in the liver and spleen. These special chemical factors are extremely important in activating the white blood cells to destroy cancer cells and viruses. Several chemical mediators of our immune system (e.g. interferon and interleukin) are being investigated in the treatment of cancer, AIDS and other conditions involving the immune system.

Several nutrients are known to enhance the body's production of these compounds including beta-carotene, zinc, manganese and vitamin C.[1,2] However, numerous herbs have demonstrated far greater effect.[1,10,11] For example, the herb *Echinacea angustifolia* is remarkable in its ability to stimulate the production and action of a number of chemical mediators of immunity, but especially interferon.[1,10,11] This leads to significant antiviral activities, as interferon binds to cell surfaces and stimulates the synthesis of proteins that prevent viral infection. Several other herbs have been shown to share many of the same effects of echinacea.[10,11] Specifically, extracts of *Eupatorium perforliatum* (boneset), *Astragalus spp.* (the vetches), *Ligustrum lucidum* and *Glycyrrhiza glabra* (liquorice) have also been shown to enhance the synthesis and secretion of interferon. [1,10,11,12,22]

Stress and the immune system

The term 'stress-induced illness' is certainly not a misnomer, since many studies have clearly demonstrated that stress, personality, attitude and emotion are causative factors in many diseases. Reaction to stress is entirely individual, reinforcing the fact that people differ significantly in their perceptions and responses to various events. The variations in response help account for the wide diversity of stress-induced illnesses. Stress causes increases in the adrenal gland hormones including corticosteroids and catecholamines. Among other things, these hormones inhibit white blood cells and cause the thymus to shrink (involute). This leads to a significant suppression of immune function, leaving the host susceptible to infections, cancer and other illnesses. The level of immune suppression is usually proportional to the level of stress.

Stress results in stimulation of the sympathetic nervous system, which is responsible for the fight or flight response. The immune system functions better under para-sympathetic nervous system tone; this portion of our nervous system assumes control over bodily functions during periods of rest, relaxation, visualisation, meditation and sleep. During the deepest levels of sleep, potent immune enhancing compounds are released and many immune functions are greatly increased.[23] The value of good quality sleep and relaxation techniques for counteracting the effects of stress and enhancing our immune system cannot be overemphasised.

Many nutritional factors have been shown to prevent the effect of stress on the thymus. Specifically, vitamins A and C, beta-carotene, zinc and other antioxidants prevent stress and free-radical induced damage to the thymus, and enhance immune functions.[1-5]

Nutritional factors in immune function

Undernourishment is generally regarded as the most frequent cause of immuno-deficiency in the world.[1] Although, historically, research relating nutritional status to immune function has concerned itself with severe malnutrition states (i.e. kwashiorkor and marasmas), attention is now shifting towards marginal deficiences of single or multiple nutrients and the effects of overnutrition. There is ample evidence to support the conclusion that a single nutrient deficiency can profoundly impair the immune system.

Nutrient deficiency is not limited to third world countries. In 1965 a randomly selected sample of the US population was analysed for vitamin levels. Even though the extremely conservative recommended dietary allowance (RDA) was used as the standard for adequacy, the survey demonstrated that 88 per cent of the group had at least one deficiency and 59 per cent had two or more deficiencies.[24] These results have been repeatedly supported by population studies conducted by the US Department of Agriculture. Several studies have estimated that 19–66 per cent of the elderly population in parts of North America consume two-thirds or less of the RDA for various nutrients.[25] The significance of these findings is substantial, as demonstrated by the following examination of nutrient effects on the immune system.

General Factors

Protein The importance of adequate protein intake to proper immune function has been extensively studied.[26] The most severe effects of protein-calorie malnutrition

(PCM) are on cell mediated immunity, although all facets of immune function are ultimately affected. PCM is not, however, a single nutrient deficiency. It is normally associated with multiple nutrient deficiencies, and some immune dysfunctions attributed to PCM are most likely due to these other factors. Partial deficiencies of dietary vitamins produce a comparatively greater depression in immune functions than do partial protein deficiencies. None the less, adequate protein is essential for optimal immune function.

Sugar   The ingestion of 100-gram portions of carbohydrate as glucose, fructose, sucrose, honey and orange juice all significantly reduced the ability of neutrophils to engulf and destroy bacteria.[27,28] In contrast, the ingestion of 100 grams of starch had no effect. These effects started less than 30 minutes after ingestion and lasted for over five hours. Typically there was at least a 50 per cent reduction in neutrophil activity two hours after ingestion. Since neutrophils constitute 60–70 per cent of the total circulating white blood cells, impairment of their activity leads to depressed immunity.

In addition, ingestion of 75 grams of glucose has also been shown to depress lymphocyte activity.[29] Other parameters of immune function are also undoubtedly affected by sugar consumption. It has been suggested that the ill effects of high glucose levels are a result of competition between blood glucose and vitamin C for membrane transport sites into the white blood cells.[30,31] This is based on evidence that vitamin C and glucose appear to have opposite effects on immune function and the fact that both require insulin for membrane transport into many tissues.

Considering that the average American consumes 150 grams of sucrose, plus other refined simple sugars, each day, the inescapable conclusion is that most Americans have chronically depressed immune systems. It is clear, particularly during an infection, that the consumption of simple sugars, even in the form of fruit juice, is deleterious to the hosts' immune status. In addition, fasting should be encouraged, particularly during the first 36 to 60 hours of an acute infectious illness, since this results in a significant (up to 50 per cent) increase in the phagocytic index.[27] The fast should not be continued for an excessive period, however.

Obesity   Obesity is associated with such conditions as atherosclerosis, hypertension, diabetes mellitus and joint disorders. It is also associated with decreased immune status, as evidenced by the decreased bacteria killing activity of neutrophils, and increased morbidity and mortality from infections.[1,32] Cholesterol and lipid levels are usually elevated in obese individuals, which may explain their impaired immune function (see below).

Lipids   Increased blood levels of cholesterol, free fatty acids, triglycerides and bile acids inhibit various immune functions, including the ability of lymphocytes to proliferate and produce antibodies, and the ability of neutrophils to migrate to areas of infection and engulf and destroy infectious organisms.[1,32] Optimal immune function is therefore dependent on control of these serum components. L-carnitine, even at minimal concentrations, has been shown to neutralise lipid induced immunosuppression.[33,34] This is probably due to carnitine's role in the removal of fats from the blood.

Alcohol   Alcohol increases the susceptibility to experimental infections in animals, and alcoholics are known to be more susceptible to pneumonia. Studies of human neutrophils show a profound depression after alcohol ingestion, even in nutritionally normal people.[1]

Selected vitamins and minerals important in immune system enhancement

Vitamin A and beta-carotene   Vitamin A plays an essential role in maintaining the integrity of the epithelial and mucosal surfaces and their secretions. These systems constitute a primary nonspecific host defence mechanism. Vitamin A has been shown to stimulate and/or enhance numerous immune processes, including induction of cell mediated immunity against tumours, natural killer cell activity, monocyte phagocytosis and antibody response.[2,4,35,36] These effects are not due simply to reversal of vitamin A deficiency, since many of them are further enhanced by the administration of (supposedly) excessive levels of vitamin A.[28,35,36] In addition, vitamin A prevents and reverses stress-induced thymic involution and can actually promote thymus growth.[4] Vitamin A also demonstrates potent antiviral activity.[37]

Considerable research is directed at the relationship between both vitamin A and carotenes and the incidence of epithelial cancer, i.e. cancer of the lungs, gastrointestinal tract, genito-urinary tract and skin. Carotenes are plant pigments which protect the plant cell from being destroyed during the process of photosynthesis by acting as potent antioxidants. About 30 of the 400 or so carotenes so far characterised are able to be converted into vitamin A by the human body. Studies have demonstrated an inverse relationship between carotene intake and cancer incidence, i.e. the higher the intake of carotenes the lower the incidence of cancer. Most of the research has focused on beta-carotene.

Beta-carotene has been shown to potentiate interferon's stimulatory action on the immune system.[38-40] In addition, as carotenes are better antioxidants than vitamin A,[41] they may be more advantageous in protecting the thymus gland, since the thymus gland is particularly susceptible to free radical and oxidative damage. A study on normal human volunteers demonstrated that oral beta-carotene (180 mg/day, approximately 300,000 iu) significantly increased the frequency of helper T cells by approximately 30 per cent after seven days and all T cells after 14 days.[42] As helper T cells play a critical role in determining host immune status, this study indicates that oral beta-carotene may be effective in increasing the immunological competence of the host in conditions that are characterised by a selective lowering of the helper subset of T cells, such as AIDS. Oral beta-carotenes may also be useful for boosting anti-tumour immunity in cancer patients (in proper conjunction with other treatments).

In summary, there is much evidence that vitamin A and carotenes significantly affect the immune function and can be used preventively as well as therapeutically to improve the status of the immune system. Particularly good sources of carotenes include all green leafy vegetables, coloured root vegetables like carrots, sweet potatoes and yams, apricots, cantaloupe melons, broccoli and squash.

Vitamin C   Many claims have been made about the role of vitamin C (ascorbic acid) in enhancing the immune system, especially in regard to the prevention and treatment of the common cold. However, despite numerous positive clinical[43-46] and experimental studies,[2,3,47,48] for some reason this effect is still hotly debated. From a biochemical viewpoint there is considerable evidence that vitamin C plays a vital role in many immune mechanisms. The high concentration of vitamin C in white blood cells, particularly lymphocytes, is rapidly depleted during infection, and a relative vitamin C deficiency may ensue if ascorbic acid is not regularly replenished.

Although vitamin C has been shown to be antiviral and antibacterial, its main effect is via improvement in host resistance. Immune enhancing effects have been demonstrated in many different immune functions, including white blood cell function and activity, and increasing interferon levels, antibody responses, antibody levels, secretion of thymic hormones and integrity of connective tissue (ground substance).[2,3,47,48] Vitamin C has many biochemical effects very similar to interferon.[47]

It is important that flavonoids be administered at the same time with vitamin C, since these compounds raise the concentration of vitamin C in some tissues and potentiate vitamin C's effects.[43] These compounds also have properties of their own, useful in enhancing immune function and preventing viral infection.

Zinc   Zinc is perhaps the critical nutrient of immunity as it is involved in so many immune mechanisms, including both cell-mediated and antibody-mediated immunity, thymus gland function and thymus hormone action. When zinc levels are low the number of T cells is reduced, thymic hormone levels are lower and many white blood functions critical to the immune response are severely lacking. All of these effects are reversible upon adequate zinc administration and absorption.[49,50]

Adequate zinc levels are particularly important in the elderly and in young children. Zinc supplementation in elderly subjects results in increased number of T cells and enhanced cell mediated immune responses.[50,51] Children prone to upper respiratory tract infections typically have low levels of zinc and other trace minerals. Zinc has also been shown to inhibit the growth of several viruses including rhino, picorna and toga viruses, and *Herpes simplex* and vaccinia virus.[52]

One double-blind clinical study demonstrated that zinc gluconate lozenges significantly reduced the average duration of common colds by seven days.[53] The lozenges contained 23 milligrams of elemental zinc, which the patients were instructed to dissolve in their mouths every two waking hours after an initial double dose. After seven days, 86 per cent of the 37 zinc treated subjects were without cold symptoms, compared to 46 per cent of the 28 placebo treated subjects. Similarly impressive results were obtained by other researchers, who were also able to demonstrate that zinc lozenges had a protective effect against the development of colds.[54] The authors hypothesised that the local zinc concentration as a result of the lozenge was high enough to inhibit the replication of cold viruses.

Pyridoxine (vitamin B6)   A pyridoxine deficiency results in depressed immunity, noted by a reduction in the quantity and quality of antibodies produced, shrinkage of lymphatic tissues including the thymus gland, decreased thymic hormone activity and a reduction in the number and activity of lymphocytes.[2,55] Factors predisposing to deficiency are low dietary intake, excess protein intake and alcohol and oral contraception use.

Iron   Iron deficiency is a commonly encountered isolated nutritional deficiency which causes immune dysfunction in large numbers of patients. Marginal iron deficiency, even at levels that do not lower haemoglobin values, can influence the immune system. Lymphatic tissue shrinkage, defective macrophage and neutrophil function, and decreased proportion of T cell to B cell ratios are common findings as a result of iron deficiency.[2,55]

Iron is an important nutrient for bacteria as well as humans. During infection, one of the body's defence mechanisms to limit bacterial growth is to reduce plasma iron.[56] There is much scientific evidence to support the conclusion that iron supplementation is not indicated during acute infection, especially in young children. However, in patients with impaired immune function, chronic infections and low iron levels, adequate supplementation is essential.

Botanicals and the immune system

Many herbs have significant antibiotic action against bacteria, viruses and fungi. However, herbs are much more than 'natural' antibiotics. Many herbs show remarkable effects in stimulating our own immune mechanisms. Modern research is upholding what herbal practitioners have known for thousands of years, that herbs work with our body's systems to affect health. Perhaps the three herbs most widely used by naturopaths for enhancing immune functions are *Echinacea angustifolia* (purple coneflower), *Hydrastis canadensis* (goldenseal) and *Glycyrrhiza glabra* (liquorice).

Purple coneflower (Echinacea angustifolia)

This perennial plant is native to the midwestern states in the US and was used by the American Indian tribes as a blood purifier, analgesic, antiseptic and snake bite remedy. Recently, this herb has been shown to have significant immuno-enhancing activity.[10,11,19,20,21,57]

Its major component, inulin, is an activator of the alternative complement pathway. This pathway is responsible for increasing non-specific host defence mechanisms like neutralisation of viruses, destruction of bacteria and increasing the migration of white blood cells to areas of infection.

Echinacea has also been shown to increase properdin levels.[10,11] This compound is the body's natural activator of the alternative complement pathway. This double activation of complement may be responsible for much of echinacea's antibiotic and anticancer effects. However, further studies have shown that echinacea has other components with profound immunostimulatory effects.[10,11,19,20,21,57] The components responsible for these effects are polysaccharides that are able to bind to carbohydrate receptors on the cell surface of T lymphocytes and other white blood cells. This binding results in non-specific T cell activation including increased production and secretion of interferon.

The resultant effect is enhanced T cell mitogenesis (reproduction), macrophage phagocytosis (the engulfment and destruction of bacteria or viruses), antibody binding, and natural killer cell activity, and increased levels of circulating neutrophils (white blood cells primarily responsible for defence against bacteria).

Root extracts of echinacea have been shown to possess interferon-like activity and specific antiviral activity against influenza, herpes and vesicular stomatitis viruses.[57] Echinacea also prevents the spread of the organism via its ability to inhibit hyaluronidase. This enzyme is secreted by organisms and increases the permeability of the surrounding connective tissue. At one time hyaluronidase was termed the spreading factor.

In summary, echinacea has potent immunostimulatory activity via the alternative complement pathway, activation of T lymphocytes and other white blood cells, promotion of interferon production and secretion, antiviral activity and its ability to decrease the infectivity of the organism.

Goldenseal (Hydrastis canadensis)

This perennial herb is native to eastern North America, and was also used by the American Indian for a wide variety of conditions including infections. The pharmacologic activity of goldenseal has been largely attributed to its high content of biologically active alkaloids – berberine, hydrastine and canadine. The antibiotic activity of goldenseal's alkaloids is well documented in the literature; berberine is an effective antibiotic against a wide range of harmful organisms, including *Staphylococcus spp., Streptococcus, spp., Chlamydia spp., Corynebacterium diphtheria, Salmonella typhi, Vibrio cholerae, Diplococcus pneumonia* and *Candida albicans.*[58–60]

Goldenseal has shown remarkable immunostimulatory activity. Foremost is its ability to increase the blood supply to the spleen, thus promoting optimal activity of the spleen and the release of immunopotentiating compounds.[18] Berberine has also been shown to be a potent activator of macrophages,[16] which you will remember are responsible for engulfing and destroying bacteria, viruses, fungi and tumour cells.

Liquorice (Glycyrrhiza glabra)

This perennial temperate zone herb has been used for its medicinal properties in both western and eastern cultures for several thousand years. It is reported to be especially effective in treating respiratory tract infections (bronchitis, pharyngitis and pneumonia).[1,58]

Recent scientific evidence supports liquorice's use in treating infections. Its major components have been shown to induce interferon production.[12]; this leads to significant antiviral activities, as interferon binds to cell surfaces and stimulates the synthesis of proteins that prevent viral infection. The major liquorice components have also been shown to inhibit directly the growth of several human viruses in cell cultures, including *Herpes simplex* type 1.[61] Liquorice prevents the suppression of immunity by stress and cortisone,[13] and liquorice extracts have displayed antibiotic activity against staphylococcus, streptococcus and *Candida albicans.*[62]

A healthy immune system

This chapter has detailed the immune system, its components and natural ways to enhance its function. Perhaps the most important determinant of immune status is lifestyle – adopting a healthy lifestyle and the dietary guidelines described in Chapter 2 is certainly the first step in improving one's immune system. Specific recommendations for an acute infectious process are listed below. In addition, depending on the individual, those recommendations in such chapters as Chapter 12, AIDS, Chapter 28, Common cold, Chapter 26, Chronic fatigue, and Chapter 69, Sore throat, may be appropriate.

What to do during an infection

General measures
- Rest (bed rest better).
- Drink large amounts of fluids, preferably diluted vegetable juices, soups and herb teas.
- Limit simple sugar consumption (including fruit sugars) to less than 50 grams a day.

Supplements
- Vitamin C, 500 mg every two hours.
- Bioflavonoids, 1,000 mg per day.
- Vitamin A, 25,000 iu per day.
- Beta-carotene, 200,000 iu per day.
- Zinc lozenges, one lozenge containing 23 mg elemental zinc every two waking hours for one week. (Note: prolonged supplementation at this dose is not recommended as it may lead to immunosuppression.)
- Thymus extract, 500 mg twice daily.

Botanical medicines
Echinacea angustifolia, Hydrastis canadensis (goldenseal) and *Glycyrrhiza glabra* (liquorice) can be taken at the following doses during an infectious process (three times a day doses):
- Dried root (or as tea), 1 to 2 g.
- Freeze-dried root, 500 to 1,000 mg.
- Tincture (1:5), 4 to 6 ml (1 to 1.5 tsp).
- Fluid extract (1:1), 0.5 to 2.0 ml (¼ to ½ tsp).
- Powdered solid extract (4:1), 250–500 mg.

(Note: if liquorice is to be used over a long time it is necessary to increase the intake of potassium-rich foods – see page 98).

7

Life extension

Life extension – longevity – has been a goal of humans since long before Ponce de Leon's search for the mythical fountain of youth. More recently, a number of authors have written books advocating the use of vitamins, minerals, drugs and other compounds as a 'practical scientific approach' to life extension.[1-3] Whether or not following such recommendations will have an impact on human longevity remains to be seen, but some of the recommendations to slow down the aging process do make sense and appear to be sound. This chapter will focus on such recommendations.

Current life expectancy amd maximum life span

Life expectancy refers to the average numbers of years a person in a given population is expected to live, while life span refers to the maximal obtainable age by a member of a species.[4,5] In the United States impressive gains in extending life from birth have been made this century – from 45 years in 1900 to 71 years for men and 78 for women in 1983.[4] However this increase in expectancy is due almost entirely to decreased infant mortality; in contrast to the increase in life expectancy, life span has remained constant during this period. Increasing life expectancy involves reducing causes of premature death. Since cardiovascular disease due to atherosclerosis is the number one killer of Americans and cancer is number two, every effort should be made to reduce the risk of these diseases.

Myths still circulate about certain groups of people (the Hunzas of Pakistan, Georgian Russians and the inhabitants of Andean villages in Ecuador for example) who are reported to live to an extreme age, between 125 and 150 years. However, detailed scientific reports have refuted many of these claims.[5-7] For example, one group of investigators studying the people of Vilcabamba, Ecuador, to determine whether the degree of bone loss that occurred during aging was different in that population compared to the US population, made a revealing discovery.[6] They did an initial survey and five years later went back for a follow-up. After this five year interval a number of individuals reported being ten years older than they had been during the first survey.

Table 7.1 Causes of death in US, and rank order (1985 data)

Rank	Disease	Incidence (%)
1	Heart diseases	37.0
2	Cancer	22.1
3	Cerebrovascular disease	7.3
4	Accidents	4.5
5	Chronic lung diseases	3.6
6	Pneumonia and influenza	3.2
7	Diabetes mellitus	1.8
8	Suicide	1.4
9	Liver disease	1.3
10	Other	17.8

From studying birth records it became obvious that there was considerable exaggeration of age. In this society, as well as in the other societies associated with longevity, social standing increases with age. In the Georgia region of Russia it has been demonstrated that the majority of reported centenarians (people older than 100 years) are actually in their 70s and 80s; they just look like they are 140 years old as a result of their arduous existence.[7]

The official world record of longevity which is considered valid in scientific journals belonged to a Japanese man, Shigechiyo Izumi, who died at the age of 120 years in 1986.

What causes aging?

When a person ages, structural and physiological changes become apparent.[8] However, the reason for these changes remains the centre of controversy, although answers to the question 'What causes aging?' are developing rapidly as a result of research in gerontology, the science of aging.

There are many interesting theories of aging. However, only the most significant will be briefly discussed below. There are basically two types of aging theories: programmed theories and damage theories. Programmed theories believe there is some sort of genetic clock ticking away which determines when old age sets in, while damage theories believe aging is a result of cumulative damage to cells and genetic materials.[2,9]

The Hayflick limit

In 1912 in a laboratory at the Rockefeller Institute, Dr Alexis Carrel, one of the foremost biologists of his time, began an experiment that would last over 34 years. Dr Carrel set out to find out how long he could keep chicken fibroblasts dividing. Fibroblasts are connective tissue cells which manufacture collagen. Fed with a special broth containing an extract of chick embryo, the chicken fibroblasts grew quite well in flasks. They would divide and form new cells, with the excess cells being periodically discarded. This 'tissue culture' system kept dividing for 34 years until two years after the death of Dr Carrel, when his co-workers discarded the culture. Dr Carrel's work prompted the idea that cells are inherently immortal if given an ideal environmnt.[2,9]

This idea was not discarded until the early 1960s when Dr Leonard Hayflick observed that human fibroblasts in tissue culture wouldn't divide more than about 50 times.[2,9,10] Why the discrepancy? It appears Dr Carrel has inadvertently added new 'fresh' fibroblasts contained in his embryo broth used as nutrition for the tissue culture – new cells had repeatedly been added to the tissue cultures.

Hayflick did find that if he froze cells in culture after 20 divisions, they would 'remember' that they had 30 doublings left when they were thawed and refed. Fifty cell divisions or doublings is called the Hayflick limit. As fibroblasts approach 50 divisions, they begin looking old; they become larger and accumulate an increased amount of lipofuscin, the yellow pigment responsible for age-spots.

The programme theory

Based on the Hayflick limit, some gerontologists have theorised that there is a genetic clock ticking away within each cell which determines when old age sets in. Another programme theory involves the endocrine system. In the most popular version of this offshoot theory, it is thought that the 'clock' of aging resides in the hypothalamus, a pea-sized area of the brain that controls the pituitary gland and thus the endocrine system. The hypothalamus may trigger the pituitary to release certain hormones which induce aging.[2,9]

DNA repair theory

The genetic material, DNA, is responsible for transmitting the characteristics of one generation of species or cells to another. Damage to the DNA structure results in mutations (expression of different genetic material), or the cells simply die or are destroyed. Damage to DNA is largely due to free radicals (discussed in detail below).

DNA is constantly bombarded by free radicals and other compounds which can cause damage. However, the body has enzymes which repair damaged DNA, and the differences in life spans among mammals is largely a result of an animal or human's ability to repair damaged DNA. For example, human maximal life span (about 120 years) is more than twice as long as a chimpanzee (about 50 years) because DNA repair is much more effective.[2,11]

Research has shown that old cells are not able to repair DNA as rapidly as young cells. It appears that nature has set the rate of DNA repair at less than the rate of damage, so that animals can accumulate mutations and evolve. If repair were perfect, not only would there be no aging but there would also be no evolution.[2]

The free radical theory

The free radical theory of aging postulates that damage caused by free radicals contributes to aging and age-associated disease.[2,9,12] Free radicals are defined as highly reactive molecules which can bind to and destroy cellular compounds. Free radicals may be derived from our environment (sunlight, X-rays, radiation, chemicals), ingested foods or drinks, or produced within our bodies during chemical reactions. The majority of free radicals present within the body are actually produced within the body. However, exposure to environmental and dietary free radicals greatly increases the free radical load of the body.

Cigarette smoking is a good example of how to increase free radical load. Much of the deleterious health effects of smoking are related to extremely high levels of free radicals being inhaled. Other external sources of free radicals include radiation, air pollutants, pesticides, anaesthetics, aromatic hydrocarbons (petroleum based products), fried, barbecued and char-broiled foods, solvents, alcohol, coffee, and solvents like formaldehyde, toluene and benzene found in cleaning fluids, paints and furniture polish. Obviously reduced exposure to these sources of free radicals is recommended for life extension.

Most free radicals in the body are toxic oxygen molecules. It is ironic that the oxygen molecule is the major source of free radical damage in our bodies; oxygen sustains our lives in one sense, yet in another it is responsible for much of the destruction and aging of the cells of our bodies. Similar to the formation of rust (oxidised iron), oxygen in its toxic state is able to oxidise molecules in our bodies. (Compounds which prevent this type of damage are referred to as antioxidants.)

In addition to aging, free radicals have been linked to a number of human diseases including atherosclerosis, cancer, Alzheimer's disease, cataracts, osteoarthritis and immune deficiency.[12,13]

Extending life span

Can life span be increased and the aging process slowed? The answer is definitely yes. Specific interventions commonly recommended for reducing the aging process are discussed below.

Calorie restriction

Severe restriction of calories coupled with administration of essential nutrients is a consistent and reproducible way of increasing life span in laboratory rats and mice.[2,4,14] However, it is not known if calorie restriction has any value for humans. All we do know is that population studies accumulated by insurance companies and others show that individuals who are either overweight or severely underweight have the shortest life span while those whose weight is just below the average weight for height have the longest life span.

Exercise

The effects of exercise on longevity can be examined more easily in laboratory animals than in humans. When exercise is started early in life, animals live significantly longer.

However, exercise begun later in life has not been found to have a consistent effect on increasing life span in these animals.[2,4]

Exercise is extremely important in a healthy lifestyle, for a variety of reasons, in addition to its possible effect on increasing life span. For example, exercise helps prevent cardiovascular disease, the number one killer of Americans. Exercise can reverse or at least retard many age-related phenomena including increased bone mineral loss, decreased immunity, increased serum cholesterol and triglyceride levels, and decreased cardiovascular performance.

Dietary antioxidants

At the time of writing the only aging theory that really lends itself to intervention is the free radical theory. Compounds which prevent free radical damage are known as 'antioxidants' or free radical 'scavengers'. The body has several enzymes which prevent the damage induced by specific types of free radicals; for example, superoxide dismutase (SOD) prevents the damage caused by the toxic oxygen molecule known as superoxide. Catalase and glutathione peroxidase are two other antioxidant enzymes found in the human body.

The level of antioxidant enzymes as well as the level of dietary antioxidants like beta-carotene determine the lifespan of mammals. Human beings live longer than chimpanzees, cats, dogs and many other mammmals because we have a greater quantity of antioxidants within our cells.[2,4,11,15] Some strains of mice live longer than other strains because they have higher levels of antioxidant enzymes. Presumably, the reason why some people outlive others is that they have higher levels of antioxidants in their cells. This line of thinking is largely the reason many life extension experts recommend increasing the level of antioxidant mechanisms within cells.[1-3]

It is unlikely that antioxidant enzyme levels within cells can be increased by taking antioxidant enzymes like SOD and glutathione peroxidase orally. Human subjects taking a tablet containing SOD do not appear to increase the levels of SOD in their blood or tissues. Enzyme levels may be increased, however, by taking a number of dietary antioxidants. A large number of studies in animals have demonstrated that dietary antioxidants can definitely increase life expectancy as well as decrease cancer.[1-5] Dietary antioxidants of extreme significance in life extension include vitamins C and E, selenium, beta-carotene, flavonoids, sulphur containing amino acids and coenzyme Q_{10}. Not surprisingly, these same nutrients are also of extreme significance in cancer prevention, as aging and cancer share many common mechanisms. (Dosage recommendations are given below.)

Vitamin C Vitamin C is a very important nutritional antioxidant. Numerous experimental, clinical and population studies have shown increased vitamin C intake to possess a number of beneficial effects including reducing cancer rates, boosting immunity, protecting against pollution and cigarette smoke, enhancing wound repair and, of most significance to this chapter, increasing life expectancy.[3,4]

Vitamin E and selenium These two nutritional antioxidants work together in many instances. They are extremely important in preventing free radical damage to cell membranes. Low levels of either nutrients put people at higher risk of cancer, cardio-vascular disease, inflammatory diseases and other conditions associated with increased free radical damage, including premature aging.[3]

Carotene   Perhaps the most important dietary antioxidants are carotene molecules. Carotenes represent the most widespread group of naturally occurring pigments in plant life. For many people (physicians included) the term carotene is synonymous with provitamin A, but only 30–50 of the more than 400 carotenoids which have been char-acterised are believed to have vitamin A activity.[16]

Recent evidence demonstrates that carotenes have many more activities than serving as a precursor to vitamin A. Included in these effects is the most potent quenching of the single-oxygen free radical noted to date (many times more potent than vitamin E).[16] Although research has primarily focused on beta-carotene, other carotenes are more potent in their antioxidant activity and are deposited in tissues to a greater degree.

While research is focusing on beta-carotene intake, when one consumes a diet rich in beta-carotene it is also high in the many other carotenoids. With this in mind, it has been shown that a high intake of beta-carotene is associated with a reduced rate of cancers involving epithelial cells (lung, skin, uterine cervix, respiratory tract, gastro-intestinal tract, etc.).[3,16] As mentioned earlier, cancer and aging share a number of common characteristics, including an association with free radical damage. This has led to the idea that what prevents cancer should also promote longevity. There is some good evidence to support this claim. It appears that tissue carotenoid content is the most significant factor in determining life span in mammals, including humans.[11] Since tissue carotenoids appear to be the most significant factor in determining a species' life span potential it seems logical that individuals within the species with the optimum carotenoid content in their tissues would be the ones that would live the longest.

Consumption of foods rich in carotene (green leafy vegetables, yams, sweet potatoes, carrots, etc.) or supplementation with concentrated plant extracts rich in carotenes are the best methods of increasing tissue carotenoid levels. High carotene intake may also offer significant benefit to the immune system as the thymus gland is largely composed of epithelial cells. The thymus gland undergoes a process of involution (shrinking) during normal aging and stress. This is largely a result of free radical damage. Since carotenes are concentrated in the epithelial cells of the thymus, they are significantly able to prevent thymus gland involution. In addition, a recent study indicated that thymus gland-mediated immune functions could be improved with carotene supple-mentation.[18]

Flavonoids   Another group of plant pigments with remarkable protection against free radical damage are the flavonoids. These compounds are largely responsible for the colours of fruits and flowers. However, these compounds serve other functions in plant metabolism besides contributing to their aesthetic quality; in plants, flavonoids serve as protectors against environmental stress, while in humans flavonoids appear to function as 'biological response modifiers.'

Flavonoids appear to modify the reaction to other compounds such as allergens, viruses and carcinogens, as evidenced by their anti-inflammatory, anti-allergic, antiviral and anti-carcinogenic activity.[19-22] Flavonoid molecules are also quite unique in their antioxidant and free radical scavenging activity in that they are active against a wide variety of oxidants and free radicals.

Recent research suggests flavonoids may have significant effects in the treatment of a wide variety of conditions, including those common to aging.[19,21,22] In fact, much of the medicinal actions of many herbs, pollens and propolis are now known to be directly related to their flavonoid content. Over 4,000 flavonoid compounds have been characterised and classified according to chemical structure. The antioxidant and free radical scavenging activities of flavonoids are quite remarkable, but the fact that different flavonoids have a preference for specific tissues means that different flavonoid-rich plants should be used for different conditions. As amazing as this tissue specificity is, what is even more amazing is the fact that the historical use of a particular herb for a specific organ often mirrors the deposition pattern of its flavonoid contents.

For an example, the plant *Silybum marianum* (milk thistle), which has a long folk use in the treatment of conditions of the liver, has flavonoid molecules that have very strong affinity for the liver.[23,24] In fact, these flavonoids are some of the most potent liver protecting substances known. The flavonoids in *Silybum marianum* protect the liver by acting primarily as antioxidants. *Silybum marianum* therefore contains the types of flavonoids that should be used to protect and improve the function of the liver.

In another example, *Ginkgo biloba* extract contains flavonoids that appear to have a very strong affinity for the adrenal and thyroid gland, and the central nervous system.[25] Ginkgo flavonoids are extremely potent antioxidants that are also capable of improving the flow of blood to the brain.[26] *Ginkgo biloba* flavonoids are therefore the most appropriate for conditions involving the brain and circulation. In addition, *Ginkgo biloba* extract may eventually be shown to improve age-related decreases in the function of the adrenal and thyroid glands.

Ginkgo biloba extract is extremely useful in increasing the quality of life in the elderly. Many symptoms common in the elderly are a result of insufficient blood and oxygen supply. *Ginkgo biloba* extract has demonstrated remarkable effects in improving blood and oxygen supply to tissues, and is particularly effective in treating insufficient blood and oxygen supply to the brain associated with a number of common symptoms of aging including short-term memory loss, dizziness, headache, ringing in the ears, hearing loss, lack of vigilance (get up and go) and depression.[27]

The best way to ensure an adequate intake of flavonoids is to eat a varied diet rich in fruits and vegetables.

Sulphur-containing amino acids   The sulphur-containing amino acids methionine and cysteine are important components of a life extension plan. Typically, as people age the content of these amino acids in the body decreases.[4] Since supplementing the diets of mice and guinea pigs with cysteine increases life span considerably, it has been suggested that maintaining optimum levels of methionine and cysteine may promote longevity in humans.[1-4]

Dietary methionine and cysteine levels are a major determinant in the concentration of sulphur-containing compounds such as glutathione within cells. Glutathione assumes a critical role in defence against a variety of injurious compounds by acting as part of the free radical scavenging enzyme glutathione peroxidase and by combining directly with these toxic substances to aid in their elimination. When increased levels of toxic compounds or free radical are present in the body, the body needs higher levels of methionine and cysteine. (The importance of sulphur amino acids to the liver is thoroughly discussed in Chapter 8, Liver support.)

Good dietary sources of methionine and cysteine are beans, fish, liver, eggs, brewer's yeast and nuts.

Recommendations

Specific recommendations and dosages of supplements recommended for slowing the aging process are given below. These include high, but not excessive, doses of dietary antioxidants. Higher doses of these nutrients, especially vitamin E and selenium, may be detrimental.

Diet

A high intake of vegetables and fruits is essential to a life extension programme due to the high content of vitamins, minerals, carotenes, flavonoids and dietary fibres in these foods. It is especially important to follow the dietary recommendations for reducing risk of heart disease (atherosclerosis), such as increasing the intake of dietary fibre, especially the gel-forming or mucilaginous fibres (flax seed, oat bran, pectin, etc.), cold-pressed vegetable oils and fish, while reducing the consumption of saturated fats, cholesterol, sugar and animal proteins.

Nutritional supplements

- Broad spectrum multivitamin and mineral.
- Beta-carotene or mixed carotenes, 200,000 iu.
- Vitamin C, 1–3 grams daily.
- Vitamin E, 600 iu.
- Selenium, 200 micrograms.
- Cysteine, 250 mg.
- Methionine, 250 mg.

Summary

At this time there are no 'magic bullets' to halt the aging process. However, rather than trying to lengthen life span (quantity), one should be more concerned with increasing the quality of life. The best way to ensure a long and healthy life is to adopt those guidelines described in Chapter 2.

8

Liver support

The liver is truly an intricate, complex and remarkable organ. It is, without question, the most important organ of metabolism. To a very large extent the health and vitality of an individual is determined by the health and vitality of the liver.

It is amazing how well the liver survives the constant onslaught of toxic chemicals it is responsible for detoxifying. Some of the toxic chemicals known to pass through the liver include the polycyclic hydrocarbons that are components of various herbicides and pesticides, including DDT, dioxin, 2,4,5-T, 2,4-D and the halogenated compounds PCB and PCP. Although the exact degree of exposure of people to these compounds is not known, it is probably quite high, as yearly US production of synthetic organic pesticides alone exceeds 600,000 tons.[1] The health effects of chronic exposure to these compounds, as well as many others, has not been fully determined (other than the known association with various cancers). As the liver is responsible for detoxifying these chemicals and many others, every effort should be made to promote optimal liver function.

Optimising liver function focuses on protecting the liver and the use of lipotropic factors. Liver protecting substances include many nutritional and herbal compounds which prevent damage to the liver associated with detoxifying harmful chemicals while lipotropic factors are, by definition, substances that hasten the removal or decrease the deposit of fat in the liver through their interaction with fat metabolism. Compounds commonly employed as lipotropic agents include choline, methionine, betaine, folic acid and vitamin B12, along with herbal cholagogues and choleretics. (Cholagogues are agents that stimulate gallbladder contraction to promote bile flow, while choleretics are agents that stimulate bile secretion by the liver, as opposed to the expulsion of bile by the gallbladder.)

Formulas containing lipotropic agents have been used for a wide variety of conditions by naturopathic physicians, particularly in hepatic conditions, such as hepatitis, cirrhosis and alcohol-induced fatty infiltration of the liver. They have also been used in treating premenstrual tension syndrome, as they are believed to aid the liver in its ability to conjugate and excrete oestrogens. But perhaps the most widespread use of lipotropic factors has been in the condition labelled 'congested liver', 'sluggish liver' and other equally ill-defined terms. Before discussing this condition, let's establist a reference point by reviewing several of the liver's important functions in the body.

The liver's important roles

The liver's basic functions are threefold: vascular, secretory and metabolic. Its vascular functions include being a major blood reservoir and filtering over a litre of blood per minute. The liver effectively removes bacteria, endotoxins, antigen–antibody complexes and various other particles from the circulation.

The liver's secretory functions involve the synthesis and secretion of bile. Each day the liver manufactures about 1 litre of bile. Bile is necessary for the absorption of fat soluble substances, including many vitamins. Although the majority of the bile secreted into the intestines is reabsorbed, many toxic substances are effectively eliminated from the body by the bile.

The metabolic functions of the liver are immense, as the liver is intricately involved in carbohydrate, fat and protein metabolism; the storage of vitamins and minerals; the formation of numerous physiological factors; and the detoxification or excretion into the bile of various chemical compounds including hormones such as thyroxine, cortisol, oestrogen and aldosterone, histamine, drugs and pesticides.

The 'sluggish' or congested liver

The term 'sluggish liver' probably reflects minimal impairment of liver function. Because of the liver's important role in numerous metabolic processes, even minor impairment of liver function could have profound effects. One of the leading contributors to impaired liver function is diminished bile flow or cholestasis.

Cholestasis can be caused by a great number of factors, including obstruction of the bile ducts and impairment of bile flow within the liver. The most common cause of obstruction of the bile ducts is the presence of gallstones. Currently it is conservatively estimated that 20 million people in the United States have gallstones – nearly 20 per cent of the female and 8 per cent of the male population over the age of 40 are found to have gallstones on biopsy, and approximately 500,000 gallbladders are removed because of stones each year. The prevalence of gallstones in the US has been related to the high fat/low fibre diet consumed by the majority of Americans.[2,3]

Impairment of bile flow within the liver can be caused by a variety of agents and conditions.[4] These conditions are typically associated with alterations in laboratory tests of liver function (serum bilirubin, alkaline phosphatase, serum aspartate transaminase, alanine aminotransferase, gamma-glutamyl transpeptidase, etc.) signifying cellular damage. However, relying on these tests alone to evaluate hepatic function may not be adequate, as many of these conditions in the initial or 'subclinical' stages may have normal laboratory values, with liver dysfunction measurable only by a slight increase in serum bile acid levels, bromsulphalein (BSP) retention, or structural change noted by examination of liver biopsy sample.

Causes of cholestasis[4]

Presence of gallstones
Alcohol
Endotoxins
Hereditary disorders such as Gilbert's syndrome
Pregnancy
Natural and synthetic steroidal hormones:
    Anabolic steroids
    Oestrogens
    Oral contraceptives
Certain chemicals or drugs:
    Aminosalicylic acid
    Chlorothiazide
    Erythromycin estolate
    Mepazine
    Phenylbutazone
    Sulphadiazine
    Thiouracil
Hyperthyroidism or thyroxine supplementation
Viral hepatitis

These latter two procedures do not appear to be clinically useful due to the risk of side effects, but their use in some studies has demonstrated that liver dysfunction or injury is not always accompanied by changes in the typically used liver function tests. This is particularly true in liver dysfunction related to oral contraceptive use and exposure to various drugs and chemicals.[2,3] The use of serum bile acid assays may be a more specific and sensitive indicator for chemical liver injury, especially in detecting initial enzymatic damage to the liver, but further research is needed.

At present, it appears that clinical judgment based on medical history remains the major diagnostic tool for the 'sluggish liver'. Exposure to toxic chemicals, drugs, alcohol or hepatitis is usually apparent in the individual with a sluggish liver. Among the symptoms people with this condition may complain of are fatigue, general malaise, digestive disturbances, allergies and chemical sensitivities, premenstrual syndrome and constipation.[5]

Perhaps the most common cause of cholestasis and impaired liver function is alcohol ingestion. In some individuals as little as 1 ounce (25 g) of alcohol can produce damage to the liver which results in fat being deposited within the liver (alcohol-induced fatty liver). All active alcoholics demonstrate fatty infiltration of the liver. A result of this fatty infiltration is decreased liver function and an increased risk of further damage to the liver. Obviously, alcohol use does not promote optimal liver function.

Protecting and enhancing the function of the liver

The concept of liver protection basically reflects an appreciation of the liver's critical role in all aspects of metabolism and an attempt to improve the liver's function by protecting it from damage. Several factors offer significant liver protection – antioxidants, membrane stabilising compounds, choleretics and compounds that prevent the depletion within the liver of non-protein sulphur compounds such as glutathione. Although many compounds fulfil some these criteria, only those compounds that exhibit significant benefit to the liver and that are indicated in the majority of individuals with impaired liver function are discussed here.

Nutritional considerations

General dietary factors   A diet high in saturated fat increases the risk of developing fatty infiltration and/or cholestasis. In contrast, a diet rich in dietary fibre, particularly the water-soluble fibres, has a choleretic effect by promoting increased bile secretion.

The nutritional antioxidants, i.e. vitamin C and E, zinc and selenium, are essential in protecting the liver from free radical damage. Free radicals are highly reactive molecules that can destroy cellular structures unless they are effectively scavenged. Optimum tissue concentrations of these compounds should be maintained in the treatment of hepatic disease as well as the promotion of liver health.

Choline   A fatty liver similar in appearance to alcohol-induced fatty liver has been produced in rats, guinea pigs, dogs, pigs, monkeys and several species of poultry when these animals have been placed on a diet deficient in choline and protein.[6] These findings have promoted controversy concerning the role of choline in alcohol-induced fatty liver and cirrhosis in humans. However similar the lesions may be in these animal studies, choline has not been shown to be of any value in the treatment of alcohol-induced liver disease in humans.[6,7]

Choline can be synthesised in humans from either methionine or serine. Choline may have some direct lipotropic effects in humans but research indicates that these effects may be more related to an indirect effect via methionine metabolism. Dietary sources of choline include lecithin, egg yolk, liver and all legumes (beans).

Methionine   This essential sulphur-containing amino acid is a component of the major lipotropic compound in humans, S-adenosylmethionine (SAM).[8,9] Methionine is a major source of numerous sulphur-containing compounds, including the amino acids cysteine and taurine. Methionine administered as SAM has been shown to be quite beneficial in two common conditions indicative of cholestasis, namely oestrogen excess due to either oral contraceptive use or pregnancy, and Gilbert's syndrome.[10,11,12]

SAM is able to inactivate oestrogens (through methylation), supporting the use of methionine in conditions of presumed oestrogen excess such as PMS. Its effects in preventing oestrogen-induced cholestasis have been demonstrated in pregnant women and those on oral contraceptives.[10,11] In addition to its role in promoting oestrogen excretion, methionine has been shown to increase the membrane fluidity that is typically decreased by oestrogens, thereby restoring several factors that promote bile flow.

Gilbert's syndrome is a common syndrome characterised by a chronically elevated serum bilirubin level (1.2 to 3.0 mg/dl).[2,3] Previously considered rare, this disorder is now known to affect as much as 5 per cent of the general population. The condition is usually without symptoms, although some patients do complain about anorexia, malaise and fatigue (typical symptoms of impaired liver function). Methionine, administered as SAM, resulted in a significant decrease in serum bilirubin in patients with Gilbert's syndrome in a recent clinical study.[12] SAM has been used with favourable results in a variety of other chronic liver diseases.[13]

Methionine levels are a major determinant in the liver's concentration of sulphur-containing compounds, such as glutathione. Glutathione and other sulphur-containing peptides (small proteins) assume a critical role in defence against a variety of injurious agents by combining directly with these toxic substances, eventually to form water soluble compounds. As many of the toxic compounds are lipid (fat) soluble, conversion to water soluble compounds results in more efficient excretion via the kidneys. When increased levels of toxic compounds are present, more methionine is converted to cysteine and glutathione synthesis. Methionine itself has a protective effect on glutathione and prevents depletion during toxic overload. This, in turn, protects the liver from the damaging effects of toxic compounds.[9,14]

Carnitine Carnitine is a vitamin-like compound that we can manufacture within our own body. Since carnitine normally facilitates the conversion of fatty acids to energy, a high liver carnitine level is needed to handle the increased fatty acid load produced by alcohol consumption, a high fat diet and/or chemical exposure. While the use of lipotropic agents appears warranted in treating alcohol-induced fatty liver disease, many commonly used lipotropic agents, e.g. choline, niacin and cysteine, appear to have little value.[15,16] In contrast, carnitine significantly inhibits alcohol-induced fatty liver disease. It has been suggested that chronic ethanol (alcohol) consumption or chemical exposure results in a deficiency of carnitine due to impaired synthesis.[17,18,19] By supplementing L-carnitine, this functional deficiency state is reversed, leading to normalisation of fatty acid transport and alleviation of fatty acid infiltration within the liver.

Liver extracts The oral administration of liquid liver extracts has been used in the treatment of many chronic liver diseases since 1896.[20] Numerous scientific investigations into the therapeutic efficacy of liver extracts have demonstrated that they possess a lipotropic effect, promote liver cell regeneration and prevent scarring (fibrosis).[21,22,23] Clinical studies have demonstrated that oral administration of concentrated liver extracts (hydrolysates) can be quite effective in the treatment of chronic liver disease, including chronic active hepatitis.[24,25]

Botanical medicines which improve liver function

Dandelion root (Taraxacum officinale) While many individuals consider the common dandelion to be an unwanted weed, herbalists all over the world have revered this valuable herb for many centuries. Its common name, dandelion, is a corruption of the

French for 'tooth of the lion' (*dent de lion*) which describes the several large pointed teeth of the herb's leaves. Its scientific name, *Taraxacum officinale*, from the Greek *taraxos* (disorder) and *akos* (remedy), alludes to dandelion's ability to correct a multitude of disorders.

Although generally regarded as a liver remedy, dandelion has a long folk use throughout the world for a variety of ailments. In Europe dandelion was used in the treatment of fevers, boils, eye problems, diarrhoea, fluid retention, liver congestion, heartburn and various skin problems. In China dandelion has been used in the treatment of breast problems (cancer, inflammation, lack of milk flow, etc.), liver diseases, appendicitis and digestive ailments. Its use in India, Russia and other parts of the world revolved primarily around its action on the liver.[26,27]

The dandelion contains much more nutritional value than many other vegetables, being particularly high in vitamins, minerals, protein, choline, inulin and pectins. Its carotenoid content is extremely high, as reflected by a vitamin A content higher than that of carrots (dandelion has 14,000 iu of vitamin A per 100 grams compared with 11,000 iu for carrots).[26,27]

Dandelion is regarded as one of the finest liver remedies, both as food and medicine. Studies in humans and laboratory animals have shown that dandelion enhances the flow of bile, improving such conditions as liver congestion, bile duct inflammation, hepatitis, gallstones and jaundice.[28,29] Dandelion's action on increasing bile flow is twofold. It has a direct effect on the liver, causing an increase in bile production and flow to the gallbladder (choleretic effect), and a direct effect on the gallbladder, causing contraction and release of stored bile (cholagogue effect). Dandelion's beneficial effect on such a wide variety of conditions is probably closely related to its ability to improve the functional capacity of the liver.

Milk thistle (Silybum marianum)   The common milk thistle contains some of the most potent liver protective substances known, a mixture of three flavanolignins collectively referred to as silymarin.[30-33] The concentration of silymarin is highest in the fruit, but it is also found in the seeds and leaves.

Silymarin's effect in preventing liver destruction and enhancing liver function relates largely to its ability to inhibit the factors that are responsible for hepatic damage, i.e. free radicals and leukotrienes, coupled with an ability to stimulate liver protein synthesis.[30-33]

Silymarin prevents free radical damage by acting as an antioxidant. Silymarin is many times more potent in antioxidant activity than vitamin E. Silymarin not only prevents the depletion of glutathione (GSH) induced by alcohol and other liver toxins, but it was shown to increase the basal GSH of the liver by 35 per cent over controls in one study. This is extremely useful when exposure to toxic substances is high, due to glutathione's vital role in detoxification reactions.

The protective effect of silymarin against liver damage has been demonstrated in a number of experimental and clinical studies.[30-38] Experimental liver damage in animals can be produced by such diverse toxic chemicals as carbon tetrachloride, amanita toxin, galactosamine and praseodymium nitrate. Silymarin has been shown to protect against liver damage by all of these agents.[30-33]

Another way in which the liver can be damaged is by the action of leukotrienes. These compounds are produced by the transfer of oxygen to a polyunsaturated fatty acid. This reaction is catalysed by the enzyme lipoxygenase. Silybum components inhibit this enzyme, thereby inhibiting the formation of these damaging compounds.

Perhaps the most interesting effect of silybum components on the liver is their ability to stimulate protein synthesis.[30-33] The result is an increase in the production of new liver cells to replace the damaged old ones. This demonstrates that silymarin exerts both a protective and restorative effect on the liver.

In human studies, silymarin has been shown to have positive effects in treating liver diseases of various kinds, including cirrhosis, chronic hepatitis, fatty infiltration of the liver (chemical and alcohol induced fatty liver) and inflammation of the bile duct.[32-38] The therapeutic effect of silymarin in all of these disorders has been confirmed by histological (biopsy), clinical and laboratory data. Silymarin is especially effective in the treatment and prevention of toxic chemical or alcohol induced liver damage.[32-38]

Artichoke leaves (Cynara scolymus)   The artichoke has a long folk history in treating many liver diseases. Recent evidence supports this long-time use. The active ingredients in artichoke are caffeylquinic acids (like cynarin). These compounds are found in highest concentration in the leaves. Like silymarin, cynara extracts have demonstrated significant liver protecting and regenerating effects.[33,39] They also possess choleretic effect. This is a very important property; if the bile is not being transported adequately to the gallbladder, the liver is at increased risk of damage. Choleretics are very useful in the treatment of hepatitis and other liver diseases via the 'decongesting' effect.

Choleretics typically lower cholesterol levels, since they increase the excretion of cholesterol and decrease the synthesis of cholesterol in the liver. Consistent with its choleretic effect, cynarin has shown to lower blood cholesterol and triglyceride levels in both human and animal studies.[39-41]

Turmeric (Curcuma longa)   The common spice turmeric contains the yellow pigment curcumin which has demonstrated liver protective effects similar to those of silymarin and cynarin.[42] Curcumin's documented choleretic effects support its historical use in the treatment of liver and gallbladder disorders.[26] Like cynarin, curcumin has also been shown to lower cholesterol levels.[14]

Recommendations

Diet

For optimum liver function, a diet rich in dietary fibre and plant foods, low in refined sugar and fat, and as free from pesticides and pollutants as possible is preferred. In addition, needless to say, alcohol consumption is not advised.

Nutritional supplements

- Choline, 1 gram/day.
- L-methionine, 1 gram/day.
- S-adenosylmethionine (SAM), 200 mg three times a day.
- L-carnitine, 500 mg twice daily.
- Liquid liver extract, 500 mg three times a day.

Botanical medicines

- *Taraxacum officinale*
    Dried root, 4 grams three times a day.
    Fluid extract (1:1), 4–8 ml three times a day.
    Solid extract (4:1), 250–500 mg three times a day.
- *Silybum marianum.* The standard dose of *Silybum marianum* is based on its silymarin content, 70–210 mg of silymarin three times daily.
- *Cynara scolymus*
    Extract (15 per cent cynarin), 500 mg three times a day.
    Cynarin, 500 mg a day.
- *Curcuma longa* – can be used liberally as spice.
    Curcumin, 300 mg three times a day.

Summary

Liver protective substances, including lipotropic factors and choleretics, appear to be indicated for many liver conditions, including minimal liver impairment, i.e. a sluggish or congested liver. The use of these liver remedies may offer significant benefit when vague complaints such as malaise and fatigue are present, particularly when serum bile acids are elevated or when there are signs of altered protein, carbohydrate or fat metabolism.

Lipotropic factors appear to be very much indicated in women taking oral contraceptive agents or those with increased oestrogen levels (including pregnancy). Patients with a history of exposure to toxic compounds, especially organic solvents and polycyclic hydrocarbons such as pesticides and herbicides, may also benefit from liver protective substances.

When using choleretic substances, a looser stool may be produced as a result of increased bile flow and secretion. If higher doses of choleretics are used it may be appropriate to use bile-sequestering fibre compounds (e.g. guar gum, pectin, psyllium, oat bran, etc.) to prevent irritation of the wall of the intestine and loose stools.

9

Pain control[1]

Pain accompanies almost all diseases and is one of the most common symptoms for which patients seek relief. Although pain is an unpleasant experience, it is an important message about tissue injury or other problems within the body. Therefore, before controlling pain, it is essential first to determine why the pain exists. The best way to relieve pain is to treat the primary cause (e.g. curing an infection, splinting a broken bone, healing a stomach ulcer, eliminating the food allergy that causes the migraine headache, etc.). Modern society is so afraid of pain that we sometimes consider it a disease to be eradicated rather than a symptom to be heeded.

The experience of pain

Pain is generally acknowledged to be a complex physiological/psychological phenomenon. Each individual's perception of, and reaction to, pain is highly subjective and influenced by many personal, social, cultural and economic factors. Many models have been proposed to help researchers and physicians understand the mechanisms of pain. Although a complete discussion is beyond the scope of this work, some key elements are important for the understanding of the pain control techniques discussed here.

In general, the experience of pain can be broken down to a sequential multistage process according to Loeser's 'Seattle model' and Melzack and Wall's 'gate control theory' (this is greatly simplified).[2,3]

- Nociception – the neurological signal generated by tissue damage or other derangement of normal body function.
- Transmission of pain impulses, through the A-delta and C nerve fibres in the spinal cord.
- Pain perception – the neurological reaction in the brain.
- Suffering – the subjective experience.
- Pain behaviour – the response.

A person's perception of pain and associated behavioural responses are affected at several levels by many factors – metabolic processes at the site of pain initiation, neurological activity within the spine and brain, and psychological, cultural and situational elements. These latter factors are particularly important since the way a person conceptualises their pain has a major impact on its perception. For example, a woman in labour could consider pain as positive, functional and creative, i.e. pain with a purpose, or alternatively as part of a process involving injury.[4]

Pain control

Although the medical profession has chosen to emphasise the pharmacological methods of pain control, many non-pharmacological options are available.
- Inhibiting the initiation of pain messages.
- Limiting the magnitude of the pain message.
- Blocking the transmission of pain messages.
- Limiting the perception of pain.
- Controlling the experience of pain.

Dietary considerations

Although in general diet does not have much effect on the perception of pain, some dietary factors may be important.

Animal fats Much pain is in response to inflammatory processes. Therefore, eating patterns which restrain inflammation can be of benefit in limiting the magnitude of the pain message. Since the enzyme which produces arachidonic acid is largely lacking in man, diet is the major source of arachidonic acid, the precursor of several important inflammatory prostaglandins.[5] By decreasing animal fat intake – the only dietary source of arachidonic acid – a significant reduction in the inflammatory processes attributed to the arachidonic acid cascade can be achieved.

Eicosapentaenoic acid Eating more fatty fish (e.g. mackerel, herring and salmon) results in a significant increase of eicosapentaenoic acid in the fatty acid pools.[2,3] This is significant since eicosapentaenoic acid:
- decreases the release of membrane-bound arachidonic acid, thereby decreasing the magnitude of the arachidonic acid cascade;
- forms less potent inflammatory products than those derived from arachidonic acid; and
- decreases synthesis of mediators of inflammation.[6,7]

Coffee An interesting animal experiment found that instant coffee blocks the opiate receptors in rat brains.[8] This is significant since endorphins (the body's natural opiates) are part of the internal mechanisms for controlling pain – blocking the receptor sites makes the body more receptive to pain. Instant tea, cocoa, soup powders, stock cubes and extracts of yogurt and cream cheese did not show this blocking activity.

Nutritional considerations

D-phenylalanine   Although the use of the amino acid D-phenylalanine for the control of pain has received considerable attention in the lay press, the scientific evidence is mixed. While some double-blind studies have shown a 50 per cent reduction of pain,[9] others[10] failed to reproduce this result. D-phenylalanine appears to potentiate the analgesic effects of aspirin and acupuncture.[11]

L-tryptophan   Several double-blind studies have found tryptophan supplementation to be a mild analgesic, similar in effect to aspirin.[12] It has been found effective in the treatment of chronic facial pain, dental pain, experimental pain and after dental root canal surgery.[13–16] Its mode of action is unknown, but has been hypothesised to be an increase in pain tolerance threshold, reversal of tolerance to opiates and decreased perception of pain.

Vitamin B1   In the 1940s, shortly after thiamin (then called aneurine) was first synthesised, large oral and injected doses were used to relieve pain. It was reported to be effective for the pain of dental extraction, migraine headache, varicose ulcers, amputated limbs, incurable cancer and osteoporosis.[17] Unfortunately not all research found the same results and this promising work does not seem to have been pursued. Its mode of action was thought due to the neurological system's requirement for this nutrient and its vasodilatory properties.

Herbal therapies

Many herbs have been used throughout the centuries for the treatment of pain. Discussed below are those which have both folk and scientific support.

Red or hot pepper (Capsicum frutescens)   Capsaicin is the major pungent ingredient of hot peppers.[18] Capsaicin depletes (after an initial stimulation of release) substance P (which is involved in some aspects of pain mediation) in sensory nerves[19] and has a long history of use in the control of pain.[14] The chemical structure of capsaicin is similar to that of eugenol, the active principle of clove oil, which can induce long-lasting local anaesthesia.[20]

German chamomile (Matricaria chamomilla)   German chamomile has been reported to have anti-inflammatory, antispasmodic and analgesic properties. It appears that chamazulene, a major component of the oil, is the key component responsible for these properties.[18]

Clove oil (Syzygium aromaticum)   Clove oil has a long history of use for the relief of toothache, and local application is useful after tooth extractions. The oil contains 60 to 90 per cent eugenol which is thought responsible for its analgesic properties.[18]

Wintergreen oil (Gaultheria procumbens)   Wintergreen oil is obtained by steam distillation from this evergreen shrub and is almost entirely methyl salicylate.[18] Salicylate (the active component of aspirin) is a well-documented anti-inflammatory and analgesic.[21] It should only be used topically.

Psychological approaches

The psychological approaches aim to provide control, communication, relaxation, attention focus and support. There is considerable research supporting the use of these in the development of pain tolerance. Several strategies have been developed to assist individuals in controlling their pain.

Cognitive strategies   Research has clearly demonstrated that the greater understanding a person has about what is happening during a painful experience, particularly if there is some control over the pain, the less pain they will experience.[22,23] Similarly, information received prior to the onset of experimental or surgical pain consistently decreases the perception of pain.[24]

Much of the research that has been done in this area has studied women during childbirth. This is typified by a study conducted at the University of Wisconsin, which used ice water to test the perception and endurance of pain in subjects who had been taught methods used in childbirth education classes. Two control groups were used; one group received no training and the other was offered distraction during the tests.[25] Those who had been taught the prepared childbirth techniques reported only about half the pain of the controls and endured it 2.5 times longer. The strategies improved with practice.

Attention focusing   Researchers have found that attention focusing functions effectively as an analgesic for labour pains.[26] Such strategies are strongly supported by much psychological research. The focus may be on a competing response, as in a study showing that when attention was directed to self-presented external slides, individuals were able to increase their tolerance of the pain of cold water.[27] The effectiveness of focus on a competing response is also shown in the use of hypnosis as an analgesic and in the meditative states of raja yogis. These yogis are able to pinpoint attention on the tip of their nose or a point on the back of their skull, and thus avoid any physiological reaction to cold water, bright lights or sudden sounds.[28,29] Other adepts, in unusual feats of pain control such as tolerating spikes driven into their skin, either maintain an unfocused attitude, without evaluation, or pinpoint attention totally on the pain, but without evaluation.[30] In such cases the attitude of detachment from the pain is characterised by an undisturbed EEG pattern of alpha or beta waves throughout the performance of the feat.

Relaxation training   Relaxation training is another essential element of pain control. There is a considerable body of literature to support its importance in pain control, since a state of lowered autonomic arousal is incompatible with anxiety. While progressive muscular relaxation, systematic desensitisation and autogenic training are all well-established physiological approaches to muscular relaxation, meditation traditions provide quicker methods to achieve the relaxation response,[31] One of the simplest meditation practices is maintaining a focused awareness of the flow of the breath.

Biofeedback The psychophysiological relaxation techniques of biofeedback, which include frontalis electromyography (EMG) which determines the muscular tension of the muscles of the forehead, and finger temperature feedback, are commonly applied with success to chronic pain problems such as recurrent headaches.[32]

Acceptance Acceptance has been observed to be a key factor that assists patients in greater understanding of their pain, resulting in a decreased perception of pain.[33,34] Acceptance does not mean complacency in the face of disease, but a rational understanding of the situation and the limitations that can sometimes accompany a disease process.

Placebo A person's belief in the ability of an external agent to relieve their pain can be almost as effective as the strongest pain medications. For example, an extensive review of research into the efficacy of various pain control medications found that 35 per cent of patients suffering from pain experienced a 50 per cent reduction in their symptoms following placebo medication.[35,36] This is particularly remarkable when viewed in the context that with a standard dose of morphine only 75 per cent of the patients will get a 50 per cent reduction in pain. It has been shown that lower back pain patients given a placebo described as a new pain medication will show significant benefit, even after being told they were taking a placebo. Moreover, providing strategies to reinforce their belief in the effectiveness of the placebo further enhanced its efficacy.[37]

Hypnosis Hypnosis, or auto-hypnosis, is also utilised to induce deep relaxation. It incorporates many of the therapeutic elements already referred to – focused attention, positive expectation and a supportive or permissive attitude – in making suggestions that alleviate anxiety.

Counter stimulus methods

Transcutaneous electrical nerve stimulation (TENS) The use of TENS to control pain has been evaluated by several studies.[38,39] Generally, the electrodes are placed over the painful area in order to stimulate the skin nerves in that area. This stimulation competes with the pain impulses, thus decreasing the transmission of pain messages to the brain. TENS has been shown to be effective in several conditions – experimental pain, childbirth, arthritis and tendinitis, and, in conjunction with analgesic drugs, angina pectoris and myocardial infarction.[40-3]

Acupuncture Hundreds of studies have investigated the efficacy of acupuncture analgesia for acute and chronic pain. A review article of 24 studies found that the typical clinical trial showed a 70 per cent efficacy when compared with placebo treatment.[44]

A considerable amount of research has also focused on determining the mechanism for acupuncture analgesia. The hypothesis that acupuncture stimulates release of endorphins from the brain has been the subject of considerable attention. A typical study demonstrated that the increase in pain threshold (as measured by electrical stimulation of tooth pulp) induced by acupuncture stimulation was subsequently reversed by injection of naloxene, a potent inhibitor of endorphins.[45] However, others failed to corroborate the endorphin hypothesis in their attempt to duplicate the experiment.[46]

Summary

Although pain is a common component of disease, it is, in most cases, a symptom not a disease. As such, it is a message from the body and is best handled by treating its cause, the underlying disease. When pain must be dealt with directly, many methods other than pain medications can be utilised. This chapter has presented many of the alternative strategies for control of pain.

Since the mechanism of pain perception has been shown to involve both physiological and psychological components, the optimum treatment combines psychological factors of control of fear and anxiety, understanding, acceptance, attention focus, relaxation and supportive communication; the physical stimuli of transcutaneous electrical nerve stimulation or acupuncture; and dietary, nutritional and herbal methods.

10

Stress

Stress is a term widely used in our current fast-paced society. Often the daily demands placed on us build up and accumulate to a point where it is almost impossible to cope. Job pressures, family arguments, financial pressures, deadlines – these are common examples of 'stressors'. Actually a stressor may be almost anything which creates a disturbance, including exposure to heat or cold, environmental toxins, toxins produced by microorganisms, physical trauma and of course strong emotional reactions.

Some basic control mechanisms are geared toward counteracting the everyday stresses of life. However, if stress is extreme, unusual or long-lasting, these control mechanisms can be quite harmful. Stress triggers a number of biological changes known collectively as the general adaptation syndrome. The three phases of the general adaptation syndrome are alarm, resistance and, finally, exhaustion.[1] These phases are controlled and regulated by the adrenal glands.

Basic anatomy and physiology of the adrenal gland

The adrenal glands are responsible for maintaining the balance of many bodily functions by secreting several important hormones. An abnormal adrenal response, either deficient or excessive hormone secretion, significantly alters an individual's response to stress. Often the adrenals become 'exhausted' as a result of the constant demands placed upon them. An individual with adrenal exhaustion may feel 'stressed out', tired and be prone to allergies, while an individual with excessive adrenal activity is likely to have high blood pressure, anxiety, depression and elevated blood sugar and cholesterol levels.[1]

The adrenal glands lie just above the kidneys and are composed of two distinct parts, the adrenal medulla and the adrenal cortex. The inner portion of the adrenal gland, the medulla, is functionally related to the sympathetic nervous system, and secretes the hormones adrenaline (epinephrine) and noradrenaline (norepinephrine). These hormones stimulate many body processes related to the fight or flight response (see box). They also serve to maintain normal nervous control over many involuntary bodily functions such as heart rate, respiration, digestion, etc.[2]

The outer layer of the adrenal gland, the cortex, secretes an entirely different group of hormones called corticosteroids. These hormones are all formed from cholesterol. Although all corticosteroids have similar chemical formulas, they differ in function. The three major types of corticosteroids are mineralcorticoids, glucocorticoids and 17-ketosteroids (sex hormones).

The glucocorticoids, mainly cortisol, corticosterone and cortisone, exert a profound effect upon the metabolism of glucose. These hormones can increase serum glucose levels and induce a state very similar to diabetes. These hormones also exert a catabolic effect on skin, muscle and fat. Medicinally, cortisone and other glucocorticoids are used to suppress the immune system in the treatment of allergies and to reduce inflammation.[2]

The mineralcorticoids, of which aldosterone is the most important, have profound effects on minerals. Specifically, aldosterone increases the retention of sodium and the excretion of potassium by the body.

The 17-ketosteroids (sex hormones) are also secreted by the adrenals. The primary sex hormone produced by the adrenal is the androgen (male hormone), dehydroepian-drosterone (DHEA). This hormone has received some attention recently as a possible anti-aging hormone.

The three phases of the general adaption syndrome

Alarm reaction

The initial response to stress is the alarm reaction or 'flight or fight' response.[1,3] It is triggered by reactions in the brain which ultimately cause the adrenal medulla to secrete adrenaline and other stress-related hormones. The fight or flight response is

---

The flight or fight response

- The heart rate and force of contraction of the heart increases to provide blood to areas necessary for response to the stressful situation.
- Blood is shunted away from the skin and internal organs, except the heart and lung, while at the same time the amount of blood supplying needed oxygen and glucose to the muscles and brain is increased.
- The rate of breathing increases to supply necessary oxygen to the heart, brain and exercising muscle.
- Sweat production increases to eliminate toxic compounds produced by the body and to lower body temperature.
- Production of digestive secretions is severely reduced since digestive activity is not critical for counteracting stress.
- Blood sugar levels are increased dramatically as the liver dumps stored glucose into the bloodstream.

---

designed to counteract danger by mobilising the body's resources for immediate physical activity.

Resistance reaction

While the fight or flight response is usually short-lived, the resistance reaction allows the body to continue fighting a stressor long after the effects of the fight or flight response have worn off. Hormones secreted by the adrenal cortex (corticosteroids) are largely responsible for the resistance reaction. For example, the glucocorticoids stimulate the conversion of protein to energy so that the body has a large supply of energy long after glucose stores are depleted, and the mineralocorticoids retain sodium to maintain an elevated blood pressure.

As well as providing the necessary energy and circulatory changes required to deal effectively with stress, the resistance reaction provides those changes required for meeting emotional crises, performing strenuous tasks and fighting infection. However, while the effects of adrenal cortex hormones are necessary when the body is faced with danger, prolongation of the resistance reaction or continued stress increases the risk of significant disease and results in the final stage of the general adaptation syndrome, i.e. exhaustion.

Exhaustion

Exhaustion may manifest itself in a total collapse of body functions or a collapse of specific organs. Two of the major causes of exhaustion are loss of potassium ions and depletion of adrenal glucocorticoid hormones like cortisone.[1,3] When the cells of the body lose potassium they function less effectively and eventually die. When adrenal glucocorticoid stores become depleted, hypoglycaemia results and cells of the body do not receive either enough glucose or other nutrients.

Another cause of exhaustion is weakening of the organs. Prolonged stress places a tremendous load on many organ systems, especially the heart, blood vessels, adrenals and immune system. Exhaustion will usually manifest itself in the organ system which is inherently weak.

Conditions strongly linked to psychological stress[1]

Angina	Hypertension
Asthma	Immune suppression
Autoimmune diseases	Irritable bowel syndrome
Cancer	Menstrual irregularities
Cardiovascular disease	Premenstrual tension syndrome
Common cold	Rheumatoid arthritis
Diabetes (adult onset, Type II)	Ulcerative colitis
Depression	Ulcers
Headaches	

The social readjustment rating scale

A popular method of rating stress levels is the social readjustment rating scale developed by Holmes and Rahe.[4] As seen in Table 10.1, various events are numerically rated according to their potential for causing disease. A total of 200 or more units in one year is considered to be predictive of the likelihood of getting a serious disease.

Stress management

Stress management involves the use of techniques designed to reduce the amount of stress the body has to deal with, as well as to counteract the effects of stress. Exercise and relaxation techniques such as meditation, prayer, biofeedback and self-hypnosis are vital components of a stress management programme. In addition, the effects of stress on the body can also be reduced by supplying the body with necessary nutritional support. In particular, every effort should be made to maintain potassium levels and supply those nutrients required for adrenal hormone synthesis and function, e.g. B-complex vitamins, especially pantothenic acid, vitamin C, zinc and magnesium.

Exercise as a stress reducer

Exercise is itself a physical stressor. However, it is also a beneficial way to incorporate the fight or flight response as part of the daily routine. The benefits of exercise are discussed more completely in Chapter 2. As regards stress, though, regular exercise leads to an increased ability to cope with stress and reduces the risk of stress-related diseases.

Physiological benefits of exercise

- Improved cardiovascular function, as noted by a decreased heart rate, improved heart contraction, reduced blood pressure and decreased blood cholesterol levels.
- Reduced secretions of adrenaline and noradrenaline in response to psychological stress.
- Improved oxygen and nutrient utilisation in all tissues.
- Increased self esteem, mood and frame of mind.
- Increased endurance and energy levels.

Relaxation techniques and the relaxation response

Relaxation techniques seek to counteract the results of stress by inducing its opposite reaction – relaxation. Although an individual may relax simply by sleeping, watching television or reading a book, relaxation techniques are designed specifically to produce the 'relaxation response'.[5]

Table 10.1 The social readjustment rating scale

Rank	Life event	Mean value
1	Death of spouse	100
2	Divorce	73
3	Marital separation	65
4	Jail term	63
5	Death of a close family member	63
6	Personal injury or illness	53
7	Marriage	50
8	Fired at work	47
9	Marital reconciliation	45
10	Retirement	45
11	Change in health of family member	44
12	Pregnancy	40
13	Sex difficulties	39
14	Gain of a new family member	39
15	Business adjustment	39
16	Change in financial state	38
17	Death of a close friend	37
18	Change to different line of work	36
19	Change in number of arguments with spouse	35
20	Large mortgage	31
21	Foreclosure of mortgage or loan	30
22	Change in responsibilities at work	29
23	Son or daughter leaving home	29
24	Trouble with in-laws	29
25	Outstanding personal achievement	28
26	Wife begins or stops work	26
27	Begin or end school	26
28	Change in living conditions	25
29	Revision of personal habits	24
30	Trouble with boss	23
31	Change in work hours or conditions	20
32	Change in residence	20
33	Change in schools	20
34	Change in recreation	19
35	Change in church activities	19
36	Change in social activities	18
37	Small mortgage	17
38	Change in sleeping habits	16
39	Change in number of family get-togethers	15
40	Change in eating habits	15
41	Vacation	13
42	Christmas	12
43	Minor violations of the law	11

The physiological effects of the relaxation response are opposite to those seen with stress. With the stress response the sympathetic nervous system dominates: with the relaxation response the parasympathetic nervous system dominates. The parasympathetic nervous system controls bodily functions such as digestion, breathing and heart rate during periods of rest, relaxation, visualisation, meditation and sleep. While the sympathetic nervous system is designed to protect us against immediate danger, the parasympathetic system is designed for repair, maintenance and restoration of the body. The accompanying box, listing the various physiological features of the relaxation response should be compared with the box on page 92, listing the physiological features of the fight and flight response.

The relaxation response

- The heart rate is reduced and the heart beats more effectively; blood pressure is reduced.
- Blood is shunted towards internal organs, especially those organs involved in digestion.
- The rate of breathing decreases as oxygen demand is reduced during periods of rest.
- Sweat production decreases – a person who is calm and relaxed does not experience nervous perspiration.
- Production of digestive secretions is increased, greatly improving digestion.
- Blood sugar levels are maintained in the normal physiological range.

To achieve the relaxation response a variety of techniques may be employed, e.g. meditation, progressive relaxation, autogenic training, prayer, self-hypnosis and biofeedback.[5,6] The type of relaxation technique best for each person is totally individual. As different as these techniques may sound, they share much common ground and they all have the ability to induce the relaxation response.

Progressive relaxation   One of the most popular techniques for producing the relaxation response is progressive relaxation, as developed by Jacobson.[6] The technique is based on a very simple procedure of comparing tension against relaxation. Many people are not aware of the sensation of relaxation. In progressive relaxation an individual is educated as to what it feels like to relax by comparing relaxation to muscle tension.

A muscle is first contracted forcefully for a period of 1 to 2 seconds and then allowed to relax. Since the procedure goes progressively through all the muscles of the body, eventually a deep state of relaxation will result. The procedure begins with contracting the muscles of the face and neck, holding the contraction for a period of at least 1 to 2 seconds and then relaxing the muscles. Next the muscles of the upper arms and chest are contracted then relaxed, followed by the lower arms and hands. The process is repeated progressively down the body, i.e. the abdomen, the buttocks, the thighs, the calves and the feet. This whole practice is repeated two or three times. This technique is often used in the treatment of anxiety and insomnia.

Variations of the progressive relaxation technique include the use of verbal cues or imagery. For example, saying to yourself 'I am beginning to feel relaxed . . . My neck, my jaw, my forehead, and my entire face feels relaxed, comfortable and smooth' can substitute for the progressive tensing and relaxing of muscles.

Another way of inducing a state of relaxation is the use of imagery.[6] In this technique the individual is often asked to imagine themselves in their ideal place of physical and mental relaxation – perhaps the seashore, the mountains or some other peaceful environment. The individual is encouraged to imagine they are seeing all the colours, hearing all the sounds and smelling all the aromas of this environment. Feelings of peacefulness, calmness and relaxation are encouraged. The whole body and mind become renewed and refreshed.

There are many ways to produce the relaxation response. Three techniques have been briefly described. The important thing is that at least 5 to 10 minutes be set aside each day for the performance of a relaxation technique. These sessions remind us to breath in a relaxed effective manner. When we are confronted with stressors, sometimes simply breathing in this relaxed manner triggers tremendous relaxation and ability to cope.

Adrenal gland support

Various nutrients and herbal substances can be very useful in supporting and enhancing adrenal function, particularly during times of stress. Atrophy or shrinking of the adrenal cortex is a common side effect of continual stress, cortisone administration and aging.[1] Due to the importance of the adrenal gland, optimum health is dependent on optimum adrenal function.

Potassium   As stated earlier, it is critical to maintain potassium levels within the body. This can best be done by consuming foods rich in potassium and avoiding foods high in sodium. The daily intake of potassium should be at least 3 to 5 grams per day. Table 10.2 on the next page lists some foods having a high content of potassium.

Other nutrients   Vitamin C, vitamin B6, zinc, magnesium and pantothenic acid are necessary nutrients for the manufacture of hormones by the adrenal glands.[7] Supplementation of all of these nutrients at higher then recommended dietary allowance levels in the form of a high-potency multiple-vitamin-mineral formula may be appropriate during high periods of stress or in individuals needing adrenal support.

Particularly important for optimum adrenal function is pantothenic acid. Pantothenic acid deficiency results in adrenal atrophy, characterised by fatigue, headache, sleep disturbances, nausea and abdominal discomfort.[7] Pantothenic acid is found in wholegrains, legumes, cauliflower, broccoli, salmon, liver, sweet potatoes and tomatoes.

Ginseng, Panax ginseng   Many of the historical uses of *Panax ginseng* (Korean or Chinese ginseng), particularly as a tonic, relate to its ability to enhance adrenal gland

97

Table 10.2 Foods high in potassium (and low in sodium)

Food	Portion size	Potassium (milligrams)	Sodium (milligrams)
Fresh vegetables			
Asparagus	½ cup	165	1
Avocado	½	680	5
Carrot, raw	1	225	38
Corn	½ cup	136	trace
Lima beans, cooked	½ cup	581	1
Potato	1 medium	782	6
Spinach, cooked	½ cup	292	45
Tomato, raw	1 medium	444	5
Fresh fruits			
Apple	1 medium	182	2
Apricots, dried	¼ cup	318	9
Banana	1 medium	440	1
Cantaloupe melon	¼ melon	341	17
Orange	1 medium	263	1
Peach	1 medium	308	2
Plums	5	150	1
Strawberries	½ cup	122	trace
Unprocessed meats			
Chicken, light meat	3 ounces	350	54
Lamb, leg	3 ounces	241	53
Roast beef	3 ounces	224	49
Pork	3 ounces	219	48
Fish			
Cod	3 ounces	345	93
Flounder	3 ounces	498	201
Haddock	3 ounces	297	150
Salmon	3 ounces	378	99
Tuna, drained solids	3 ounces	225	38

function and improve reactions against a variety of stresses. Ginseng is defined as an 'adaptogen', defined as agents that:

- protect against both mental and physical fatigue;
- provide non-specific resistance against stress; and
- normalise an abnormal state caused by some excess or deficient physiological factor.

Much of ginseng's adaptogenic and anti-stress activity relates to its influence on the adrenal gland.

Numerous studies have demonstrated that ginseng possesses an ability to improve the ability of humans to withstand extremely stressful conditions (heat, noise, motion, work load increase, exercise, decompression), increase mental alertness and work output, and improve the quality of work under stressful conditions and athletic performance.[8–15]

It appears, based on extensive research, that ginseng acts via nervous system control mechanisms to adjust metabolic and functional systems that maintain homeostasis during the challenges of stress.[16,17] This is very similar to the way a thermostat maintains temperature. Ginseng improves adrenal gland function and counteracts any shrinkage of the adrenal gland due to continued stress or corticosteroid drugs.[16,17]

Ginsenosides are the active components of ginseng. The dosage of ginseng as a general tonic and anti-stress agent should reflect a ginsenoside content of 25 to 50 mg per day. For a high-quality ginseng root this would mean a dose of 1 to 2 grams per day in divided doses. Since the average ginsenoside content of the highest quality root is approximately 2 per cent, a 2 gram daily dose would contain approximately 20 to 40 mg of ginsenosides. Ginseng extracts standardised for ginsenosides are available, and provide greater quality control and therapeutic consistency.

Like Korean ginseng, Siberian ginseng (*Eleutherococcus senticosus*) is also an adaptogen that has been shown to protect against the effects of physical and mental stress.[8,10–13] Siberian ginseng is generally regarded as a more subtle adaptogen than *Panax ginseng*.

Summary

This chapter has reviewed the stress response and important components of a stress management programme. The basic approach to stress management involves regular exercise, daily use of a relaxation technique, a diet rich in potassium and the use of nutritional substances and *Panax ginseng* to support the adrenal glands. Stress management is simply one component of a healthy lifestyle.

PART THREE

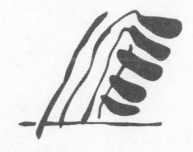

*Specific
health
problems*

11

Acne

- The presence of blackheads or white heads.
- Superficial pustules (collections of pus at the follicular opening).
- Nodules (tender collections of pus deep in the skin).
- Cysts (from nodules that fail to discharge their contents to the surface).
- Large deep pustules (from nodules that break down adjacent tissue) leading to scars.
- Most common at puberty, but may also affect adults.

General considerations

Acne is the most common of all skin problems. It occurs mostly on the face and, to a lesser extent, on the back, chest and shoulders. It is more common in males and typically begins at puberty. It occurs in two forms:

- acne vulgaris, affecting the hair follicles and oil secreting glands of the skin and manifesting as blackheads (comedones), white heads (pustules) and inflammation (papules); and
- acne conglobata, a more severe form, with deep cyst formation and subsequent scarring.

Acne has many causes, requiring an integrated therapeutic approach in order to attain the desired results. Also, because many individuals have been treated with long-term broad-spectrum antibiotics, they often develop intestinal overgrowth of *Candida albicans*; this chronic yeast infection may actually make acne worse and must be treated when present (see Chapter 21 on chronic candidiasis).

Causes

Acne has its origin in the pilosebaceous unit of the skin (see Figure 11.1). These units consist of a hair follicle and the associated sebaceous glands which are connected to the skin by the follicular canal through which the hair shaft passes. The sebaceous glands

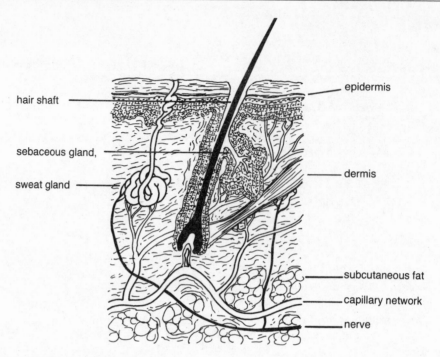

hair shaft

sebaceous gland,

sweat gland

epidermis

dermis

subcutaneous fat

capillary network

nerve

Figure 11.1   Normal pilosebaceous unit

produce sebum, a mixture of oils and waxes, which lubricate the skin and prevent the loss of water. Sebaceous glands are found in highest concentrations on the face, and, to a lesser extent, on the back, chest and shoulders.

Acne is most common in males, with the onset usually at puberty. This is due to the fact that androgens (male sex hormones), like testosterone, stimulate the cells that line the follicular canal to produce keratin as well as cause the sebaceous glands to enlarge and produce more sebum. During puberty there is an increase of androgens in both sexes, making girls just as susceptible to acne in this age group. While the onset of acne usually reflects an increase in androgens, the severity and progression of acne is determined by a complex interaction between these hormones, keratin producing cells, sebum and bacteria.

The lesions begin in the upper portion of the follicular canal with the cells that line the canal producing an excess of keratin (hyperkeratinisation). This eventually leads to blockage of the canal, resulting in ballooning and thinning. Eventually a comedo (white head or blackhead) is formed. The formation of open (blackhead) or closed comedones (white heads) is related to the degree of blockage of the duct.

With the blockage of the duct, the bacteria *Propionibacterium acnes* (*Corynebacterium acnes*) is allowed to overgrow and release enzymes which break down sebum and promote inflammation. Inflammatory acne is characterised by inflammation surrounding the comedones. The inflammatory response can result in the rupture of the follicular wall and damage to surrounding tissue. Ultimately, severe scarring can be produced.

Acne is considered to be a male hormone-dependent condition. These hormones control sebaceous gland secretion and exacerbate the development of abnormal growth of the hair follicle cells. But excessive secretion of male hormones is not necessarily the cause, since there is only a poor correlation between blood levels of these hormones and the severity of the disease.[1-3] What may be more important is that the skin of patients with acne shows greater activity of an enzyme (5-alpha-reductase) which converts testosterone to a more potent form (dihydrotestosterone).[4-6]

Another aspect of acne which is seldom recognised is the contribution of intestinal toxaemia. One study showed that 50 per cent of patients with severe acne had increased blood levels of toxins absorbed from the intestines.[7] This is important since toxins have been shown to cause an increased copper:zinc ratio (which stimulates inflammation)[8] and to enhance tissue destruction.

Acne-like lesions can occur from exposure to several agents:

- Drugs – steroids, diphenylhydantoin and lithium carbonate.
- Industrial pollutants – machine oils, coal tar derivatives and chlorinated hydro-carbons.
- Local actions – cosmetics, pomades, over-washing and repetitive rubbing.

Therapy

Nutrition

Chromium   Many dermatologists have reported that insulin is effective in the treatment of acne, suggesting impaired glucose tolerance and/or insulin insensitivity of the skin.[9,10] The insulin was given either systemically or injected directly into the lesion. Although oral glucose tolerance tests are normal in acne patients, repetitive skin biopsies reveal that their skin's glucose tolerance was significantly impaired.[11] One researcher of the role of glucose tolerance in acne coined the term 'skin diabetes' to describe the disorder of acne.[12] Considering the known immune suppressing effects of sugar and its role in the development of adult-onset diabetes, all concentrated sugars should be strictly eliminated.

High-chromium yeast is known to improve glucose tolerance and enhance insulin sensitivity[13] and has been reported to produce rapid improvement in patients with acne.[14] Although double-blind studies have yet to be done to document this effect, it is a safe nutritional supplement (except for those who are allergic to yeast or who have gout), and should be considered.

Vitamin A   Retinols, including oral vitamin A, have been shown in many studies to reduce sebum production and the hyperkeratosis of the sebaceous follicles. Retinol has been shown to be effective in treating acne, but must be used at high, potentially toxic, dosages, i.e. 300,000–400,000 iu per day for five to six months.[15] Its use at these levels is not recommended.

Although dosages of vitamin A below 300,000 iu per day for a few months rarely cause toxic symptoms, early recognition of toxicity is important and should be monitored by a physician.[15-19] The first significant toxic symptom is usually headache, followed by fatigue, emotional instability, and muscle and joint pain. Laboratory tests appear unreliable for monitoring toxicity, since serum vitamin A levels correlate poorly with toxicity, and liver enzymes are elevated only in symptomatic patients. Of far greater concern is the ability of massive doses of vitamin A to cause birth defects. Women of childbearing age should use effective birth control during treatment and for at least one month after discontinuation. Chapped lips (cheilitis) and dry skin (xerosis) will generally occur in the majority of patients, particularly in dry weather.

Large doses (above 100,000 iu per day) should be reserved for unresponsive cases and should only be used under the strict supervision of a physician, and retinol therapy should not be used alone. The major problem with many of the clinical studies using vitamin A and its analogues has been their simplistic use as isolated agents. Many other factors are of critical importance.

Zinc   Zinc is vitally important in the treatment of acne. It is involved in local hormone activation, vitamin A-binding protein formation, wound healing, immune system activity, inflammation control and tissue regeneration.

Zinc supplementation in the treatment of acne has been the subject of much controversy and many double-blind studies. The inconsistency of the results may be due to differences in absorption of the various zinc salts used. For example, studies using effervescent zinc sulphate show efficacies similar to the antibiotic tetracycline (with fewer side effects from chronic use)[20] while those using plain zinc sulphate have shown less beneficial results.[21] The majority of patients required 12 weeks' supplementation before good results were achieved, although some showed dramatic improvement immediately. There have been no studies to date using zinc picolinate, which is much more effectively absorbed than other forms.[22,23]

The importance of zinc to normal skin function is well recognised. Low levels of zinc increase the conversion of testosterone to its more active form (discussed above), while high concentrations of zinc significantly inhibit this reaction.[24] Serum zinc levels are lower in 13 and 14 year old males than in any other age group.[25]

Vitamin E and selenium   Serum vitamin A levels in rats on a vitamin E deficient diet remain low regardless of the amount of oral or intravenous vitamin A supplementation. Serum levels return to normal after vitamin E is restored to the diet. Vitamin E has also been shown to regulate vitamin A levels in humans.

Male acne patients have significantly decreased levels of red blood cell glutathione peroxidase, which normalises when vitamin E and selenium are supplemented. The acne of both men and women improves with this treatment.[26] This improvement is probably due to inhibition of lipid peroxide formation, and suggests the use of other free-radical quenchers (such as vitamin C, beta-carotene, etc.).

Vitamin B6   Women with premenstrual aggravation of acne are often responsive to vitamin B6 supplementation, reflecting its role in the normal metabolism of steroid hormones.[27] In rats, a vitamin B6 deficiency appears to cause an increased uptake and sensitivity to testosterone.[28]

Diet

Theories about direct dietary influences on acne, including those implicating chocolate, have not been proven. While a generally healthy diet is recommended, a few specifics are in order. All refined and/or concentrated carbohydrates must be eliminated, and high-fat and high-carbohydrate foods should be limited. Foods containing trans-fatty acids (milk, milk products, margarine, shortening and other synthetically hydrogenated vegetable oils) or oxidised fatty acids (fried oils) should be avoided. Foods high in iodine should be eliminated for those who are iodine-sensitive, and milk consumption (due to its high hormone content) should be limited.[29]

Botanical medicines

Purple coneflower (Echinacea angustifolia)   Purple coneflower has a long folk history of use in inhibiting inflammation, promoting wound healing, stimulating the immune system and killing bacteria – all useful in the treatment of acne. These activities are all well substantiated by experimental research. Echinacea also has some cortisone-like activity. Echinacin, a polysaccharide component of echinacea, has been shown to promote wound healing in experimental studies.[30] Other polysaccharide components of echinacea have been shown to have profound immune enhancing effects.[31,32]

Goldenseal (Hydrastis canadensis)   Goldenseal is particularly well indicated due to its detoxifying and antibacterial properties. Its antimicrobial activity is due primarily to its major alkaloid, berberine, which is effective against bacteria, protozoa and fungi.[33–40] It also stimulates the immune system[41] and detoxifies the liver.[42,43]

Other considerations

Bowel detoxification   Many factors contribute to the development of toxins in the bowel – toxic bacteria (such as *Clostridia spp.* and *Yersinia enterocolitica*), lack of lactobacilli and a low fibre diet (many toxins are eliminated by being absorbed by fibre). Equally important to consider are those factors which contribute to excessive absorption of these toxins from the bowel – inadequate secretory IgA (antibody which lines the gut and blocks the absorption of many toxins and food allergens), food allergy (which causes inflammatory damage to the gut wall) and *Candida albicans* overgrowth (which damages the gut wall).

   Proper care of the bowels requires the elimination of toxic bacteria through the use of *Hydrastis canadensis* (which selectively kills toxic bacteria while not affecting the healthy bacteria), reseeding the bowel the lactobacilli, identifying and removing allergic foods, and increasing dietary fibre (besides absorbing toxins, dietary fibre also releases short chain fatty acids which inhibit candida).

Liver detoxification   Many nutritional, dietary and botanical factors have been shown to be important in the maintenance of a healthy liver. The lipotropic factors are important for supporting the liver's enzymatic processes,[1] liver extracts promote liver regeneration,[44] *Taraxacum officinale* (dandelion) enhances bile flow,[45] and *Silybum marianum* (milk thistle) protects and detoxifies liver.[1]

Dietary fibre is also very useful since it absorbs many of the toxins excreted by the liver, including hormone breakdown products.

Treatment

The comprehensive treatment of acne involves:
- Removing excess sebum from the skin.
- Preventing closure of the follicular canal.
- Preventing overgrowth of *Propionibacterium acnes.*
- Nutritionally supporting the body.

Diet

An unrefined wholefood diet is, as always, the best. All refined carbohydrates (sugar, white flour, etc.), fried foods, milk, milk products, margarine and allergic foods should be eliminated. Dietary fibre should be increased.

Nutritional supplements

- Vitamin A, 50,000 iu per day, for three months.
- Vitamin B complex, three times the recommended dietary allowance three times a day.
- Vitamin E, 400 iu per day.
- Vitamin C, 1,000 mg per day.
- Chromium, 400 micrograms per day.
- Selenium, 200 micrograms per day.
- Zinc picolinate, 45 mg per day.
- Brewer's yeast, 1 tblsp two times a day; if susceptible to gout, use chromium chloride supplement instead.

Botanical medicines

- *Echinacea angustifolia* (purple coneflower) and *Hydrastis canadensis* (goldenseal) can be taken at the following doses for acne, three times a day:
    Dried root (or as tea), 1 to 2 g.
    Freeze-dried root, 500 to 1,000 mg.
    Tincture (1:5), 4 to 6 ml (1 to 1.5 tsp).
    Fluid extract (1:1), 0.5 to 2.0 ml (¼ to ½ tsp).
    Powdered solid extract (4:1), 250–500 mg.
- *Taraxacum officinale* (dandelion):
    Dried root, 4 grams three times a day.

Fluid extract (1:1), 4–8 ml three times a day.
Solid extract (4:1), 250–500 mg three times a day.

- *Silybum marianum* – the standard dose of *Silybum marianum* is based on its silymarin content – 70–210 mg of silymarin three times daily.

Other recommendations

- Avoid medications which contain bromides or iodides.
- Avoid exposure to oils and greases.
- Avoid the use of greasy creams or cosmetics.
- Thoroughly cleanse the face daily with sulphur-containing soap or a suitable alternative such as calendula soap.
- Extract blackheads with a comedo extractor every two to three days and have cystic lesions incised and drained by a physician every two weeks.

12

Acquired immunodeficiency syndrome

- Onset may be sudden or gradual, or may present first as an opportunistic infection.
- Sudden onset of fevers, sweats, malaise, tiredness, muscle pain, joint pain, headaches, sore throat, diarrhoea, generalised swelling of the lymph glands and a skin rash on the trunk.
- Gradual onset may present as unexplained progressive fatigue, weight loss, fever, diarrhoea and generalised swelling of the lymph glands.
- Fifty per cent first present with *Pneumocystis carinii* pneumonia, 30 per cent first present with Kaposi's sarcoma and 12 per cent first present with other opportunistic infections.

General considerations

Acquired immunodeficiency syndrome (AIDS) is a serious disease characterised by a profound defect in cell-mediated immunity. The immune system abnormality is recognised primarily by a decrease in the ratio of T-helper to T-suppressor cells – helper T cells are lymphocytes (white blood cells) which help in the immune response against viruses and bacteria, while suppressor T cells are lymphocytes which suppress the immune response. The decrease in helper T cells and the relative increase in suppressor T cells results in increased susceptibility to infections and cancer. The most serious of these are *Pneumocystis carinii* pneumonia, an infection seen in approximately 60 per cent of patients, and Kaposi's sarcoma, a connective tissue cancer. The other common infections seen in the person with AIDS include cytomegalovirus (CMV), Epstein-Barr virus (EBV), *Herpes simplex* virus (HSV), *Toxoplasma gondii*, *Mycobacterium tuberculosis*, *Mycobacterium avium-intracellulare*, salmonella, *Cryptococcus neoformans* and *Candida albicans*.[2] AIDS is thought to be due to infection by the human immunodeficiency virus (HIV).

A broad spectrum of conditions are related to AIDS: an acute mononucleosis-like syndrome; an asymptomatic state, with or without immunologic abnormalities; an AIDS related complex (ARC); and the 'full blown' AIDS syndrome. The spectrum ranges from asymptomatic presence of the virus to severe immune deficiency and life-threatening secondary infectious diseases or cancers. The mortality of the 'full blown' state is close to 100 per cent.[3]

In the United States, the vast majority of adult cases (97 per cent) are reported in persons in six major high risk groups – homosexual/bisexual men, intravenous drug users, Haitians, haemophiliacs, transfusion or blood product recipients, and hetero-sexual contacts of persons with AIDS or at risk for AIDS. There are also a number of cases reported in children born to mothers infected with the HIV virus.[4]

AIDS was first described in the summer of 1981,[5] and has since generated much fear and controversy. Once a person has been infected with the HIV virus they have a 20–38 per cent chance of developing AIDS within three years (although one report predicts that up to 99 per cent of infected homosexual men may develop the disease in an average of 7.8 years[6]). After the diagnosis has been made, 98 per cent die within three years. Of even more concern is the fact that the numbers of cases are almost doubling every year.[7]

Diagnosis

The key laboratory findings in the diagnosis of AIDS include low numbers of lympho-cytes in the blood, a quantitative deficiency in helper T cell count, elevated serum immunoglobulins (particularly IgG and IgM – specific types of antibody), and the presence of HIV antibodies in the blood.

In general, diagnosis is first suspected when the patient comes in with characteristic diseases. Fifty per cent first present with *Pneumocystis carinii* pneumonia – subacute development of a nonproductive cough and dyspnoea over several weeks. X-rays show an interstitial pneumonitis, arterial blood gases show low oxygen levels and excessive carbon dioxide build up, and biopsy shows *P. carinii* infection.

Thirty per cent first present with Kaposi's sarcoma – simultaneously appearing multiple, firm, reddish-brown or bluish plaques or nodules on the skin (primarily the lower extremities) or mucosal surfaces that may ulcerate. It may be accompanied by fever, lymphadenopathy and gastrointestinal complaints.

Twelve per cent first present with other opportunistic infections, the most common of which are recurrent mucosal candidiasis, severe progressively ulcerating perianal *Herpes simplex* infection, and disseminated cytomegalovirus.

Susceptibility factors

The host's susceptibility plays as important a role as the infective agent. In AIDS, roughly 70–90 per cent of those infected with the HIV remain asymptomatic during the first three to five years of infection. Some remain healthy carriers, while others progress to ARC, AIDS or death.[8] Attention must be focused on recognising and controlling all factors which may possibly inhibit an infected individual's immune function.

Frequent and concurrent infections

The scientific literature and the experience of those caring for ARC/AIDS patients has shown that these people have a pattern of repeated immunological stresses. These stresses include multiple sexually transmitted diseases, repeated exposure to hepatitis, frequent infections, multiple sexual partners and considerable recreational intravenous and oral drug use.

Concurrent and/or pre-AIDS infections have been documented in most ARC/AIDS patients. Cytomegalovirus (CMV), Epstein-Barr virus (EBV), *Herpes simplex* virus (HSV) and *Candida albicans* are commonly found.[5] Also, some of the immune defects observed in ARC/AIDS patients are also found in non-AIDS/ARC patients with CMV and EBV infections.This is primarily due to an increase in T suppressor cells resulting in a decreased T-helper to T-suppressor ratio, similar to that seen in patients with ARC/AIDS.[9]

Almost all people with AIDS have had a primary herpes infection prior to their AIDS diagnosis, such as genital herpes, which is very common in homosexual men.[5] One of the first infections recognised among AIDS patients was severe perianal herpes infections.

Candida infections are also prevalent in ARC/AIDS patients. Oral thrush with progression to candidal infection of the throat is common, and 'prolonged thrush in high-risk patients is thought to be a harbinger of AIDS'.[5] Candida species are common inhabitants of the human gastrointestinal tract, where their growth is kept in check by other bowel flora and normal immune function. When this balance is disturbed (as it is by the administration of antibiotics or by immune suppression from steroids, chemotherapy, CMV or EBV infection, AIDS, or other diseases) the candida can proliferate, producing toxic products which, even in healthy individuals, cause a constant challenge to the immune system.[10] In the immunodeficient patient, the results can be devastating. Since the major high-risk groups are frequently exposed to antibiotics for sexually transmitted diseases (STDs) and blood borne infections, overgrowth of gastrointestinal candida is likely and may contribute to susceptibility to HIV proliferation.

Antibiotics

The frequent use of antibiotics in the high-risk groups may also increase susceptibility to HIV infection and serve as a causative factor for AIDS. Many antibiotics have adverse effects on many aspects of immune function.[11]

Refined foods

Overconsumption of certain foods and beverages can have deleterious effects on the immune system. For instance, oral consumption of 100 grams of simple sugars such as glucose, fructose, sucrose, honey or fruit juice can significantly decrease the ability of white blood cells to kill bacteria and viruses for up to 5 hours.[12,13] The typical westerner consumes approximately 125 pounds (55 kg) of sugar a year, which works out at an average of 150 grams of sugar each day. Increased levels of cholesterol, free fatty acids, triglycerides and bile acids (all produced by the standard western diet) inhibit many aspects of immune function.[14,15] Overconsumption of alcohol and caffeine, although not nutrients, has also been demonstrated to have deleterious effects on the immune system.[16,17]

Malabsorption

Malabsorption appears to be another complicating factor in the person with AIDS.[18,19] It is usually a result of the diarrhoea, inflammation of the bowel, or intestinal infection often occurring in ARC/AIDS patients, and probably contributes significantly to their nutrient deficiencies.[20]

Bowel permeability

It has been conclusively demonstrated that the normal bowel allows the absorption of as much as 2 per cent of ingested food protein. When such intact protein reaches the blood it causes antibodies to be formed, resulting in food allergy.[21,22] If protein digestion is impaired, the protein load in the gut is increased, resulting in more antibody production. In people with AIDS, intestinal permeability may be increased, allowing even larger amounts of antigenic substances (not just food proteins, but also bacterial toxins and other antigens) to be absorbed into the circulation. Bowel trauma from anal intercourse, infectious bacteria and parasites, allergies and cancers often found in the major high-risk groups and AIDS patients can cause this increased permeability.[23] It is important to note that individuals who do not engage in anal receptive intercourse have significantly lower rates of antibody to HIV compared to those who do engage in such sexual practice.[9]

The body has several mechanisms for protecting itself from these absorbed food proteins and bacterial toxins. First it secretes an antibody (IgA) which lines the intestinal tract and binds proteins and toxins, either preventing them from entry into the body or making them more susceptible to elimination by the liver. The next line of defence is special cells that line the gut (macrophages) which dissolve or detoxify the antigens and toxins.[24] If an antigen or toxin gets absorbed, the next line of defence is the special macrophages of the liver, Kupffer cells.

Constant challenge by a particular antigen or a temporary or permanent deficiency of secretory IgA leads to a greater influx of unbound proteins and toxins, resulting in overload of the Kupffer cells. In chronic liver disease the increased levels of circulating immune complexes (antibodies bound to antigens) and toxins pose serious problems.[25]

Patients with AIDS have many predisposing factors for significant liver disease. These include frequent histories of hepatitis, intravenous drug abuse, recurrent infections and treatment with multiple antibiotics and chemotherapeutic agents for infections and neoplasms.[26] Elevated liver enzymes and enlarged livers are common laboratory and clinical findings in people with AIDS, signalling significant liver impairment. The intestinal/liver picture of the person with AIDS is one of increased gut-derived antigenic and toxic load resulting in chronic immune system challenge and stimulation.

Stress

Since Hans Selye's visionary work in the early 1950s, the diverse and numerous health damaging effects of stress on the whole organism, particularly on the human immune system, have been well documented.[27]

AIDS high-risk groups commonly have lifestyles contributing to high levels of physiological and psychological stress. Social disapproval, a positive HIV test and the loss of close friends or lovers to AIDS can stimulate emotional-psychological states of bereavement, loss, loneliness, depression, anxiety, guilt and isolation.[28] These negative emotions can have detrimental effects on cellular, humoral, natural killer cell activity, and other components of immune response, and may contribute to the progression of the disease.[29]

Positive emotional states and laughter, however, may have positive effects on immune response. One research study demonstrated that salivary IgA concentration could be significantly increased by having subjects view a humorous videotape.[30]

Smoking

Smoking contributes to host susceptibility, both directly through its local toxic effects, particularly in pneumocystis and other pneumonias, and indirectly through inhibition of cellular immunity. In heavy smokers, T-suppressor cells can increase and the T-helper cells can decrease. Fortunately, these effects are temporary, and reverse when smoking is stopped completely.[31]

Nutrient deficiencies

Animal studies have demonstrated decreased thymus hormone output under the conditions of single-nutrient dietary deficits of vitamin A, pyridoxine and zinc.[32,33]

Other animal studies have shown that lymphocyte function is impaired by deficiencies of single nutrients such as vitamin A, thiamine, riboflavin, pantothenic acid, pyridoxine, folic acid, vitamin E, iron, zinc and several amino acids.[32]

In humans, immunoglobulin levels have been depressed under the conditions of single-nutrient deficiencies of pantothenic acid and pyridoxine, as well as calorie restriction.[32]

Monocyte function in animals can be disrupted with deficits of vitamin A, vitamin C, vitamin E, iron or magnesium. Excess zinc and cholesterol can also adversely affect animal monocyte function. Iron and zinc deficiencies are known to suppress monocyte function in humans.[32]

Host resistance in humans is impaired by single-nutrient deficiencies of vitamin A, thiamine, folic acid, iron and zinc. Resistance in humans is also adversely affected by excess vitamin E (more than 600 iu per day), iron and polyunsaturated fatty acids.[32]

Inadequate sleep and exercise

Adequate sleep and exercise can relieve stress and support proper circulation, excretion and metabolism. They also have a stimulating effect on two immunological mediators (interleukin and interferon), adversely affected by the AIDS pathology.[34,35]

Therapy

At this time there is no known cure for AIDS, and many aspects of its cause are still obscure. This current lack of understanding makes the treatment of people with AIDS difficult. None the less, a comprehensive approach is recommended in an effort to affect positively all possibly relevant factors. Fundamental to this approach is the elimination of all known controllable causes of immune suppression, the utilisation of all supportive therapies which stimulate immune function, and the application of herbs and nutrients which have known antiviral activity. Due to the importance of promoting as healthy a lifestyle as possible and the lack of much direct research in this area, many of the recommendations are based on the traditional approaches to keeping well that are consistently found in a variety of cultures.

A comprehensive approach stresses lifestyle modifications (safe sex practices, elimination of recreational drug use and significant reduction or elimination of alcohol use and smoking), stress reduction and emotional support (through group support, counselling, positive imagery and visualisation), dietary modifications (high-complex carbohydrate, high-fibre, moderate protein and low fat diet of wholefoods), nutritional supplementation (with emphasis on immunologically active or supportive nutrients such as protein, zinc, carotene, ascorbic acid, selenium, etc.), botanical medicines (for immune support and antiviral activity) and exercise. This therapeutic protocol, along with the most up-to-date therapies for any acute or life-threatening complications, helps decrease susceptibility to and improve the recovery rate from the secondary infections and complications of AIDS patients and thereby slows the progression of the disease and decreases the percentage of individuals progressing to ARC or AIDS.

Unfortunately, little research has been done which directly studies the efficacy of these natural therapies in the treatment of AIDS. Much of the rationale discussed below is based on inferences from existing research, and the clinical experience of the naturopathic doctors treating people with ARC and AIDS.

Nutritional support of immune function

Current research is conclusively demonstrating the importance of optimal nutrition in maintaining immune function. As laboratory experimentation and clinical experience progress, much is being uncovered about the relationship between individual nutrients and specific components of the immune system.

Carotenes   Medical research has shown carotenes to be of immense value in supporting the immune system. In particular, large doses of beta-carotene have been found to increase the numbers of T-helper cells.[36] Unlike high doses of vitamin A, high doses of naturally occurring carotenes have been shown to be non-toxic in humans.[37] Animal studies have shown that increased vitamin A intake preserves the thymus and inhibits stress-induced thymus damage.

Vitamin C   Vitamin C is a powerful immune-stimulating and virus-inhibiting nutrient. Vitamin C is known to increase serum immunoglobulin levels and to increase thymus hormone secretion.[35] Improved host resistance in humans occurs after supplementation with vitamin C.[38] Aggressive use of vitamin C (typically to bowel tolerance) is recommended by physicians and researchers using this nutrient as part of the treatment for people with AIDS, cancer and other diseases in which optimising immune function is a critical therapeutic goal. Although controversy has raged since the late 1960s concerning theorised generation of kidney stones, the most recent literature indicates there is little risk. Nevertheless, the use of adequate amounts of magnesium and pyridoxine will minimise the possibility of kidney stones.[39]

Bioflavonoids These compounds, widely found in higher green plants, are found closely associated with vitamin C in nature and are known to enhance the effect of vitamin C in therapy. They are also directly antiviral.[40]

Zinc Zinc is widely recognised as an immune system potentiator and antiviral agent. The picolinate form seems to be the most efficiently absorbed. In order to prevent imbalances in copper metabolism, daily zinc supplementation of the picolinate form should be held to 15 mg of elemental zinc a day, with meals (copper is usually supplemented at one-eighth the dosage). Zinc supplementation has also been shown to enhance thymus hormone output and improve host resistance in humans.[35]

Catechin Catechin has antitoxin effects, is effective in the treatment of viral hepatitis and accelerates clearance of viral antigens.[41,42] Its use normalises abnormalities of the liver and decreases liver enzyme levels in alcohol-induced liver disease.[43]

Herbal support of immune function

American coneflower (Echinacea spp.) Studies with preparations made from *Echinacea purpurea* have revealed a 40–50 per cent increase in the function of several aspects of the immune system.[44,45] Plants in this family are also known for their ability to inhibit proliferation of herpes group viruses.[46] However, it is not clear at this time if echinacea is an appropriate herb in the treatment of AIDS, since laboratory research indicates that most agents that stimulate T-cells also increase replication of the HIV virus. Since echinacea stimulates T-cells, research is needed to determine if its net effects are positive.

Goldenseal (Hydrastis canadensis) Experimental use of preparations from this plant indicates enhancement of many aspects of immune function.[47] Goldenseal's most active component, berberine, is a broad spectrum antimicrobial, antiprotozoal and antifungal agent, effective against a number of organisms. It is effective in the treatment of many acute diarrhoeas, such as are typical of the patient with AIDS.[48]

Inhibiting the HIV virus

Nutrients Experiments with several nutrients indicate inhibitory effects on a number of viruses and bacteria associated with human disease. Vitamin A is known to inhibit viruses by potentiating the loss of a viral envelope protein essential to absorption to cell membranes.[49] Vitamin C has a well-established reputation for the *in vitro* inhibition of both viral and bacterial organisms.[50,51] And zinc has well-documented antiviral activity.

Radix astragalis   Astragalis species plants have a long tradition of efficacy in infectious diseases among practitioners of traditional Chinese medicine. Western experiments with mice and humans reveal the ability of these plants to enhance interferon production, a function crucial for the inhibition of viruses.[52]

Leptotania (Lomatia spp.) *and Osha root* (Ligusticum porteri)   These plants, native to the American western states, have for many years been used by practitioners of traditional native American medicine, eclectic herbology and naturopathic medicine. Although recent literature identifying the specific constituents and their effects on immune system functioning and microbial activity is unavailable, the empirical experience with virus-associated diseases strongly recommends serious consideration of these plants as elements of a protocol for virus-associated acquired immune deficiency.[53]

Liquorice (Glycyrrhiza glabra)   One of the most widely used plants in both oriental and occidental herbal medicine, liquorice has demonstrated, in animal studies, its ability to enhance many aspects of immune function.[54] Furthermore, studies have revealed it to inhibit viruses of the herpes group irreversibly. Glycyrrhizic acid from *Glycyrrhiza glabra* root inhibits growth and infectivity of several DNA and RNA viruses.[55,56]

Summary

The state of health or susceptibility of the host in the treatment of ARC/AIDS, or any other disease, is extremely important. Although we do not yet know how to cure AIDS, many traditional natural therapies significantly enhance immune function while others inhibit viruses, thus offering hope for improving the quality and length of life of the person infected with HIV. Much more research is needed.

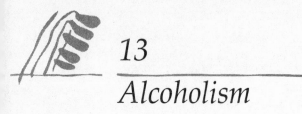

13

Alcoholism

- Alcohol dependence as manifested when alcohol is withdrawn – tremulousness, convulsions, hallucinations, delirium.
- Alcoholic binges, benders (48 hours or more of drinking associated with failure to meet usual obligations) or blackouts.
- Evidence of alcohol-induced illnesses – cirrhosis, gastritis, pancreatitis, myopathy, polyneuropathy, cerebellar degeneration.
- Physical signs of excess alcohol consumption – alcohol odour on breath, flushed face, tremor, bruises.
- Psychological/social signs of excess alcohol consumption – depression, loss of friends, arrest for driving while intoxicated, surreptitious drinking, drinking before breakfast, frequent accidents, unexplained work absences.

General considerations

Alcoholism is defined by the World Health Organisation as alcohol consumption by an individual that exceeds the limits accepted by the culture or that injures health or social relationships. As can be seen from the box on the next page, the health, social and economic consequences of alcoholism are diverse and serious. Alcoholism is a leading cause of disease and death throughout the world.

Current estimates indicate that alcoholism affects at least 10 million people in the United States and causes 200,000 deaths each year, making it one of the most serious health problems today.[1] The total number of people affected, either directly or indirectly, is much greater when one considers the disruption of family life, automobile accidents (50 per cent of fatal accidents involve a drinking driver), crime, decreased productivity, and mental and physical disease.

Often, alcoholism is a 'hidden' disease. The natural consequences of the alcoholic's behaviour may be disguised by sympathetic family and friends. This allows the alcoholic to target other factors as the 'real problem', without identifying his or her drinking behaviour. Table 13.1 has a screening questionnaire for recognising alcoholism.

Table 13.1 The brief Michigan alcoholism screening test (MAST)[1]

	Question	Answer (score)	
1	Do you feel you are a normal drinker?	Yes (0)	No (2)
2	Do friends or relatives think you are a normal drinker?	Yes (0)	No (2)
3	Have you ever attended a meeting of Alcoholics Anonymous (AA)?	Yes (5)	No (0)
4	Have you ever lost friends or girlfriends or boyfriends because of drinking?	Yes (2)	No (0)
5	Have you ever been in trouble at work because of drinking?	Yes (2)	No (0)
6	Have you ever neglected your obligations, your family or your work for two or more days in a row because you were drinking?	Yes (2)	No (0)
7	Have you ever had delirium tremens (DTs), severe shaking, heard voices, or seen things that weren't there after heavy drinking?	Yes (2)	No (0)
8	Have you ever gone to anyone for help about your drinking?	Yes (5)	No (0)
9	Have you ever been in hospital because of drinking?	Yes (5)	No (0)
10	Have you ever been arrested for drunk driving or driving after drinking?	Yes (2)	No (0)

Alcoholism is indicated by a score of greater than five.

Cause

The cause of alcoholism is unknown. It represents a multifactorial condition with genetic, physiological, psychological and social factors, all seemingly equally important. However, recent research indicates genetic factors may be very important.[2] The finding of a genetic marker for alcoholism could result in the diagnosis of the disease in its initial and more reversible stage.

A number of studies have shown that the incidence of alcoholism is four to five times more common in the biological children of alcoholic parents than those of non-alcoholic parents.[2] This suggests that a biological marker may not be necessary for the implementation of a prevention programme. The genetic basis of alcoholism has been supported by:

- genealogical studies showing that alcoholism is a family condition;
- studies of adopted children of alcoholic parents raised by foster parents showing continued higher risk of alcoholism;
- twin studies showing differences between identical and non-identical twins;
- association with genetic markers such as colour vision; and
- biochemical studies showing the importance of the enzyme differences in races susceptible to alcoholism, like Native Americans.[2]

Diagnosis

Alcoholism is one of the most commonly missed diagnoses. Physicians often do not consider alcoholism until the disease is very well established and significant health and social problems have developed. The questionnaire in Table 13.1 is a useful early screening tool.

Consequences of alcoholism[1]

Increased mortality
    10-year decrease in life expectancy
    Double the usual death rate in men, triple in women
    Six times greater suicide rate
    Major factor in the four leading causes of death in men between the ages of 25
       and 44 – accidents, homicides, suicides, cirrhosis
Economic toll (yearly in the United States)
    Lost production, $14.9 billion
    Health care costs, $8.3 billion
    Accident and fire losses, $5.0 billion
    Cost of violent crime, $1.5 billion
    Cost of response of society to above, $1.9 billion
Health effects
    Metabolic damage to every cell
    Intoxication
    Abstinence and withdrawal syndromes
    Nutritional diseases
    Cerebellar degeneration
    Cerebral atrophy
    Psychiatric disorders
    Oesophagitis, gastritis, ulcers
    Increased cancer of mouth, pharynx, larynx, oesophagus
    Pancreatitis
    Liver fatty degeneration and cirrhosis
    Arrhythmias
    Myocardial degeneration
    Hypertension
    Angina
    Hypoglycaemia
    Decreased protein synthesis
    Increased serum and liver triglycerides
    Decreased serum testosterone
    Myopathy
    Osteoporosis
    Rosacea, spiders
    Coagulation disorders
    Teratogenic effects during pregnancy

Intoxication and withdrawal

The signs of alcohol intoxication are typical of a central nervous system depressant – drowsiness, judgment errors, loss of inhibitions, poorly articulated speech, uncoordinated movement and involuntary, rhythmic movements of the eyes.[3] Fifteen millilitres of pure alcohol (the equivalent of one measure of whisky, a glass of wine, or half a pint of beer) raises the blood level of alcohol by 25 mg/dl in a 70 kg person. Table 13.2 shows the effects of varying blood levels of alcohol.

Table 13.2 Effects of varying levels of blood alcohol[4]

Blood level	Effect
< 50 mg/dl	No significant dysfunction
80	Legally intoxicated (level varies with jurisdiction)
100	Mild intoxication – decreased inhibitions, slight visual impairment, slight muscular incoordination, slowing of reaction time
150	Difficult speech, uncoordinated movement, slurring of speech, nausea and vomiting
350	Marked muscular incoordination, blurred vision, approaching stupor
500	Coma and death

Withdrawal symptoms usually occur one to three days after the last drink. They typically range from anxiety and tremulousness to mental confusion, tremor, sensory hyperactivity, visual hallucinations, autonomic hyperactivity, sweating, dehydration, electrolyte disturbances, seizures and cardiovascular abnormalities.[3]

Metabolic effects of alcohol and alcoholism

Alcohol metabolism The rate at which alcohol is broken down in normal individuals is dependent on several factors, such as how quickly it is consumed and absorbed, the concentration and activity of specific liver enzymes (alcohol dehydrogenase and aldehyde dehydrogenase), and the availability of certain nutrients.[5] As alcohol is broken down it is converted to acetaldehyde. Acetaldehyde is believed responsible for many of the harmful effects of alcohol consumption, as well as the addictive process itself. Higher than normal blood aldehyde levels have been found in alcoholics and their relatives after alcohol consumption.[6] This suggests either increased production or depressed elimination of aldehyde in people susceptible to alcoholism. Most aldehyde is eventually converted to long chain fatty acids.[5]

Fatty liver All active alcoholics display fatty infiltration of the liver, with the severity roughly proportional to the duration and degree of alcohol excess.[3] Even as little as the equivalent of 1 ounce of alcohol can produce both acute and chronic fatty liver infiltrates.

Hypoglycaemia Alcohol induces reactive hypoglycaemia.[8,3] The resultant drop in blood sugar produces a craving for food, particularly foods which quickly elevate blood sugar, e.g. sugar and alcohol. Increased sugar consumption aggravates the reactive hypo-glycaemia, particularly in the presence of alcohol, due to alcohol-induced impairment of normal glucose production in the body.[5] Hypoglycaemia aggravates the mental and emotional problems of the alcoholic and the withdrawing alcoholic with such symptoms as sweating, tremor, rapid heart beat, anxiety, hunger, dizziness, headache, visual disturbance, decreased mental function, confusion and depression.[1]

Therapy

Nutrition

While many of the nutritional problems of alcoholics directly relate to the effects of alcohol, a major contributing factor is that alcoholics tend not to eat. They substitute alcohol, a calorie-rich, nutrient-poor substance, for food.

Zinc The primary enzymes necessary for detoxification of alcohol are zinc dependent enzymes.[5,9] Alcohol consumption results in zinc deficiency.[9–11] Several factors contri-bute to the development of zinc deficiency in alcoholics:
- decreased dietary intake;
- decreased absorption, probably due to interference with the zinc binding (by picolinic acid secreted by the pancreas) and non-specific gastrointestinal damage; and
- excessive urinary loss.

Low serum zinc levels are associated with impaired alcohol metabolism, a pre-disposition to cirrhosis, impaired gonadal function, and other complications of alcohol abuse.[9,12] Zinc supplementation, particularly when combined with vitamin C, greatly increases alcohol detoxification and survival in rats.[13]

Vitamin A A vitamin A deficiency is also common in alcoholics and appears to work along with the zinc deficiency to produce the major complications of alcoholism.[12] The mechanism has been hypothesised as follows. Reduced intestinal absorption of zinc and vitamin A, in conjunction with impaired liver function, results in reduced blood levels of zinc, vitamin A, retinol binding protein and transport proteins. This causes, in the tissues, reduced concentrations of zinc and vitamin A, abnormal enzyme activities and protein synthesis, and impaired DNA metabolism. In the kidneys there is increased loss of zinc. These metabolic abnormalities then lead to the common disorders of alcohol-ism, i.e. night blindness, skin disorders, cirrhosis of the liver, reduced skin healing, decreased testicular function, impaired immune function, etc.[12]

Vitamin A supplementation inhibits alcohol consumption in female, but not male, rats, an effect that is inhibited by testosterone administration.[14] Rats who have had their ovaries and adrenal glands removed show decreased preference for alcohol.[15]

Antioxidants   Alcohol consumption causes an increase in the free radical lipoperoxide in both the liver and serum. These levels require two weeks of abstinence before they normalise in alcoholics. There is a significant correlation between serum lipoperoxide levels and liver cell necrosis.[16] Antioxidant administration, either prior to or simultaneous with ethanol intake, inhibits lipoperoxide formation and prevents fatty infiltration of the liver.[17] Effective antioxidants include vitamins C and E, zinc, selenium and cysteine.

Carnitine   Although the use of lipotropic agents appears warranted in treating alcoholic fatty liver disease, many commonly used lipotropic agents, e.g. choline, niacin and cysteine, appear to have little value.[18,19] One lipotropic agent, carnitine, does significantly inhibit alcohol-induced fatty liver disease. It has been suggested that chronic ethanol consumption results in a functional deficiency in carnitine.[20-22] Since carnitine normally facilitates fatty acid transportation and oxidation, a high liver carnitine level may be needed to handle the increased fatty acid load produced by alcohol consumption. Supplemental carnitine reduces serum triglyceride levels while elevating the blood HDL-cholesterol.[20]

Amino acids   Serum amino acid levels are abnormal in alcoholics, and restoration to normal levels greatly aids the alcoholic patient.[23-26] Since the liver is the primary site for amino acid metabolism, it is not surprising that alcoholics develop abnormal amino acid patterns. Normalisation of amino acids is particularly indicated in those patients showing signs or symptoms of hepatic cirrhosis or depression. The branched chain amino acids, i.e. valine, isoleucine and leucine, inhibit the hepatic brain dysfunction and increased protein breakdown that are the common consequences of cirrhosis.[26] Derangement of brain neurotransmitter ratios, particularly due to the very low plasma levels of tryptophan typically seen in withdrawing alcoholics, can result, leading to depression, brain damage and coma.[24,26] These problems are aggravated by the low-protein diet used as standard therapy for cirrhosis, but can be avoided through the use of free form amino acids without the risk of hepatic encephalopathy.[24,26]

Vitamin C   In one study a deficiency of ascorbic acid was found in 91 per cent of patients with alcohol-related diseases.[27] Supplemental vitamin C helped reduce the effects of acute and chronic ethanol toxicity in experimental studies involving both humans and guinea pigs, two species unable to synthesise their own vitamin C.[13,28] There is a direct correlation between white blood cell vitamin C levels (a good index of actual body vitamin C status), the rate of alcohol clearance from the blood and the activity of the liver enzymes involved in alcohol detoxification.[13] The evidence suggests that vitamin C can increase the further elimination of acetaldehyde.[13,28]

B vitamins   Alcoholics are classically deficient in most of the B vitamins.[2,29] These deficiencies result from a variety of mechanisms – low dietary intake, deactivation of the active form, impaired conversion to the active form by ethanol or acetaldehyde, impaired absorption and decreased storage capacity. A thiamine (B2) deficiency is both the most common (55 per cent in one study[29]) and the most serious of the B-vitamin deficiencies; a deficiency causes beri-beri and the Wernicke-Korsakoff syndrome. A functional pyridoxine (B6) deficiency is also common in alcoholics, due not so much to inadequate intake as impaired conversion to its active form and increased breakdown.[30]

Magnesium A magnesium deficiency is common in alcoholics and commonly demonstrated in electrocardiograms.[1,31] This deficiency is due primarily to alcohol-induced increased loss of magnesium through the kidneys,[1,31] which continues during withdrawal, despite low serum magnesium levels.

Selenium The trace mineral selenium is an important antioxidant and works synergistically with vitamin E to prevent alcohol-induced lipoperoxidation. Low dietary intake and plasma and urinary levels have been reported in alcoholics, resulting in lower levels of glutathione peroxidase and increased lipoperoxidation.[32]

Essential fatty acids Alcohol induces essential fatty acid deficiency, particularly of the omega-6 series. In rats, the mechanism appears to be an increased renal excretion of prostaglandins, particularly cyclo-oxygenase products.[33]

Glutamine Glutamine supplementation (1 gram per day) has been shown to reduce voluntary alcohol consumption in uncontrolled human studies and experimental animal studies.[8,34-37]

Botanical medicines

Any of the botanical medicines discussed in Chapter 8, Liver support, are suitable in the treatment and prevention of alcoholic liver disease; however, silymarin (from *Silybum marianum*) is perhaps the most important component in the treatment and prevention of toxic chemical or alcohol induced liver damage. Clinical studies have shown silymarin to have positive effects in treating liver diseases of various kinds, including alcohol induced fatty liver and cirrhosis.[38-42]

Psychosocial considerations

Psychological and social measures are critical in the treatment of the alcoholism. Alcoholism should be viewed as a chronic, progressive, addictive and potentially fatal disease, although many aspects of the alcoholic's behaviour may make it difficult to maintain this objectivity.[1]

Social support for both patient and family is very important, and success often appears proportional to the involvement of Alcoholics Anonymous (AA), counsellors and other social agencies.[3] Since most physicians have not had adequate training or experience in handling the psychosocial aspects of this problem, it is important to establish a close working relationship with an experienced counsellor and AA. Al-Anon and Ala-Teen are useful resources for family members.

Successful initiation of treatment requires:
- the patient's agreement that they have an alcohol problem;

- education of the patient and their family about the physical and psychosocial effects of alcoholism; and
- immediate involvement of the patient in a treatment programme.

Successful programmes (such as AA) usually include strict control of drinking and replacement of the alcohol addiction with another addiction that is non-chemical, time consuming and heavily supported by family, friends and peers. Although strict abstinence may not be absolutely necessary, at this time it appears the safest and most effective choice.[1]

Depression   Depression is common in alcoholics and contributes to the high suicide rate.[23,24,43] Many alcoholics are depressed first and later become alcoholic (primary depressives), while others become alcoholic first and later develop depression in the context of their alcoholism (secondary depressives). Alterations in the metabolism of the brain neurotransmitter serotonin, and the availability of its precursor, tryptophan, catecholamines, and their tyrosine precursor have been implicated in the development of depression.[24,29]

Alcoholics have severely depleted levels of tryptophan, which may explain both the depression and sleep disturbances common in alcoholism, since brain serotonin levels are dependent on circulating tryptophan levels.[23,24,43] Alcohol impairs tryptophan transport into the brain. In one study, five out of six chronic alcoholics had no detectable plasma tryptophan upon withdrawal.[23] The tryptophan levels returned to normal after six days of treatment and abstinence.

Another factor influencing tryptophan uptake into the brain is competition from amino acids which share the same transport – tyrosine, phenylalanine, valine, leucine, isoleucine and methionine – many of which are elevated in malnourished alcoholics.[23,24] Alcoholics have significantly depressed ratios of tryptophan to these amino acids when compared with normal controls, with depressed alcoholics having the lowest ratios.[24]

The amino acid taurine is also low in depressed alcoholics, with the lowest levels being reported in psychotic alcoholics.[23]

Miscellaneous considerations

Intestinal flora   The intestinal microflora is severely deranged in alcoholics.[44] Growth of toxin-producing bacteria in the small intestine may lead to malabsorption of fats, carbohydrates, protein, folic acid and vitamin B12. This is probably the cause of the abnormalities of the small intestine commonly found in alcoholics. Alcohol ingestion also increases intestinal permeability to toxins and incompletely digested foods, allowing increased toxic and food allergy effects.[45] The subsequent allergic reactions and formation of immune complexes which can be deposited in body tissues probably contribute to the many complications of alcoholism, and, considering the addictive tendency of food allergies, may also contribute to alcoholic cravings.

Exercise   The involvement of the alcoholic patient in a graded, individually-tailored fitness programme has been shown to improve the likelihood of maintaining abstinence.[46] Research has shown that regular exercise is effective in alleviating anxiety and depression and enables individuals to respond better to stress. Improved fitness may allow more effective responses to emotional upset, thereby reducing the likelihood of resorting to alcohol when involved in conflict.

Treatment

Alcoholism is a difficult disease to treat. Although many therapeutic regimes have been attempted, there has been little documented long-term success, except for that of Alcoholics Anonymous. The approach presented here is unique in that it is an integrated, whole-person, stage-oriented programme.

The treatment of the alcoholic patient must be optimised for the four stages of alcoholism – active alcohol consumption, withdrawal, recovery and recovered. The recovery stage is defined here as the period between withdrawal and full re-establishment of normal metabolic function. All alcoholics, at whatever stage, need a number of counselling, lifestyle and metabolic balancing therapies. What follows are the recommended therapies for all alcoholics, followed by additional recommendations for each stage. A complete diagnostic check-up is also necessary, due to the high risk that the alcoholic patient will develop a wide variety of clinical and subclinical diseases.

Diet   Stabilisation of blood sugar levels is critical to successful treatment. Although a strict hypoglycaemic diet may not be warranted, most of the dietary guidelines must be followed. These include elimination of all simple sugars (foods containing added sucrose, fructose or glucose; fruit juice; dried fruit; and low-fibre fruits such as grapes and citrus fruits), limitation of processed carbohydrates (white flour, instant potatoes, white rice, etc.), and an increase in complex carbohydrates (whole grains, vegetables, beans, etc.). Protein levels should be moderate, and fat intake low.

Nutritional supplements
- Vitamin A, 25,000 iu per day.
- Vitamin B complex, 20 times the recommended dietary allowance.
- Vitamin C, 1 g two times per day.
- Vitamin E (d-alpha-tocopherol), 400 iu per day.
- Magnesium, 250 mg two times per day.
- Selenium, 200 µg per day.
- Zinc (picolinate), 15 mg per day.
- Carnitine (L-carnitine), 500 mg two times per day.
- Glutamine, 1 g per day.
- *Lactobacillus acidophilus*, 1 tsp per day.

Botanical medicines   *Silybum marianum*, of which the standard dose is based on its silymarin content – 70–210 mg of silymarin three times daily.

Exercise   Establish a graded programme using heart rate response to determine intensity. The patient should exercise five to seven times per week, for 20–30 minutes, at an intensity sufficient to raise the heart rate to 60–80 per cent of maximum for the age group.

Counselling Establish a good working relationship with AA and an experienced counsellor who has particular expertise in working with alcoholics.

Additional recommendations

Active alcohol consumption Work with family, peers, social group and whoever else is involved with the patient to elicit the patient's recognition of his/her alcohol problem and willingness to enter a treatment programme. Supplements include:
- Pyridoxal-5-phosphate, 20 mg per day.
- Riboflavin, 100 mg per day.
- Vitamin A, 50,000 iu per day.
- Zinc, 30 mg per day.
- Silymarin, 140–210 mg three times a day.

Withdrawal Severity of symptomatology varies widely, although it is usually proportional to the degree of physiological dependence and the duration of the disease. Milder cases usually start within a few hours after cessation of drinking and typically resolve within 48 hours. More severe cases usually occur only in patients over 30 years of age and usually develop after about 48 hours of abstinence. These patients should be admitted to a hospital or other inpatient facility. Some institutions may not allow the use of supplements; this should be checked beforehand. Additional supplements:
- Tryptophan, 3 g per day.
- Riboflavin, 100 mg per day.
- Electrolyte replacement as necessary.

Recovering Establish a strong network of caring family, friends and peers to support the patient regularly. Get the patient involved and busy with intense, people-oriented activities. Help the patient recognise that alcohol is no answer to the stresses of life; aid him or her in developing more effective ways of handling adversity. An additional supplement at this stage is:
- Flax seed oil, 1 tblsp three times a day.

Recovered The patient's support group must always be maintained. Continued total abstinence is the best policy, although carefully controlled drinking may be possible. Slowly reduce supplement doses after a period of six months of abstinence to 25 per cent of the above.

14
Alzheimer's disease

- Progressive mental deterioration, loss of memory and cognitive function; inability to carry out daily activities.
- Definitive diagnosis can be made only by post mortem study of brain.

General considerations

Is a progressive loss of mental function part of the normal aging process and is senility the reward of an increased lifespan? Can anything be done to prevent Alzheimer's disease and other causes of senile dementia? The basic answers are optimistic. Senility and senile dementia may be viewed as abnormal.

Dementia refers to a general mental deterioration. In the elderly this is referred to as senile dementia. It can be marked by progressive mental deterioration, loss of recent memory, moodiness and irritability, self-centredness and childish behaviour. This is often due to Alzheimer's disease, although there are many other causes of senile dementia.

Although much remains to be known about aging, it is safe to say that Alzheimer's disease and other senile dementias are not necessarily a normal process, and do not have to be the reward of a ripe old age. Much can be done, even though the incidence of senile dementia is likely to increase alarmingly for a time as the median age of the population grows.

Currently 1.3 million elderly in the US suffer severe dementia and approximately 3 million endure mild to moderate dementia – roughly 15 per cent of all the US elderly have some degree of dementia, while two-thirds of their 1.5 million nursing home patients have dementia. As staggering as these figures may seem, they are expected to increase.

Senile dementia: a 20th-century epidemic?

Best known and most feared of the dementias is Alzheimer's disease. This disease can occur at any age, but most commonly after 50. Symptoms occurring before 65 are designated presenile dementia of the Alzheimer's type (PDAT); after 65 it's senile dementia of the Alzheimer's type (SDAT). Current diagnosis of Alzheimer's disease is extremely difficult as the only definitive diagnosis is a post mortem biopsy of the brain.

Alzheimer's disease is characterised by the general destruction of nerve cells in several key areas of the brain devoted to mental functions. This results in neuro-fibrillary tangles (tangles of nerve fibres) and plaque formation. The disease's clinical features are believed to be related to a decrease in acetylcholine which functions as a transmitting agent in the brain, although there is a general reduction in the concentration of all neurotransmitting substances.

Post mortem studies have demonstrated that about 50 per cent of all cases of dementia, in both the presenile and senile periods, are the result of Alzheimer's disease. This means approximately 50 per cent of dementia patients do not have Alzheimer's. It is not known to what degree patients are erroneously diagnosed as having Alzheimer's, or some other dementia, but it is estimated to be a significant number.[1,2] The diagnostic process – a diagnosis of exclusion – is extremely difficult.

A comprehensive diagnosis by a skilled physician is paramount in the approach to the demented patient. The first step is the diagnosis of dementia. Error rates of 10 to 50 per cent have been reported when diagnosis is based only on the first evaluation. Most of those misdiagnosed are found on further examination to have nothing more than depression, which can mimic dementia in the elderly. Complete evaluation by a competent physician includes:

- A detailed history.
- Neurological and physical examination.
- Psychological evaluation, with emphasis on the detection of subtle metabolic, toxic or cardiopulmonary disorders that can precipitate confusion.
- A series of neurophysiological tests to document the type and severity of mental impairment.
- Appropriate laboratory studies, including an electrocardiogram (ECG), electro-encephalogram (EEG) and computerised tomography (CAT scan).[1,3]
- Evaluation by a social worker or other qualified individual who can mobilise community resources.

The value of a complete diagnostic check-up for people with dementia cannot be over-emphasised. Many cases of dementia are entirely reversible. Every effort should be made to rule out these reversible factors. Over 80 per cent of the elderly are deficient in one or more vitamins or minerals, which, if levels get too low, may induce dementia. In addition, over 30 per cent of the elderly use eight or more prescribed drugs daily.[4] Drugs and drug interactions probably play a greater role in dementia and confusional states than is currently realised. Table 14.1 provides a detailed list of the majority of causes of senile dementia.

Table 14.1 Causes of senile dementia[2]

Degenerative etiology (disturbances of gene expression and thus of protein metabolism)
    Altered genetic code
    Alzheimer's disease
    Huntington's chorea
    Idiopathic dementia
        Localised form
        Parkinson's disease
        Pick's disease
        Loss of neuronal redundancy
    Cerebrovascular disease
        Chronic meningitis
        Encephalomyelitis
        Encephalopathy following head injury (boxers)
        Epileptic dementia
        Virus encephalopathy

Nutritive etiology
    Chronic alcoholism
    Diabetes mellitus
    Disturbances of electrolyte metabolism
        Hypoglycaemia
        Hyponatraemia
        Hypothyroidism
        Korsakoff syndrome
        Nicotinamide deficiency
        B vitamin deficiency

Toxic etiology
    Addiction to barbiturates, psychotropic drugs, etc.
    Chronic carbon monoxide intoxication
    Chronic sulphite intoxication
    Mycotoxins
    Renal/hepatic encephalopathy
    Drug reaction

Causative factors

Primary treatment of Alzheimer's disease is prevention. Appropriate measures can be instituted from the limited knowledge that we have of the disease:

- There is a curious and persistent association between Alzheimer's disease and Down's syndrome.
- There is more than a casual relationship between high body aluminium and silicon levels and Alzheimer's disease.
- Serum vitamin B12 levels are significantly lower in patients with Alzheimer's disease.
- Degeneration of the central nervous system may be secondary to a decreased blood and oxygen supply to the brain.

- Increasing cholinergic neurotransmission may offer some benefit to patients already showing some signs of dementia.

Association with Down's syndrome

Down's syndrome (trisomy 21, mongolism) is a genetic condition due to an extra 21st chromosome, characterised by both physical and mental retardation. If Down's syndrome victims are fortunate enough to survive into their 30s and 40s, they are invariably rewarded with Alzheimer's disease.[3,5] Although not much of a reward, this process provides many valuable clues about the cause of Alzheimer's disease.

Free radicals   Central to these similarities may be a susceptibility to free radical damage. Free radicals are highly reactive compounds that bind to and destroy other molecules, while antioxidants are compounds which prevent free radical damage. Examples of natural antioxidant compounds are vitamins C and E, carotenes, flavonoids, zinc and selenium. Free radical related processes are thought by many to be involved in the development of Alzheimer's disease and are definitely involved in the accelerated aging processes observed in Down's syndrome. Dietary supplementation with antioxidants may offer some protection against Alzheimer's disease and accelerated aging.

Immune system dysfunction and low zinc levels   Free radical damage is particularly detrimental to our immune system. Down's syndrome studies have revealed numerous deficits in the immune systems of patients. These alterations and deficits are consistent with the decline in immunity that occurs in normal aging.[6] However, many of these abnormalities in immune function can be reversed by zinc supplementation.[6]

Zinc absorption in the elderly is marginal at best.[7] Even an adequate dietary intake does not mean adequate levels of zinc absorption, which seems to be dependent on adequate picolinic acid secretion by the pancreas.[8,9] Since elderly individuals usually have some degree of pancreatic insufficiency, zinc picolinate is probably the best form of zinc supplementation for a majority of the elderly.

As well as normalising immune defects, zinc, a component of more enzymes than any other trace mineral, may also play a role in normalising cell replication. Included in the list of zinc-containing enzymes are most enzymes involved in DNA replication, repair and transcription.

DNA is the genetic core that serves as the blueprint for cellular functions and cell replication. It has been suggested that dementia, possibly because of a long-term zinc deficiency, may represent the long-term cascading effects of error-prone or ineffective DNA-handling enzymes in nerve cells. The end result could be the destruction of nerve cells and the formation of the neurofibrillary tangles and plaques. Further research is needed to determine if low zinc levels in the brain could be responsible for Alzheimer's disease. In any event zinc supplementation will result in improved immune status in elderly patients.

Thyroid abnormalities   Another finding in patients with Alzheimer's disease and/or Down's syndrome is a high rate of thyroid disease.[5,10] Although the correction of thyroid abnormalities has resulted in improvement to patients with Down's syndrome, there have been no studies concerning Alzheimer's.[10] Thyroid abnormalities may increase the risk of developing dementia.

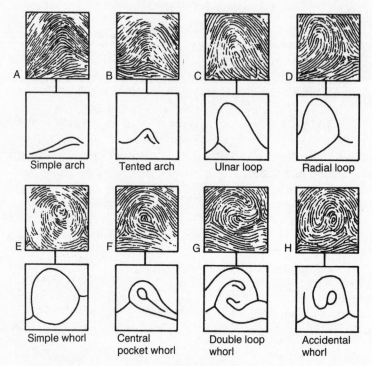

Figure 14.1   Fingerprint patterns in Alzheimer's disease

Fingerprint patterns   Abnormal fingerprint patterns are associated with both Alzheimer's disease and Down's syndrome.[11] Compared to the normal population, Alzheimer's and Down's patients show an increased number of ulnar loops (see Figure 14.1) on the fingertips, with a concomitant decrease in whorls, radial loops and arches. Ulnar loops (loop pointing toward the ulnar bone, away from the thumb) are frequently found on all ten fingertips. Radial loops (loops pointing toward the thumb), when they do appear, tend to be shifted away from the index and middle fingers, where they most commonly occur, to the ring and little fingers. If you have the fingerprint pattern characteristic of Alzheimer's disease, it is recommended that you initiate an aggressive preventive approach immediately.

Aluminium and silicon

The relevance of aluminium as a causative factor in the development of Alzheimer's disease has been hotly debated in the scientific literature.[2,3,12,13,14] Most research seems to support a role for aluminium and another mineral, silicon, as causative. Increased levels of silicon and aluminium have been detected in the neurofibrillary tangles and senile plaques of Alzheimer's patients. Environmental sources of aluminium and silicon are included in many antacids, many processed foods, underarm deodorants, bentonite clay, cooking pans and drinking water.

Perhaps the most convincing argument for the role of aluminium as a dementia villain is the 'dialysis dementia' developed in patients undergoing haemodialysis for kidney failure. Increased aluminium levels have been the result of using antacids containing aluminium and elevated aluminium levels in the water used for dialysis. The latter factor is effectively dealt with by using aluminium-free water in the artificial kidney, while the antacids containing aluminium are thought of as a necessity at this time. Magnesium carbonate may prove to be an acceptable antacid for these patients, thereby greatly reducing the risk of aluminium toxicity and dementia.

Further support is offered by the following:

- When rabbits injest aluminium, neurofibrillary tangles similar to those in Alzheimer's disease appear.
- Aluminium at levels commonly found in Alzheimer's disease inhibits choline transport and the synthesis of the neurotransmitter acetylcholine.
- Aluminium leads to a decreased synthesis of other neurotransmitters (dopamine, serotonin, epinephrine, norepinephrine) as well.[2,3,12,13,14]

Although the role of aluminium and silicon in Alzheimer's disease has not been definitely demonstrated, there is enough evidence at this time to support the recommendation that aluminium and silicon exposure be kept as low as possible.

Chronic subclinical vitamin B12 deficiency

Serum vitamin B12 levels are significantly low, and vitamin B12 deficiency significantly common, in Alzheimer's disease patients.[15,16] There is often mistaken reliance on the presence of anaemia to diagnose vitamin B12 or folic acid deficiency. However, deficiencies of either vitamin is associated with mental symptoms, including dementia, long before changes occur in the blood.[1,17] In addition, changes in the blood may never occur, despite the fact that severe deficiencies are occurring in other tissues.

Despite these facts, there is often reluctance to measure serum vitamin B12 and folate levels when there are no changes occurring in the blood. Supplementation of B12 and/or folic acid may result in complete reversal in some patients, but generally there is little improvement in the majority. It has been hypothesised that prolonged low levels may lead to irreversible changes that will not respond to supplementation.

Cerebrovascular insufficiency and senile dementia

Dementia in the elderly is often a result of insufficient blood and oxygen flow to the brain. Also associated with these insufficiencies are short-term memory loss, vertigo, headache, ringing in the ears, lack of vigilance and depression. Much of this is due to the presence of atherosclerotic cardiovascular disease. Now, an extract from the leaves of a remarkable tree, *Ginkgo biloba*, offers great hope.

In a large open trial involving 112 geriatric patients with chronic cerebral insufficiency, the administration of *Ginkgo biloba* extract (GBE), at 120 mg per day, resulted in a statistically significant ($P > 0.001$) regression of the major symptoms of vascular insufficiency mentioned above.[18] The regression of these symptoms induced by *Ginkgo biloba* suggests that a reduced blood and oxygen supply to the brain may indeed by the major causative factor of the so-called age-related cerebral disorders, including senility, rather than a true degenerative process of nerve tissue. It appears *Ginkgo biloba* extract, by increasing blood flow to the brain, resulting in an increase in oxygen and glucose utilisation, offers relief of these presumed side effects of aging and may offer significant protection against the development of these symptoms and strokes.

Increasing mental performance in patients already demonstrating dementia

As mentioned earlier, the first step in the treatment of dementia is diagnosis. Once other factors have been ruled out, supplements designed to improve mental performance are necessary.

Ginkgo biloba *extract*

As well as improving blood supply to the brain, it has been demonstrated in clinical studies that *Ginkgo biloba* extract also increases the rate at which information is transmitted at the nerve cell level.[19,20] In one double-blind study (one group received GBE, the other a placebo), the time of reaction in healthy young women performing a memory test was improved significantly after the administration of GBE.[19] In another double-blind study, *Ginkgo biloba* extract induced in elderly patients vigilance approaching normal levels and improved mental performance.[20]

The findings at the behavioural level correlated with improvements in brain wave patterns as demonstrated by electroencephalograph (EEG) tracings. Patients with a more unfavourable initial situation, as measured in resting EEG activity, displayed the greatest improvement. 'The results show,' the study concluded, 'that chronic G.B.E. medication has a positive effect in geriatric subjects with deterioration of mental performance and vigilance, and this effect is reflected at the behavioural level.'

Ginkgo biloba extract may be of great benefit in many cases of senility, including Alzheimer's disease. It has been shown to normalise the acetylcholine receptors in the brain of aged animals and to increase transmission of nerve impulses.[20] Both of these factors are decreased in Alzheimer's disease.

Phosphatidylcholine

Since phosphatidylcholine as found in lecithin can increase acetylcholine levels in the brain in normal patients, and since Alzheimer's disease is characterised by a decrease in cholinergic transmission, it seems reasonable to assume phosphatidylcholine supplementation would be of benefit to Alzheimer patients. However, clinical trials using phosphatidylcholine have been disappointing.[21] Studies have shown inconsistent improvements in memory from choline supplementation in both normal and Alzheimer patients.[21,22,23] The studies have been criticised for small sample size, low dosage of phosphatidylcholine and poor design.

Most commercial lecithin contains only 10–20 per cent phosphatidylcholine, while most 'phosphatidylcholine' supplements contain only 35 per cent. There are preparations available containing up to 90 per cent phosphatidylcholine, and ideally these are the preparations which should be used since they are associated with fewer side effects (anorexia, nausea, abdominal bloating, gastrointestinal pain and diarrhoea are associated with high doses of lecithin). Since large doses of phosphatidylcholine are often required, i.e. 25 grams, if a preparation contains only 25 per cent phosphatidylcholine, 100 grams would have to be used. This is just not feasible due to the side effects noted above, along with the expense of the supplement.

In a patient with mild to moderate dementia, the use of a high-quality phosphatidylcholine preparation may be worth a try. However, if there is no noticeable improvement within two weeks, supplementation should be halted. The basic defect in cholinergic transmission in Alzheimer's disease relates to impaired activity of the enzyme acetylcholine transferase. This enzyme combines choline (as provided by phosphatidylcholine) with an acetyl molecule to form acetylcholine, the neurotransmitter. Since providing more choline will not necessarily increase the activity of this key enzyme, phosphatidylcholine supplementation will not be beneficial in the majority of patients with Alzheimer's disease.

Treatment

Prevention of Alzheimer's disease at this time remains only speculative, but some preventive measures seem reasonable:
- Avoidance of exposure to aluminium and silicon.
- Consuming supplemental antioxidants such as carotenes, flavonoids, vitamins C and E, zinc and selenium.
- Correction of any underlying thyroid abnormality.
- Maintenance of adequate blood and oxygen flow to the brain. The latter measure is particularly indicated if such symptoms of cerebrovascular insufficiency exist as ringing in the ears, dizziness, depression, lack of vigilance and headache. An extract of *Ginkgo biloba* has been shown to be especially effective in the treatment of these symptoms and capable of improving brainwave patterns in elderly individuals with dementia.

The standard dose of GBE (containing 24 per cent ginkgo heterosides) is 40 mg three times a day; a higher dose is required for less concentrated extracts. There have been no reports of significant adverse reactions to GBE at the prescribed dose. Mild adverse reactions, although quite rare, have been reported and include gastrointestinal upset and headache.

The use of phosphatidylcholine or lecithin does not appear to be effective at this time, due to the necessity of having to use very large doses, although in the future it may be shown to offer some benefit when used in combination with a more powerful drug. This has already been demonstrated with the drug physostigmine. This drug (originally isolated from a plant) increases cholinergic transmission in the brain, but unfortunately the rest of the body as well. At this time the side effects of the drug are thought to outweigh the benefits.

15

Anaemia

- Pallor, weakness and a tendency to tire easily.
- Low level of total red blood cells, volume of blood, or abnormal size or shape of red blood cells.

General considerations

Anaemia refers to a condition in which the blood is deficient in red blood cells or the haemoglobin (iron containing) portion of red blood cells. The primary function of the red blood cell (RBC) is to transport oxygen from the lungs to the tissues of the body in exchange for carbon dioxide. The symptoms of anaemia, such as extreme fatigue, reflect a lack of oxygen being delivered to tissues and a build-up of carbon dioxide.

There are three major classifications of anaemias:
- Anaemias due to excessive blood loss.
- Anaemias due to excessive RBC destruction.
- Anaemias due to deficient RBC production.

Anaemias due to excessive blood loss

Anaemia can be produced during acute (rapid) or chronic (slow but constant) blood loss. Acute blood loss can be fatal if more than one-third of total blood volume is lost (roughly 1.5 litres). Since acute blood loss is usually quite apparent, there is little difficulty in diagnosis. Often blood transfusion is required.

Chronic blood loss, e.g. from a slowly bleeding peptic ulcer, haemorrhoids or menstruation, can also produce anaemia. This highlights the importance of a thorough diagnosis in individuals with anaemia.

Anaemias due to excessive red blood cell destruction

Old RBCs, as well as abnormal RBCs, are removed from the circulation primarily by the spleen. If destruction of old or abnormal RBCs exceeds the body's ability to manufacture new RBCs, anaemia can result. The most common cause of excessive destruction of RBCs is abnormal RBC shape.

A number of things can lead to abnormal RBC shape, including defective haemoglobin synthesis, as seen in hereditary conditions like sickle cell anaemia, mechanical injury due to trauma or turbulence within arteries, hereditary RBC enzyme defects and vitamin or mineral deficiency.

Anaemias due to deficient red blood cell production

This is the most common category of anaemia. The most common causes of deficient RBC production are nutritional deficiencies. Although a number of vitamins and minerals can produce anaemia, only the most common – iron, vitamin B12 and folic acid – are discussed here. Iron deficiency anaemia is characterised as a microcytic anaemia because the RBC's become very small, while folic acid and B12 deficiency anaemias are classified as macrocytic anaemias because the RBCs become quite large.

The anaemias

Iron deficiency anaemia

Iron deficiency is the most common cause of anaemia; however, anaemia is the last stage of iron deficiency. Studies in several developed countries have found evidence of iron deficiency in 30–50 per cent of the population.[1] The groups at highest risk for iron deficiency are infants under two years of age, teenage girls, pregnant women and the elderly. Iron deficiency may be due to an increased iron requirement, decreased dietary intake, diminished iron absorption or utilisation, blood loss, or a combination of factors.[1,2]

Increased requirements for iron occur during the growth spurts of infancy and adolescence, and during pregnancy and lactation. Currently, the vast majority of pregnant women are routinely given iron supplements during their pregnancy.[2]

Inadequate intake of iron is common in many parts of the world, especially areas which consume primarily a vegetarian diet. Typical infant diets in developed countries (high in milk and cereals) are also low in iron. The adolescent consuming a junk food diet is at high risk of iron deficiency. However, the population at greatest risk for a diet deficient in iron is the low-income elderly population.[3] This is complicated by the fact that decreased absorption of iron is extremely common in the elderly.[4]

Decreased absorption of iron is often due to a lack of hydrochloric acid secretion in the stomach.[1,2] This is an extremely common condition in the elderly.[4] Other causes of decreased absorption include chronic diarrhoea or malabsorption, the surgical removal of the stomach and antacid use.[1]

Blood loss is the most common cause of iron deficiency in women of childbearing age. This is most often due to excessive menstrual bleeding (see Chapter 43, Heavy periods). Other common causes of blood loss include bleeding from peptic ulcers, haemorrhoids and donating blood.[1,2]

The diagnosis of iron deficiency can best be made by measuring serum ferritin, the iron storage protein. This is by far the most sensitive test. Other measures of iron stores such as serum iron, total iron binding capacity and RBC haemoglobin are less sensitive, but are often performed on a routine basis. Long-term iron deficiency is characterised by low RBC levels, a low haematocrit (volume of red blood cells), small RBCs and low serum ferritin levels.[1]

Vitamin B12 deficiency anaemia

Vitamin B12 deficiency is most often due to a defect in absorption and not a dietary lack. In order for vitamin B12 to be absorbed it must be liberated from food by hydrochloric acid and bound to a substance known as intrinsic factor within the small intestine.[5] Intrinsic factor is secreted by the parietal cells of the stomach, cells which are also responsible for the secretion of hydrochloric acid. Hence the secretion of intrinsic factor parallels that of hydrochloric acid. The B12-intrinsic factor complex is absorbed in the small intestine with the aid of the pancreatic enzyme trypsin.

In order for vitamin B12 to be absorbed an individual must secrete enough hydrochloric acid and intrinsic factor, adequate pancreatic enzymes including trypsin, and have a healthy and intact ileum (the terminal portion of the small intestine where the vitamin B12-intrinsic factor complex is absorbed).

Lack of intrinsic factor results in a condition known as pernicious anaemia. The defect is rare before the age of 35 and it is more common in individuals of Scandinavian, English and Irish descent; it is much less common in southern Europeans, orientals and blacks. Pernicious anaemia is frequently associated with iron deficiency as well.[6]

A dietary lack of vitamin B12 is most often associated with a strict vegetarian diet. Since normal body stores of vitamin B12 may last an individual three to six years, deficiency of vitamin B12 is usually not apparent in a vegetarian until after many years. Fermented foods such as soy sauce, miso and tempeh contain some vitamin B12.

The diagnosis of vitamin B12 deficiency is best made by measuring the vitamin B12 level in the blood. Most physicians, however, simply rely on the presence of large red blood cells and characteristic symptoms. Symptoms of severe B12 deficiency can include paleness, tiring easily, shortness of breath, a sore, beefy red and swollen tongue, diarrhoea and heart and nervous system disturbances.[1,2] The nervous system disturbances of a vitamin B12 deficiency can be quite serious; common nervous system symptoms include numbness and tingling of the arms or legs, depression, mental confusion, loss of vibration sense and loss of deep tendon reflexes.[1,2] In the elderly a vitamin B12 deficiency can mimic Alzheimer's disease.

Folic acid deficiency anaemia

Folic acid deficiency is the most common vitamin deficiency in the world. Unlike vitamin B12, the body does not store a large surplus of folic acid; folic acid stores in the body are only sufficient to sustain the body for one to two months.

Folic acid deficiency is extremely common in alcoholics, as alcohol impairs folic acid absorption, disrupts folic acid metabolism and causes the body to excrete folic acid.

Folic acid deficiency is also common in pregnant women. This is due to an increased demand for folic acid. Folic acid is vital to cell reproduction within the foetus; if the foetus does not have a constant source of folic acid, birth defects like neural tube defects will result. Pregnant women may become deficient in folic acid because of the high demand of the developing foetus. If alcohol is consumed during pregnancy, the lowering of folic acid levels by the alcohol may lead to the foetal alcohol syndrome.[7]

In addition to alcohol, there are a number of drugs which can induce a folic acid deficiency, including anti-cancer drugs, drugs for epilepsy and oral contraceptives.[1,2]

Folic acid deficiency is quite common in patients with chronic diarrhoea or malabsorptive states such as coeliac disease, Crohn's disease and tropical sprue. Since a deficiency of folic acid will result in diarrhoea and malabsorption, often a vicious circle ensues. The administration of folic acid as a preventive measure is warranted in anyone experiencing chronic diarrhoea. Often this has a therapeutic effect as well.[2]

Folic acid deficiency will result in the same type of anaemia as a vitamin B12 deficiency – a macrocytic anaemia. The most sensitive test to determine folic acid deficiency is determining the folic acid content of the serum and RBC. In addition to anaemia, other symptoms of folic acid deficiency include diarrhoea, depression and a swollen/red tongue.[1]

Therapy

The treatment of anaemia is dependent on proper clinical evaluation by a physician. It is imperative that a comprehensive laboratory analysis of the blood is performed. Do not be satisfied with the diagnosis of 'anaemia'; it is critical that the underlying cause for the anaemia be uncovered if appropriate therapy is to be employed.

Recommended therapy in this chapter will be divided into five categories – general nutritional support, iron deficiency anaemia, vitamin B12 deficiency anaemia, folic acid deficiency anaemia and botanicals indicated in anaemia.

General nutritional support

Perhaps the best food for an individual with any kind of anaemia is calf liver. It is not only rich in iron, but also all B-vitamins. Care must be taken not to eat more than 4 oz (100 g) of liver on a routine basis due to its high content of vitamin A. Hydrolysed (liquid) liver extracts are perhaps an even better source of highly bio-available nutrients than regular liver; these extracts have the benefit of liver, but are free of fats, cholesterol and fat soluble vitamins.

The use of liver or liver extracts has fallen out of favour in mainstream medicine. Instead isolated vitamin B12, folic acid or iron is used. The use of liver therapy in the treatment of anaemia was viewed as a 'shotgun' approach, since liver contains such a large number of factors which can stimulate normal RBC production, in addition to vitamins and minerals. In the authors' opinion, though, liver or hydrolysed liver extracts still represent an effective natural treatment of all types of anaemia.

Green leafy vegetables are also of great benefit in individuals with any kind of anaemia. These vegetables contain natural fat-soluble chlorophyll as well as other important nutrients including iron and folic acid. The chlorophyll molecule is very similar to the haemoglobin molecule. Fat-soluble (but not water-soluble) chlorophyll products may be used in an anaemic individual. (Water-soluble chlorophyll is not absorbed from the gastrointestinal tract and therefore it has no use in the treatment of anaemia.)

Since a large percentage of individuals with anaemia do not secrete enough hydrochloric acid, it is often appropriate to supplement hydrochloric acid with meals. (See Chapter 5, Digestion, for more information and dosage instructions.)

Iron deficiency anaemia   Again, treatment of any type of anaemia should focus on underlying causes. For iron deficiency anaemia, this typically involves finding a reason for chronic blood loss or why an individual is not absorbing sufficient amounts of dietary iron. Lack of hydrochloric acid is a common reason for impaired iron absorption, especially in the elderly.

Iron is absorbed best on an empty stomach; however, it also causes the greatest gastric irritation when given on an empty stomach. Ferrous sulphate is the most widely used iron supplement, but will often cause gastrointestinal upset including nausea, heartburn, bloating and diarrhoea or constipation. Other ferrous salts also produce these types of complaints. Ferrous succinate is absorbed 30 per cent better than ferrous sulphate, while other iron salts, e.g. ferrous lactate, fumarate, aspartate, etc., are absorbed about as well as ferrous sulphate.[1]

Recently several preparations have been shown to enhance iron absorption and utilisation without causing gastrointestinal upset.[8,9,10] Perhaps the best iron supplement is ferritin. Ferritin is a protein in the body which complexes with iron and stores it in tissues. Studies in humans have shown that ferritin produces a greater effect in improving RBC counts, haemoglobin and haematocrit levels, without causing gastric upset.[10] Hydrolysed (liquid) calf liver and spleen extracts are good sources of ferritin.

Foods rich in iron, in addition to liver and green leafy vegetables, include dried beans, blackstrap molasses, lean meat, organ meats, dried apricots and other dried fruits, almonds and shellfish. Vitamin C supplementation has been shown to enhance the absorption of dietary iron greatly; in fact, vitamin C is regarded as the most potent enhancer of iron absorption.[1] Vitamin C alone will often increase body iron stores – 500 milligrams with each meal is a suitable dose for this effect.

Several foods and beverages contain substances which inhibit iron absorption, including tea, coffee, wheat bran and egg yolk. Antacids and over-use of calcium supplements also decrease iron absorption. These items should be restricted in the diet in individuals with iron deficiency.[1]

Vitamin B12 deficiency anaemia   In 1926 Minot and Murphy reported the effectiveness of liver therapy in the treatment of pernicious anaemia.[11] Soon after, active concentrates of liver were available for intramuscular as well as oral administration. As mentioned earlier, the use of liver and liver extracts has fallen out of favour in mainstream medicine; as regards pernicious anaemia, standard medical treatment involves injecting vitamin B12 at a dose of 1 microgram daily for one week.

Oral doses of vitamin B12 in individuals with pernicious anaemia have to be quite large since these individuals lack intrinsic factor. An appropriate oral dose of vitamin B12 in these individuals would be 1 mg, preferably as a sublingual tablet or liquid.

Meats, eggs, milk and milk products are particularly rich in vitamin B12. Fermented vegetable foods like tempeh, miso and soy contain small amounts of vitamin B12.

Folic acid deficiency anaemia   It is always necessary to differentiate folic acid deficiency anaemia from vitamin B12 deficiency anaemia. Administration of folic acid in a vitamin B12 deficiency could correct the anaemia, but it would not correct the vitamin B12 deficiency. The result would be continuation of the vitamin B12 deficiency and progression of nervous system damage. For this reason, vitamin B12 should always be given along with folic acid.

To replenish folic acid stores, 1 mg of folic acid should be taken every day for up to one month. The folic acid content of the diet should be at least 400 µg per day. Foods rich in folic acid include liver, asparagus, dried beans, brewer's yeast, dark green leafy vegetables and grains. Since folic acid is destroyed by heat and light, fruits and vegetables should be eaten fresh or with very little cooking. Poor sources of folic acid include most meats, milk, eggs and root vegetables.

Botanical medicines

Many botanicals have a long folk history of use in the treatment of anaemia; however, as the condition is generally a result of nutritional deficiency, botanicals should be used in combination with nutritional therapy.

Gentian (Gentiana lutea)   Gentian root is the standard 'bitter', against which all others are measured; at dilutions of 1:12,000 it still has a bitter taste. Gentian has been shown to stimulate digestion by increasing the secretion of digestive juices and enzymes. This could lead to better absorption of those nutrients necessary to reverse the anaemia. Administration of gentian preparations has been shown to be most effective if it precedes meals by about half an hour.[12,13]

Dandelion (Taraxacum officinale)   Dandelion contains more vitamins, iron and other minerals, protein and other nutrients than any other herb. It has a long history of use in the treatment of anaemia, presumably due to its high nutritive content.[13]

Treatment

Effective treatment of anaemia is dependent on proper classification as to its cause. The following recommendations are given with this in mind. Blood tests should be performed monthly to determine when the blood returns to normal.

Diet

The ingestion of 4 oz (100 g) of calf liver per day is recommended, along with the liberal consumption of green leafy vegetables.

Supplements

- Iron (elemental), 30 mg three times per day.
- Vitamin C, 1 gram three times per day with meals.
- Folic acid, 400 micrograms three times per day.
- Vitamin B12, 1 mg per day.
- Liver extracts, as directed on product label.

Botanical medicines

- *Gentiana lutea*
    Dried root, 1–2 grams before meals.
    Fluid extract (1:1), 2–4 ml before meals.
- *Taraxacum officinale*
    Dried root, 4 grams three times a day.
    Fluid extract (1:1), 4–8 ml three times a day.
    Solid extract (4:1), 250–500 mg three times a day.

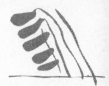

16

Angina pectoris

- Squeezing or pressure-like pain in the chest that appears quickly after exertion. Pain may radiate to the left shoulderblade, left arm or jaw. The pain typically lasts for only one to twenty minutes.
- Stress, anxiety and high blood pressure usually accompany angina.
- The majority of individuals with angina will demonstrate an abnormal electro-cardiograph reading in response to light exercise (stress test).

General considerations

Angina pectoris is characterised by the signs and symptoms described above. It is caused by an insufficient supply of oxygen to the heart muscle, usually as a result of atherosclerosis. The primary lesion of atherosclerosis is the atheromatous plaque, which progressively narrows and ultimately blocks the coronary artery, resulting in a decreased blood and oxygen supply to the heart tissue. When this occurs, significant pain or angina results.

A special type of angina exists that is not related to a build up of plaque on the coronary arteries. It is known as Prinzmetal's variant angina and is caused by spasm of a coronary artery. This form of angina is more apt to occur at rest, may occur at odd times during the day or night, and is more common in women under the age of 50.

Therapy

Angina is a serious condition that requires strict medical supervision. The recommendations given below are specific for angina, but are meant to be part of a comprehensive plan containing the guidelines and recommendations in Chapter 18, Atherosclerosis, and possibly prescription medications.

From a natural perspective, there are two primary therapeutic goals in the treatment of angina: improvement of the blood supply to the heart (which is covered primarily in

Chapter 18, Atherosclerosis); and improving energy metabolism within the heart (dealt with below).

Free fatty acids are the major metabolic fuel for the heart. Defects in fatty acid metabolism greatly increase the risk of atherosclerosis, heart attacks and angina pains. Impaired utilisation of fatty acids by heart tissue results in accumulation of high concentrations of fatty acids within the heart muscle. This is thought to be one of the major factors responsible for producing the cellular damage to the heart muscle which ultimately leads to a heart attack.

Carnitine, pantethine and coenzyme Q10 are essential compounds in normal fat and energy metabolism and are of extreme benefit to sufferers of angina. These three nutrients prevent the accumulation of fatty acids within the heart muscle by improving the breakdown of fatty acids and other compounds into energy. Extracts of hawthorn berries or flowering tops also have an effect in improving heart function in individuals with angina.

Nutrition

Carnitine   Carnitine, a vitamin-like compound, stimulates the breakdown of long-chain fatty acids by the mitochondria (energy producing units in cells). Carnitine is essential in the transport of fatty acids into the mitochondria; a deficiency in carnitine results in a decrease in fatty acid concentrations in the mitochondria and reduced energy production.[1]

Since long-chain fatty acids are the preferred energy source in well-oxygenated heart tissue, normal heart function is dependent on adequate concentrations of carnitine. The normal heart stores more carnitine than it needs, but if the heart does not have a good supply of oxygen, carnitine levels quickly decrease. Supplementation with carnitine normalises heart carnitine levels and allows the heart muscle to utilise its limited oxygen supply more efficiently.[2-7]

Several clinical trials have demonstrated that carnitine improves angina and heart disease.[3-7] Improvements have been noted in exercise tolerance and heart function. These results indicate that carnitine may be an effective alternative to other antianginal agents such as beta-blocking drugs, calcium-channel antagonists and nitrates, especially in cases of chronic stable angina pectoris. In Kamikawa *et al.*'s study of patients with stable angina, 900 mg of L-carnitine administered orally increased mean exercise time and the time necessary for abnormalities to occur on a stress test (6.4 minutes in the placebo group compared to 8.8 minutes in the carnitine group).[5]

The ability to enhance physical performance may not be limited to patients with heart disease, as carnitine supplementation (2 g three times a day) has also been shown to be of benefit in normal human subjects.[8] The carnitine-treated group showed significant improvements in cardiovascular function in response to exercise. Compared to the control group, the subjects on L-carnitine showed lower ventilation values and consequently lower oxygen consumption and a rapid return of heart rate to resting values. It appeared that carnitine was able to mimic improvements in heart function produced by training.

Carnitine, by improving fatty acid utilisation and energy production in the heart muscle, may also prevent the production of toxic fatty acid metabolites.[2,9] These compounds are extremely deleterious as they activate various phospholipases and disrupt cellular membrane structures. The changes in the properties of cardiac cell membranes induced by fatty acid metabolites are thought to contribute to impaired heart muscle contractility and compliance, increased susceptibility to irregular beats and eventual death of heart tissue. Supplemental carnitine increases heart carnitine levels and prevents the production of fatty acid metabolites. This has been demonstrated clinically; the early administration of L-carnitine (40 mg/kg per day) in patients having heart attacks reduced damage to the heart considerably.[10]

It appears that carnitine, along with pantethine and coenzyme Q10, should be considered in all heart disorders including angina. Carnitine's ability to lower cholesterol and triglyceride levels are highlighted in Chapter 18, Atherosclerosis.

Pantethine　Pantethine is the stable form of pantetheine, the active form of pantothenic acid, which is the fundamental component of coenzyme A (CoA). CoA is involved in the transport of fatty acids to and from cells, and to the mitochondria. The synthetic pathway from pantethine to CoA is much shorter than that of pantothenic acid, making pantethine the preferred therapeutic substance. In addition, pantethine has significant lipid-lowering activity, while pantothenic acid has very little (if any) effect in lowering cholesterol and triglyceride levels.

Pantethine administration (standard dose 900 mg per day), like carnitine, has been shown to reduce serum triglyceride and cholesterol levels significantly while increasing HDL-cholesterol levels in clinical trials.[11-16] Its lipid lowering effects are most impressive when its toxicity (virtually none) is compared to conventional lipid lowering drugs. Its mechanism of action is due to inhibiting cholesterol synthesis and acceleration of fatty acid breakdown in the mitochondria.

Pantethine is very much indicated in angina. Like carnitine, heart pantethine levels decrease during times of reduced oxygen supply. Pantethine has demonstrated effects in animals that would indicate that it would be of great benefit to individuals with angina.[17]

Coenzyme Q10　Coenzyme Q10 (CoQ10), also known as ubiquinone, is an essential component of the mitochondria, where it plays a major role in energy production. Like carnitine and pantethine, CoQ10 can be synthesised within the body. None the less, deficiency states have been reported. Deficiency could be a result of impaired CoQ10 synthesis due to nutritional deficiencies, a genetic or acquired defect in CoQ10 synthesis, or increased tissue needs.[18]

Cardiovascular diseases, including angina, hypertension, mitral valve prolapse and congestive heart failure, are examples of diseases which require increased tissue levels of CoQ10.[18,19,20] In addition, the elderly in general may have increased CoQ10 requirements as the decline of CoQ10 levels that occurs with age may be partly responsible for age-related deterioration of the immune system.

CoQ10 deficiency is common in individuals with heart disease. Heart tissue biopsies in patients with various heart diseases showed a CoQ10 deficiency in 50–75 per cent of cases.[18,19,21-3] Being one of the most metabolically active tissues in the body, the heart may be unusually susceptible to the effects of CoQ10 deficiency. Accordingly, CoQ10 has shown great promise in the treatment of heart disease.

In one study, 12 patients with stable angina pectoris were treated with CoQ10 (150 mg/day for four weeks) in a double-blind, crossover trial.[24] Compared to the placebo, CoQ10 reduced the frequency of anginal attacks by 53 per cent. In addition, there was a significant increase in treadmill exercise tolerance (time to onset of chest pain and time to development of electrocardiogram abnormalities) during CoQ10 treatment. The results of this study and others suggest that CoQ10 is a safe and effective treatment for angina pectoris.[18,24,25]

Magnesium   Magnesium deficiency may play a major role in some cases of angina. A magnesium deficiency has been shown to produce spasms of the coronary arteries and is thought to be a cause of non-occlusive heart attacks.[26] Furthermore, it has been observed that men dying suddenly of heart attacks have significantly lower levels of heart magnesium, as well as potassium, than matched controls.[27]

Magnesium administration has been found to be helpful in the management of irregular heart beats, and several reports have suggested that its administration should become the treatment of choice for angina due to coronary artery spasm.[26-29]

Hawthorn (Crataegus monogyna)   Hawthorn berry and flowering tops extracts are widely used in Europe for their cardiovascular activities. Studies have demonstrated hawthorn extracts are effective in reducing angina attacks as well as lowering blood pressure and serum cholesterol levels.[30,31,32]

The beneficial effects of hawthorn extracts in the treatment of angina are a result of improvement in the blood and oxygen supply to the heart by dilating the coronary vessels,[30-36] as well as improvement of the metabolic processes in the heart.[30,31,37-39] Hawthorn's ability to dilate coronary blood vessels has been repeatedly demonstrated in experimental studies.[30-36] This effect appears to be due to relaxation of vascular smooth muscle by the various flavonoid components in hawthorn.[30] This is extremely important in the treatment of angina.

Improvement in heart metabolism has been demonstrated in humans and animals to whom hawthorn extracts have been given.[2,14,20,21] The improvement is a result not only of increased blood and oxygen supply to the heart muscle, but also a result of hawthorn flavonoids interacting with key enzymes.

Hawthorn extracts thus exhibit a combination of effects that are of great value to sufferers of angina or other heart problems.

Treatment

The primary therapy for angina is prevention, since angina is usually a result of atherosclerosis. Once angina has developed, restoring proper blood supply to the heart and enhancing energy production within the heart are necessary. Particularly important nutrients for accomplishing these are carnitine, pantethine, coenzyme Q10 and magnesium. Magnesium is of additional benefit because of its ability to relax spastic coronary arteries and improve heart function. Hawthorn berries or extracts offer a number of benefits to individuals with angina, including dilating coronary arteries and improving metabolism within heart muscle.

Diet

Increase dietary fibre, especially the gel-forming or mucilaginous fibres (flax seed, oat bran, pectin, etc.), onions and garlic (both raw and cooked), vegetables and fish, while reducing the consumption of saturated fats, cholesterol, sugar and animal proteins. All fried foods should be avoided.

Lifestyle

The individual with angina should stop smoking and drinking alcohol and coffee. Stress should be decreased by using stress management techniques such as progressive relaxation or guided imagery. A carefully graded, progressive, aerobic exercise programme (30 minutes three times a week) is a necessity. Walking is a good exercise to start with.

Supplements

- Carnitine, 300 mg
- Pantethine, 300 mg
- Coenzyme Q10, 20 mg
- Magnesium (aspartate or orotate), 250 mg

All three times a day.

Botanical medicines

Doses three times a day.

- *Crataegus monogyna*
    Berries or flowers (dried), 3–5 grams or as a tea
    Tincture (1:5), 4–6 ml (1–1.5 tsp)
    fluid extract (1:1), 1–2 ml (0.25–0.5 tsp)
    Solid extract (10 per cent procyanidins), 100–250 mg

17

Asthma and hayfever

Asthma
- Recurrent attacks of shortness of breath, cough and expectoration of tenacious mucoid sputum.
- Prolonged expiration phase with generalised wheezing and musical râles (rattly wheezing).
- Increased eosinophils in the blood, increased serum IgE; positive food and/or inhalant allergy tests.

Hayfever
- Watery nasal discharge, sneezing, itchy eyes and nose.
- Usually associated with a particular season.

General considerations

Asthma and hayfever are discussed together since the mechanisms responsible for the development, as well as treatment, are similar in both. Asthma is an allergic disorder characterised by spasm of the bronchial tubes and excessive excretion of a viscous mucous in the lungs that can lead to difficult breathing. It occurs as recurrent attacks, which range from mild wheezing to a life-threatening inability to breathe.

Asthma has typically been divided into two categories, extrinsic and intrinsic. Extrinsic or atopic asthma is generally considered an allergy-related condition with a characteristic increase in the serum immunoglobulin IgE. Intrinsic asthma is associated with a bronchial reaction that is due, not to antigen–antibody stimulation, but rather to such factors as chemicals, cold air, exercise, infection and emotional upset.[1,2]

Asthma affects approximately 3 per cent of the United States population. Although it occurs at all ages, it is most common in children under 10. There is a 2:1 male:female ratio in children, which equalises by the age of 30.

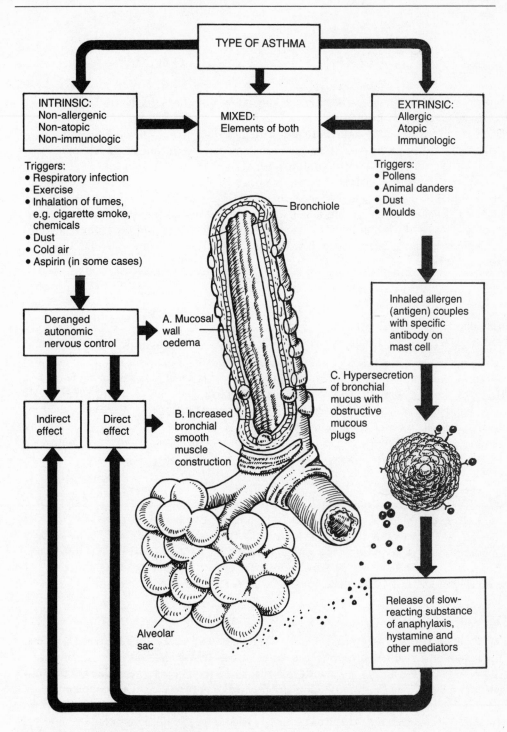

Figure 17.1 Mechanisms of asthma

Causes

The major causes of asthma are:

- allergy;
- hypersensitivity of the airways; and
- excessive release of inflammatory chemicals from mast cells (cells containing histamine-like chemicals).

The effective treatment of asthma requires the determination of the specific underlying defects and initiating factors, since many diverse defects and metabolic abnormalities result in the same clinical picture of bronchospasm.

Hayfever (seasonal allergic rhinitis) is an allergic reaction to wind-borne pollens. Significant pollens inducing hayfever include various grass and tree pollens. If the hayfever develops in the spring it is usually due to tree pollens; if it develops in the summer grass and weed pollens are usually the culprits. Some people develop hayfever in response to airborne fungus spores. These spores are most common in mid-March to late November.

Causative factors

Food allergy

Many studies have indicated that food allergies play an important role in asthma and hayfever.[3-6] Adverse reactions to food may be immediate or delayed. Double-blind food challenges in children have shown that immediate onset sensitivities are usually due (in decreasing order of frequency) to eggs, fish, shellfish, nuts and peanuts; while foods most commonly associated with delayed onset reactions include (in decreasing order of frequency) milk, chocolate, wheat, citrus and food colourings.[5] Elimination diets have been successful in treating asthma, particularly in infants and children (see Chapter 38, Food allergy, for full description of elimination diets).

Low stomach acid

Stomach hydrochloric acid analyses in 200 asthmatic children by Bray in 1931 showed that 80 per cent of them had below normal amounts of stomach acid.[7] This is very important to those for whom food allergy causes their asthma. Inadequate stomach acid has a major impact on the success of rotation and/or elimination diets, since, if not corrected, it will lead to the development of allergies to new foods.[8]

Food additives

Vitally important in the control of asthma is the elimination of food additives.[9] Artificial dyes and preservatives are widely used in foods, beverages and drugs. The most common colouring agents are azo dyes – tartrazine (orange), sunset yellow, amaranth and the new coccine (both red) – and the non-azo dye pate blue. The most commonly used preservatives in food are sodium benzoate, 4-hydroxybenzoate esters and sulphur dioxide. Various sulphites are also commonly used in prepared foods.

Tartrazine, benzoates, sulphur dioxide and, in particular, sulphites have been reported to cause asthma attacks in susceptible individuals.[9,10] Tartrazine is found in most processed foods and can even be found in vitamin preparations and anti-asthma prescription drugs, e.g. aminophylline, while it is estimated that 2–3 mg of sulphites are consumed each day by the average US citizen, while an additional 5–10 mg are ingested by wine and beer drinkers.[10] The main sources are the salads, vegetables (particularly potatoes) and avocado dip served in restaurants. A customer can ingest 25–100 mg of metabisulphite in as little as one restaurant meal.

Therapy

Diet

Vegan diet In a long-term trial, a vegan diet (elimination of all animal products) provided significant improvement in 92 per cent of the 25 treated patients who completed the study (nine dropped out).[11] The researchers also found a reduction in the tendency to infectious disease. It is important to recognise, however, that while 71 per cent of the patients responded within four months, one year of therapy was required before the 92 per cent level was reached.

The diet excluded all meat, fish, eggs and dairy products. Drinking water was limited to spring water (chlorinated tap water was specifically prohibited), and coffee, ordinary tea, chocolate, sugar and salt were excluded. Herbal spices were allowed, and water and herbal teas were allowed, up to 1.5 litres per day. Vegetables used freely were lettuce, carrots, beets, onions, celery, cabbage, cauliflower, broccoli, nettles, cucumber, radishes, Jerusalem artichokes and all beans except soya and green peas. Potatoes were allowed in restricted amounts. A number of fruits were also used freely – blueberries, cloudberries, raspberries, strawberries, blackcurrants, gooseberries, plums and pears. Apples and citrus fruits were not allowed, and grains were either very restricted or eliminated.

The beneficial effects of this dietary regime are probably related to two areas:
- elimination of common food allergens; and
- altered fatty acid metabolism.

The production of leukotrienes that contribute to the allergic and inflammatory reactions found in asthma are derived from arachidonic acid, a fatty acid found exclusively in animal products.

Leukotrienes are 1,000 times more potent as stimulators of bronchial constriction than histamine. It has been observed that people with asthma have an imbalance in fatty acid metabolism, leading to a relative increase in leukotriene production.[12-14] This implies that eliminating animal products may be of significant importance in the treatment of asthma, a hypothesis confirmed in the study described above.

Tryptophan Children with asthma have been shown to have a defect in tryptophan metabolism and reduced platelet transport of serotonin.[15-16] Tryptophan is converted to serotonin, a known broncho-constricting agent in asthmatics. Double-blind clinical studies have shown that patients benefit from either a tryptophan-restricted diet[15] or vitamin B6 supplementation[16] to correct the blocked tryptophan metabolism.

Nutritional supplements

Vitamin B6   Pyridoxine, vitamin B6, may be of direct benefit to asthmatic patients, since it is a key cofactor in the synthesis of all major neurotransmitters. In one study, plasma and red cell pyridoxal phosphate (the active form of vitamin B6) levels in 15 adult patients with asthma were significantly lower than in 16 controls. Oral supplementation with 50 milligrams of vitamin B6 twice daily to seven of the patients failed to produce a substantial elevation of these low levels. However, all patients reported a dramatic decrease in frequency and severity of wheezing and asthmatic attacks while taking the supplements.[17]

Vitamin B12   Jonathan Wright MD believes 'B12 therapy is the mainstay in childhood asthma'.[18] In one clinical trial, weekly intramuscular injections of 1 mg of vitamin B12 produced definite improvement in asthmatic patients. Of 20 patients, 18 showed less shortness of breath on exertion, as well as improved appetite, sleep and general condition.[18] Vitamin B12 appears to be especially effective in sulphite-sensitive individuals. It offers the best protection when given orally prior to challenge, compared to other pharmacological agents, e.g. cromolyn sodium, atropine and doxepin.[19] The mode of action is the formation of a sulphite-cobalamin complex, which blocks sulphite's effect. A vitamin B12 deficiency is not surprising considering the high degree of correlation between hypochlorhydria and B12 deficiency since the cells in the stomach which secrete hydrochloric acid are also responsible for secreting a substance (intrinsic factor) which binds to vitamin B12 and facilitates B12 absorption.

Vitamin C   Both treated and untreated asthmatic patients have been shown to have significantly lower levels of ascorbic acid in serum and white blood cells.[20] Vitamin C inhibits experimentally-induced bronchial constriction in both normal and asthmatic subjects.[21,22] Ascorbic acid appears to normalise fatty acid metabolism.[23]

Vitamin C has a wide variety of effects that appear important in treatment of the person with asthma. In double-blind controlled studies, moderately high doses (1 gram per day) alone have been shown to be an effective, but not curative, preventive measure for some patients with bronchial asthma.[24] However, studies using smaller doses or smaller numbers of patients have not shown statistically significant effects.

Vitamin C and other antioxidants are thought to provide an important defence, since oxidising agents can both stimulate bronchoconstriction and increase allergic reactions to other agents.[25]

Carotenes   Carotenes are powerful antioxidants which increase the integrity of the epithelial lining of the respiratory tract and decrease leukotriene formation.[26]

Vitamin E   Vitamin E's activity as an antioxidant and inhibitor of the formation of inflammatory compounds makes it a useful agent in asthma treatment.[27]

Selenium   A selenium containing enzyme, glutathione peroxidase, is very important for reducing leukotriene formation. Supplemental selenium may reduce the production of leukotrienes by ensuring optimal activity of this enzyme.[28]

Magnesium Magnesium relaxes bronchial smooth muscle.[29] Uncontrolled clinical studies have demonstrated that magnesium is beneficial in the treatment of patients with acute attacks of bronchial asthma.[30] A double-blind clinical study reconfirmed that magnesium (administered other than by mouth in this research) significantly improves breathing in asthmatics.[31] The degree of improvement correlated with serum magnesium levels.

Botanical medicines

Ephedra (Ephedra sinica) The Chinese have long treasured ephedra for allergy, asthma, hayfever, colds and inflammatory conditions.[32,33] In fact, the medicinal use of ephedra can be traced back to over 5,000 years ago. Its use in modern medicine began in 1923 with the 'discovery' of the alkaloid compound ephedrine. Synthetic manufacture of ephedrine began very shortly thereafter (1927). Synthetic ephedrine and related compounds are still widely used in many prescription medications for asthma, emphysema, hay fever and nasal congestion.[34] There are, however, other components in the crude plant besides ephedrine that possess significant anti-inflammatory and anti-allergy activities.[35]

Ephedra and its alkaloids have proved effective in the treatment of mild to moderate asthma and hayfever. However, the therapeutic effect of ephedra will diminish if used over a long time due to weakening of the adrenal glands caused by ephedrine. It is therefore often necessary to use ephedra in combination with adrenal gland supportive herbs like liquorice (*Glycyrrhiza glabra*) and *Panax ginseng*, as well as nutrients which support the adrenal glands like vitamin C, magnesium, zinc, vitamin B6 and pantothenic acid.

The old herbal treatment of asthma and hayfever involves the use of ephedra in combination with herbal expectorants. Expectorants are herbs that modify the quality and quantity of secretions of the respiratory tract, resulting in the expulsion of the secretions and improvement in respiratory tract function. Examples of commonly used expectorants include lobelia (*Lobelia inflata*, *Lobelia urens* and *Lobelia dortmanns*) liquorice (*Glycyrrhiza glabra*), grindelia (*Grindelia camporum*), euphorbia (*Euphorbia hirta*), sundew (*Drosera rotundifolia*) and senega (*Polygala senega*).

Chinese skullcap (Scutellaria baicalensis) Chinese skullcap has confirmed anti-arthritic and anti-inflammatory actions, comparable to nonsteroid anti-inflammatory drugs like aspirin, indomethacin, ibuprofen and phenylbutazone. However, while these drugs are associated with toxicity and adverse effects, Chinese skullcap does not appear to have any adverse effects at therapeutic levels.

Its therapeutic action appears to be related to its high content of flavonoid molecules.[37] These flavonoids inhibit the formation of compounds that are over 1,000 times more potent in their allergic and inflammatory effect than histamine. These flavanoids function similarly to the flavonoid drug disodium cromoglycate (Intal) which is used as an anti-asthmatic. In addition these flavanoids are extremely potent antioxidants and free-radical scavenging compounds.

Angelica (Angelica sinensis)   Angelica has been shown to have significant effects in conditions in which individuals are sensitive to a variety of substances (pollens, dust, animal dander, food, etc.).[38,39] These conditions include hayfever, asthma and eczema. Angelica also has a long history of use by Chinese herbalists in the prevention and relief of allergic symptoms. Its action is related to its ability to inhibit the production of allergic antibodies (IgE) in a selective manner. IgE levels are typically elevated three to ten times greater than the upper limit of normal in patients with allergic conditions.

Liquorice (Glycyrrhiza glabra)   Liquorice root is one of the most extensively investigated plants. Its anti-inflammatory and anti-allergy activities are well known, having been demonstrated in many studies.[32,33,40–44] Much of its activity in these types of conditions relates to its ability to increase the half-life of cortisol, resulting in increased anti-inflammatory action of this hormone.

Liquorice also acts to prevent some of the significant side effects associated with cortisone, the most widely utilised drug in the treatment of asthma. The net effect of liquorice is an increase in the anti-inflammatory activity of this hormone while decreasing some of its undesirable effects on the other areas of the body. In addition, liquorice has many similar actions to cortisone in reducing inflammation via its inhibition of several key enzymes involved in the promotion of inflammation.

Onions and garlic (Allium spp.)   Onions and garlic inhibit the lipoxygenase enzyme which generates an important inflammatory chemical.[45] Oral pretreatment of guinea pigs with 1 ml of an alcohol/onion extract markedly reduced their asthmatic response to inhalant allergens.[46] Onion contains the flavonoid quercetin, which may account for some of its effect,[47] but the major protective actions appear to be related to its content of mustard oils. Although the mechanism of action is unknown, it has been suggested that it is due to inhibition of the manufacture of leukotrienes.

Indian tobacco (Lobelia inflata)   Indian tobacco contains the alkaloid lobeline, a very efficient expectorant with a long history of use in asthma. It also promotes the release of adrenal hormones which help relax the bronchial muscle.[48] Although effective when used alone, it has traditionally been used in combination with other botanical agents.[49] Typically, it is combined with *Capsicum frutescens* and *Symphlocarpus factida*.

Chilli pepper (Capsicum frutescens)   Experimental evidence has shown that capsaicin, cayenne pepper's major active component, induces long-lasting desensitisation of airway mucosa to various mechanical and chemical irritants.[50] Clinical experience has shown capsicum to be useful in breaking an asthma attack.

Skunk cabbage (Symphlocarpus factida)   Skunk cabbage is an expectorant and respiratory sedative and has a long history of use, in conjunction with lobelia and capsicum, in acute asthmatic attacks.[49]

Green tea (Thea sinensis)   Green tea is useful as a supportive measure in asthma treatment due to its theophylline content and antioxidant components.

Treatment

Eliminate all food allergens and food additives, and bananas if they aggravate the condition. The person who has many food allergies may need to utilise a four-day rotation diet. In the early stages of treatment, mild tryptophan reduction should be useful, but not critical, unless there is a metabolic defect in tryptophan metabolism. Garlic and onions should be liberally used unless the patient is allergic to them. If the patient is willing, or his or her asthma is unresponsive to this therapy, a vegan diet should be tried (for a minimum of four months).

It is important to avoid the use of aspirin and other non-steroidal anti-inflammatory drugs as these drugs can induce an asthma attack.[51,52]

Nutritional supplements

These are all adult doses; decrease for children in proportion to their weight. Carefully evaluate the content of all supplements to ensure avoidance of allergens and food additives.
- Vitamin B6, 25 mg twice a day.
- Vitamin B12, 1 mg per day (oral) or weekly injection. Evaluate for efficacy after 6 weeks.
- Vitamin C, 1–2 g per day.
- Vitamin E, 400 iu per day.
- Carotenes, 50,000 iu per day.
- Eicosapentaenoic acid, 3 g per day.
- Calcium, 500 mg per day.
- Magnesium, 400 mg per day.
- Selenium, 250 μg per day.

Botanical medicines

Doses three times a day.
- *Ephedra sinica*, crude herb or as tea, 0.5 to 1 gram or the equivalent of 12.5 to 25 mg ephedrine.
- *Lobelia inflata* (Indian tobacco)
    Crude herb or as tea, 0.5 to 1 gram.
    Tincture (1:5), 1–4 ml (¼ to 1 tsp).
    Fluid extract (1:1), 0.5 to 1 ml (½ to 1 tsp).
- *Glycyrrhiza glabra* (liquorice), *Scuttelaria baicalensis* (Chinese skullcap) and *Angelica sinensis* (Dong quai) can be taken at the following dosages:
    Dried root (or as tea), 1 to 2 g.
    Tincture (1:5), 4 to 6 ml (1 to 1.5 tsp).
    Fluid extract (1:1), 0.5 to 2.0 ml (¼ to ½ tsp).
    Powdered solid extract (4:1), 250–500 mg.
If liquorice is to be used over a long time it is necessary to increase the intake of potassium-rich foods.

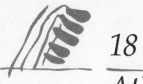

18
Atherosclerosis

- Characteristically associated with high blood pressure, weak pulse and wide pulse pressure.
- Symptoms and signs depend on arteries involved and degree of obstruction – angina, leg cramps (intermittent claudication), gradual mental deterioration, weakness or dizziness. May also be without symptoms.
- Diagonal earlobe crease.

General considerations

Atherosclerosis and its complications are the major causes of death in the United States and have reached epidemic proportions throughout the western world. Heart attacks alone account for 20 per cent of all deaths in the US while degenerative and arterio-sclerotic heart disease account for 33 per cent. Cerebral vascular disease is the third most common cause of death.

Atherosclerosis is a degenerative condition of the arteries, characterised by accumu-lation of lipids (mainly cholesterol, usually complexed to proteins, and cholesterol eshers) within the artery. The atherosclerotic plaque, or atheroma, represents the endpoint of a complex insidious process. Although any artery may be affected, the aorta, coronary and cerebral vascular systems are most frequently involved.[1,2]

Atherosclerosis begins at a very early age – even one-year-old infants show lesions in the aorta, which progress to coronary artery abnormalities by the age of ten. Due to the silent nature of the disease, an atheromatous plaque will develop quietly over a period of several years. Atherosclerosis is usually not diagnosed until the lesions suddenly precipitate a serious, and often lethal, clinical condition. As the plaque increase in size, they begin to narrow the lumen of the artery, progressively reducing the blood flow, leading to insufficient blood flow and the formation of blood clots.

Earlobe crease

Recently, the presence of a diagonal crease on the earlobe has been shown to correlate very well with the degree of atherosclerosis. If you have this crease, begin a programme to reverse the atherosclerotic process immediately.

The earlobe is richly vascularised, and a decrease in blood flow over a period of time is believed to result in collapse of the vascular bed. This leads to a diagonal earlobe crease, which has been recognised as a sign of cardiovascular disease since 1973. Since then, over 30 studies have been reported in the medical literature, with the largest to date involving 1,000 unselected patients.[3]

The crease is seen more commonly with advancing age, until the age of 80, when the incidence drops dramatically. However, the association with atherosclerosis is age-independent.

The earlobe appears to be a better predictor of heart disease than any other known risk factor, including age, smoking, sedentary lifestyle, elevated cholesterol levels and others. While the presence of an earlobe crease does not prove heart disease, it strongly suggests it, and examination of the earlobe should be a useful screening procedure. The correlation does not work with orientals, native Americans, and children with Beckwith's syndrome.[3]

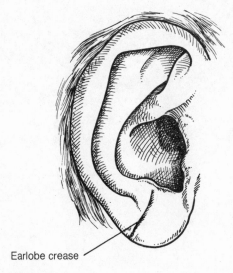

Earlobe crease

Figure 18.1   Earlobe crease

The development of Atherosclerosis

To understand fully the development of atherosclerosis, it is necessary to examine closely the structure of an artery. An artery is divided into three major layers:

- The intima of the artery consists of a layer of endothelial cells lining the vessel's interior surface. Beneath these surface cells there is a layer of connective tissue which provides support to the endothelial cells as well as separates the intima from the media. Mesoglycan is the term used to describe the mucopolysaccharide or glyucosaminoglycan (GAG) complex contained within the arteries of humans and other mammals. Simply stated, mesoglycan is responsible for holding the cells of the artery together and providing structural support. Mesoglycan is also naturally present on the surface of the vessel where it protects the endothelial cells from damage as well as promotes repair.

- The media consists primarily of smooth muscle cells. Interposed among the cells is mesoglycan and other ground substance structures which provide support and elasticity to the artery.
- The adventitia consists primarily of connective tissue providing structural support and elasticity to the artery.

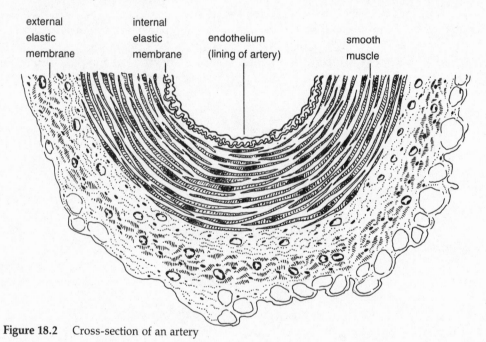

Figure 18.2 Cross-section of an artery

Reaction to injury hypothesis

No single theory of the development of atherosclerosis (AS) has been formulated that satisfies all investigators. However, the most widely accepted theory is the reaction to injury hypothesis, which theorises that the lesions of AS are initiated as a response to injury to the cells lining the inside of the artery, the arterial endothelium.[1,2] Figure 18.3 details the progression of atherosclerosis according to the reaction to injury hypothesis.

A   The initial step in the development of atherosclerosis is damage to the endothelium. Immune, physical, mechanical, viral, chemical and drug factors have all been shown to induce damage to the endothelium that can lead to AS.

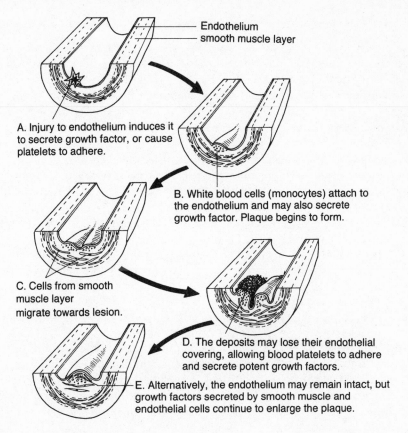

Endothelium
smooth muscle layer

A. Injury to endothelium induces it to secrete growth factor, or cause platelets to adhere.

B. White blood cells (monocytes) attach to the endothelium and may also secrete growth factor. Plaque begins to form.

C. Cells from smooth muscle layer migrate towards lesion.

D. The deposits may lose their endothelial covering, allowing blood platelets to adhere and secrete potent growth factors.

E. Alternatively, the endothelium may remain intact, but growth factors secreted by smooth muscle and endothelial cells continue to enlarge the plaque.

Figure 18.3   Progression of atherosclerosis

B   Once the endothelium has been damaged, sites of injury become more permeable to plasma constituents, especially lipoproteins (fat-carrying proteins). The binding of lipoproteins to glycosaminoglycans leads to a breakdown in the integrity of the connective tissue matrix and causes an increased affinity for cholestrol. Once significant damage has occurred, monocytes (large white blood cells) and platelets adhere to the damaged area where they release growth factors which stimulate smooth muscle cells to migrate from the media into the intima and replicate.

C   The local concentration of lipoproteins, monocytes and platelets leads to the migration of smooth muscle cells from the media into the intima, where they undergo proliferation. The smooth muscle cells dump cellular debris into the intima, leading to further development of the atheroma.

D   The formation of a fibrous cap (consisting of collagen, elastin and glycosamino-glycans) over the intimal surface occurs. Fat and cholesterol deposits accumulate.
    The atheroma continues to grow until eventually it blocks the artery. Blockage is usually around 90 per cent before symptoms of atherosclerosis are apparent.

E   Alternatively, the endothelium may remain intact, but growth factors secreted by smooth muscle and endothelial cells continue to enlarge the plaque.

Homocysteine theory and pyridoxine deficiency

Of particular interest to the nutritionally oriented is the homocysteine theory of athero-sclerosis, a chemical form of endothelial damage due to a vitamin B6 (pyridoxine) deficiency. Since the first report in 1948 by Rinehart and Greenberg of an association of AS with pyridoxine deficiency, numerous studies have further substantiated the role of pyridoxine in preventing atherosclerosis.[4] Homocysteine is derived from methionine during protein breakdown and converted with the help of pyridoxine to a non-toxic derivative. A deficiency of pyridoxine leads to the accumulation of homocysteine, which is damaging to endothelial cells, leading to atherosclerosis.[4]

Pyridoxine may also be important in other aspects of atherosclerosis. Lysyl oxidase, a copper-dependent enzyme responsible for normal cross-linking of both collagen and elastin (constituents of connective tissue and muscle) is also pyridoxine-dependent. It has been hypothesised that since the earliest visible lesion of atherosclerosis is a focal splitting of the internal elastic lamina, this lesion may be the result of imperfect cross-linking of the arterial elastin and collagen. Such a defect could be due to impaired lysyl oxidase activity, secondary to either a copper or pyridoxine deficiency.[5] Pyridoxine also inhibits platelet aggregation.[6]

Monoclonal hypothesis

This hypothesis states that intimal plaque originates as the result of benign cancerous growth initiated by mutation. The mutagens may be chemicals from the environment (e.g. hydrocarbons), body metabolites (e.g. cholesterol byproducts) or viruses.[2,7]

The aryl hydrocarbons, including benzypyrene and methylcholanthrene, found in cigarette smoke are extremely potent mutagens which directly damage arteries as well as evoke cancerous growth of vascular cells.[7]

Therapy

The only effective treatment of atherosclerosis appears to be prevention by diet and lifestyle modification. This contention is supported by the well accepted fact that the major risk factors of atherosclerosis (elevated blood cholesterol levels, high blood pressure, cigarette smoking and diabetes) are all induced by the western diet and lifestyle, and most of the other risk factors are also related to lifestyle (genetic factors, obesity, stress, personality type and physical inactivity).[1,2]

In order to understand fully the dietary recommendations given below it is important first to examine the role of cholesterol and platelets in the development of athero-sclerosis.

Cholesterol and atherosclerosis

Foremost in the prevention and treatment of atherosclerosis is the reduction of serum cholesterol levels. The evidence overwhelmingly associates elevated cholesterol levels with heart disease. In men and women 33 to 44 years of age, those with serum cholesterol levels of 256 mg/dl or over have a five times greater risk of developing coronary artery disease than those whose levels are below 220 mg/dl.

Further analysis of serum lipoproteins (fat-carrying proteins) has refined this risk to show that the serum levels of low density lipoproteins (LDL) and very low density lipoproteins (VLDL) are directly related to risk in both men and women, while high density lipoprotein levels (HDL) are protective against atherosclerosis.[1,2]

LDL transports cholesterol to the tissues. HDL, on the other hand, transports cholesterol to the liver for metabolism and excretion. Therefore the HDL-to-LDL ratio largely determines whether cholesterol is being broken down or deposited in tissues. The HDL-to-LDL ratio also affects other balances in the body; for instance, as the HDL/LDL ratio increases platelet aggregation decreases proportionally.[8]

Platelets and atherosclerosis

The importance of platelet activity in the development of atherosclerosis cannot be overemphasised. Once platelets aggregate, they release potent compounds that cause migration and proliferation of smooth muscle cells into the intima of the artery.[9] Atherosclerosis can be prevented by inhibition of platelet function. Saturated fats increase platelet aggregation, while polyunsaturated fats, particularly lineoleic and linolenic acids, have the opposite effect.[10] These effects are mediated through prostaglandin metabolism.

Prostaglandins Prostaglandins and related compounds are hormone-like molecules derived from 20-carbon-chain fatty acids that contain three, four or five double bonds. The number of double bonds in the fatty acid determines the classification of the prostaglandin. For example, di-homo-linolenec acid contains three double bonds and is known as the prostaglandin-1 (PG1) series; arachidonic acid contains four double bonds and is known as the PG2 series; and eicosapentaenoic acid (EPA) contains five double-bonds and is known as the PG3 series. Subdivision into various prostaglandin subtypes is made according to changes in the structure.[11]

The prostaglandin I class (PGI or prostacyclin) is produced by the vascular endothelium and has anti-aggregating effects, while thromboxane A_2 (a product of arachidonic acid metabolism) is produced by platelets and stimulates aggregation. The balance of these two compounds is greatly affected by dietary fatty acids. Arachidonic acid increases aggregation via conversion to thromboxane A_2, while linoleic, linolenic and eicosapentaenoic (EPA) acids inhibit the conversion of arachidonic acid to thromboxane.

Arachidonic acid and linoleic acid are classified as omega-6 oils. This means that the first unsaturated bond is at the sixth carbon atom of the carbon chain. Linolenic acid, from flaxseed or linseed oil, and EPA are termed omega-3 oils because their first unsaturated bonds are at the third carbon atom. By manipulating prostaglandin metabolism through the use of dietary oils, not only can platelet aggregation be inhibited but a significant anti-inflammatory and anti-allergy effect can be produced. In addition to atherosclerosis, other conditions can be improved by increasing the omega-3 oils, including psoriasis, eczema, menstrual cramps and rheumatoid arthritis.

EPA and platelets   There has been considerable research into the effects of EPA (from fish oils) on prostaglandin metabolism and platelet function.[12-15] Eskimo and Japanese diets are rich in EPA and are associated with a lower incidence of cardiovascular disorders, more favourable plasma lipid and lipoprotein levels, and reduced platelet aggregation.[16] In contrast, western diets are rich in arachidonic acid and linoleic acid and are relatively poor in EPA and linolenic acid.

It has been demonstrated in population studies that fish consumption is protective against mortality from heart disease,[17] while meat consumption is causative.[18] Death due to heart disease is 50 per cent lower among those who consume an average of 30 g of fish per day compared with those who eat meat daily. Meat eaters have a 300 per cent increase in risk for heart disease.

Clinical studies have shown that the daily ingestion of 10–20 grams of commercially produced EPA results in reduced total cholesterol, increased HDL and reduced platelet aggregation in individuals with very high blood lipids.[12,14,15] The effects of EPA are largely due to alteration of prostaglandin ratios. Increased consumption of EPA results in decreased production of PG2 series prostaglandins and increased levels of the PG3 series.

How to decrease platelet aggregation   In summary, decreasing platelet aggregation (particularly excessive aggregation) is an extremely important factor in the prevention and treatment of atherosclerosis. An increased consumption of fish oils and linolenic acid and a decreased consumption of saturated fat and arachidonic acid (found only in animal products) will significantly reduce platelet aggregation and hence athero-sclerosis.

Dietary considerations

Most authorities now agree that the level of plasma cholesterol is largely determined by the dietary intake of total calories of cholesterol, saturated fat and polyunsaturated fat.[1,2] The dietary and lifestyle guidelines discussed below will effectively lower cholesterol levels.

Vegetarian diet   It is well established that vegetarians have a much lower risk of developing heart disease.[19] A vegetarian diet has been shown to be quite effective in lowering cholesterol levels and reducing the risk for atherosclerosis. Such a diet is rich in a number of protective factors such as fibre, essential fatty acids, vitamins and minerals.

The importance of even simple alterations in diet can be quite significant. For example, in one study 200 grams of raw carrots (two medium sized) were eaten daily at breakfast by (supposedly) normal subjects. After three weeks the significant results included an 11 per cent reduction in cholesterol levels, a 50 per cent increase in faecal bile and fat excretion, and a 25 per cent increase in stool weight.[20]

However, strict vegetarianism is not as important as consuming a diet high in fibre and complex carbohydrates, low in fat and low in cholesterol.[21]

Table 18.1 Fatty acid constitution of common domestic fats and oils

Source	Per cent of total fatty acids*					
	18:2 ω-6 Linoleic	20:4 ω-6 Arachidonic	18:3 ω-3 Linolenic	20:5 ω-3 Eicosa-pentaenoic	22:6 ω-3 Docosa-hexaenoic	Saturated
Predominantly ω-6						
Safflower oil	73	—	0.5	—	—	9
Corn oil	57	—	1.0	—	—	13
Cottonseed oil	50	—	0.4	—	—	26
Sunflower seed oil	56	—	0.3	—	—	10
Peanut oil	29	—	1.0	—	—	19
Predominantly ω-3						
Linseed oil	15	—	55.0	—	—	13
Salmon oil	1	—	1.0	8	5	26
Cod liver oil	2	—	1.0	12	12	19
Channel catfish oil	6	2.0	0.7	4	9	26
Mackerel	2	2.0	1.0	10	16	35
Whale oil	1	4.0	—	3	7	19
Both ω-3 and ω-6						
Soybean oil	51	—	7.0	—	—	15
English walnut oil	55	—	11.0	—	—	11
Low in both ω-6 and ω-3						
Cow milk fat	2	—	1.0	—	—	62
Human milk fat	7	0.2	0.7	0.6	0.3	50
Lard	10	—	1.0	—	—	36
Chicken fat	17	—	1.0	—	—	33
Beef tallow	4	—	0.5	—	—	48
Egg yolk	11	6.0	0.2	—	—	53
Beef liver	10	6.0	0.5	.	.	39
Coconut oil	2	—	—	—	—	88
Olive oil	8	—	0.7	—	—	14
Cocoa butter	3	—	0.2	—	—	60
Palm oil	9	—	0.3	—	—	48

* Monounsaturated fatty acids constitute the remaining fatty acids. They are thought to have neutral effects upon plasma lipid levels. Adapted from: Goodnight, S.H., *et al.*, 'Polyunsaturated fatty acids, hyperlipidemia, and thrombosis', *Arteriosclerosis*, 1982, 2, p. 87.
ω: omega.

Fibre   Fibre sources which gel or form a mucilaginous mass (psyllium seed, guar gum, pectin, oat bran, etc.) bind bile and cholesterol in the intestines and promote their excretion. Because of this action, these water-soluble fibres have potent cholesterol lowering effects and further improve the situation by decreasing LDL levels while increasing HDL levels.[22-24] In contrast, the water-insoluble fibres (wheat bran) do not affect serum cholesterol levels to any significant degree. (For a more detailed discussion of the effects of dietary fibre see Chapter 4, Dietary fibre.)

Dietary protein   Vegetable proteins have been shown to lower cholesterol levels, whereas equivalent diets containing milk protein and other animal proteins raise cholesterol levels.[25] This evidence provides further support for a diet rich in vegetables in the prevention of atherosclerosis.

Sucrose   Common sugar promotes increased concentrations of plasma cholesterol, triglycerides and uric acid; and increase platelet aggregation, all of which are known to be involved in the development of atherosclerosis.[26]

Fatty acids   Saturated fats, fats which have been heated at high temperatures in the presence of oxygen (deep frying), and processed trans-partially-saturated fats and oils (e.g. margarine) are all believed to contribute greatly to the development of athero-sclerosis.[1,2,27,28] Sources of saturated fats are usually also sources of cholesterol; while processed, heated or trans-partially-saturated fats and oils are sources of lipid peroxides which interfere with normal essential fatty acid metabolism and, as they are incorpor-ated into cell membranes, alter membrane structure and function.[28,29]

Instead, the diet should be composed of vegetable oils containing the essential fatty acids linoleic (18:2 omega-6) and linolenic (18:3 omega-3) acids. Essential fatty acids lower cholesterol and triglyceride levels and decrease platelet aggregation.[30-35]

Men with coronary artery disease have significantly lower levels of linoleic acid in their diet, fatty tissue and platelets.[35] When all fatty acids were assayed in these men, a stronger correlation was demonstrated between atherosclerosis and low dihomo-gamma-linolenic acid (GLA, 20:3 omega-6) levels. Linoleic acid is converted to GLA by the enzyme delta-6-desaturase. This zinc-and-vitamin-B6-dependent enzyme is inhibited by trans-fatty acids (found in margarine and dairy products), aging, diabetes mellitus, alcohol and catecholamines.[34] GLA is the precursor for PGE1, one of the most potent inhibitors of platelet aggregation. Evening primrose oil (9 per cent GLA and 72 per cent linoleic acid) has been shown to lower high cholesterol levels effectively, with the GLA portion being 170 times more potent than the linoleic acid fraction.[34]

The diet should also be rich in the fish oil eicosapentaenoic acid (EPA). EPA is present in high concentrations in cold-water fish such as salmon, mackerel and herring, or available in supplement form.[12-15] In humans the essential fatty acid linolenic acid can be elongated and desaturated to form EPA.[36] The best source of linolenic acid is flaxseed oil which contains over 50 per cent linolenic acid and 15 per cent linoleic acid. As little as 20 ml (two tablespoons) of flaxseed oil a day can, in only two weeks, double lipid and platelet levels of EPA, resulting in a marked decrease in platelet aggregation.

Despite the clear importance of polyunsaturated fatty acids (PUFA) in preventing atherosclerosis and coronary heart disease, it is important to be aware of their negative effects when they become rancid and, therefore, sources of free radicals. Fresh oils and adequate intake of vitamin E are essential to prevent complications of a diet high in PUFA.

Vitamins

Vitamin C   Strong clinical and experimental evidence suggests that a chronic low intake of vitamin C can lead to elevated cholesterol levels and the accumulation of cholesterol in certain tissues.[37,38] Vitamin C helps prevent atherosclerosis directly through its important roles in cholesterol and fat metabolism, and through its regulation of arterial wall integrity.[39,40]

Vitamin E   A vitamin E deficiency results in significantly higher levels of lipid peroxides (free radicals), significantly reduced release of prostacyclin and lower levels of the antioxidant enzymes superoxide dismutase (SOD), glutathione peroxidase and catalase, resulting in increased free radical damage, particularly of the vascular endothelium.[41,42]

Supplemental vitamin E has been shown to prevent atherosclerosis through its inhibition of the platelet-releasing reaction, which produces a marked rise in lipid peroxides,[43] its actions as a free radical scavenger, inhibition of platelet aggregation[44-6] and its elevation of HDL levels.[47]

Vitamin B6   The important role that B6 plays in preventing atherosclerosis has been discussed above. More recent studies cast a doubt on whether vitamin B6 deficiency is responsible for the atherosclerosis in most individuals.[48]

Niacin   Niacin has long been used to lower cholesterol levels; however, the dose required (1 gram three times per day) often results in toxicity, i.e. liver damage and glucose intolerance.[11] Because of these side effects, niacin therapy for atherosclerosis must be supervised by a physician. Safer more effective natural measures exist.

Minerals

Magnesium   Magnesium offers significant protection against atherosclerosis.[49] It has been observed that individuals dying suddenly of heart attacks have significantly lower levels of heart tissue magnesium and potassium than people dying of other causes.[49,50] Such a deficiency may be due to inadequate magnesium intake or excessive vitamin D intake, which intensifies magnesium deficiency.[51] A magnesium deficiency has been shown to produce spasms of the coronary arteries, and is thought to be a cause of heart attacks not due to a build up of plaque but rather to coronary artery spasm.[50]

Magnesium contributes greatly to the strength of contraction by heart muscle.[49] Magnesium supplementation has been found to be helpful in the management of cardiac arrhythmias and high blood pressure, and many reports have suggested that its administration should become the treatment of choice for coronary artery spasm and heart beat irregularities.[49,50,52] Magnesium supplementation also increases HDL levels,[53] decreases platelet aggregation[54] and prolongs clotting time.

Population studies have yielded a number of interesting associations. Milk consumption is linked to heart disease and is apparently related to its magnesium lowering effects rather than to any other factor.[51] The rate of heart disease is inversely correlated with the magnesium content of the water supply.[49] Although the low incidence of cardiovascular disease in Greenland eskimos has been attributed to the high levels of EPA in their diet, their diets also contain high serum magnesium levels.[55]

Calcium   The daily administration of 2 grams of calcium carbonate (800 mg elemental calcium) resulted in a 25 per cent decrease in serum cholesterol in men with high cholesterol levels, over a period of one year.[56]

Zinc and copper   The zinc-to-copper ratio appears to affect lipoprotein levels.[57] Zinc administration (160 mg per day) has been shown to lower serum HDL levels in men (but not in women)[58] and to induce atherosclerosis in experimental animals.[59]

A deficiency of copper produces marked elevation of cholesterol.[57,60] A deficiency of copper has been suggested to play a major role in the development of atherosclerosis. Copper is important both in lipid metabolism and in production of normal connective tissue via induction of lysyl oxidase.[61]

These findings are significant, since zinc and copper compete for binding sites, and copper levels are commonly marginal in western diets. Obviously, a balanced zinc-to-copper ratio is necessary for optimal function.[62]

Chromium   Chromium chloride supplementation (200 mg per day) results in a decrease in serum triglycerides and total cholesterol, while increasing HDL levels and improving glucose tolerance.[63] These results have also been duplicated with chromium-rich brewer's yeast, but not chromium-poor torula yeast.[44] The chromium content of the western diet is generally quite low.

Selenium   Low selenium levels are associated with an increased risk of heart disease.[65] This observation is based on a study of 11,000 case-controlled pairs from Finland. Restricted selenium intake reduces the levels of the antioxidant enzyme glutathione peroxidase, which may lead to increased lipid peroxide-induced vascular endothelial damage. These effects would be aggravated by a vitamin E deficiency. Selenium also influences prostaglandin metabolism and decreases platelet aggregation.[66]

Special foods and food factors

Carnitine   Carnitine, a vitamin-like compound, stimulates the breakdown of long-chain fatty acids by mitochondria (energy producing units in cells). Carnitine is essential in the transport of fatty acids into the mitochondria. A deficiency in carnitine results in a decrease in fatty acid concentrations in the mitochondria and reduced energy production.

Carnitine is synthesised from lysine in the liver, kidney and brain. It requires alpha-ketoglutarate, iron and vitamin C as cofactors. A deficiency of any of these factors will lead to a deficiency of carnitine. The normal heart stores more carnitine than it needs, but if the heart does not have a good supply of oxygen, carnitine levels quickly decrease. Supplementation with carnitine normalises heart carnitine levels and allows the heart muscle to utilise its limited oxygen supply more efficiently.

Carnitine has been shown to be effective therapeutically in the treatment of atherosclerotic heart disease.[67,68] Since long chain fatty acids are the preferred energy source in well-oxygenated heart tissue, normal heart function is dependent on adequate concentrations of carnitine within the heart.[68,69]

Carnitine also increases HDL levels, while decreasing triglyceride and cholesterol levels.[69–71] Carnitine deficiency is linked to a large number of heart disorders (familial endocardial fibroelastosis, cardiac enlargement, congestive heart failure and cardiac myopathies), all of which respond to carnitine supplementation.[72]

Bromelain   This proteolytic enzyme of the pineapple plant has been shown to inhibit platelet aggregation, improve angina pain, reduce blood pressure and break down atherosclerotic plaques.[73,74] Pancreatic enzyme preparations would have similar effects to bromelain.

Onions and garlic   Onions have been shown to counteract the increased platelet aggregation seen after a high-fat meal and to increase fibrinolytic activity as well.[75] Fibrin is the major constituent of most occlusive thrombi (blood clots) and has a platelet-aggregating effect. The inhibition of fibrin formation is critical in the prevention of atherosclerosis. Crude extracts of onion have been shown to have antihypertensive and cholesterol lowering effects.[76]

Garlic oil, in doses equivalent to 1 gram of raw garlic per kilogram of body weight, increases the breakdown of fibrin by over 100 per cent in humans and inhibits platelets from aggregating.[77,78] Additionally, garlic has been shown to lower total serum cholesterol and triglycerides significantly, while increasing HDL levels.[78]

Ginger   Common ginger has been shown to lower cholesterol levels[79] and inhibit platelet aggregation.[80] Its effects on platelet aggregation has been shown to be greater than that of both garlic and onion.[80]

Alfalfa   Alfalfa leaf decreases cholesterol levels and has a 'shrinkage' effect on atherosclerotic plaque. Supplementation in monkeys has been shown to dissolve cholesterol feeding-induced plaques.[81]

Lecithin   Lecithin (phosphatidyl-choline) has many important functions in the body, including increasing the solubility of cholesterol, thereby decreasing its ability to induce atherosclerosis. Lecithin also aids in removal of cholesterol from tissue deposits and inhibits platelet aggregation.[82] This effect is seen only with the polyunsaturated forms, such as that from the soybean, and not with the relatively saturated lecithin from eggs.

Mesoglycan   As mentioned earlier, mesoglycan is the term used to describe the mucopolysaccharide or glycosaminoglycan (GAG) complex contained within the arteries of humans and other mammals. Simply stated, glycosaminoglycans are the ground substance components responsible for holding cells of the body together and providing structural support. Mesoglycan functions as structural support in blood vessels.

Mesoglycan is essential for maintaining the health of arteries and other blood vessels. In addition, mesoglycan has many important effects including preventing damage to the surface of the artery, formation of damaging blood clots, migration of smooth muscle cells into the intima and formation of fat and cholesterol deposits, as well as lowering total cholesterol levels while raising HDL-cholesterol.[83-8]

Studies of animals have indicated that mesoglycan is effectively absorbed orally and is incorporated into vessels, where it dramatically improves integrity and function.[89] As for human use, a number of clinical studies have demonstrated that supplementing the diet with mesoglycan has a remarkable effect in improving the structure, function and integrity of arteries.[90-2]

Pantethine   Pantethine is the stable form of pantetheine, the active form of pantothenic acid, which is the fundamental component of coenzyme A (CoA). CoA is involved in the transport of fatty acids to and from cells, and to the mitochondria. Pantethine has significant lipid-lowering activity while pantothenic acid has very little (if any) effect in lowering cholesterol and triglyceride levels.

Panthethine administration (standard dose 900 mg per day), like carnitine, has been shown to reduce serum triglyceride and cholesterol levels significantly, while increasing HDL-cholesterol levels in clinical trials.[93-98] Its lipid lowering effects are most impressive when its toxicity (virtually none) is compared to conventional lipid lowering drugs. Its mechanism of action is due to inhibiting cholesterol synthesis and accelerating fatty acid breakdown in the mitochondria.

Pantethine is very much indicated in angina. Like carnitine, heart pantethine levels decrease during times of reduced oxygen supply. Pantethine has demonstrated effects in animals that would indicate that it would be of great benefit to individuals with angina.[99]

Lifestyle

Physical exercise   Many studies have shown a direct relationship between physical activity and cholesterol levels.[100-3] One study investigated various lipoprotein parameters in middle-aged marathon runners, joggers and inactive men.[103] It demonstrated that HDL increases and total cholesterol decreases in direct proportion to the distance run. Physical exercise is also associated with a decreased incidence of coronary artery disease.[93-104]

Smoking   Cigarette smoking is a potent risk factor for atherosclerosis. Statistical evidence reveals a mean increase of about 70 per cent in the death rate and a three-to-fivefold increase in the risk of coronary artery disease in smokers compared to non-smokers. Women over the age of 35 who smoke and who also take oral contraceptives are at very high risk for coronary artery disease. The more cigarettes smoked and the longer the period of years smoked the greater risk of dying from a heart attack or other complication of atherosclerosis.

Coffee   A strong association exists between coffee consumption (six cups a day) and serum cholesterol.[105] The incidence of acute myocardial infarction has been found to correlate with coffee, but not tea, consumption.[106]

Alcohol   Alcohol ingestion elevates serum cholesterol triglycerides and uric acid levels, as well as blood pressure, and greatly increases the risk of atherosclerosis.

Treatment

There is no doubt that atherosclerosis is a disease directly caused by the western diet and lifestyle. Treatment and prevention include reducing serum cholesterol levels, reducing factors that damage the vascular endothelium and preventing platelet aggregation. Eliminating, or at least reducing, all known risk factors requires a major change in diet and lifestyle.

Since so many factors are known to be involved in atherosclerosis, any treatment plan must be individualised. What follows is a general approach which needs to be tailored to each individual.

Diet

Increase the intake of vegetables and fruits. Increase the intake of dietary fibre, especially the gel-forming or mucilaginous fibres (flax seed, oat bran, pectin, etc.), cold-pressed vegetable oils and fish, while reducing the consumption of saturated fats, cholesterol, sugar and animal proteins. All fried foods should be avoided. Ginger, garlic and onions can be used liberally.

Lifestyle

The individual with angina should stop smoking and drinking alcohol and coffee. Stress should be decreased by using stress management techniques such as progressive relaxation or guided imagery. A carefully graded, progressive, aerobic exercise programme (30 minutes three times a week) is a necessity. Walking is a good exercise to start with.

Supplements

- Broad spectrum multivitamin and mineral.
- Vitamin C, 2 g per day.
- Vitamin E, 200 iu per day.
- Fibre supplement (guar gum, psyllium seed or other water soluble fibre), a minimum of 5 grams daily.
- Flaxseed (linseed) oil, 1–2 tblsp a day.
- EPA, 5–10 g a day.

If significant atherosclerosis is already apparent, it may be appropriate to take the following supplements:

- Mesoglycan, 100 mg a day.
- Carnitine, 900 mg a day.
- Pantethine, 900 mg a day.

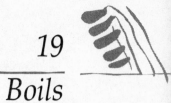

19
Boils

- Painful inflammatory swelling of a hair follicle that forms an abscess which typically appears as rounded or conical 1-cm-diameter red nodule surrounded by redness, progressing to localised pus pockets with white centres.
- There is tenderness and pain and, if severe, mild fever.
- *Staphylococcus aureus* is cultured from the abscess.

General considerations

A boil (furuncle) is a deep-seated infection (abscess) involving the entire hair follicle and adjacent subcutaneous tissue. The most commonly involved sites are the hairy parts exposed to friction, pressure or moisture. Plugging the hair follicles with petroleum-based products also increases the risk of boil formation. Since the lesion can spread, several are often found at one location.[1] When several furuncles join together they are called a carbuncle.

There is no particular cause of boils, although occasionally they may be an indication of an underlying disease such as diabetes mellitus, obesity, nephritis, blood disorders or other debilitating disease. It is at times epidemic. Most lesions will resolve within one to two weeks. Recurrent boils can indicate a highly infective form of bacteria, poor hygiene, industrial exposure to chemicals or depression of the immune system.

The exact number of people with boils is difficult to determine since most people with boils will usually not consult a physician. Recurrent boils are usually more common in young men.

Therapy

Recurrent attacks of boils can indicate a depressed immune system caused by nutritional deficiencies, food allergies and/or excessive consumption of sugar and other concentrated refined carbohydrates (see Chapter 6, Immune support, for further discussion). Zinc and vitamin A are especially important in the treatment of boils. One clinical trial demonstrated zinc supplementation to be quite effective in the treatment of recurrent boils.[2]

Botanical medicines

Goldenseal (Hydrastis canadensis) Berberine, the most active alkaloid of goldenseal, is a well-documented antimicrobial agent.[3,4] It is toxic to the bacteria commonly associated with boils, particularly *Staphylococcus aureus*. It has also been found to stimulate immune system function[5] and decrease inflammatory processes.[6]

Poultices Various herbal poultices are commonly used in the treatment of abscesses. Folk healers have used burdock root, castor oil, chervil, liquorice root and others.[7] They are simple and effective. A poultice commonly used with great success by naturopathic physicians is a paste made out of goldenseal root powder.[8,9] It will typically clear an abscess in two to three days. Its high degree of efficacy is probably due to the properties of berberine mentioned above, i.e. antimicrobial and anti-inflammatory. An advantage of goldenseal poultices as compared to hot packs and other types of poultices is that they usually will not rupture.

Treatment

Eliminate all dietary factors which may suppress immune function, i.e. sugar, refined simple carbohydrates and food allergens. If the lesion does not resolve within two to three days, a physician should be consulted since the infection can spread through the subcutaneous tissues (cellulitis) or into the bloodstream (bacteraemia). Cleanliness should be rigorously maintained.

Supplements

- Vitamin C, 1 g three times a day.
- Beta-carotene, 100,000 iu a day.
- Vitamin A, 50,000 iu daily for two weeks.
- Zinc, 45 mg a day.

Botanical medicine

Doses three times a day.
- *Hydrastis canadensis,* ½ tsp per cup.
     Dried root (or as tea) 1 to 2 g.
     Freeze-dried root, 500 to 1,000 mg.
     Tincture (1:5), 4 to 6 ml (1 to 1.5 tsp).
     Fluid extract (1:1), 0.5 to 2.0 ml (¼ to ½ tsp).

Powdered solid extract (4:1), 250–500 mg.

Poultice – 1 tblsp root powder mixed with water or egg white to form a paste. Apply to abscess and cover with an absorbant bandage.

Other recommendations

The infected area should be immobilised and not handled, except when necessary to change the poultice. If hydrastis packs are unavailable, or localisation, rupture and drainage are preferred, hot Epsom salt packs (two tblsp Epsom salt per cup of hot water) will bring an abscess to a head.

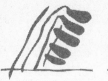

20

Bronchitis and pneumonia

- Bronchitis and pneumonia are usually preceded by upper respiratory tract infection.
- Sudden onset of shaking, chills, fever and chest pain.
- Pneumonia shows classic signs of lung involvement (shallow breathing, cough, abnormal breath sounds, etc.).
- X-ray shows infiltration of fluid and lymph in lungs.

General considerations

Bronchitis refers to an infection or irritation of the bronchial tree (the tubes leading down into the lungs) while pneumonia refers to infection or irritation of the lungs. Both of these conditions are much more common in the winter as they usually follow an upper respiratory tract infection (cold).

Acute pneumonia is still the fifth leading cause of death in the US, as it is particularly dangerous in the elderly. Although pneumonia may appear in healthy individuals, it is usually seen in individuals with low immune function, particularly drug and alcohol abusers. The growing population of individuals with chronic lung diseases primarily due to smoking and immunosuppressive drugs has contributed to a further increase of chronic bronchitis as well as serious pneumonias, which have very high mortality rates.[1]

In healthy individuals, pneumonia and bronchitis most often follow an insult to the host defence mechanisms – viral infection (especially influenza), cigarette smoke and other noxious fumes, impairment of consciousness (which depresses the gag reflex, allowing aspiration), cancer and hospitalisation.

The airway below the larynx is normally sterile due to several protective mechanisms, both mechanical and immune related. The mucus-covered lining of the lower respiratory tract propels sputum to the larger bronchi and trachea with the aid of cilia (microscopic fingerlike projections). The respiratory secretions contain a number of substances which exert nonspecific antimicrobial actions.

Table 20.1 Causes of common pneumonias

Type	Percentage
Viral	20
Influenza	3
Mycoplasmal	10–20
Bacterial	12
Bacterial superimposed on viral	6
Chlamydia	10
Unknown cause (legionnaires, toxic)	38

Antibodies of the IgA class are present in high concentrations in the secretions of the upper respiratory tract, protecting against viral infection. In the lower respiratory tract (below the larynx) IgA along with IgG antibodies aid in neutralising bacteria and microbial toxins, reducing bacterial attachment to respiratory tract surfaces and activating immune mechanisms which destroy the bacteria. In the lung, potent defence mechanisms are present, including macrophages, a rich blood supply capable of rapidly delivering white blood cells and an efficient lymphatic drainage network.

Therapy

Specific therapy will depend on the type of pneumonia or bronchitis (bacterial, viral or other). Since bacterial pneumonia can be quite serious, any individual with symptoms suggestive of pneumonia should be seen by a physician. The recommendations given below are for all types of pneumonia and bronchitis. They are of a general nature, to be used along with the recommendations given in Chapter 6, Immune support.

Expectorants

Botanical expectorants have a long history of use in bronchitis and pneumonia. They act to increase the quantity, decrease the viscosity and promote expulsion of the secretions of the respiratory mucous membranes. Many also have antibacterial and antiviral activity. It is important to note that they are not cough suppressants, whose use is contraindicated in pneumonia; many commonly used herbal expectorants actually promote the cough reflex.

Commonly used herbal expectorants include lobelia (*Lobelia urens*, *Lobelia dortmanns* and *Lobelia inflata*), liquorice (*Glycyrrhiza glabra*), gumweed (*Grindelia camporum*), wild cherry bark (*Prunus spp.*), white horehound (*Marrubium vulgare*), coltsfoot (*Tussilago farfara*) and sundew (*Drosera rotundifolia*).

Vitamin C

In the early part of this century, before the advent of effective antibiotics, many controlled and uncontrolled studies demonstrated the positive effects of large doses of vitamin C in the treatment of pneumonia, but only when started on the first or second day of infection.[2] If administered later, vitamin C tended only to lessen the severity of the disease. Researchers also demonstrated that in pneumonia, as well as other infectious conditions, white blood cells take up large amounts of vitamin C.[3]

Treatment

The general approach to all infectious bronchial conditions and pneumonias includes stimulation of the immune system and support of respiratory tract drainage (for a full discussion of immune system stimulation see Chapter 6, Immune support). Drainage is supported by the use of local heat, massage and expectorants.

General measures

- Rest (bed rest better).
- Drink large amounts of fluids (preferably diluted vegetable juices, soups and herb teas).
- Limit simple sugar consumption (including fruit sugars) to less than 50 grams a day.

Supplements

- Vitamin C, 500 mg every two hours.
- Bioflavonoids, 1 g per day.
- Vitamin A, 25,000 iu per day.
- Beta-carotene, 200,000 iu per day.
- Zinc lozenges, one lozenge containing 23 mg elemental zinc every two waking hours for one week. (Prolonged supplementation at this dose is not recommended as it may lead to immunosuppression.)
- Thymus extract, 500 mg twice daily.

Botanical medicines

Echinacea angustifolia, Hydrastis canadensis (goldenseal) and *Glycyrrhiza glabra* (liquorice) can be taken at the following doses during an infection (doses three times a day):
- Dried root (or as tea), 1 to 2 g.
- Freeze-dried root, 500–1,000 mg.
- Tincture (1:5), 4 to 6 ml (1 to 1.5 tsp).
- Fluid extract (1:1), 0.5 to 2.0 ml (¼ to ½ tsp).
- Powdered solid extract (4:1), 250–500 mg.

Cough syrups

Onion cough syrup   Put six chopped white onions in a double boiler and add half a cup of honey. Cook slowly over low heat for two hours and strain. Take at regular intervals, preferably warm.

Expectorant mixture Mix the following ingredients: 2 oz liquorice root, 1 oz wild cherry bark, 1 oz coltsfoot, 1 oz lobelia and 1 oz horehound. Boil the mixture slowly in four cups of water for two minutes. Let steep for ten minutes more. Strain and take one cup every two hours if an adult, half a cup for children. Sweeten with honey if necessary.

Physical therapy

A heating pad or hot water bottle can be applied to the chest and back, 30 minutes daily.

Mustard poultice A mustard poultice is made by mixing one part dry mustard with three parts flour and adding enough water to make a paste. The paste is then spread on thin cotton (old pillow casing works well) or cheesecloth, folded, and then placed on the chest. Leave on for up to 20 minutes. However be sure and check periodically, as it will cause blisters if left on too long.

Postural drainage

This should be performed three times per day. As Figure 20.1 indicates, postural drainage is performed by lying with the top half of the body off the bed, using the forearms as support. The position should be assumed for a 5 to 15 minute period while the individual is urged to cough and expectorate into a basin or newspaper on the floor. This procedure imposes hard work on an individual, so it is a good idea to have a helper.

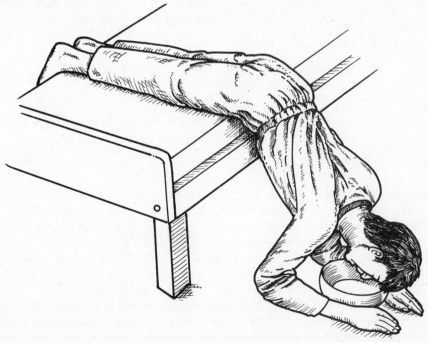

Figure 20.1 Postural drainage

21
Candidiasis

- Overgrowth of *Candida albicans* in stool culture.
- Presence of high levels of antibodies against *Candida albicans*.
- Common symptoms attributed to the intestinal overgrowth of *Candida albicans* can affect any system of the body, but primarily it affects the gastrointestinal, nervous, endocrine and immune systems.
- General symptoms – chronic fatigue, loss of energy, general malaise, decreased libido.
- Gastrointestinal symptoms – thrush (candida overgrowth of the mouth), bloating, gas, intestinal cramps, rectal itching and altered bowel function.
- Genitourinary system complaints – vaginal yeast infection and frequent bladder infections.
- Endocrine system complaints – primarily menstrual complaints.
- Nervous system complaints – depression, irritability and inability to concentrate.
- Immune system complaints – allergies, chemical sensitivities and low immune function.

General considerations

The common yeast *Candida albicans* is present in every individual. Normally, the yeast lives harmlessly in the gastrointestinal tract. However, occasionally the yeast will overgrow and lead to significant disease. Candida overgrowth is believed to cause a wide variety of symptoms (see above) as part of a complex medical syndrome (the yeast syndrome or chronic candidiasis). The major body systems most sensitive to the yeast are the gastrointestinal, genitourinary, endocrine, nervous and immune systems. Allergies have also been attributed to candida overgrowth.[1-3]

Candida overgrowth is most often associated with chronic antibiotic use. Antibiotics kill off the friendly bacteria which help keep candida in check. When antibiotic use first became widespread it was noted immediately that yeast infections increased. Initially, antifungal drugs were often given along with the antibiotic to prevent this problem, but for some reason this practice fell out of favour.

The yeast syndrome or chronic candidiasis has thus been around for a long time. However, it was not until Orion Truss published *The Missing Diagnosis* and William Crook published *The Yeast Connection* that the public and many physicians became aware of the magnitude of the problem.[2,3]

In addition to antibiotic use, the overgrowth of candida in the intestinal tract is often the result of other drugs such as corticosteroids, anti-ulcer drugs, oral contraceptive (birth control) pills, lack of digestive secretions or too much sugar in the diet.[1]

Typical patient profile

Individuals with chronic candidiasis will have different symptoms depending on such factors as age, sex, host resistance and environmental exposure to various factors promoting candida overgrowth. The typical clinical patient with chronic candidiasis is summarised in the accompanying box.

Typical chronic candidiasis patient profile

- Sex: adult female.
- Age: 15–50.
- Presenting symptoms: any of those listed at the beginning of the chapter.
- Past history: chronic vaginal yeast infections; chronic antibiotic use for infections or acne; oral birth control usage; oral steroid hormone usage.
- Associated conditions: premenstrual syndrome; sensitivity to foods, chemicals and other allergens; endocrine disturbances; psoriasis; irritable bowel syndrome; etc.
- Other: craving for foods rich in carbohydrates or yeast.

Diagnosis

The diagnosis of candidiasis is often quite difficult. The questionnaire on the following pages is a useful screening tool to determine an individual's likelihood of having the yeast syndrome.[3] Definitive diagnosis usually involves a positive stool culture for candida or elevated antibody levels to candida.[1]

Therapy

The successful treatment of chronic candidiasis involves reducing predisposing factors to candida overgrowth. Figure 21.1 on page 184 illustrates a vicious cycle which exists in many people with chronic candidiasis and highlights the importance of a comprehensive approach to the problem.

Chronic candidiasis may play a role in other health conditions, most notably hives,

Candida questionnaire

Section A: History

		Point score
1.	Have you taken tetracyclines or other antibiotics for acne for 1 month (or longer)?	25
2.	Have you at any time in your life taken other broad spectrum antibiotics for respiratory, urinary or other infections (for 2 months or longer, or in shorter courses 4 or more times in a 1-year period)?	20
3.	Have you taken a broad spectrum antibiotic drug, even a single course?	6
4.	Have you, at any time in your life, been bothered by persistent prostatitis, vaginitis or other problems affecting your reproductive organs?	25
5.	Have you been pregnant:	
	2 or more times?	5
	1 time?	3
6.	Have you taken birth control pills:	
	For more than 2 years?	15
	For 6 months to 2 years?	8
7.	Have you taken prednisone or other cortisone-type drugs:	
	For more than 2 weeks?	15
	For 2 weeks or less?	6
8.	Does exposure to perfumes, insecticides, fabric shop odours and other chemicals provoke:	
	Moderate to severe symptoms?	20
	Mild symptoms?	5
9.	Are your symptoms worse on damp, muggy days or in mouldy places?	20
10.	Have you had athlete's foot, ring worm, other chronic fungal infections of the skin or nails? Have such infections been:	
	Severe or persistent?	20
	Mild to moderate?	10
11.	Do you crave sugar?	10
12.	Do you crave breads?	10
13.	Do you crave alcoholic beverages?	10
14.	Does tobacco smoke really bother you?	10

Total score Section A

Section B: Major symptoms

For each of your symptoms, enter the appropriate figure in the point score column:

If a symptom is occasional or mild	score 3 points
If a symptom is frequent and/or moderately severe	score 6 points
If a symptom is severe and/or disabling	score 9 points

Add total score and record it at the end of this section.

Point score

1. Fatigue or lethargy
2. Feeling of being 'drained'
3. Poor memory
4. Feeling 'spacey' or unreal
5. Depression
6. Numbness, burning or tingling
7. Muscle aches
8. Muscle weakness or paralysis
9. Pain and/or swelling in joints
10. Abdominal pain
11. Constipation
12. Diarrhoea
13. Bloating
14. Troublesome vaginal discharge
15. Persistent vaginal burning or itching
16. Prostatitis
17. Impotence
18. Loss of sexual desire
19. Endometriosis
20. Cramps and/or other menstrual irregularities
21. Premenstrual tension
22. Spots in front of eyes
23. Erratic vision

Total score, Section B

Section C: Other symptoms

For each of your symptoms, enter the appropriate figure in the point score column:

If a symptom is occasional or mild	score 1 point
If a symptom is frequent and/or moderately severe	score 2 points
If a symptom is severe and/or disabling	score 3 points

Add total score and record it at the end of this section.

Section 3 (continued)   *Point score*
1. Drowsiness
2. Irritability or jitteriness
3. Uncoordination
4. Inability to concentrate
5. Frequent mood swings
6. Headache
7. Dizziness/loss of balance
8. Pressure above ears, feeling of head swelling and tingling
9. Itching
10. Other rashes
11. Heartburn
12. Indigestion
13. Belching and intestinal gas
14. Mucus in stools
15. Haemorrhoids
16. Dry mouth
17. Rash or blisters in mouth
18. Bad breath
19. Joint swelling or arthritis
20. Nasal congestion or discharge
21. Postnasal drip
22. Nasal itching
23. Sore or dry mouth
24. Cough
25. Pain or tightness in chest
26. Wheezing or shortness of breath
27. Urgency or urinary frequency
28. Burning on urination
29. Failing vision
30. Burning or tearing or eyes
31. Recurrent infections or fluid in ears
32. Ear pain or deafness

    Total score, Section C
    Total score, Section A
    Total score, Section B'
Total score

The total score will help you and your physician decide if your health problems
are yeast-connected. Scores in women will run higher as seven items in the
questionnaire apply exclusively to women, while only two apply exclusively to
men.
*   Yeast-connected health problems are almost certainly present in women with
    scores over 180 and in men with scores over 140.

- Yeast-connected health problems are probably present in women with scores over 120 and in men with scores over 90.
- Yeast-connected health problems are possibly present in women with scores over 60 and in men with scores over 40.
- With scores of less than 60 in women and 40 in men, yeasts are less apt to cause health problems.

irritable bowel syndrome, psoriasis, AIDS and depression. Brief discussions of candida's role in these diseases are contained in the individual chapters dealing with these conditions.

Reducing predisposing factors

Decreased digestive secretions   Digestive secretions such as hydrochloric acid, pancreatic enzymes and bile normally prevent the overgrowth of candida and its penetration into the absorptive surfaces of the intestine. A lack of any one of these digestive factors will allow the yeast to overgrow. Restoration of normal digestive secretions with the aid of hydrochloric acid supplements, pancreatic enzymes and substances which promote bile flow is critical in the treatment of chronic candidiasis.

Pancreatic enzymes are especially important therapeutic agents. Incomplete digestion of proteins and other food components creates a number of problems for the body, including the development of food allergies and formation of toxic substances. As well as being necessary for digestion, the pancreatic enzymes are largely responsible for keeping the small intestine free from parasites (including bacteria, yeast, protozoa and intestinal worms[4]) and help the body break down immune complexes.[5]

Diet   A number of dietary factors appear to promote the overgrowth of candida. A special diet must therefore be employed in the treatment of candidiasis.[1-3]

The diet should be free of refined sugar, including sucrose, fructose, fruit juices, honey and maple syrup, since candida thrives in a high sugar state. Foods with a high content of yeast or mould, including alcoholic beverages, cheeses, dried fruits and peanuts, also promote candida overgrowth and therefore should also be eliminated.

Milk and milk products should be avoided due to their high content of lactose (milk sugar) and trace levels of antibiotics. All known allergens should also be eliminated since allergies can weaken the immune system and provide a more hospitable environment for the yeast.

Impaired immunity   When the immune system is impaired, candida will overgrow rapidly (see Chapter 12, AIDS for example). Therefore a healthy immune system is critical in preventing the overgrowth of candida.

A number of things can weaken the immune system, including frequent antibiotic use, chemotherapy, steroids, radiation, various environmental chemicals, nutrient deficiencies, various diseases like cancer, diabetes and hypothyroidism, alcohol and stress. Chapter 6 provides information on how to maintain a healthy immune system.

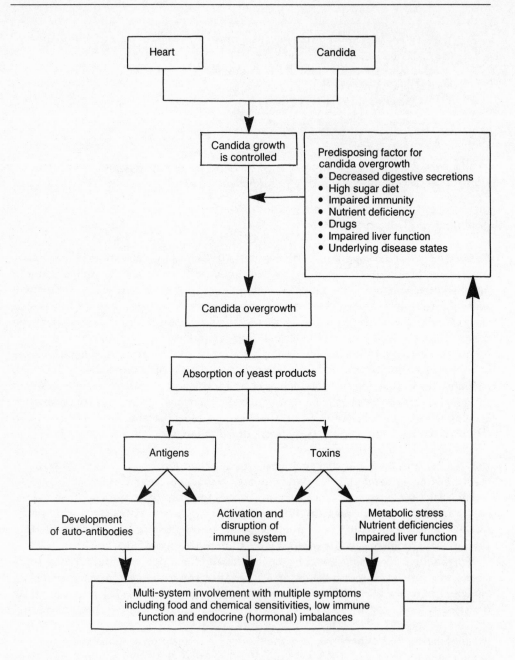

Figure 21.1, The cycle of candidiasis

Nutrient deficiency   Virtually any nutrient deficiency can result in the overgrowth of candida since all known nutrients are critical to optimum immune function. Those nutrients of particular significance in chronic candidiasis include vitamin A, vitamin B6, zinc, selenium, magnesium, essential fatty acids, folic acid and iron. Deficiencies of these nutrients have been documented in patients with chronic candidiasis and are thought to contribute significantly to the candida overgrowth.[1,6-9]

Reversing any nutrient deficiency is of upmost importance in the treatment of chronic candidiasis. To ensure against nutrient deficiency a high potency multiple vitamin-mineral preparation is indicated.

Drugs   Prolonged antibiotic use is believed to be the most important factor in the development of chronic candidiasis. Antibiotics, through suppressing normal intestinal bacteria which prevent yeast overgrowth and suppression of the immune system, strongly promote the overgrowth of candida.[1] This results in a positive feedback cycle or vicious circle. A person with low immune function is more susceptible to chronic *Candida albicans* infection. This low immune function also increases the likelihood of developing an acute bacterial infection that will be treated with antibiotics. This in turn increases the overgrowth of candida, which in turn further suppresses immunity, and the individual begins to spiral downwards.

Other drugs which strongly promote the overgrowth of candida include corticosteroids, oral contraceptives and anti-ulcer medications.[1-3] Patients on the anti-ulcer drugs Tagamet (cimetidine) or Zantac (ranitidine) actually develop candida overgrowth in the stomach, thus highlighting the importance of hydrochloric acid in the prevention of candida overgrowth.[10]

Impaired liver function   Impaired liver function as a result of chemical damage promotes candida overgrowth in mice.[11] Presumably the same phenomenon occurs in humans. It appears the liver is a key organ in the battle against candida.

The toxins of candida absorbed from the gut are filtered from the blood by the liver. Impaired detoxification mechanisms of the liver are thought to be responsible for the high sensitivity to chemicals in individuals with candida overgrowth. Symptoms of chronic candidiasis occurring outside the gastrointestinal tract, such as psoriasis, PMS, etc., are very strong indication that the liver is not filtering the blood sufficiently.

Individuals with candida often experience the 'die off' or Herxheimer reaction when placed on compounds which kill the yeast. This reaction is produced when the candida dies and releases its toxins into the blood. If the liver is not filtering the blood adequately, the toxins released by the dying candida will not be filtered from the blood and the individual will have a worsening of symptoms. It is therefore important to support the liver before, during and after employing measures designed to destroy the yeast.

Underlying disease states   Any disease which can suppress the immune system can increase susceptibility to candida overgrowth. Common diseases which predispose to candidiasis include diabetes mellitus, thyroid diseases, cancers and any disease requiring the use of corticosteroids.[1-3]

Nutritional and herbal compounds

Caprylic acid Caprylic acid, a naturally occurring fatty acid, has been reported to be an effective antifungal compound in the treatment of candidiasis.[12,13] Since caprylic acid is readily absorbed in the intestines,[14] it is necessary to take timed-released or enteric coated caprylic acid formulas to allow for gradual release throughout the entire intestinal tract.

Lactobacillus supplementation *Lactobacillus acidophilus* is the type of bacteria found in natural yogurt. It has been shown to retard the growth of candida in culture media.[15] Since many individuals may react to traditional sources of *L. acidophilus* (milk products), many health practitioners recommend commercial *L. acidophilus* supplements. Addition of high-potency *L. acidophilus* supplement to the diet may be helpful in controlling the yeast.

Garlic Garlic has demonstrated significant antifungal activity against a wide range of fungi.[16–20] Garlic is especially active against *C. albicans*, being more potent than nystatin, gentian violet and six other reputed antifungal agents.[15,18–20]

Barberry (Berberis vulgaris) The common barberry plant has been used as a valuable antidiarrhoeal and anti-infective agent in folk medicine. Its therapeutic action is related to its high content of the alkaloid berberine. The antibiotic activity of berberine is well documented.[21–24] It is an effective antimicrobial agent against a wide range of organisms, including *Candida albicans*. Its action on *Candida albicans*, as well as on disease-causing bacteria, prevents the overgrowth of yeast that commonly follows antibiotic use. It appears to be effective in normalising the bacterial content of the gut by acting against both disease-causing bacteria and the yeast. Its activity against the yeast is quite potent.[24]

Diarrhoea is a common symptom in patients with chronic candidiasis. Berberine has shown remarkable antidiarrhoeal activity in even the most severe cases. It has shown positive clinical results in relieving diarrhoea in cases of cholera, amoebiasis, giardiasis and other causes of acute gastrointestinal infection, e.g. *E. coli*, shigella, salmonella and klebsiella, and may also relieve the diarrhoea seen in patients with chronic candidiasis.[25,26]

Another common symptom in patients with chronic candidiasis is decreased immune function. Berberine has shown remarkable immune stimulating activity. Foremost is its ability to increase the blood supply to the spleen, thus promoting optimal activity of the spleen and the release of compounds that potentiate our immune system.[27] Berberine has also been shown to be a potent activator of macrophages,[28] cells responsible for destroying bacteria, viruses, yeast and tumour cells.

Other berberine-containing plants such as goldenseal root (*Hydrastis canadensis*) and Oregon grape root (*Berberis aquifolium*) have similar properties to barberry.

Pau d'arco (La Pacho or taheebo) This South American tree has a long folk history of use in the treatment of infections and cancer. Much of its pharmacologic action is thought to be a result of its high content of the compound lapachol. This compound is considered among the most important antitumour agents from plants. Lapachol and another compound from pau d'arco, xyloidine, have shown anti-candida effects.[29]

*German chamomile (*Matricaria chamomilla*)* German chamomile contains several compounds that kill candida. Its folk use is in the treatment of colic, diarrhoea and indigestion, common symptoms in candida sufferers.[21,22]

Common spices Ginger (*Zingiber officinale*), cinnamon (*Cinnamomum zeylanicum*), thyme (*Thymus vulgaris*), balm (*Melissa officinale*) and rosemary (*Rosmarinus officinalis*) contain some of the most powerful candida killing substances available.[21,22]

Treatment

There are seven important steps in the successful control of *Candida albicans* outlined below.

- Eliminate the use of antibiotics, steroids, immune-suppressing drugs and birth control pills (unless there is absolute medical necessity).
- Follow the candida control diet given below.
- Enhance digestion (see Chapter 5, Digestion, for guidelines.)
- Enhance immune function (see Chapter 6, Immune support, for guidelines).
- Enhance liver function (see Chapter 8, Liver support, for guidelines).
- Use nutritional and herbal supplements which help control yeast overgrowth and promote a healthy bacterial flora.
- Eliminate candida toxins by using a water-soluble fibre source such as guar gum, psyllium seed or pectin which can bind to toxins in the gut and promote their excretion.

Diet

- Avoid foods high in simple carbohydrate content such as refined sugars (sucrose, fructose, corn syrup), fruit juices, honey and maple syrup.
- Avoid foods with a high content of yeast or mould, including alcoholic beverages, cheeses, dried fruits, melons and peanuts. These foods also promote candida overgrowth and therefore should be eliminated.
- Avoid milk and milk products, due to their high content of lactose (milk sugar) and antibiotics.
- Limit intake of high carbohydrate vegetables such as potatoes, corn and parsnip.
- Avoid all known or suspected allergens, since allergies can weaken the immune system and provide a more hospitable environment for the yeast.
- Foods which can be eaten freely include all vegetables, protein sources (legumes, fish, poultry and meat) and whole grains. Two to three one-cup servings of the following fruit can be eaten per day as well – apples, bilberries, cherries, other berries and pears.

Nutritional supplements

- Multiple vitamin-mineral formula (yeast-free, hypoallergenic formulas are better tolerated), daily.
- Iron, 45 mg per day.
- Zinc (picolinate), 45 mg per day.
- Selenium, 200 μg a day.
- Caprylic acid (delayed release formula), 1 gram with meals.
- Lactobacillus product, as directed on label.
- Fibre (guar gum, pectin or psyllium seed) supplement, 1 tablespoon at night before retiring.

Botanical medicines

Liberal consumption of garlic, ginger, cinnamon and other aromatic herbs with potent antifungal activity.

- *Berberis vulgaris* (barberry), doses three times a day:
    Dried bark of root (or as tea), 1 to 2 g.
    Tincture (1:5), 4 to 6 ml (1 to 1.5 tsp).
    Fluid extract (1:1), 0.5 to 2.0 ml (¼ to ½ tsp).
    Powdered solid extract (4:1), 250–500 mg.
- *Hydrastis canadensis*, doses three times a day:
    Dried root (or as tea), 1 to 2 g.
    Tincture (1:5), 4 to 6 ml (1 to 1.5 tsp).
    Fluid extract (1:1), 0.5 to 2.0 ml (¼ to ½ tsp).
    Powdered solid extract (4:1), 250–500 mg.
- Pau d'arco, 15–20 grams of bark boiled in 500 ml or 1 pint of water for 5 to 15 minutes, three to four times daily.

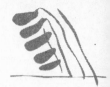

22

Carpal tunnel syndrome

- Numbness, tingling and/or burning pain of the first three fingers of the hand, particularly at night.
- Appearance or worsening of symptoms caused by flexion of the wrist for 60 seconds and relieved by extension.

General considerations

Carpal tunnel syndrome is a common painful disorder caused by compression of the median nerve as it passes between the bones and ligaments of the wrist. Compression of the nerve causes weakness, pain when gripping and burning, tingling or aching which may radiate to the forearm and shoulder. Symptoms may be occasional or constant, and usually occur most at night. Carpal tunnel syndrome is found most commonly in people who perform repetitive, strenuous work with their hands, e.g. carpenters. It may also follow injuries of the wrist. More frequently, however, there is no history of significant trauma.

Causes

The swelling of the tissues of the wrist which results in the carpal tunnel syndrome may be initiated by a variety of factors, including inflammation, overuse, trauma, swelling, rheumatoid arthritis and, less commonly, several systemic diseases (leukaemia, multiple myeloma, hypothyroidism, acromegaly and sarcoidosis). The symptoms are caused by pressure on the median nerve as it passes through the space formed by the inelastic wrist bones and the transverse carpal ligament (the carpal tunnel). Carpal tunnel syndrome is more common in women, particularly those who are pregnant, taking oral contraceptives or menopausal, and in patients on haemodialysis.[1] All these conditions are associated with an increased need for pyridoxine or pyridoxine deficiency.[2,3] Others at risk are those performing unaccustomed repetitive manual activity.

Therapy

Vitamin B6 deficiency is a common finding in carpal tunnel syndrome. In fact, except when due to direct trauma or systemic disease, Ellis and co-workers have never found an exception to this correlation.[4-6] A person's vitamin B6 status can be determined by measuring the activity of an enzyme in the red blood cells (erythrocyte glutamic oxalo-acetic transaminase, EGOT[4]) or by measuring plasma pyridoxal phosphate levels.[7] Several clinical and double blind studies have conclusively demonstrated that vitamin B6 supplementation (usually 50–100 mg per day) relieves all symptoms of the carpal tunnel syndrome in patients with low levels of vitamin B6.[4-7] Typically, 80 per cent of those with the condition have low B6 levels. Even Phalen (who pioneered the surgical treatment for carpal) agrees that, in the future, pyridoxine (in doses of 100–200 mg per day) may be the treatment of choice.[2] A therapeutic response may require up to three months supplementation.

The increased rate of carpal tunnel syndrome since its initial description by Phalen in 1952[2] parallels the increased levels of vitamin B6 antagonists found in the food supply and drugs during the same period. These antagonists include the hydrazine dyes, drugs (isoniazid, hydralazine, dopamine and penicillamine), oral contraceptives and excessive protein intake.[8] Although no particular diet has been tested for the treatment of carpal tunnel syndrome, it is appropriate to avoid foods containing yellow dyes and to limit protein consumption to 50 grams per day.

Botanical medicines

During the acute inflammatory stage of carpal tunnel syndrome, herbs which limit the inflammatory process may be of assistance. However, since none have been specifically tested for efficacy in this condition, these recommendations have not been substantiated.

Turmeric (Curcuma longa) Turmeric (also known as Indian saffron) has been used in both the Indian (ayurvedic) and Chinese systems of medicine for the treatment of many forms of inflammation. Its efficacy is probably due to its well-documented anti-inflammatory properties and vitamin C content.[9]

The volatile oil fraction of the spice has been demonstrated, in a variety of animal studies, to possess anti-inflammatory activity comparable to the primary medical anti-inflammatory drugs, hydrocortisone and phenylbutazone.[10,11] Even more potent in acute inflammation is the yellow pigment of turmeric, curcumin.[12-14] Curcumin and the alcoholic extract of the curcuma root are used in several indigenous systems of medicine for the treatment of sprains and inflammation. Curcumin is as effective as cortisone or phenylbutazone in models of acute inflammation, but only half as effective in chronic models. While phenylbutazone is associated with significant toxicity (ulcer formation, leucopenia, lymphocytopenia), curcumin displays no significant toxicity.

A potent ancient household remedy for sprains, muscular pain, and inflamed joints is a poultice made from turmeric mixed with slaked lime.[14]

Bromelain   For patients whose carpal tunnel syndrome is due to injury or who don't respond to vitamin B6 (about 20 per cent) and require surgical intervention, the proteolytic enzyme of pineapple (*Ananas comosus*) may be of benefit. Bromelain has well-documented effects in virtually all inflammatory conditions, regardless of etiology.

The effect of orally administered bromelain on the reduction of swelling, bruising, healing time and pain following various injuries and surgical procedures has been demonstrated in several clinical studies.[15-17] For example, Tassman's studies of patients undergoing oral surgery concluded that, while post-surgical medication alone is effective, a regimen of pre- and post-surgical medication is recommended.[15,16] In a double-blind study of patients undergoing oral surgery, bromelain was found to be significantly superior to placebo; swelling decreased in 3.8 days with bromelain, compared with 7 days for the placebo, and the duration of pain was reduced to 5.1 days in the bromelain group, compared with 8.1 in the placebo.[16] Similar observations were made in studies of episiotomy cases. Bromelain reduced oedema, inflammation and pain, and pre-operative administration potentiated the effects.[17,18]

Treatment

As with all diseases, finding and removing the cause is important. However, with carpal tunnel syndrome the cause can be difficult to determine. All known contributing factors, e.g. strenuous repetitive use of the hands, excessive consumption of protein or foods high in yellow dyes, etc., should be controlled.

Supplements

- Pyridoxine, 100–200 mg a day.
- Vitamin B complex, 10 times the recommended dietary allowance per day.

Botanical medicines

- Curcumin (from turmeric), 250 to 500 mg between meals.
- Bromelain, 250 to 500 mg between meals.

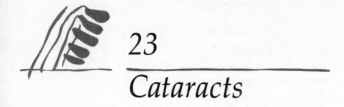

23

Cataracts

- Clouding or opacity in the crystalline lens of the eye.
- Absence of or altered red reflex (small cataracts stand out as dark defects).
- Gradual loss of vision.

General considerations

Cataracts are the leading cause of impaired vision and blindness in the United States[1] – approximately 4 million people have some degree of vision-impairing cataract, and at least 40,000 people in the US are blind due to cataracts.

Cataracts may be classified by location and appearance, by cause or significant contributing factor, and by age of onset.[1] Many factors may cause or contribute to the progression of cataracts, including ocular diseases, injury or surgery, systemic diseases (e.g. diabetes mellitus, galactosaemia), toxin, ultraviolet and near-ultraviolet light or radiation exposure, and hereditary disease.[1] Aging-related (or senile) cataracts are discussed in this chapter and diabetic and galactose-induced cataracts (sugar cataracts) are discussed in Chapter 33, Diabetes.

The crystalline lens is, obviously, a vital component of the optical system due to its ability to focus light (via changes in shape) while maintaining transparency. Unfortunately, this transparency decreases with age. The majority of the elderly population display some degree of cataract formation. In the normal aging eye there is a progressive increase in size, weight and density of the lens throughout life.

Therapy

The origin of cataract formation is ultimately related to an inability to maintain normal concentrations of sodium, potassium and calcium within the lens. These abnormalities are apparently the result of the decreased cellular pump which pumps sodium out and potassium into the cell (the sodium-potassium pump).[2–7] This defect is usually due to free radical damage to some of the sulphur-containing proteins in the lens, including the sodium-potassium pump.

Free radicals

In cataract formation the normal protective mechanisms are unable to prevent free radical damage. Free radicals are highly reactive molecules which can react with and destroy lens proteins. The lens, like many other tissues of the body, is dependent on adequate levels and activities of superoxide dismutase (SOD), catalase and glutathione (GSH), and adequate levels of the accessory antioxidants vitamins E and C and selenium. These compounds all aid in preventing free radical damage, and are discussed individually below.

Antioxidants

Vitamin C   The concentration of vitamin C or ascorbic acid in the aqueous humour of man is 30 to 50 times that of the serum.[2] The vitamin C concentration in the normal lens is second only to that in the adrenal glands,[2,3] while in the lens with a cataract it is absent or greatly reduced.[8] Vitamin C functions primarily as a superoxide free-radical scavenger, thus having a sparing effect on the antioxidant enzyme SOD.[2-4]

Clinical studies have demonstrated that vitamin C does indeed halt cataract progression.[9,10] In one study, 450 patients with cataracts were placed on a nutritional programme that included 1 gram of vitamin C per day, resulting in a significant reduction in cataract development.[9] More recent information indicates that a dose of at least 1,000 milligrams of vitamin C is needed to increase levels in the aqueous humour and lens.

Glutathione   This compound is composed of three amino acids – glycine, glutamic acid and cysteine. Glutathione (GSH) is found at very high concentrations in the lens. GSH plays a vital role in maintaining a healthy lens and has been postulated as a key protective factor against toxins.

Glutathione functions as an antioxidant, maintains reduced sulphur bonds within the lens proteins, acts as a coenzyme of various enzyme systems and participates in amino acid and mineral transport.[2,6] GSH levels are diminished in virtually all forms of cataracts.[2,6,11]

Levels of glutathione can be increased by providing the amino acid precursors (cysteine, glutamine and glycine), which have been shown to be of some benefit in cataract treatment.[2,9] The ancient Chinese herbal formula *hachimijiogan* has been shown to increase glutathione levels in the lens, which may explain its historical use in preventing the progression of cataracts.[12,13]

Selenium and vitamin E   These antioxidants are known to function synergistically and are therefore discussed together. Human lens glutathione peroxidase is selenium-dependent,[2,14] suggesting that a selenium deficiency would greatly promote cataract formation. In fact, the selenium content in human lens with a cataract is only 15 per cent of normal levels.[15] This suggests that a decreased selenium level may be significantly involved in the progression of the cataract. Vitamin E is known to protect against free radical damage.[16]

Superoxide dismutase   The activity of SOD in the human lens is lower than it is in other tissues as a result of the increased ascorbate and glutathione levels.[2,4,5] A progressive decrease in SOD is encountered in cataract progression. Oral supplementation is probably of little value, as it has been demonstrated that orally administered SOD does not affect tissue SOD activity.[14] It is also significant that the trace mineral cofactors of SOD are greatly reduced in the cataractous lens (copper over 90 per cent, manganese 50 per cent and zinc over 90 per cent).[15]

Catalase   Catalase is concentrated in the front portion of the lens (anterior surface), with very low levels found in the rest of the lens.[2] Its primary function is to reduce hydrogen peroxide to water and oxygen.

Hachimijiogan   As mentioned earlier, this ancient Chinese herbal formula has been shown to increase the glutathione content of the lens.[12] It has long been used in the clinical treatment of cataracts in both China and Japan. Its therapeutic effect is quite impressive in the early stages of cataract formation. Fujihira's clinical study displayed improvement in 60 per cent of the subjects on *Hachimijiogan*, while 20 per cent of the group showed no progression and only 20 per cent of the group displayed progression of the cataract.[13] *Hachimijiogan* appears to have both protective and therapeutic effects on senile cataracts.

Other nutritional factors

Riboflavin   Deficiency of riboflavin is believed to enhance cataract formation.[11,17] While riboflavin deficiency is fairly common in the geriatric population (33 per cent), original studies demonstrating an association between riboflavin deficiency and cataract formation were followed by studies demonstrating no association.[11,17] Although correction of the deficiency is warranted, more than 10 mg per day of riboflavin should not be used in individuals with cataracts since riboflavin is a photosensitising substance, i.e. superoxide radicals are generated by the interaction of light, oxygen and riboflavin. Riboflavin and light have been used experimentally to induce cataracts.[3,4] The evidence appears to suggest that excess riboflavin does more harm than good in the cataract patient.

Amino acids   Methionine is a component of the lenticular antioxidant enzyme methionine sulphoxide reductase and a precursor of cysteine, a component of GSH.[2,7] Cysteine, along with the other amino acid precursors of GSH, has been shown to be of some aid in cataract treatment.[2,18]

Zinc, vitamin A and beta-carotenes   These nutrients are known antioxidants and vital for normal lens function and integrity. In addition, beta-carotene may act as a filter, protecting against light-induced damage to the fibre portion of the lens.[19]

Dairy products   Cataracts often develop in infants with a homozygous deficiency of either galactokinase or galactose-1-phosphate uridyl transferase and in laboratory animals fed a high galactose diet. Abnormalities of galactose metabolism can be identified by measurements of the activity of these enzymes in red blood cells. It has been suggested that this is an important mechanism in approximately 30 per cent of cataract patients.[17] However, this mechanism of cataract formation appears only significant in diabetic cataract formation and is probably not relevant to senile cataract formation (for further discussion see Chapter 33, Diabetes).

Heavy metals   A number of heavy metals have been shown to have increased concentrations in both the aging lens and the lenses with cataracts. Although the levels are higher in the latter, the significance of this is unknown.[15]

The cadmium concentration in the lens with a cataract is two to three times higher than in the normal lens. Since cadmium displaces zinc from binding in enzymatic proteins, it may contribute to deactivation of antioxidant enzymes and other protective/repair mechanisms. Other elevated elements of unknown significance include bromine, cobalt, iridium and nickel.[15]

Drugs and surgery   In cases of severe vision impairment, cataract removal and a lens implant may be the only alternative. Recently a Japanese drug, phenoxazine carboxylic acid, has been shown to be effective in inhibiting, as well as reversing, cataract formation.[2,20,21]

Treatment

As with most diseases, prevention or treatment at an early stage is most effective. Since free radical damage appears to be the primary factor in senile cataracts, individuals with cataracts should avoid direct sunlight, bright light, and wear protective lenses (sunglasses) when outdoors. They should also greatly increase their intake of antioxidant nutrients.

Progression of the disease can be stopped and early cataracts can be reversed. However, significant reversal of well-developed cataracts does not appear possible at this time.

Diet

Avoid rancid foods and other sources of free radicals. Increase consumption of legumes (high in sulphur-containing amino acids), yellow vegetables (carotenes) and vitamin E and C rich foods (fresh fruits and vegetables).

Supplements

- Vitamin C, 1 g three times a day.
- Vitamin E, 600 to 800 iu a day.
- Selenium, 400 µg a day.
- Beta-carotene, 200,000 iu a day.
- L-cysteine, 400 mg a day.
- L-glutamine, 200 mg a day.
- L-glycine, 200 mg a day.

Botanical medicine

Hachimijiogan contains the following eight herbs per 22 grams: alismatis rhizome (3 g), rehmanniae root (6 g), cornus fruit (3 g), dioscoreae rhizome (3 g), hoelen (3 g), mountain bark (2.5 g), cinnamon bark (1 g) and aconite root (0.5 g). The standard dose is 150–300 mg per day.

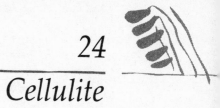

24
Cellulite

- Demonstration of the 'mattress phenomenon', i.e. pitting, bulging and deformation of the skin.
- Ninety to ninety-eight per cent of cases occur in women.
- Symptoms may include feeling of tightness and heaviness in areas affected (particularly the legs).
- Tenderness of the skin is quite apparent when the skin is pinched, pressed upon or vigorously massaged.

General considerations

The term cellulite is used to describe a cosmetic defect that is the cause of great distress for millions of European and American women. This French word was adopted by the lay public in the United States before American physicians and medical literature were educated in a condition that European physicians had been dealing with for over 150 years.[1]

The correct English translation of the French word *cellulite* would be cellulitis. However, in English, cellulitis is used solely to describe an inflammatory or infectious process involving the connective tissue of the skin. In cellulite there is no inflammatory or infectious process occurring. This difference in meaning in the translated term was just one source of confusion for American physicians. Researchers have suggested that the terms dermo-panniculosis deformans or adiposis oedematosa be used to designate the clinical condition.[2] In this chapter, however, the term cellulite will be used.

Structural features of cellulite

The subcutaneous tissue is the tissue just below the surface of the skin that binds the skin loosely to underlying tissue or bones. The subcutaneous tissue contains fat cells which vary in size and number from individual to individual, and it is this subcutaneous tissue that is disturbed in cellulite. Since the thighs are the prime area of involvement in cellulite, the structure of the subcutaneous tissue of the thighs will be discussed in greatest detail.

The subcutaneous tissue of the thighs is composed of three layers of fat, with two planes of connective tissue (ground substance) between them. The basic construction of the subcutaneous tissue of the thigh differs in men and women, as shown in Figure 24.1. In women, the uppermost subcutaneous layer consists of what are termed large standing fat-cell chambers, which are separated by radial and arching dividing walls of connective tissue anchored to the overlying connective tissue of the skin (corium or dermis). In contrast, the uppermost part of the subcutaneous tissue of men is thinner and has a network of crisscrossing connective tissue walls. In addition, the corium (the connective tissue structure between the skin and subcutaneous tissue) is thicker in men than in women.[1,2]

These basic differences in subcutaneous tissue structure are the reason cellulite is seen almost exclusively in women. A simple test to illustrate these differences is the pinch test. Pinching the skin and subcutaneous tissue of the thighs of women will result in the 'mattress phenomenon', i.e. pitting, bulging and deformation of the skin, while in most men the skin will fold or furrow, but will not bulge or pit. These structural differences between men and women are responsible for most women producing the mattress phenomenon in response to the pinch test.[1,2]

As women age, the corium, which is already thinner in women than in men, becomes progressively thinner and looser.[3] This allows fat cells to migrate into this layer. In addition, the connective tissue walls between the fat-cell chambers also become thinner, allowing the fat-cell chambers to enlarge excessively (hypertrophy).

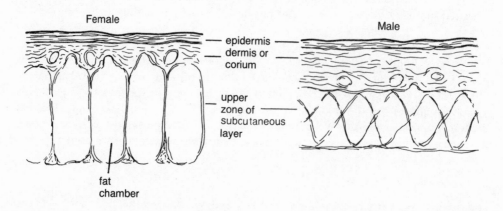

Figure 24.1   Anatomical basis of cellulite

The breaking down or thinning of connective tissue structures is a major contributor to the development of cellulite and is responsible for the granular 'buckshot' feel of cellulite.[1,2]

The mattress phenomenon is brought about by alternating depressions and protrusions in the upper compartment systems of fat tissue. The vertical orientation of women's fat cell compartments, in conjunction with the weakening of the tissues noted above, is apparently what allows the protrusion of the fat cells into the lower corium.[2] The anatomical differences between men and women are summarised in Table 24.1.

Histological examination (microscopic examination of the cells) also reveals distension of the lymphatic vessels of the upper corium and a decrease in the number of important elastic fibres.

Clinical features

The basic clinical features of cellulite are well known and described above as the mattress phenomenon. Women comprise 90–98 per cent of the cases, reflecting histological differences between men and women. Symptoms of cellulite include feeling of tightness and heaviness in areas affected (particularly the legs) and tenderness of the skin is quite apparent when the skin is pinched, pressed or vigorously massaged.[1,2] The areas of the body involved are typically the buttocks, thighs and, to a lesser extent, the lower part of the abdomen, the nape of the neck and the upper parts of the arms. These are the areas of the body usually affected in gynecoid (female) obesity.

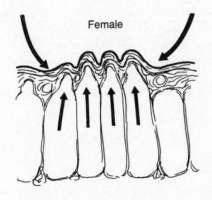
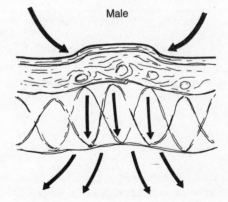

Figure 24.2   The Pinch Test

Table 24.1 Sex-typical differences of the skin of the lateral thighs of men and women (16–50 years old)[2]

Cutis and subcutis	Of men	Of women
Epidermis	Thicker (58–77 μm)	Thinner (47–62 μm)
Corium/dermis	Thicker (1,159–1,798 μm)	Thinner (994–1,349 μm)
Border zone of corium and subcutis	Fewer papillae adiposae	More papillae adiposae
Subcutis	Variably thinner	Variably thicker
Upper zone	Small polygonal fat-cells, criss-crossing septa of connective tissue	Large, standing fat-cells with chambers with radially running septa of connective tissue
Status protrusis cutis (so-called mattress phenomenon)	Does not develop	Develops

Cellulite is classified in four major stages:

- Stage 0 is the stage in which the skin on the thighs and buttocks has a smooth surface when the subject is standing or lying. When the skin is pinched (pinch test) it folds and furrows but does not pit or bulge. This stage is the normal stage of most men and slim women.
- Stage 1 is the stage in which the skin surface is smooth while a subject is standing or lying, but the pinch test is clearly positive for the mattress phenomenon (pitting, bulging and deformity of the affected skin surfaces). This is normal for most females, but in a male may be a sign of deficiency of androgenic hormones.
- Stage 2 is the stage in which the skin surface is smooth while a subject is lying, but when standing there is pitting, bulging and deformity of the affected skin surfaces. This stage is common in women who are obese or past 35–40 years of age.
- Stage 3 is the stage in which the mattress phenomenon is apparent when a subject is lying or standing. It is very common after menopause and in obesity.

Although most women consider stage 0 the cosmetic ideal, stage 1 is the best classification most can expect, due to structural predisposition.

Therapy

As usual, the best approach is prevention. However, since the number and size of fat cells an individual has are largely determined by maternal prenatal nutrition, many people have a significant predisposition. The next step is maintaining a slim subcutaneous fat layer. This is best done by exercising and maintaining a normal body weight throughout life – slim women and female athletes have little or no cellulite.[1,2]

Weight reduction and exercise

Weight reduction and exercise can be employed in the treatment of cellulite: indeed they should always be the primary method of treatment. However, weight reduction should be gradual, especially in women over the age of 40. A rapid loss of weight in individuals whose skin and connective tissues are already undergoing changes from aging will often make the mattress phenomenon more apparent.

Massage

Massage is very beneficial, particularly self administered massage with the hand or brush. The physical and mechanical effects of massage improve circulation of blood and lymph. The direction of the massage should always be from the periphery to the heart.

Botanical medicines

There are many cosmetic formulas and herbal preparations on the market that claim to be effective in 'curing' cellulite. However, the majority of these formulas have no scientific basis to support their use. In addition, long-term double-blind studies of some of the more popular cellulite treatments demonstrates them to be no more effective than placebos.[3,4] However, several botanical compounds do have confirmed effects in the treatment of cellulite.

The comprehensive herbal treatment of cellulite involves both the oral and topical administration of botanical medicines which enhance connective tissue structures. As stated earlier, the breaking down or thinning of connective tissue structures is a major contributor to the development of cellulite.

Centella asiatica An extract of centella containing the triterpenic acids asiatic acid and asiatoside has demonstrated impressive clinical results when given orally in the treatment of cellulite, venous insufficiency of the lower limbs and varicose veins.[5–9]

Several experimental studies have demonstrated that centella exerts a normalising action on the metabolism of connective tissue. Specifically, it enhances connective tissue integrity by stimulating glycosaminoglycan synthesis without promoting excessive collagen synthesis or cell growth.[5] Glycosaminoglycans are the major components of the ground substance in which collagen fibres are embedded. The net outcome is the development of normal connective tissue that is rich in glycosaminoglycans.

The effect of centella in the treatment of cellulite appears to be related to its ability to enhance connective tissue structure and reduce sclerosis, while its action in venous insufficiency and varicose veins is a combination of its connective tissue effects and its ability to improve the blood flow through the affected limbs.

Aescin Aescin is a compound isolated from the seeds of the *Aesculus hippocastanum* (horse-chestnut). It has anti-inflammatory and anti-oedema properties, and it decreases capillary permeability by reducing the number and size of the small pores of the capillary walls.[10–12] Investigators have also demonstrated that aescin has venotonic activity.[13] This has been confirmed in clinical trials that demonstrate a positive effect in the treatment of varicose veins and thrombophlebitis.[11,14]

In the treatment of cellulite, aescin can be given orally, or an aescin/cholesterol complex can be applied topically. The topical application of aescin is also of benefit in the treatment of bruises, due to aescin's ability to decrease capillary fragility and swelling.

*Bladderwrack (*Fucus vesiculosus*)* *Fucus vesiculosus* is a seaweed that has been used in the treatment of obesity since the 17th century. Its high iodine content is thought to stimulate thyroid function. Bladderwrack has also been used in toiletries and cosmetics for its soothing, softening and toning effects.[15]

Another major topical application of bladderwrack has been in the treatment of cellulite. Its effects in this application have not been confirmed by careful scientific investigation, but bladderwrack's general actions may be of benefit.

Cola species Cola is a very rich source of caffeine and related compounds. These compounds potentiate the effect of catecholamine-induced lipolysis. Topical administration of caffeine is preferable to oral administration in the treatment of cellulite, since its effects will be primarily local.

Treatment

It must be kept in mind that cellulite is not a disease *per se*. Instead, it is primarily a cosmetic disorder due to anatomical changes. Excessive subcutaneous adipose tissue or degeneration of subcutaneous connective tissue leads to fat chamber enlargement and greater visibility of the mattress phenomenon. The basic therapeutic approach is straightforward, i.e. reduce subcutaneous fat and enhance connective tissue integrity.

Varicose veins are often found in conjunction with cellulite, and the two conditions share much in common. In particular, both appear to result largely from a loss of integrity of supporting connective tissue (see Chapter 73, Varicose veins, for further discussion).

It must be stated again that demonstration of the mattress phenomenon in men is a highly probable sign of androgen (male hormones) deficiency.[1]

Diet

A diet high in complex carbohydrates and low in refined carbohydrates and fats is very important. Weight loss should be promoted in obese individuals.

Physical measures

- Exercise – 20–30 minutes of aerobic exercise, a minimum of five days per week
- Massage – regular self massage of the affected area with hand or brush.

Botanical medicines

- Oral administration of *Centella asiatica* extract (70 per cent triterpenic acid content), 30 mg three times a day.
- *Aesculus hippocastanum*
    Bark of root, 500 mg three times a day.
    Aescin, 10 mg three times a day.
- Topical application of salves, ointment, etc., two times a day:
    Cholesterol aescin complex, 0.5–1.5 per cent.
    Cola vera extract (14 per cent caffeine), 0.5–1.5 per cent.
    Fucus vesiculosis, 0.25–0.75 per cent.

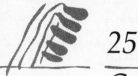

25

Cervical dysplasia

- Cervical dysplasia is usually diagnosed upon gynaecological examination through inspection and the Pap smear. It is confirmed by the finding of dysplasic cells on biopsy of the lesion.

General considerations

Cervical dysplasia is an abnormal condition of the cells of the cervix. It is generally regarded as a precancerous lesion, and has risk factors similar to those of cervical cancer.[1] There are several lifestyle and nutritional factors that appear to play a prominent role in the development of cervical dysplasia and cervical carcinoma. These include early age of first intercourse, multiple sexual partners, *Herpes simplex* type-II and papilloma viruses, lower socioeconomic class, smoking, oral contraceptive use and many nutritional factors.[1,2] All risk factors appear to be closely related, as is common in other multifactorial diseases.

Although the death rate due to invasive cervical cancer has dropped remarkably since the early 1950s (due primarily to improved screening via the Pap smear), cervical cancer still accounts for approximately 7,500 deaths per year in the United States.[1] Approximately 16,000 cases of invasive cervical cancer and 45,000 cases of cervical carcinoma *in situ* occur annually in the United States.[1,2] The peak incidence of invasive lesions occurs at age 45, while *in situ* lesions peak at around age 30. In contrast to invasive carcinoma, the incidence of carcinoma *in situ* is increasing dramatically, probably as a result of the increase in risk factors (e.g. early age at first intercourse, multiple sexual partners, oral contraceptive use and cigarette smoking).

Risk factors

Sexual activity Early age at first intercourse and/or multiple sexual partners are associated with an increased risk of cervical dysplasia/carcinoma.[1,2] From this and other evidence it has been suggested that cervical cancer is in some respects a venereal disease, since the implicated infectious agents appear to be sexually transmitted. Furthermore, some of the substances released by sperm while it breaks down in the vagina could be mild stimulants of cancerous-type changes in the cervical cells.[2]

Viruses   Two classes of virus are currently suspected of playing a causative role in cervical cancer, *Herpes simplex* type II and the human papilloma (wart) virus. The possible relationship with herpes infection has been demonstrated in many studies, using a variety of methods:

- in one study, 23 per cent of women with herpes infection had cervical dysplasia or cancer, compared with 2.6 per cent of those without infection;
- herpes antibody levels are significantly higher in women with cervical cancer or dysplasia than in controls; and
- women with herpetic cervicitis have a 4- to 16-fold increased risk of cervical cancer and dysplasia.

The human papilloma virus is the etiological agent in venereal warts, and has been detected by various techniques in the cervix of patients with cervical dysplasia.

Although these agents have been shown to be related to cervical dysplasia, it has not been determined whether they reflect decreased resistance or are themselves the causative agents.[1,2]

Smoking   A major risk factor for cervical cancer and/or cervical dysplasia is cigarette smoking: smokers have a two- to three-fold increased incidence compared with non-smokers (one study[3] found the increase to be as high as 17-fold in women aged 20–9).[3–6]

Many hypotheses have been proposed to explain this association:

- smoking may depress immune functions, allowing a sexually transmitted agent to promote abnormal cellular development, leading to the onset of cervical dysplasia;
- smoking is known to cause a vitamin C deficiency, as vitamin C levels are significantly depressed in smokers[7];
- vaginal or uterine cells may concentrate carcinogenic compounds from inhaled smoke; and
- unrecognised associations between smoking and sexual behaviour.[3–6]

Oral contraceptives   The long-term use of oral contraceptives is associated with an increased risk of cancer of the cervix.[6–10] Oral contraceptives are known to potentiate the adverse effects of cigarette smoking and to decrease the levels of numerous nutrients, including vitamins C, B6 and B12, folic acid, riboflavin and zinc.[11]

Therapy

Many nutritional factors have been found to be possibly involved in the development of cervical dysplasia.[14] Many single nutrients may play a significant role (particularly beta-carotene and other retinoids, folic acid, pyridoxine and vitamin C). Significant abnormalities have also been found to be indicators of dietary imbalances, such as height-to-weight ratios, skin-fold thickness, mid-arm muscle circumference, serum

Table 25.1 Risk factors in cervical dysplasia cancer*

Risk factor	Relative risk
Smoking (10+ cigarettes a day)	3.0[6]
Multiple sexual partners (2–5)	3.4[6]
Age at first intercourse (< 18)	2.7[6]
Oral contraceptive use (5–8 years)	3.6[6]
Deficient dietary beta-carotene (< 5,000 iu a day)	2.8[12]
Deficient dietary vitamin C (<30 mg a day)	6.7[13]

*The actual values for the risk of the various risk factors are as yet somewhat unclear. The numbers listed here are summarised from the literature. These risks are not necessarily additive, since they are usually closely related, and more involved multivariant analysis is necessary to determine the actual relative risk of each.

protein levels, haemoglobin levels, blood clotting time and white cell count. Many other patients have marginal but 'normal' nutritional status.[15] These suggest that multiple nutrient deficiencies are probably the rule rather than the exception.

Vitamin assessment by blood tests in patients with untreated cervical cancer shows that at least one abnormal vitamin level was present in 67 per cent of patients, while 38 per cent had abnormal vitamin levels.[16] If mineral levels are also included, it is clear that nutrition plays a major role in the onset of cervical dysplasia/carcinoma.

General dietary factors are also important. A high-fat intake has been associated with increased risk for cervical cancer, while a diet rich in fruits and vegetables is believed to offer significant protection against cancer, probably due to the higher intake of fibre, beta-carotenes and vitamin C.[5]

Vitamin A and beta-carotene   There appears to be a strong relationship between low beta-carotene intake and the risk of cervical cancer/dysplasia.[12,17,18] While only 6 per cent of patients with untreated cervical cancer have below-normal serum vitamin A levels, 38 per cent have abnormal blood levels of beta-carotene in proportion to the seriousness of their cervical disease.[16] Low serum beta-carotene levels are associated with a three-fold greater risk for severe dysplasia,[18] and serum vitamin A levels in patients with cervical dysplasia are half those found in a control group.[19]

Vitamin C   There is a significant decrease in vitamin C intake and plasma levels in patients with cervical dysplasia, and it has been documented that inadequate vitamin C intake is an independent risk factor for the development of cervical dysplasia and carcinoma *in situ*.[13,20]

Folic acid   Although macrocytic anaemia is the most commonly recognised sign of folic acid deficiency, abnormalities in the cervical cells are seen many weeks earlier.[21,22] As folic acid is the most common vitamin deficiency in the world, and quite common in women who are pregnant or taking oral contraceptives,[11,23] it is probable that many abnormal Pap smears reflect folate deficiency rather than true dysplasia.[21,22,24,25] This is particularly true in women taking oral contraceptives.

It has been hypothesised that oral contraceptives interfere with folate metabolism and, although serum levels may be increased, tissue levels of the cervix may be deficient.[24,25] This is consistent with the observation that tissue status, as measured by red blood cell folate levels, is typically decreased (especially in women with cervical dysplasia), while serum levels may be normal or even increased.[25] Oral contraceptives are believed to stimulate the synthesis of a molecule that inhibits folate uptake by cells.

Folic acid supplementation (10 mg per day) has resulted in improvement or normal-isation of Pap smears in patients with cervical dysplasia in placebo-controlled[25] and clinical studies.[24] The rate of normalisation for women with untreated cervical dysplasia is typically 1.3 per cent for mild and 0 per cent for moderate dysplasia. When treated with folic acid, the regression-to-normal rate was observed to be 20 per cent in one study and 100 per cent in another.[24] Furthermore, the progression rate of cervical dysplasia in untreated patients is typically 16 per cent at four months, a figure matched in the placebo group in one study, while none of the folate-supplemented group progressed.[25] All these figures were observed despite the fact that the women remained on the birth control pills.

Since the average time for progression from cervical dysplasia to carcinoma *in situ* in untreated women ranges from 86 months for patients with very mild dysplasia, to 12 months for patients with severe dysplasia, and improvement is very uncommon, it is suggested that a trial of folate supplementation (along with other considerations discussed) be instituted in mild-to-moderate dysplasia, with a follow-up Pap smear and colposcopy at three months. Vitamin B12 supplementation should always accompany folate supplementation.

Pyridoxine Vitamin B6 status, as determined by a red blood cell enzyme test, is decreased in one-third of women with cervical cancer.[26] Decreased pyridoxine status would have a significant effect on the metabolism of oestrogens and tryptophan, as well as impairing immune response.

Selenium Low serum, dietary and soil selenium levels have been found with all skin and mucous membrane cancers,[14] and in patients with cervical dysplasia.[19] Increased glutathione peroxidase activity resulting from increased selenium intake is believed to be responsible for selenium's anti-carcinogenic effect, although other factors may be of equal significance. Many toxic elements, such as lead, cadmium, mercury and gold, antagonise selenium.[14] The role these heavy metals may play in cervical disease has not been determined.

Treatment

For women with a class IV Pap, proper treatment of cervical dysplasia involves first determining if carcinoma *in situ* is present, and usually requires surgical treatment. Since this can be determined only through biopsy, consultation with a gynaecologist is necessary. A woman with recurrent class III Paps should also be biopsied if she has had recurrent abnormal Paps, has significant risk factors or has been unresponsive to therapy. Patients with carcinoma *in situ* or a class V Pap should undergo a cone biopsy.

The basic approach is to eliminate all factors known to be associated with cervical dysplasia and to optimise one's nutritional status, in particular, eliminate smoking and oral contraceptive use and supplement with folic acid, beta-carotenes and vitamin C. For most women, the vaginal depletion pack will accelerate the rate of normalisation of the cervix. For those who undergo a cone biopsy, treatment is still necessary since the causes of cervical dysplasia are not treated by this approach. Pap smears should be repeated every one to three months, according to severity.

Diet

Animal product consumption should be decreased, particularly animal fats and foods contaminated with oestrogens. High-fibre foods are also useful.

Supplements

- Folic acid, 2 mg a day for three months, then 0.5 mg a day.
- Pyridoxine, 50 mg three times a day.
- Vitamin B12, 1 mg four times a day.
- Beta-carotene, 200,000 iu a day.
- Vitamin C, 1 g a day.
- Vitamin E, 200 iu four times a day.
- Selenium, 400 μg a day.
- Zinc (picolinate), 30 mg a day.

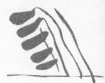

26

Chronic fatigue syndrome¹

- Chronic fatigue.
- Recurrent sore throats.
- Low-grade fever.
- Lymph node swelling.
- Headache.
- Muscle and joint pain.
- Intestinal discomfort.
- Emotional distress, and/or depression.
- Loss of concentration.

General considerations

Chronic fatigue syndrome (also called myalgic encephalomyelitis [ME] chronic mononucleosis-like syndrome or chronic EBV syndrome) is a newly established syndrome that describes varying combinations of symptoms including recurrent sore throats, low grade fever, lymph node swelling, headache, muscle and joint pain, intestinal discomfort, emotional distress and/or depression and loss of concentration. The cause is not known although some believe it to be due to a chronic infection with Epstein-Barr virus (EBV).[2-6] The syndrome may persist for months to years, and its occurrence appears to be increasing.

Chronic Epstein-Barr virus infection

EBV is a member of the herpes group of viruses, which includes *Herpes simplex* types 1 and 2, *Varicella zoster* virus, cytomegalovirus and pseudorabies virus. A common aspect of these viruses is their ability to establish a lifelong latent infection after the initial infection. This latent infection is kept in check by a normal immune system, but when the immune system is compromised in any way, these viruses can become active as viral replication and spread is increased. This is commonly observed with herpes virus infections in AIDS, cancer and drug-induced immunodeficient patients.

Infection with EBV is inevitable among humans. By the end of early adulthood almost all individuals demonstrate detectable antibodies in their blood to the Epstein-Barr virus, indicating past infection. When the primary infection occurs in childhood there are usually no symptoms, but when it occurs in adolescence or early adulthood the clinical manifestations of infectious mononucleosis develop in approximately 50 per cent of the cases.[7]

Although reports of a prolonged or recurrent mononucleosis-like syndrome began appearing in the 1940s and 1950s, the chronic mononucleosis-like syndrome/chronic fatigue syndrome is not yet a clearly defined syndrome within the medical literature.[8-10] It has been only since the mid-1980s that evidence has implicated EBV in this broad clinical spectrum of chronic fatigue and associated symptoms.[2-6] Several studies have demonstrated persistently elevated levels of serum antibodies against the Epstein-Barr virus in a number of patients presenting with the symptom pattern of this syndrome.[2-5].

A careful study of 134 patients who had undergone EBV antibody testing because of suspected chronic mononucleosis-like syndrome found mixed results about the importance of EBV infection. Fifteen patients identified as having severe, persistent fatigue of unknown origin were compared with the remaining 119 with less severe illness and with 30 age- and race-matched controls.[11] The more seriously ill patients generally had higher levels of EBV antibodies than did the comparison groups and, interestingly, they also demonstrated higher antibody levels to cytomegalovirus, *Herpes simplex* viruses types 1 and 2 and measles. This led the researchers to conclude that 'some patients with these illnesses [syndromes of chronic fatigue] may have an abnormality of infectious and/or immunologic origin', and that there remained 'questions concerning the relationship between the chronic fatigue syndromes and EBV'.

Current (1988) knowledge about EBV infection can be summarised:

- EBV and the herpes group of viruses produce latent lifelong infections.
- The host's immune system normally holds the latent infection in check.[12-14]
- Any compromise in the immune system, especially the cellular components, can lead to the reactivation of the virus and recurrent infection.[15,16]
- The infection itself can compromise and/or disrupt immunity, thereby leading to other diseases.[7,15-21]
- Elevated EBV antibody levels are observed in a significant number of diseases characterised by immunological dysfunction.[22]
- Elevated antibody levels to the herpes group viruses and measles have been observed in patients suspected of having a chronic fatigue or mononucleosis-like syndrome who also display elevated EBV antibody levels.[11]

Cytomegalovirus

Cytomegalovirus infection can produce a clinical picture almost identical to an EBV-associated infection. An enlarged spleen, liver involvement and abnormal lymphocytes are also common features of this viral infection. However, it usually involves an older age group, around 20–30 years old, and generally does not include sore throat and enlargement of the throat lymph nodes.[7]

Susceptibility

The importance of susceptibility is too often overlooked in the disease/infection orientation which continues to dominate conventional medicine. This is not meant to deny the value of this approach; over the short term it saves many lives and reduces much suffering. However, in many instances the symptoms recur and the agent reinfects, because this approach does not change the host's susceptibility and primarily results in relief of acute symptoms, which are not always synonymous with cure.

Support and enhancement of immune system function is perhaps the most important and vital step in achieving host resistance, reducing susceptibility and, hence, achieving any degree of cure. The chronic fatigue syndrome appears to be indicative of a chronically disturbed or compromised immune system (whether or not it is due to an EBV infection or other factors) and the symptoms are manifested on all levels, from psycho-emotional to physiological/biochemical.

Candidiasis An important consideration in determining susceptibility is the role played by *Candida albicans*. Candida species are common inhabitants of the intestinal tract, where their growth is kept in check by other bowel bacteria and normal immune function. When this balance is disturbed (as it is by the administration of antibiotic drugs or by immune suppression from steroids, chemotherapy, CMV or EBV infection, AIDS and other diseases) the candida can proliferate. These organisms produce antigenic products and byproducts which cause a constant challenge to the immune system (see Chapter 21, Candidiasis, for complete discussion).

Conditions causing elevation of Epstein-Barr virus antibodies[22]

- AIDS
- AIDS-related complex
- Ankylosing spondylitis
- Cancer chemotherapy
- Chronic kidney failure
- Endemic Burkitt's lymphoma
- Hodgkin's disease
- Kidney transplantation
- Leukaemias
- Nasopharyngeal carcinoma
- Multiple sclerosis
- Non-Hodgkin's lymphoma
- Non-lymphomatous malignant tumours
- Primary immunodeficiency states (e.g. ataxia telangiectasia)
- Rheumatoid arthritis
- Secondary immunodeficiency states (e.g. steroid therapy, antithymocyte globulin therapy)
- Systemic lupus erythematosus

Table 26.1 Clinical findings of chronic mononucleusis-like syndrome[8]

Findings	% of patients
History	
Chief complaint is the fatigue syndrome	30
Severity of the fatigue at its worst	
Bedridden, can do virtually nothing	28
Shut in, cannot do even light housework or its equivalent	13
Can do all the things usually do at home or work, but feel much more easily fatigued from it, no energy left for anything else	60
Description of the frequency of the fatique	
Consistent fatigue that does not change	15
Always some fatigue that may get better but never goes away completely	23
The fatigue alternates with feeling normal	63
Associated recurrent pharyngitis	60
Associated recurrent muscle aches	80
Severity of muscle aches at their worst (N=31)	
Need to stop all normal activities and rest	39
Can continue normal activities but muscle aches make it hard	23
Not aware of muscle aches during normal activities, only at rest	39
Associated recurrent headaches	83
Severity of headaches at their worst (N=33)	
Need to stop all normal activities and rest	55
Can continue normal activities but headaches make it hard	33
Not aware of headaches during normal activities, only at rest	12
Fatigue plus sore throat, plus myalgias, plus headaches	45
Associated symptoms	
Depression or unusual mood changes	78
Difficulty in sleeping	73
Difficulty in concentrating	65
Anxiety	60
Nausea	55
Swollen lymph glands (N=39)	44
Stomach ache	40
Diarrhoea	38
Cough	38
Rash	35
Odd sensations in skin	33
Loss of appetite	30
Joint pain	30
Vomiting	25
Recurrent fevers at home	25
Intermittent swelling of fingers (N= 30)	20
Weight loss	15
Weight gain	5
Have seen a physician for this problem before	55
Have seen more than one physician for this problem	25
The problem has caused problems or stress at home and at work	60
Patient has sometimes thought these symptoms 'might just all be in my head'	58
Past history	
Mononucleosis (N=39)	26

Oral herpes	38
Genital herpes	0
Herpes zoster (shingles)	0
Allergies (to food or drugs, or hay fever)	53
Physical examination	
Tonsillar/pharyngeal exudate	0
Cervical adenopathy (enlarged or tender)	
Anterior	15
Posterior	3
Submandibular gland enlarged or tender (*N*=38)	13
Hepatomegaly or splenomegaly	0
Temperature > 37.5 °C	0

This table is of findings in 40 patients, aged 17–50, with symptoms suggestive of chronic mononucleosis-like syndrome and without any known chronic disease.

Depressed immune system in chronic fatigue syndrome

The information given in the preceding test supports the hypothesis that the chronic fatigue syndrome is indicative of a chronically disturbed or depressed immune system, resulting in decreased host resistance and low vital energy. This information also suggests that EBV antibody testing (and antibody testing for other herpes group viruses and measles) may be useful as a measure of immunological function and overall host resistance. Elevated antibody levels may precede by months or years (especially if chronically elevated) the onset of a more serious immunological disease such as those listed in the box on page 211.

Diagnosis

Since the cause(s), as well as the exact characteristics, of the chronic fatigue syndrome are still unclear, diagnosis is difficult and often made by the exclusion of other diseases. At this time, the diagnosis is probably best made according to the symptom pattern, as shown in Table 26.1. The presence of elevated antibodies to the Epstein-Barr virus (see below) is probably the best way to confirm the diagnosis.

Elevated levels of antibodies to EBV, suggestive of chronic mononucleosis or recurrent EBV infection, have also been found in a number of other conditions (listed in the box on page 211), most of which are related to immunologically stressed and/or immuno-compromised conditions, including some 'healthy' people.[7,15,16,18–25] The relationship of elevated EBV antibodies to these diseases raised questions about the involvement of EBV in their development. It is unknown whether EBV is a causative agent creating depressed immunity, or whether its reactivation is a manifestation of a previously existing malfunctioning immune system.

Diagnosis of chronic EBV infection   In acute Epstein-Barr virus infection (i.e. infectious mononucleosis), several antibodies become detectable in the blood. They normally decrease to low levels after several months. However, when the levels of an antibody designated anti-EA(R) rise above the normal range, recurrent or reactivated EBV infection is likely.[2,22,26]

Therapy

The treatment of chronic fatigue syndrome involves a comprehensive host-centred approach. Every attempt should be made to enhance resistance by optimising overall health and immunity, thereby significantly reducing susceptibility to reactivation of the Epstein-Barr or other virus.

The approach outlined below focuses on three basic processes – detoxification, supportive therapy and stimulation of host defence mechanisms.

Detoxification

The first therapeutic intervention in potentiating the immune system and optimising overall health is based on Hahnemann's principle of 'first and foremost, remove all obstacles to cure'[27] or, as stated by naturopathic pioneer Benedict Lust, 'eliminate the poisonous products in the system, and so raise the vitality of the patient'.[28] Reduction and/or elimination of those factors (i.e. toxins) deleterious to proper immune function and health is important. This approach entails reducing exposure to external toxins (e.g. chemicals, drugs, dietary toxins, food allergies, etc.) and detoxification and elimination of internal toxins (e.g. toxins from the bowel, *Candida albicans* and other pathogens, free radicals, heavy metals, etc.).

A good detoxification programme should include stimulating the eliminative organs (bowel, liver and biliary tract, kidneys, lymph and reticuloendothelial systems, lungs and skin) in a functional, supportive and regenerative manner. Detoxification of the liver and lymphatic system is of primary importance when a possible EBV-related condition is suspected. This is due to the fact that most of the manifestations and complications of such conditions (lymph gland swelling, enlargement of the spleen and liver, hepatitis, jaundice and Burkitt's lymphoma) involve these tissues.[7,17] Therefore, protection from inflammatory damage and supporting and stimulating normal function, flow and elimination is of utmost importance, especially when any of these complications or manifestations are present.

Enhancing liver function Stimulating bile production and bile flow are the traditional routes to liver detoxification. Other aspects include protection of liver cells from inflammatory and free radical damage, stimulation and support of liver cell regeneration, and stimulation of the liver macrophages (Kupffer cells). Table 26.2 summarises the methods of liver detoxification.

Spleen and lymphatic system Enhancement of lymphatic flow, blood flow to the spleen and lymphatic tissue and lymphocyte activity are used when detoxifying these tissues.

Table 26.2 Liver detoxification

Action	Agent
Lipotropic	Methionine[29-35]
Bile production and flow stimulation	Carnitine[29,36-8]
	Cheledonium majus[39]
	Chionanthus virginicus[39]
	Curcuma longa[29,40]
	Cynara scolymus[29,41]
	Hydrastis canadensis[39]
	Taraxacum officinalis[29,39,42]
Liver protective	*Silybum marianum*[29,43-5]
	Catechin[29,46-9]
Anti-inflammatory	*Silybum marianum*[29,43-5]
	Scutellaria baicalensis[50,51]
Liver regenerative	*Silybum marianum*[29,43-5]
	Cynara scolymus[29,52]
	Glycyrrhiza glabra[53]
	Liver extracts[29,54-6]
Kupffer cell stimulation	*Echinacea angustifolia*[57,58]
	Baptisia tinctoria[58]

Lymphatic flow and prevention of lymph-stasis is readily encouraged and stimulated by several methods, as summarised in the accompanying box.

Methods for stimulating lymphatic flow

- Muscle action (exercise and stretching)
- Elevation of extremities
- Massage (especially lymphatic massage)
- Hydrotherapy with hot and cold applications

Blood flow to the spleen can be enhanced by berberine, the alkaloid found in the berberidaceae family of plants which includes barberry (*Berberis vulgaris*), Oregon grape (*Berberis aquifolium*), and goldenseal (*Hydrastis canadensis*).[59] This increased blood flow could promote the release of immuno-potentiating substances from the spleen.

Immune support

Optimal immune function requires good health, i.e. a good diet (a diet of whole, natural, unprocessed, living foods which are high in fibre and complex carbohydrates, low in fats and moderate in protein), eight to ten glasses of water (preferably pure) per day, a good basic multivitamin-mineral supplement (in the most bioavailable and easily absorbable form and including adequate amounts of trace minerals), an exercise programme of at least 30 minutes of aerobic exercise and 15–30 minutes of passive stretching daily (may be modified according to tolerance and condition), daily deep breathing and relaxation exercises, daily reflection (meditation, prayer, etc.), time to play and enjoy family and friends, and six to eight hours of sleep daily.

The immune system can also be significantly potentiated by several nutritional factors and plant compounds. Since it is well established that the cellular arm (especially the T lymphocytes, interferons, macrophages and natural killer cells) of the immune system is involved in antiviral, antifungal and antitumour activity,[7] support of this aspect of the immune system is the primary goal. Defects in cellular immunity are commonly observed in diseases or conditions causing aberrations of EBV-specific serologic tests (see box on page 211) as well as in the geriatric population.

It is interesting to note that nutritional supplementation has been shown to reverse some of the age-related defects in cell mediated immunity commonly found in the elderly.[60] This is particularly significant since the elderly have increased levels of antibodies to EBV due to decreased cellular immune response.[61]

Nutritional support of immune function

A basic high-quality multivitamin and mineral supplement high in B complex vitamins (particularly B6, B12, folate and pantothenic acid) and trace minerals (particularly zinc, selenium, chromium and manganese) is an essential supplement baseline. In addition, three specific nutrients, discussed below, should be emphasised for their immune-enhancing activity.

Carotenes   Beta-carotene is a potential natural antioxidant and an effective immuno-potentiator, demonstrating notable antitumour and antiviral actions.[62–72] Beta-carotene supplementation in humans can enhance the action of interferon,[73] stimulate macrophage cytotoxicity and production of tumour necrosis factor[69] and increase the number of circulating helper T lymphocytes.[74]

Vitamin C   Vitamin C has been demonstrated to reduce both the occurrence and the intensity of symptoms of the common cold,[75,76] to have interferon-like[77] and antiviral activity[78] and to enhance white cell destruction of viruses and bacteria.[79,80] Many clinicians have found vitamin C to be effective in increasing general host resistance to, and recovery from, infection.

Zinc   Zinc is very important for proper function of the thymus gland and thymus hormones,[81,82] as well as cellular immunity.[80,83] The optimal functional activity of natural killer cells, important in viral infections, may be dependent on a zinc intake higher than that needed to support normal growth and development.[84]

Glandular support of immune function

Although comparatively few studies have investigated the use of glandular extracts (usually from beef) to enhance human glandular function, 'protomorphogen' therapy is quite popular. Like zinc supplementation, the administration of thymus gland extracts (injectable extracts were used in these studies) has been shown to reverse some of the age-related defects in cell mediated immunity and to enhance immune function.[85,86] Studies with calf thymus administered orally have demonstrated impressive clinical results in a variety of infectious conditions.[85-8] In EBV infections this extract has been shown to normalise altered T-cell subset ratios.[85,87] In particular, administration of the lysate has resulted in clinical improvement and partial correction of the T-cell defects of acquired immunodeficiency syndrome and lymphadenopathy syndrome.[85,87] Positive results have also been demonstrated in patients with food allergy, chronic bronchitis and recurrent upper respiratory tract infections, all common features of chronic EBV.[85,86,88]

Spleen extracts may also be of benefit, as many of the potent immune system enhancing molecules secreted by the spleen are small-molecular-weight peptides that would be easily absorbed. Orally administered spleen extracts have been shown to increase white blood cell counts in extreme leucopenia and neutropenia and to be of some benefit in patients with malaria and typhoid fever.[89]

Botanical support of immune fuction

Goldenseal (Hydrastis canadensis)   Goldenseal, due primarily to its high content of the alkaloid berberine, is of particular importance in the treatment of possible EBV-related infections. Berberine has been shown to increase splenic blood flow, improve liver function and increase white cell activity.[90,91] As the liver and spleen are often involved in EBV functions, hydrastis appears to be extremely well indicated.

*Purple coneflower (*Echinacea angustifolia *and* purpurea)   Purple coneflower, long used for infectious conditions, contains the polysaccharides inulin and echinacin. These poly-saccharides are primarily responsible for the immunostimulatory activities (listed in the accompaning box) of echinacea. These actions make it especially effective in viral infections and cancerous conditions.

Immunostimulatory activities of echinacea polysaccharides[92-6]

- Activation of the alternate complement pathway.
- Promotion of macrophage cytotoxicity.
- Stimulation of T lymphocytes.
- Enhanced T lymphocyte transformation.
- Increased macrophage phagocytosis (including Kupffer cells).
- Stimulation of interferon production.

Baptisia tinctoria   Baptisia has traditionally been used in the treatment of infectious conditions, particularly of the upper respiratory tract. It is a specific for tonsillitis, pharyngitis, lymphadenitis and septic conditions.[39,97,98] Recent studies have demonstrated its immunostimulatory activity. It can enhance white cell destruction of viruses and bacteria, production and activation of lymph cells and the production of antibodies.[58,94,99] Since it can be toxic in high does, dosages must be carefully controlled.

Other botanicals have polysaccharides that have exhibited immune-enhancing effects similar to echinacea and baptisia, including *Eupatorium perfoliatum* (boneset), *Matricaria chamomilla* (German chamomile), *Arctium lappa* (burdock) and *Achillea millefolium* (yarrow).[92] These herbs may be suitable alternatives to baptisia due to their much lower toxicity and can be included in the therapeautic regime as infusions.

*Pokeweed (*Phytolacca decandra-Americana*)* Pokeweed has traditionally been used as a specific in the treatment of upper respiratory tract infections, pharyngitis, rheumatism and, especially, lymphatic disease.[39] It appears, through traditional clinical experience, to have specificity to lymphatic tissue.[97,98] It is well known that extracts of the roots, leaves and berries of phytolacca are potent activators of B and T lymphocytes and are commonly used in research and laboratory investigations (as pokeweed mitogen or PWM) for this activity. Phytolacca can enhance the immunologic response in humans and has antiviral activity against many viruses, such as *Herpes simplex*.[100,101] Caution should be used while employing phytolacca since it can be toxic in high and/or prolonged doses.

*Liquorice root (*Glycyrrhiza glabra*)* Liquorice root has a long history of use in both Chinese and western traditional medicine, especially in the treatment of upper respiratory tract infections and gastrointestinal disorders.[39,102] Glycyrrhiza and some of its natural compounds have demonstrated antiviral activity against many viruses including *Herpes simplex*,[103] an ability to induce interferon production[104] and efficacy in the treatment of viral hepatitis.[53]

Radix astragalus Astragalus has a well respected history of use in Chinese medicine as a valuable tonic specific for strengthening the body's resistance, especially in wasting and exhausting diseases. This therapeutic activity is particularly valuable in the treatment of the chronic fatigue syndrome. Recent studies have shown that astragalus can enhance the production of interferon, increase the lifespan of human lung cells in culture, and reduce the incidence and shorten the course of the common cold.[105]

Lomatium dissectum and Ligusticum porteri These plants are members of the umbellifereae family and are native to the American western states, where they have been used for many years by practitioners of native American medicine, herbalists and naturopathic physicians in the treatment of viral infections. Although there has been little specific research done on these plants' immunostimulatory and antiviral activity, their successful empirical use in the treatment of viral-related infectious diseases suggests their usefulness in the treatment of the chronic fatigue syndrome.[106] These plants are rich sources of coumarin compounds which may result in photosensitivity or skin eruptions and should be used under the supervision of a herbalist or naturopathic physician.

Shitake mushroom (Lentinus edodes) The Shitake mushroom has been used in traditional Chinese medicine to increase resistance to disease. It has been found to contain a polysaccharide complex, lentinan, which is a nontoxic, yet potent, immuno-stimulating agent.[107-13] Its immunostimulating activity (listed in the accompanying box) is specific for macrophages and T lymphocytes.

Immune-stimulating activity of the Shitake mushroom[107-13]

- Stimulation of macrophages, increasing their production of interleukin-1.
- Induction of T lymphocyte production of interleukin-2.
- Increased T lymphocyte proliferation.
- Enhanced T helper cell function.
- Increased cytotoxic activity of macrophages.

Stress reduction

Over the last few years a large body of information has accumulated documenting the multitude of adverse effects that psychological and physiological stress inflicts on an organism, specifically the immune system (see Chapter 6, Immune support). These data implicate stress as a major factor in the etiology and progression of the chronic fatigue syndrome. The chronic mononucleosis-like syndrome is very similar to other ill-defined syndromes, particularly 'adrenal exhaustion'.

There is considerable information available on the many techniques and therapies used for stress reduction, ranging from biofeedback and visualisation to counselling and psychotherapy. In addition to stress reduction techniques, various nutritional and botanical approaches can be utilised. Appropriate nutritional therapy to normalise adrenal function may include a broad-spectrum multiple vitamin and mineral supplement, along with additional vitamin C, pantothenic acid and bovine adrenal extracts.

Those guidelines and recommendations in Chapter 10, Stress, are especially important in the treatment of the chronic fatigue syndrome.

Treatment

The chronic mononucleosis-like syndrome may or may not be directly related to reactivation of an Epstein-Barr virus infection. The fact that the elevation of EBV antibody levels (and of *Herpes simplex* virus 1 and 2, CMV and measles antibodies) has also been found in a number of other conditions, most of which are related to immunologically stressed or compromised conditions, suggests that this syndrome may be indicative of a chronically disturbed immune system and is perhaps a harbinger of future serious immunological disease. Therefore, in addition to antiviral agents, the therapy should support and potentiate the immune system, reduce stress and build up overall health.

Diet

Eliminate all allergic foods and, if highly allergic, rotate non-allergenic foods. Eliminate all simple sugars and refined foods. Emphasise whole, unprocessed foods, particularly those which inhibit viruses, e.g. fruits, garlic and onions.

Nutritional supplements

- Beta-carotene, 100,000 iu a day.
- Vitamin C, 3,000 mg a day.
- Pantothenic acid, 150 mg a day (do not take close to bedtime).
- Zinc, 15 mg a day (picolinate form).
- Multiple vitamin and mineral supplement.
- Adrenal extract, 1–2 tablets three times a day.
- Thymus gland extract, 1–2 tablets three times a day.

Botanical medicines

The indications for botanicals are categorised according to the stage of disease process, i.e. acute infection or exacerbation, convalescence and recovery.

Acute infection or exacerbation   *Echinacea angustifolia, Hydrastis canadensis* (goldenseal) and *Glycyrrhiza glabra* (liquorice) can be taken at the following doses during an infectious process (three times a day doses):
- Dried root (or as tea), 1 to 2 g.
- Freeze-dried root, 500 to 1,000 mg.
- Tincture (1:5), 4 to 6 ml (1 to 1.5 tsp).
- Fluid extract (1:1), 0.5 to 2.0 ml (¼ to ½ tsp).
- Powdered solid extract (4:1), 250–500 mg.

If liquorice is to be used over a long time it is necessary to increase the intake of potassium rich foods.
- *Phytolacca decandra-Americana* (dried root), 100–400 mg three times a day.
- *Baptisia tinctoria* (dried root), 0.5–1.0 g three times a day.

Convalescent or chronic phase
- *Hydrastis canadensis*, as above.
- *Astragalus membranaceus* (dried root), 5–15 g three times a day.
- *Glycyrrhiza glabra*, as above.
- *Eleutherococcus senticosus:*
  - Dried root or as tea, 2–4 g three times a day.
  - Fluid extract (1:1), 2.0–4.0 ml (½ to 1 tsp) three times a day.
  - Solid extract (20:1), 100–200 mg three times a day.

Recovery phase
- *Panax ginseng*:
    Dried root, 1.5–2.0 g three times a day.
    Extracts, equivalent to 25 to 50 mg ginsenosides daily.
- *Eleutherococcus senticosus* (dried root), as above.

Stress reduction

The method of stress reduction used should be tailored to the individual's needs. It should include some combination of counselling, relaxation techniques and exercise. The importance of this aspect of therapy cannot be overstated.

27

Coeliac disease

- A chronic intestinal malabsorption disorder caused by an intolerance to gluten.
- Bulky, pale, frothy, foul-smelling, greasy stools with increased faecal fat.
- Weight loss and signs of multiple vitamin and mineral deficiencies.
- Increased levels of serum gliadin antibodies.
- Diagnosis confirmed by jejunal biopsy.

General considerations

Coeliac disease, also known as non-tropical sprue, gluten-sensitive enteropathy or coeliac sprue, is characterised by malabsorption and an abnormal small intestine structure which reverts to normal on removal of dietary gluten. The protein gluten and its polypeptide derivative, gliadin, are found primarily in wheat, barley and rye grains.

Symptoms of coeliac disease most commonly appear during the first three years of life, after cereals are introduced into the diet. A second peak incidence occurs during the third decade. Breastfeeding appears to have a preventive effect as breastfed babies have a decreased risk of developing coeliac disease.[1-3] The early introduction of cow's milk is also believed to be a major causative factor.[1-4] Research in the past few years has clearly indicated that breastfeeding, along with delayed administration of cow's milk and cereal grains, are primary preventive steps that can greatly reduce the risk of developing coeliac disease.

Coeliac disease also appears to have a genetic cause.[3,5] The frequency of individuals having the genetic trait for coeliac disease is much higher in northern and central Europe and the northwest Indian subcontinent.[3,6] Wheat cultivation in these areas is a relatively recent development (1,000 BC). The prevalence of coeliac disease is much higher in these areas compared with other parts of the world, e.g. 1:300 in southwest Ireland compared with 1:2,500 in the United States (estimated).

Chemistry of grain proteins

Gluten, a major component of the wheat endosperm, is composed of gliadins and glutenins. Only the gliadin portion has been demonstrated to activate coeliac disease. In rye, barley and oats the proteins that appear to activate the disease are termed secalins, hordeins and avenins respectively, and prolamines collectively. Cereal grains belong to the family gramineae. The closer a grain's taxonomic (classification) relationship to wheat, the greater its ability to activate coeliac disease. Rice and maize, two grains that do not appear to activate coeliac disease, are further removed taxonomically from wheat.[3,7] The classification of the grains is shown in Figure 27.1.

Gliadins are proteins consisting of single polypeptide chains with a very high glutamine and proline content. Gliadins have been divided into four major electrophoretic fractions, alpha, beta, gamma and omega. Alpha-gliadin is believed to be the fraction most capable of activating coeliac disease, although beta- and gamma-gliadin are also capable. Omega-gliadin does not appear to activate the disease at all, although it has the highest content of glutamine and proline. Gliadin that has been subjected to complete digestion does not activate coeliac disease in susceptible individuals, suggesting a possible relation to deficient enzymes involved with protein digestion.[3]

Opioid activity

Wheat gluten components have demonstrated opioid (opium-like) activity.[8,9] This activity is believed to be the factor responsible for the association between wheat consumption and schizophrenia.[10,11,12] The hypothesis that gluten is a causative factor in the development of schizophrenia is substantiated by epidemiological, clinical and experimental studies.

Immune defects

Various hypotheses have been proposed to explain the development of coeliac disease. Currently, the most likely hypothesis relates to abnormalities in the immune response rather than some 'toxic' property of gliadin.[13] In animals, immune mediated mechanisms can produce the characteristic intestinal damage seen in coeliac disease.

Associated conditions

Conditions such as thyroid abnormalities, insulin-dependent diabetes mellitus, psychiatric disturbances (including schizophrenia), dermatitis herpetiformis and urticaria have also been linked to gluten intolerance.[14] A more ominous association is the increased risk of malignant cancers seen in coeliac patients.[3,15,16]

This may be a result of decreased vitamin and mineral absorption, particularly vitamin A and carotenoids. However, it may also be a result of gliadin suppressing immune function.[17] Alpha-gliadin has demonstrated immune suppressing activity in coeliac patients but has no effect in healthy controls.

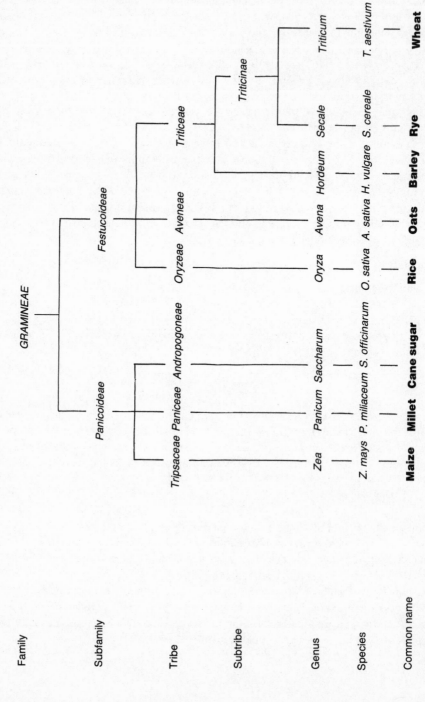

Figure 27.1 Relationship of major cereal grains

Diagnosis

Biopsy of the small intestine is the only definitive procedure available at present. However, several easily performed blood tests may be available soon which will aid in the diagnosis.[18–21]

Therapy

Diet

Once the diagnosis has been established, a gluten-free diet is indicated. This diet does not contain any wheat, rye, barley, triticale or oats. Buckwheat and millet are often excluded as well. Although buckwheat is not in the grass family, and millet appears to be more closely related to rice and corn, they do contain prolamines with similar antigenic activity to the alpha-gliadin of wheat.

In addition, milk and milk products should be eliminated until the patient redevelops milk tolerance as intestinal structure and function return to normal.

Patient response

Usually clinical improvement will be apparent within a few days or weeks (30 per cent respond within three days, another 50 per cent within one month and 10 per cent within another month). However, 10 per cent of patients only respond after 24–36 months of gluten avoidance.[22]

If the patient does not appear to be responding, the following should be considered:
- incorrect diagnosis;
- the patient is not adhering to the diet or is being exposed to hidden sources of gliadin; and
- the presence of an associated disease or complication, such as zinc deficiency.[3,23]

Table 27.1 Gluten and gliadin content of selected foods[27]

Food	Total protein (% dry weight)	Prolamines* (% of total protein)	Glutelins** (% of total protein)	Cross-reactivity with gliadin
Wheat	10–15	40–50	30–40	++++
Rye	9–14	30–50	30–50	+++
Oats	8–14	10–15	approx. 5	++
Maize	7–13	50–55	30–45	+
Rice	8–10	1–5	85–90	—
Sorghum	9–13	>60		
Millet	7–16	57	30	—

* Primarily gliadin
** Primarily gluten

The last reason highlights the importance of multi-vitamin and mineral supplementation in these patients. In addition to treating any underlying deficiency, supplementation provides the necessary cofactors for growth and repair. Coeliac disease will be unresponsive to dietary therapy if an underlying zinc deficiency is present.[3,23]

Papain

The protein-digesting enzyme from papaya, papain, has been shown to be able to digest wheat gluten and render it harmless in coeliac disease subjects.[24,25] Taking a papain supplement (500–1,000 mg) with meals may allow some individuals to tolerate gluten.[26]

Treatment

The therapeutic approach is quite straightforward:
- Eliminate all sources of gliadin.
- Eliminate dairy products initially.
- Correct underlying nutritional deficiencies.
- Treat any associated conditions.
- Determine and eliminate all food allergens.

If the individual with coeliac disease does not begin to respond within one month, search for hidden sources of gliadin.

Maintenance of a strict gluten-free diet is quite difficult in the west, due to the wide distribution of gliadin and other activators of coeliac disease in processed foods. Individuals with coeliac disease must be encouraged to read labels carefully in order to avoid hidden sources of gliadin, such as are found in some brands of soy sauce, modified food starch, ice cream, soup, beer, wine, vodka, whisky, malt, etc. Individuals should also be encouraged to consult resources for patient education and information on gluten-free recipes.

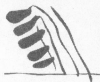

28

Common cold

- Nasal discomfort with watery discharge and sneezing.
- Dry, sore throat.
- Red, swollen nasal mucosa.
- Swollen cervical lymph nodes.

General considerations

The common cold can be caused by a wide variety of viruses that are capable of infecting the upper respiratory tract. We are all constantly exposed to many of these viruses, yet the majority of us only experience the discomfort of a cold once or twice a year. This implies that a decrease in resistance is the major factor in catching a cold.

In general, the individual with a cold will experience a general malaise, fever, headache and upper respiratory tract congestion. Initially there is usually a watery nasal discharge and sneezing, followed by thicker secretions containing mucus, white blood cells and dead organisms. The throat may be red, sore and quite dry.

Usually a cold can be differentiated from other conditions with some similar symptoms (influenza and allergies for example) by commonsense. Influenza is much more severe in symptoms and usually occurs in epidemics, so contacting the local public health department is all that is needed to rule this out. Allergies may be an underlying factor, decreasing resistance and allowing a virus to infect the upper airways, but usually allergies can be differentiated from the common cold by the fact that no fever occurs with allergies, there is usually a history of seasonal allergic episodes and there is no evidence of infection.

Therapy

Prevention

Maintaining a healthy immune system is the prime way of protecting against an excessive number of colds. If an individual catches more than one or two colds a year it may be indicative of a weak immune system. Nutrition is the major determinant in having a healthy immune system.

Another important factor in reducing resistance and allowing a virus to infect is stress, whether it be physical, emotional or mental. During the stress response, compounds are released by the adrenal glands that cause the thymus gland to shrink and reduce its activity. Many nutritional factors have been shown to prevent this effect of stress on the thymus, our major gland of immunity. Specifically, vitamins A and C, beta-carotene, zinc and other antioxidants prevent stress and free radical induced damage to the thymus and enhance immune functions.[1] Individuals who are under a lot of stress, have weak immune systems or who are exposed to high levels of pollutants (virtually all of us) should supplement their diets with these important nutrients.

There are several other factors to consider besides nutrient deficiency and stress. Alcohol and tobacco consumption, prescribed, non-prescribed and recreational drug use, elevated glucose, triglycerides and cholesterol levels in the blood, excessive sugar consumption, environmental factors (chemical exposure) and allergies can all significantly weaken our immune system.[1]

For a more detailed account of how to enhance the immune system please read Chapter 6, Immune support.

What to do once a cold is caught

Once a cold develops there are several things that can be done to speed up recovery. It should be noted, however, that with a healthy functioning immune system a cold should not last more than two or three days. Even utilising a wide variety of natural healing methods, once a cold is underway it is very difficult to throw off the cold completely within two days. Do not expect immediate relief in most instances when using natural substances. In fact, since most natural therapies for colds involve assisting the body, as opposed to suppressing the symptoms, often the symptoms of the cold temporarily worsen.

Many of the symptoms of the cold are a result of our body's defence mechanisms. For example, the potent immune-stimulating compound interferon released by our blood cells and other tissues during infections is responsible for many flu-like symptoms. Another example is the beneficial effect of fever on the course of infection; while an elevated body temperature can be uncomfortable, suppression of fever is thought to counteract a major defence mechanism and prolong the infection. In general, fever should not be suppressed during an infection unless it is dangerously high (> 104 °F, 40 °C). For these and other reasons it is not uncommon for the individual treating themselves for the common cold with natural medicines to experience a greater degree of discomfort, due to the immune enhancing effects of these compounds. Of course the illness is generally much shorter lived.

Sleep and rest   Our immune system functions better under parasympathetic nervous system tone.[1] This portion of our autonomic nervous system assumes control over bodily functions during periods of rest, relaxation, visualisation, meditation and sleep. During the deepest levels of sleep, potent immune enhancing compounds are released and many immune functions are greatly increased. The value of sleep and rest during a cold cannot be overemphasised.

Liquids   Liquid consumption offers several benefits. When the mucous membranes that line the respiratory tract get dehydrated it provides a much more hospitable environment for the virus. Consuming plenty of liquids and/or using a vaporiser maintains a moist respiratory tract that repels viral infection. Drinking plenty of liquids will also improve the function of white blood cells by decreasing the concentration of solutes in the blood.

It should be noted that the type of liquid consumed is very important. Studies have shown that consuming concentrated sources of sugars like glucose, fructose, sucrose, honey or orange juice greatly reduces the ability of the white blood cells to kill bacteria.[2,3,4] Before being consumed, fruit juices should be greatly diluted. Drinking concentrated orange juice during a cold probably does more harm than good.

Sugar   As mentioned above, sugar consumption, even if derived from 'natural' sources like fruit juices and honey, can impair immune functions.[2,3,4] This impairment appears to be due to the fact that glucose (blood sugar) and vitamin C compete for transport sites into the white blood cells. Decreased vitamin C levels due to excessive sugar consumption may result in a significant reduction in white blood cell function.

Nutrition

Vitamin C   For the common cold, the recommendation of 500 to 1,000 mg of vitamin C every two hours seems appropriate to ensure tissue saturation. Vitamin C supplementation has been shown to shorten the course of the common cold in several clinical studies.[5–8]

Although vitamin C has been shown to be antiviral and antibacterial, its main effect is via improvement in host resistance. Immunostimulatory effects have been demonstrated on many different immune functions, including enhancing white blood cell production and increasing interferon levels, antibody responses, secretion of thymic hormones and increasing the integrity of connective tissue.

Zinc   Zinc is a critical nutrient for optimum immune system function.[9] Like vitamin C, zinc also possesses direct antiviral activity, including antiviral activity against several viruses that can cause the common cold.[10] In a double-blind clinical trial, zinc gluconate lozenges significantly reduced the average duration of common colds by seven days.[11] The lozenges contained 23 milligrams of elemental zinc, which the patients were instructed to dissolve in their mouths every two waking hours after an initial double dose. After seven days, 86 per cent of the 37 zinc-treated subjects were symptom free, compared to 46 per cent of the 28 placebo-treated subjects. The authors of the study hypothesised that the local zinc concentration was high enough to inhibit replication of the cold viruses. The use of zinc supplementation, particularly as a lozenge, appears to be of much value during a cold.

Beta-carotene or vitamin A   Beta-carotene (provitamin A) supplementation (180 mg a day) has demonstrated significant immune enhancing action.[1,12] Being a potent anti-oxidant, beta-carotene probably offers the greatest protection to the thymus gland of any nutrient. Vitamin A does not have nearly the antioxidant action of beta-carotene, yet it too has a significant effect on the immune system. Originally known as the 'anti-infective' vitamin, vitamin A plays an essential role in maintaining the integrity of the lining of the respiratory tract and its secretions.[1] Vitamin A also demonstrates potent virus killing activity.[13]

Botanical medicines

Many herbs have significant antibiotic action against bacteria, viruses and fungi. However, herbs are much more than 'natural' antibiotics. Several herbs have shown remarkable effects in stimulating our own immune mechanisms. Modern research is upholding what herbal practitioners have known for thousands of years – herbs work with our body's systems to promote health. The following herbs represent some of the most potent herbal enhancers of immune system function – *Echinacea angustifolia* (purple coneflower), *Hydrastis canadensis* (goldenseal), *Glycyrrhiza glabra* (liquorice) and *Astragalus membranaceus* (astragalus root). The first three are discussed in detail in Chapter 6. Astragalus is discussed below.

Astragalus membranaceus   The Chinese value astragalus as an immune system enhancer, a specific tonic for strengthening the body's resistance to disease. In clinical studies in China, astragalus has been shown to reduce the incidence and shorten the course of the common cold.[14]

Astragalus significantly increases interferon production and secretion. Interferon binds to cell surfaces and stimulates the synthesis of proteins that prevent viral infection. Several other herbs have been shown to share many of the same effects of astragalus, including extracts of *Echinacea spp.*, *Eupatorium perforliatum* (boneset), *Ligustrum lucidum,* and *Glycyrrhiza glabra* (liquorice).[15,16,17]

Treatment

Although the focus of this chapter is on the use of natural methods to assist the body in recovering from the common cold, nutritional and lifestyle factors offer the most logical approach to treatment by their preventive effect. The old adage 'an ounce of prevention is worth a pound of cure' is true for the common cold as well as the majority of other conditions afflicting human health.

General measures

- Rest (bed rest better).
- Drink large amount of fluids (preferably diluted vegetable juices, soups and herb teas).
- Limit simple sugar consumption (including fruit sugars) to less than 50 grams a day.

Nutritional supplements

- Vitamin C, 500 to 1,000 mg every two hours (decrease if diarrhoea results).
- Bioflavonoids, 1,000 mg per day.
- Vitamin A, 25,000 iu per day.
- Beta-carotene, 200,000 iu per day.
- Zinc lozenges, one lozenge containing 23 mg elemental zinc every two waking hours for one week. Prolonged supplementation (more than one week) at this dose is not recommended as it may lead to immunosuppression.

Botanical medicines

Echinacea angustifolia, Hydrastis canadensis (goldenseal), *Glycyrrhiza glabra* (liquorice) or *Astragalus radix* can be taken at the following doses during an infectious process (doses three times a day):
- Dried root (or as tea), 1 to 2 g.
- Freeze-dried root, 500 to 1,000 mg.
- Tincture (1:5), 4 to 6 ml (1 to 1.5 tsp).
- Fluid extract (1:1), 0.5 to 2.0 ml (¼ to ½ tsp).
- Powdered solid extract (4:1), 250–500 mg.

If liquorice is to be used over a long time it is necessary to increase the intake of potassium-rich foods.

29

Constipation

- Difficulty in passing stools.
- Incomplete or infrequent passage of stools.

General considerations

The frequency of defaecation and the consistency and volume of stools vary so greatly from individual to individual that it is difficult to determine what is normal. Familial, social and dietary customs have a major effect on bowel habits.

There are many causes of constipation, most of which are listed in Table 29.1. In general, inappropriate diet, inadequate exercise and laxative/enema abuse are the most common causes, although more serious disease must always be borne in mind.

Therapy

Proper elimination is very important as the bowel is a potential source of many toxins. For example, antigens and toxins from bowel bacteria have been found to be possibly related to the development of diabetes mellitus.[2] meningitis,[3] myasthenia gravis,[4] thyroid disease,[5] ulcerative colitis[6] and other diseases.[7] Naturopathic physicians have long stressed the importance of proper bowel health.

Although a healthy bowel is important, the exact treatment goal is somewhat unclear since there is no generally agreed upon frequency of bowel movements. In general, most nutritionally-oriented physicians recommend two to three bowel movements per day, as is typically found in healthy people eating a high-fibre diet and getting adequate exercise. Some suggest that more frequent movements are appropriate since each time food is consumed, a peristaltic action is initiated which, in infants, will result in a bowel movement.

Table 29.1 Causes of constipation[1]

Cause	Examples
Dietary	Highly refined and low-fibre foods; inadequate fluid intake.
Physical inactivity	Inadequate exercise; prolonged bed rest.
Pregnancy	
Advanced age	
Drugs	Anaesthetics, antacids (aluminium and calcium salts), anticholinergics (bethanechol, carbachol, pilocarpine, physostigmine, ambenonium), anticonvulsants, antidepressants (tricyclics, monoamine oxidase inhibitors), antihypertensives, anti-Parkinsonism drugs, antipsychotics (phenothiazines), beta-adrenergic blocking agents (propanolol), bismuth salts, diuretics, iron salts, laxatives and cathartics (chronic use), muscle relaxants, opiates, toxic metals (arsenic, lead, mercury).
Metabolic abnormalities	Hypokalaemia, hyperglycaemia, uraemia, porphyria, amyloidosis.
Endocrine abnormalities	Hypothyroidism, hypercalcaemia, panhypopituritarism, pheochromocytoma, glucagonoma.
Structural abnormalities	
Bowel diseases	Diverticulosis, irritable bowel syndrome (alternating diarrhoea and constipation), tumour.
Neurogenic abnormalities	Nerve disorders of the bowel (aganglionosis, autonomic neuropathy), spinal cord disorders (trauma, multiple sclerosis, tabes dorsalis), disorders of the splanchnic nerves (tumours, trauma), cerebral disorders (strokes, Parkinsonism, neoplasm).
Psychogenic disorders	
Enemas (chronic use)	
Insecticide exposure	Organophosphates.

Bowel retraining

After the causes of constipation have been eliminated, the bowels need to be retrained to establish healthy habits. Listed in the box overleaf are recommended rules for bowel regularity. The recommended procedure will take four to six weeks.

High fibre diet

It is well established that a low-fibre diet causes constipation.[8] Equally well established is the efficacy of dietary changes which increase fibre in the treatment of chronic constipation. Increased dietary fibre increases the frequency and quantity of bowel movements, decreases the transit time of stools, decreases the absorption of toxins from the stool and appears to be a preventive factor in several diseases. Particularly effective are the foods containing the water-insoluble hydrophilic fibres such as cellulose (e.g. bran) which increase stool weight as a result of their water-holding properties.[9,10] Table 29.2 lists the primary fibres found in high-fibre foods.

Rules for bowel retraining

- Find and eliminate known causes (see Table 29.1).
- Never repress an urge to defaecate.
- Eat a high-fibre diet, particularly fruits and vegetables.
- Drink six to eight glasses of fluid per day.
- Sit on the toilet at the same time every morning (even when the urge to defaecate is not present), preferably immediately after breakfast or exercise.
- Exercise at least 20 minutes, three times per week.
- Stop using laxatives (except as discussed below to re-establish bowel activity) and enemas.

  Week one: every night before bed take three herbal laxative tablets (determine actual number needed by amount needed reliably to ensure a bowel movement every morning).

  Weekly: each week decrease dosage by half a tablet. If constipation recurs, go back to the previous week's dosage. Decrease by one tablet if diarrhoea occurs.

Table 29.2 Dietary fibre constituents of the food groups

Food group	Main dietary fibres
Fruits and vegetables	Cellulose, hemicellulose, lignin, pectic substances, cutin, waxes
Grains	Cellulose, hemicellulose, lignin, phenolic esters
Seeds (other than grains)	Cellulose, hemicellulose, pectic substances, guar endosperm
Seed husk of *Plantago ovata*	Arabinogalacturonosyl-rhamno-xylan (mucilage)
Food additives	Gum arabic, alginate, carrageenan, carboxymethylcellulose

When high-fibre foods are being used to increase bulk, the typical recommendation is half a cup of bran cereal, increasing to one and a half cups over several weeks.[11] Corn bran is more effective than wheat bran, while oat bran is less irritating and a better absorber of fats. For best results, adequate amounts of fluids must be consumed. If bran alone is being used, a quarter to half a cup per day is the recommended dosage. (For a more complete discussion, see Chapter 4, Dietary fibre.)

Folic acid

One study found that women with a folic acid deficiency presented with chronic constipation as well as the typical signs and symptoms of restless legs, depression, tiredness, depressed ankle jerks and impaired vibratory sensation. The symptoms all resolved with folic acid supplementation.[12]

Botanical medicines

Basically, most laxatives act through one of the mechanisms listed in the box below. Lubricants such as mineral oil are not recommended since not only do they not treat the cause of the disorder, but they also interfere with the absorption of fat soluble vitamins,[13] and deposits of mineral oil have been found in the lymph system of chronic users.[14] Although most herbs are popularly considered always to be safe, excess dosages can cause toxic reactions. It is important to recognise that any agent which causes a physiological response can also cause a toxic response. Most of the herbal laxatives (e.g. castor oil, cascara, aloe, senna and rhubarb) are active due to their anthraquinone content. Excessive dosages of any of these can cause purging, griping, collapse and blood in the stools.[14]

Mechanisms of laxative action[15]

- Hydrophylic and osmotic
- Contact stimulants
- Lubricant
- Increase bulk of intestinal contents
- Increase intestinal mucosa secretion
- Softener

Cascara sagrada (Rhamnus purshiana *or* Rhamnus catharticus *in the UK*)   Cascara (buckthorn) has long been used as a laxative. Its anthraglycosides are responsible for most of its activity. They act on the large intestine by increasing peristalsis (the muscular activity of the colon).[16] Its bitter principles (from its content of aloins) probably also help by stimulating digestion. It is available in many forms – dried herb, crude extract, fluid extract, solid extract, etc. It is generally considered to be safe with a minimum of side effects except, as noted above, when used in excessive dosages or over long periods of time.

Cassia senna   Senna leaves are also commonly used for their laxative properties. Its activity is due to its anthracene derivatives which are probably formed during the drying process. Its use, properties and toxicity are similar to cascara.[14]

Aloe vera   There are at least 120 known species of aloe, many of which have been used as laxatives. Its anthraglycosides are primarily responsible for its activity. Aloe is not considered as good a laxative as cascara and senna since it produces more griping and irritation.[14]

*Psyllium seed (*Plantago ovata*)*   Psyllium seed husks are a commonly used mucilaginous bulk laxative. The typical dose is one to two rounded teaspoons after meals in a full glass of water.

Treatment

Constipation is a common symptom, not a true disease. Treatment starts by first eliminating all known causes of constipation (see Table 29.1 above). A healthy high-fibre diet should be instituted, and then bowel retraining (see box on page 234) begun. Laxative herbs are only to be used as part of the bowel retraining programme. Bulking agents such as oat bran and psyllium seed husks can be very useful.

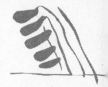

30

Crohn's disease and ulcerative colitis

Crohn's disease

- Intermittent bouts of diarrhoea, low-grade fever.
- Anorexia, weight loss, flatulence and malaise.
- Abdominal tenderness, especially in the right lower quadrant, with signs of peritoneal irritation and an abdominal or pelvic mass.
- X-rays show abnormality of the terminal ileum.

Ulcerative colitis

- Bloody diarrhoea, with cramps in the lower abdomen.
- Mild abdominal tenderness, weight loss and fever.
- Rectal examination may show perianal irritation, fissures, haemorrhoids, fistulas and abscesses.
- Diagnosis confirmed by X-ray and sigmoidoscopy (internal examination of the colon).

General considerations

Inflammatory bowel disease (IBD) is a general term for a group of chronic inflammatory disorders of the bowel. It is divided into two major categories, Crohn's disease and ulcerative colitis. Clinically, IBD is characterised by recurrent inflammatory involvement of specific intestinal segments, resulting in diverse clinical manifestations.

Crohn's disease

Crohn's disease is characterised by an inflammatory reaction throughout the entire thickness of the bowel wall. In approximately 40 per cent of cases, however, the granulomas are either poorly developed or totally absent. The original description in

1932 by Crohn and his colleagues localised the disease to segments in the ileum, the terminal portion of the small intestine. However, the same granulomatous process may involve the mucosa of the mouth, oesophagus, stomach, duodenum, jejunum and colon. Crohn's disease of the small intestine is also known as regional enteritis, while involvement of the colon is known as Crohn's disease of the colon, or granulomatous colitis.

Ulcerative colitis

In ulcerative colitis there is a non-specific inflammatory response limited largely to the lining of the colon. Crohn's disease and ulcerative colitis do share many common features and, where appropriate, will be discussed together. Otherwise they will be discussed as separate entities.

Common features

- The colon is frequently involved in Crohn's disease and is invariably involved in ulcerative colitis.
- Although rare, patients with ulcerative colitis who have total colon involvement may develop a so-called backwash ileitis. Thus, both conditions may cause changes in the small intestine.
- Patients with Crohn's disease often have close relatives with ulcerative colitis, and vice versa.
- When there is no granulomatous reaction in Crohn's disease of the colon, the two lesions may resemble each other clinically as well as pathologically.
- There are many epidemiological similarities between the two diseases, including age, race, sex and geographic distribution.
- Both conditions are associated with similar extra-intestinal manifestations.
- There appear to be etiological parallels between the two conditions.
- Both conditions are associated with an increased frequency of colonic cancer.

The rates of the two diseases differ slightly, with most studies showing ulcerative colitis to be more common than Crohn's disease. The current estimate of the yearly rate of newly diagnosed cases of ulcerative colitis in western Europe and the United States is approximately 6–8 cases per 100,000, and the estimated rate of the total number of cases is approximately 70–150 cases per 100,000. The estimate of the yearly rate of newly diagnosed cases of Crohn's disease is approximately 2 cases per 100,000, while the total number of cases is estimated at 20–40 per 100,000. The rate of Crohn's disease is increasing in western cultures.[1,2]

Inflammatory bowel disease (IBD) may occur at any age, but most often it occurs between the ages of 15 and 35. Females are affected slightly more than males. Caucasians develop the disease two to five times more often than blacks or orientals, while Jews have a three- to six-fold higher incidence compared with non-Jews.[1-4]

Theories about the cause of IBD can be divided into several groups:

- Genetic predisposition.
- Infectious agent or agents.

- Immunologic abnormality.
- Dietary factors.
- An assortment of miscellaneous concepts implicating psychosomatic, vascular, traumatic and other mechanisms.[3,4]

Genetic predisposition   Although the search for a specific genetic marker for IBD has been futile, several factors suggest a genetic predisposition. As already mentioned, IBD is two to four times more common in Caucasians than non-Caucasians, and four times more common in Jews than in non-Jews. In addition, multiple members of a family have Crohn's disease or ulcerative colitis in 15 to 40 per cent of the cases.[3,4]

Infectious etiology   Many microorganisms have been hailed as potential causes of IBD, but in spite of numerous attempts to confirm a bacterial, mycobacterial, fungal or viral cause, the idea that a microbial agent is responsible for IBD is still a hotly debated subject. Viruses such as rotavirus, Epstein-Barr virus and cytomegalovirus, and myco-bacteria, continue to be favoured candidates. Other candidates include pseudomonas-like organisms, chlamydia and *Yersinia enterocolitica*.[3-7]

Immune mechanisms   An overwhelming amount of evidence points to immune system disturbances in IBD, but whether these disturbances are causal or secondary phenomena remains unclear. Theories linking immune system derangements with IBD have been proposed, but the current evidence seems to indicate that these derange-ments are probably secondary to the disease process.[3,4]

Dietary factors   Despite the fact that a dietary cause of Crohn's disease is hardly considered (if mentioned at all) in most standard medical and gastroenterology texts, several lines of evidence strongly support dietary factors as being the most important causative factor.[8-20]

The incidence of Crohn's disease is increasing in cultures consuming the 'western' diet, while it is virtually non-existent in cultures consuming a more primitive diet.[8-13] As food is the major factor in determining the intestinal environment, the considerable change in dietary habits over the last century could explain the rising rates of Crohn's disease.

Several studies which analysed the pre-illness diet of patients with Crohn's disease have found that people who develop Crohn's disease habitually eat more refined sugar, and less raw fruit and vegetables and dietary fibre than healthy people.[8-12] In one study, the pre-illness intake of refined sugar in Crohn's disease patients was nearly twice that of controls (122 g/day versus 65 g/day).[12] One researcher found that before the onset of disease, Crohn's disease patients had eaten corn flakes more frequently than controls.[21] Although other researchers could not verify this specific finding, corn flakes are high in refined carbohydrates and are derived from a very common allergen (corn).

Much of the controversy over the role of pre-illness diet in the etiology of Crohn's disease is largely due to the fact that the only way to assess this diet is from post-diagnostic interviews. Studies where the interview has taken place within the first six months of diagnosis tend to be more supportive than studies done more than seven months after diagnosis. In contrast, patients with ulcerative colitis do not show an increased consumption of refined carbohydrate when compared with controls.[22]

Another important dietary factor that is entirely overlooked in the standard texts is the role of food allergy. Support for this hypothesis is offered in clinical studies which have utilised an elemental diet, total parenteral nutrition (nutrition other than by mouth) or an exclusion diet with great success in the treatment of IBD.[14–20] The role of food allergy is discussed in greater detail below, as is the effect of dietary fibre in the etiology and treatment of IBD.

Miscellaneous factors   Psychosomatic factors, vascular disturbances and chronic trauma have received consideration in the origin of IBD, but at present are not considered significant mechanisms.[3,4] While there is little evidence directly relating psychological factors to the initiation of IBD, there is little doubt that emotional factors are important in modifying the course of the disease.

Therapy

Natural history of Crohn's disease

Little is known concerning the natural course of Crohn's disease, as virtually all patients with the disease undergo standard medical care (drugs and/or surgery) or alternative therapy. The only exceptions are those patients in clinical trials who are assigned to the placebo group.[23–25] However, even these patients do not represent the natural course of the disease, since they are frequently seen by physicians and other members of a healthcare team and are taking medication, even if it is only in the form of a placebo. If proper evaluation of therapies for IBD is to occur, there must be a greater understanding of its natural history.

This is particularly important for alternative practitioners, as it is commonly believed that standard medical care often interferes with the normal efforts of the body to restore health. Some aspects of the 'natural' course of Crohn's disease support this idea, especially when coupled with the limited efficacy of current medications and surgery and their known toxicity. However, heroic measures do have their place in many instances and should be used when appropriate.

Researchers in the National Cooperative Crohn's Disease Study (NCCDS) reviewed 77 patients who received placebo therapy in part one of the 17-week study.[23,24] They all had active disease, as defined by a Crohn's disease activity index (CDAI, see box on page 251) of above 150. Of the patients completing the study:

- No patient died.
- Only seven (9 per cent) suffered a major worsening of their disease, i.e. either they developed a major fistula or required abdominal surgery.
- Twenty-five (32 per cent) suffered a lesser worsening (increase in the CDAI to over 450 or presence of fever of 100 °F, 38 °C, for two weeks).
- Twenty-five (32 per cent) were considered failures, as their CDAI remained at over 150.

- And 20 patients (26 per cent) achieved clinical remission.

On at least one occasion during the 17 weeks of therapy, 49 per cent of the patients were found to have a CDAI of under 150.

The patients who responded favourably to the placebo continued to be observed on placebo therapy for up to two years (part one, phase two). It is interesting to note that while none of these patients' X-rays worsened during phase one or phase two, 18 per cent showed improvement on their intestinal X-rays. Of the patients responding to placebo (20, 26 per cent, of the 77) the majority (70 per cent) remained in remission at one year, and a fair number (45 per cent) remained in remission at two years. These results indicate that many patients will undergo spontaneous remission, approximately 20 per cent at one year and 12 per cent at two years. However, when another factor is considered, the success of placebo therapy rises dramatically. In patients having no previous history of steroid therapy, 41 per cent achieved remission after 17 weeks. In addition, 23 per cent of this group continued in remission after two years, compared to only 4 per cent of the group with a prior history of steroid use.

The European Cooperative Crohn's Disease Study (ECCDS), although different in some details of method, is quite similar to the NCCDS.[23,25] In the ECCDS, 110 patients constituted the placebo group, 68 patients with prior treatment and 42 patients with no prior treatment. The result of the study indicated that 55 per cent of the total placebo group achieved remission by 100 days, 34 per cent remained in remission at 300 days and 21 per cent remained in remission at 700 days. Like the NCCDS, the ECCDS demonstrated that patients with no prior therapy have an increased likelihood of remission.

While one group of researchers did not advocate placebo therapy, they did carefully point out that once remission is achieved, 75 per cent of the patients will continue in remission at the end of one year and up to 63 per cent by two years, regardless of the maintenance therapy used. These results would suggest that the key is achieving remission, which, once attained, can be maintained by conservative non-drug therapy rather than the 'medicines we are currently using with their limited efficacy and known toxicity'.[23]

Abnormalities found in inflammatory bowel disease

Prostaglandin metabolism Prostaglandin levels are greatly increased in the colonic mucosa, serum and stools of patients with IBD. Specifically, these patients show an increase in the synthesis of the inflammatory leukotrienes.[26–9] These compounds are produced by neutrophils and are known to amplify the inflammatory process and cause intestinal cramping and pain.

As in other inflammatory conditions, manipulation of dietary oils is indicated. Dietary arachidonic acid should be reduced considerably, while the consumption of omega-3 oils (alpha-linolenic acid and eicosapentaenoic acid as found in flaxseed oil and fish oils respectively) should be encouraged. The omega-3 oils lead to significantly fewer inflammatory leukotrienes and have been shown to reduce inflammatory processes.[30,31]

Mucin defects   Mucins are glycoproteins (proteins with sugar molecules attached) that are largely responsible for the viscous and elastic characteristics of secreted mucus. Alterations in mucin composition and content in the colonic mucosa have been reported in patients with ulcerative colitis.[31-34] The factors responsible for this appear to be a dramatic decrease in the mucus content of the mucus producing cells or goblet cells (proportional to the severity of the disease) as well as a decrease in the major sulphur-containing mucin.

In contrast, these abnormalities are not found in patients with Crohn's disease. It is significant that while the mucin content of the goblet cells return to normal during remission of ulcerative colitis, the sulphur-containing mucin deficiency does not. The specific components of the sulphur-containing mucin and the cause of its lower concentration have not yet been determined. These mucin abnormalities are also thought to be a major factor in the increased risk of colon cancer in these patients.

Many of the herbs used historically in the treatment of ulcerative colitis are demulcents, i.e. agents that soothe irritated mucus membranes and promote the secretion of mucus. This effect appears to be very much indicated and supports the use of demulcents in ulcerative colitis.

Intestinal microflora   The intestinal microflora is extraordinarily complex and contains over 400 distinct microbial species.[5,6] The faecal flora of patients with Crohn's disease has been found to be greatly disturbed.[5] Studies have indicated that these alterations in faecal flora are not secondary to the disease, and alterations in the metabolic activity of the various bacteria are thought to be more important than alterations in the number of bacteria *per se*. In addition, it is thought that specific bacterial cell components (which vary even within the same species) are responsible for promoting destruction of the intestinal cells.[5,6]

Carrageenan   It is very interesting to note that researchers investigating ulcerative colitis often use the carrageenan (a compound extracted from red seaweeds) model to induce the disease experimentally in animals. In the initial experiments reported by Marcus and Watt in 1969, 1 per cent and 5 per cent carrageenan solutions were provided as the exclusive source of oral fluids for guinea pigs.[35] Over a period of several days the animals lost weight, developed anaemia, had bloody diarrhoea, and developed ulcerative colitis. These results have since been confirmed by numerous investigators and in studies involving other animal species, including primates.[5,36-8]

In its native state carrageenan has a molecular weight of 100,000 to 800,000, but in the studies it is degraded by mild acidic hydrolysis to yield products with weights in the vicinity of 30,000. Carrageen compounds are used by the food industry as stabilising and suspending agents, with different molecular weight polymers being used for a variety of purposes. Typically, carrageenans used in the food industry have a molecular weight greater than 100,000. Carrageenan is widely used in milk and chocolate milk products (ice cream, cottage cheese, milk chocolate, etc.) due to its ability to stabilise milk proteins.

As suggestive as the animal studies are in linking ulcerative colitis with carrageenan, and despite the increased consumption of carrageenan in western diets, there appears to be no correlation between human consumption of carrageenan and development of ulcerative colitis at this time. No lesions of IBD were observed in healthy human subjects fed enormous quantities of degraded carrageenan.[39] However, differences in intestinal bacterial flora are probably responsible for this discrepancy, as germ-free animals do not display carrageenan-induced damage.

Upon further examination, it was discovered that the bacteria that has been linked to facilitating the carrageenan induced damage in animals is a strain of *Bacteroides vulgatus*.[5] This organism is found in much higher concentrations (six times as high) in the faecal cultures of patients with Crohn's disease. When all the data is evaluated, it appears to imply that, while carrageenan can be metabolised into non-damaging components in most human subjects, those individuals with an overgrowth of *Bacteroides vulgatus* may be at risk. Strict avoidance of carrageenan appears warranted at this time for patients with IBD until further research clarifies its safety for these patients.

Extra-gastrointestinal manifestations

Over 100 disorders, known as extra-intestinal lesions (EIL), constitute a diverse group of systemic complications of IBD.[4,40,41] The most common EIL in adults is arthritis, which is found in about 25 per cent of patients. Two types are typically described, the more common being peripheral arthritis affecting the knees, ankles and wrists. Arthritis is more frequently found in patients with colon involvement. Severity of symptoms is typically proportional to disease activity.[4,40,41]

Less frequently, the arthritis affects the spine. Symptoms are low back pain and stiffness with eventual limitation of motion. This EIL occurs predominantly in males and is fairly indistinguishable from typical ankylosing spondylitis. In fact, it may precede the bowel symptoms by several years. There is probably a consistent underlying factor in both the progression of ankylosing spondylitis and IBD.[4,40,41]

Skin manifestations are also common, being seen in approximately 15 per cent of patients. Typical lesions are erythema nodosum, pyoderma gangrenosum and canker sores. Recurrent canker sores occur in approximately 10 per cent of the patients.[4,40,41] Serious liver disease (i.e. sclerosing cholangitis, chronic active hepatitis, cirrhosis, etc.) is also a common EIL, affecting 3–7 per cent of the patients with IBD. If patients are demonstrating liver enzyme abnormalities, substances such as liquorice, silymarin and curcumin are indicated[42–4] (see Chapter 8, Liver support).

Other common EIL are thrombophlebitis, finger clubbing, eye manifestations (episcleritis, iritis and uveitis), kidney stones, gallstones and, in children, failure to grow, thrive and mature normally.[4,40,41]

General nutrition

Many nutritional complications occur during the course of IBD.[45–7] As these can have a significant influence on the well-being, and perhaps also the mortality, of these patients, every effort should be made to ensure optimal nutritional status. The major mechanisms that contribute to nutritional depletion in these patients are listed in the accompanying box.

Causes of malnutrition in inflammatory bowel disease

- Decreased oral intake.
- Disease-induced (pain, diarrhoea, nausea, anorexia).
- Doctor-induced (restrictive diets without supplementation).
- Malabsorption.
- Decreased absorptive surface due to disease or resection.
- Bile salt deficiency after surgical resection.
- Bacterial overgrowth.
- Drugs (e.g. corticosteroids, sulphasalazine, cholestyramine).
- Increased secretion and nutrient loss.
- Protein-losing enteropathy.
- Electrolyte, mineral and trace mineral loss in diarrhoea.
- Increased utilisation and increased requirements.
- Inflammation, fever, infection.
- Increased intestinal cell turnover.

A decreased food intake is the most important mechanism of nutritional deficiency in these patients, and deficient calorie intake is the most common nutritional deficit in patients requiring hospitalisation. Often the patient feels significant pain, diarrhoea, nausea and/or other symptoms after a meal, resulting in a subtle diminution in dietary intake. Weight loss is prevalent in 65 to 75 per cent of IBD patients.[45]

Malabsorption can be anticipated in patients with extensive involvement of the small intestine and in patients who have had surgical resection of segments of the small intestine. Particularly common is fat malabsorption, resulting in significant calorie loss and loss of fat-soluble vitamins and minerals. Involvement of the ileum or resection of that area typically results in bile acid malabsorption. Because of the laxative effect of bile acids on the colon, this may result in a chronic watery diarrhoea. Electrolyte and trace mineral deficiency should be suspected in patients with a history of chronic diarrhoea, while calcium and magnesium deficiency may be a result of chronic steatorrhoea (fatty stools).

Increased secretion and nutrient loss due to the exudative and inflammatory nature of IBD often occur. In particular, there is a significant loss of plasma proteins across the damaged and inflamed mucosa. The loss of protein may exceed the ability of the liver to replace plasma proteins, despite a high protein intake. The chronic loss of blood often leads to iron depletion and anaemia.

The most common drugs used in the allopathic treatment of IBD are corticosteroids and sulphasalazine, both of which increase nutritional needs. Corticosteroids are known to stimulate protein catabolism, depress protein synthesis, decrease the absorption of calcium and phosphorus, increase the urinary excretion of vitamin C, calcium, potassium and zinc, increase blood glucose, serum triglycerides and serum cholesterol, increase the requirements for vitamin B6, ascorbic acid, folate and vitamin D, decrease bone formation and impair wound healing. Sulphasalazine has been shown to inhibit the absorption and transport of folate, decrease serum folate and iron, and increase the urinary excretion of ascorbic acid.[48]

The last consideration in the causes of nutrient deficiency in IBD patients is the nutritional consequences of a chronic inflammatory and/or infectious disease. This topic has not been fully investigated, and the only conclusion that currently can be made is that protein requirement may be increased in patients with acute worsening of IBD. Typically, patients with IBD require perhaps as much as 25 per cent more protein than the usual recommended allowance.[45–7]

Dietary considerations

Principles of nutritional therapy　The importance of correcting nutritional deficiencies in patients with IBD cannot be overstated. Nutrient deficiencies, both macro- and micro-, lead to altered gastrointestinal function and structure, which may result in the patient entering a vicious circle, i.e. the secondary effects of malnutrition on gastrointestinal tract function and structure may lead to a further increase in malabsorption, with a further decrease in nutrient status.

Foremost in nutritional therapy is the provision of an adequate calorie intake. It should be assumed that the majority of patients suffer from micronutrient deficiency, although often the deficiency is subclinical and can only be detected by appropriate laboratory investigation. In general, patients with inflammatory bowel disease should be placed on therapeautic vitamin supplements of at least five times the recommended dietary allowance. Several minerals may also need to be supplemented at equally high levels. Dietary treatment involves the use of either an elemental or an elimination diet (described below).

Elemental diets　The elemental diet has been shown to be an effective non-toxic alternative to corticosteroids as the primary treatment of acute IBD.[14–17] An elemental diet is one that is purported to contain all essential nutrients, with protein being provided only as predigested or free-form amino acids. The improvements noted on an elemental diet are, however, probably not primarily related to nutritional improvement. Although the improvement could be a result of alterations in the faecal flora (which have been noted to occur in patients consuming an elemental diet), a stronger case could be made for a secondary immune mechanism being bypassed during elemental feeding – the elemental diet is serving as an allergy elimination diet.

Hospitalisation is often required for satisfactory administration of elemental diets. Relapse is quite common when patients resume normal eating. An elimination diet, rather than an elemental diet, may be a more acceptable alternative in the treatment of IBD, particularly when treating chronic IBD.

Elimination (oligoantigenic) diets　Although food allergy has long been considered an important causative factor in the development of IBD, it is only recently that there have been studies utilising an elimination diet in the treatment of IBD.[18–20] (Elimination diets are described in Chapter 38, Food allergy.) These studies demonstrate that elimination is the primary therapy of choice in the treatment of chronic IBD. The most common offending foods were found in the studies to be wheat and dairy products.

An alternative approach is to determine the actual allergens by laboratory methods, preferably a method that measures both IgG- and IgE-mediated reactions (IgG and IgE are different types of antibody). The allergens are then either avoided or a rotary diversified diet is used as appropriate (see Chapter 38, Food allergy).

High-complex carbohydrate, high-fibre diet Treatment with a high-fibre diet has been shown to have a favourable effect on the course of Crohn's disease.[13] This is in direct contrast to one of the oldest allopathic dietary treatments of IBD, i.e. a low-fibre diet. Although some foods may be too 'rough' to handle, the dietary treatment of IBD should utilise an unrefined-carbohydrate fibre-rich diet combined with an avoidance or rotary-diversified diet. This latter combination is much more effective than just a high-fibre diet alone.[19]

Dietary fibre has a profound effect on the intestinal environment and is thought to promote a more optimal intestinal flora composition.[49] However, considering the high degree of intolerance to wheat found in patients with IBD, and the known roughness of wheat bran, supplemental wheat bran is not the fibre of choice for these patients.

Nutritional deficiencies

As shown in Table 30.1, the number of nutritional deficiencies is quite high in hospital-ised patients with IBD. Although it is generally agreed that a greater rate of nutritional deficiencies exist in hospitalised patients than outpatients (as these patients typically have a more severe condition), a great number of non-hospitalised patients with Crohn's disease display one or more nutrient deficiency as well.[50] In addition to the deficiencies listed in the table, low levels of vitamin K, copper, niacin and vitamin E have been reported.[45]

Table 30.1 Prevalence of nutritional deficiency in hospitalised patients with inflammatory bowel disease[49]

Deficiency	Prevalence (%)
Hypoalbuminaemia	25–80
Anaemia	60–80
Iron deficiency	40
Low serum vitamin B12	48
Low serum folate	54–64
Low serum magnesium	14–33
Low serum potassium	6–20
Low serum retinol	21
Low serum ascorbate	12
Low serum 25-OH-vitamin D	25–65
Low serum zinc	40–50

Zinc Zinc deficiency is a well known complication of Crohn's disease, due to low dietary intake, poor absorption and excess faecal losses.[45,46,51] Evidence of zinc deficiency occurs in approximately 45 per cent of Crohn's disease patients.[51] Low zinc concentrations in the blood, low hair zinc levels, malabsorption of zinc, altered urinary excretion of zinc and impaired taste acuity are commonly found in Crohn's disease patients.[45,51] In addition, many of the complications of the disease may be a direct result of zinc deficiency – the complications of poor healing of fissures and fistulas, skin lesions, hypogonadism, growth retardation, retinal dysfunction, depressed immunity and anorexia.[51-3]

Many patients will not respond to oral or intravenous zinc supplementation, as there appears to be a defect in tissue transport. Intravenous supplementation results in a tremendous increase in urinary excretion but insignificant clinical results. Several clinical trials using oral zinc sulphate have shown the same lack of results.[54]

Supplying zinc as a picolinate may be more advantageous, possibly improving both intestinal absorption and tissue transport. Zinc citrate may also be an appropriate alternative. In any event, every attempt should be made to ensure adequate tissue stores of zinc are maintained, as disease activity is correlated with zinc deficiency. This may necessitate administration by injection in some cases. Although less than ideal, intravenous zinc is often the only way to attain even marginal zinc levels in patients with Crohn's disease.[54]

Magnesium Magnesium deficiency is quite prevalent in patients with IBD.[45,55,56] Patients with low magnesium levels may present with weakness, anorexia, low blood pressure, confusion, hyperirritability, tetany, convulsions and electrocardiographic or electroencephalographic abnormalities.[45]

A daily intravenous dose of 200–400 mg elemental magnesium may be necessary for those not responding to oral supplementation. Individuals with IBD may require this route of supplementation due to magnesium's laxative action. Oral supplementation should be with magnesium chelates (i.e. citrate, aspartate, etc.), rather than inorganic magnesium salts (i.e. carbonate).

Iron Iron deficiency anaemia is very frequent in IBD, largely because of chronic blood loss through the gut.[45] There should be an attempt to increase iron stores by improving absorption, as with supplemental vitamin C, rather than through direct iron supplementation, since iron promotes intestinal infection.[57]

Calcium Patients with IBD are also at risk of developing calcium deficiency. This is probably due to several factors – loss of absorptive surfaces, malabsorption, corticosteroid use and vitamin D deficiency.[45]

Potassium Diarrhoea is often associated with potassium and other electrolyte deficiencies. Although symptoms of potassium deficiency are quite rare in patients with IBD, levels are probably below optimum. In one study, nutritional support to correct potassium deficiency resulted in significantly reduced rates of surgical complications.[58]

Vitamin A   Low serum vitamin A levels are found in approximately 20 per cent of Crohn's disease patients and are correlated with the activity of the disease.[45,53] Vitamin A can profoundly affect the metabolism of the intestinal mucosa, since it can increase the number of mucus-producing goblet cells, increase the production of mucins, increase the secretion of mucus and restore normal barrier function.

Preliminary case reports have indicated that vitamin A may be useful therapeutically in Crohn's disease.[59,60] However, long-term controlled trials have indicated that vitamin A (50,000 iu twice daily) had no therapeautic effect in the majority of Crohn's disease cases.[61,62] It should be kept in mind, however, that certain patients may respond to vitamin A therapy, and that zinc supplementation will often normalise disturbances of vitamin A metabolism.[53]

Vitamin D   There is evidence that vitamin D deficiency is quite common in IBD patients, particularly in those patients with other signs of nutritional deficiency.[45,63] Patients with IBD are at an increased risk for the development of metabolic bone diseases, such as osteoporosis and osteomalacia. This relates to previously mentioned factors regarding calcium.

Vitamin E   Vitamin E deficiency can occur in IBD, as observed in one case report.[64] The patient had a 25-year history of Crohn's disease, with multiple small bowel resections. Presenting symptoms relating to vitamin E deficiency included visual disturbances, generalised motor weakness and nervous system abnormalities. Supplementation with 270 iu per day eventually brought complete recovery over a period of two years. Vitamin E supplementation is also indicated due to its ability to inhibit inflammation and reduce free radical damage.[65]

Vitamin K   Vitamin K deficiency is quite common in patients with IBD.[66,67]

Folic acid   Low serum concentrations of folic acid are quite common in IBD, with reports of occurrence ranging between 25 and 64 per cent.[45,68–70] The drug sulphasalazine worsens the condition by interfering with folate absorption and metabolism.[48] A folate deficiency promotes further malabsorption due to altered structure of the intestinal mucosal cells.[71] These cells have a very rapid turnover (one to four days) and need to have a constant supply of folic acid.

Vitamin B12   Since vitamin B12 is absorbed at the portion of the intestine most commonly affected with Crohn's disease, i.e. the terminal ileum, deficiency is quite common.[45,72] Overall, abnormal B12 absorption is found in 48 per cent of patients with Crohn's disease. Often the terminal ileum is surgically removed (resected). If the length of the resection is less than 60 cm, or the extent of the inflammatory lesion is less than 60 cm, adequate absorption may occur.

Vitamin C   A low vitamin C intake is common in patients with IBD, particularly in those patients on a low fibre diet.[45,73] Vitamin C levels in the blood and tissues are significantly lower in patients with Crohn's disease than in matched controls.[45,73]

Vitamin C is thought to be particularly important in the prevention of fistula formation (a fistula is an abnormal passageway between two organs, e.g. the colon and the bladder). It has been shown that patients with fistulas have lower ascorbic acid levels than patients without fistulas.[74]

Other nutrients   Obviously, patients with IBD are at risk of developing any nutrient deficiency, including nutrients not discussed above. However, there is probably no real need for laboratory investigation to determine micronutrient deficiencies, other than for those nutrients discussed above.[45]

Botanical medicines

Flavonoids   Several plant flavonoids appear to be particularly indicated in the treatment of IBD. Flavonoids, in general, are considered natural biological response modifiers.[75,76] Quercetin, perhaps the most pharmacologically active flavonoid, has remarkable effects on a variety of enzyme systems.[75,76] Pharmacokinetic studies with radioactive quercetin in rats have shown that absorbed quercetin is concentrated in lung tissue (12 per cent of the oral dose) and in the wall of the large intestine (3 per cent of dose).[77] Many of the enzymes affected by quercetin and other flavonoids are important in processes associated with the inflammatory response, i.e. the release of histamine and other inflammatory mediators from mast cells, basophils, neutrophils and macrophages, migration and infiltration of leucocytes, and smooth muscle contraction.

Composition of Bastyr's Formula

8 parts *Althaea officinalis*
4 parts *Baptisia tinctora*
8 parts *Echinacea angustifolia*
8 parts *Geranium maculatum*
8 parts *Hydrastis canadensis*
8 parts *Phytolacca americana*
8 parts *Ulmus fulva*
8 parts cabbage powder
2 parts pancreatin
1 part niacinamide
2 parts duodenal substance

Bastyr's Formula (modified Robert's Formula)   Although no research has been done to document its efficacy, an old naturopathic remedy, Robert's Formula, has a long history of use in IBD. It is composed of several botanical medicines:

- *Althaea officinalis*, marsh mallow root, a demulcent with soothing properties on the mucous membranes.
- *Baptisia tinctora*, wild indigo, used for gastrointestinal infections.
- *Echinacea angustifolia*, purple coneflower – antibacterial and used to promote normalisation of the immune system.
- *Geranium maculatum*, a gastrointestinal haemostatic.
- *Hydrastis canadensis*, goldenseal – inhibits the growth of many disease-causing bacteria.
- *Phytolacca americana*, poke root – used for healing ulcerations of the intestinal mucosa.
- *Symphytum officinale*, comfrey – anti-inflammatory, as well as promoting tissue growth and wound healing.
- *Ulmus fulva*, slippery elm, for its demulcent effect.
- Cabbage powder is included because of its documented ability to heal gastro-intestinal ulcers (see Chapter 71, Ulcers).
- Pancreatin is used to assist in the digestive process.
- Niacinamide is used for its anti-inflammatory effects.
- And duodenal substance is used because it too heals gastrointestinal ulcers.[78–80]

Monitoring and evaluation

Crohn's disease activity index (CDAI)

The Crohn's disease activity index was developed as a monitoring tool in the National Cooperative Crohn's Disease Study.[48] It met the basic requirements necessary for the study, i.e. it provided uniform clinical parameters which could be assessed, and produced a consistent numerical index for recording the results of the study from several centres over a period of several years.

The CDAI is calculated by adding together eight variables (see box). It incorporates both subjective and objective information in determining relative disease activity. When the patient returns with the completed form, the calculation of disease activity can be completed. Generally speaking, CDAI scores below 150 indicate a better prognosis than higher scores. The CDAI is a very useful way to monitor therapeutic progress.

Monitoring of the paediatric patient

The paediatric patient with IBD presents a particularly difficult problem in that it is often very difficult to achieve normal growth and development. Growth failure occurs in 75 per cent of Crohn's disease paediatric patients, while ulcerative colitis causes growth failure in 25 per cent.[47] The paediatric patient with IBD should be evaluated at least twice yearly. Evaluation should include the pertinent history, clinical anthro-pometry, Tanner staging (a system of noting sexual development) and appropriate laboratory testing. The box on page 252 outlines the necessary components of a comprehensive bi-yearly nutritional evaluation in paediatric patients with IBD. An

---

Independent variables and formula used to calculate the CDAI[48]

x_1 Number of liquid or very soft stools in 1 week.

x_2 Sum of 7 daily abdominal pain ratings:
         0 = none, 1 = mild, 2 = moderate, 3 = severe.

x_3 Sum of 7 daily ratings of general well-being:
         0 = well, 1 = slightly below par, 2 = poor, 3 = very poor,
         4 = terrible.

x_4 Symptoms or findings presumed related to Crohn's disease:
- Arthritis or arthralgia.
- Iritis or uveitis.
- Erythema nodosum, pyoderma gangrenosum, aphthous stomatitis.
- Anal fissure, fistula or perirectal abscess.
- Other bowel-related fistula.
- Febrile episode > 100 °F, 38 °C during past week.

         Add 1 for each category corresponding to patient's symptoms.

x_5 Taking Lomotil or opiates for diarrhoea:
         0 = no, 1 = yes.

x_6 Abdominal mass:
         0 = none, 0.4 = questionable, 1 = present.

x_7 47 minus haematocrit, males; 42 minus haematocrit, females.

x_8 100 × (Standard weight − Body weight)/Standard weight.

$$CDAI = 2x_1 + 5x_2 + 7x_3 + 20x_4 + 30x_5 + 10x_6 + 6x_7 + x_8$$

aggressive nutritional programme should be instituted, including supplements (it may be necessary to use enteral or parenteral methods in some patients), that is similar to the approach outlined for the adult patient, with the doses adjusted as appropriate.

The CDAI is not as accurate in monitoring the disease in children as it is in adults. To overcome this shortcoming, Lloyd-Still and Green devised a clinical scoring system for IBD in children.[65] The scoring system is divided into five major divisions (the maximum score in parentheses): general activity (10), physical examination and clinical complications (30), nutrition (20), X-rays (15) and laboratory (25). An elevated score (i.e. scores in the 80s) represents good status, while scores in the 30s and 40s represent severe disease. Table 30.2 outlines the determination of clinical score.

Treatment

It is important to recognise that in some individuals these are life threatening diseases which at times require emergency treatment. A small percentage of patients who have severe disease may experience severe worsenings requiring hospitalisation. This is more common in patients with ulcerative colitis, who typically present with a fever of

> **Monitoring the paediatric patient with IBD**
>
> - Type and duration of inflammatory bowel disease, frequency of relapses.
> - Severity and extent of ongoing symptoms.
> - Medication history.
> - Three-day diet diary.
> - Physical examination
>   Height, weight, arm circumference, triceps skinfold measurements.
>   Loss of subcutaneous fat, muscle wasting, oedema, pallor, skin rash, hepatomegaly.
> - Laboratory tests
>   CBC and differential, reticulocyte and platelet count, sedimentation rate, urinalysis.
>   Serum total proteins, albumin, globulin and retinol binding protein.
>   Serum electrolytes, calcium, phosphate, ferritin, folate, carotenes, tocopherol and B12.
>   Leucocyte ascorbate, magnesium and zinc.
>   Creatinine height index, BUN: creatinine ratio.

101 °F, 38.5 °C, or higher, profuse, constant, loose, bloody stools, anorexia, apathy and prostration, and a distended abdomen.

For the typical patient, IBD is a chronic disease requiring long-term therapy and follow-up. The first step is to identify and remove all factors which may be initiating or aggravating the inflammatory reaction, i.e. food allergens and carrageenan. The patient is put on a diet which maximises macro- and micro-nutrients while minimising aggravating foods/non-foods.

A broad-based individualised nutritional supplementation plan constructed by a trained professional is necessary for all patients with IBD. Particularly important are the nutrients zinc, magnesium, folic acid and vitamin A. As appropriate, nutritional supplements are utilised to correct deficiencies, normalise the inflammatory process and promote healing of the damaged mucosa. Botanical medicines are used to promote healing and normalise the intestinal flora.

Diet

All allergens, wheat, corn and dairy products, and carrageenan-containing foods should be eliminated. The diet should be high in complex carbohydrates and fibre and low in sugar and refined carbohydrates.

Supplements

- Multivitamin and mineral supplement.
- Magnesium, 600 mg a day in divided doses.

Table 30.2 Clinical score in chronic IBD in children

Category	Score	
General activity	10	Normal school attendance < 3 bowel movements per day
	5	Lacks endurance 3–5 bowel movements per day Misses < 4 weeks school/year
Physical examination and complications		
Abdomen	10	Normal
	5	Mass
	1	Distension, tenderness
Proctoscope	10	Normal, no fissures
	5	Friability, 1 fissure
	1	Ulcers, bleeding, fistulas, multiple fissures
Arthritis	5	Nil
	3	One joint/arthralgia
	1	Multiple joints
Skin/stomatitis/eyes	5	Normal
	3	Mild stomatitis
	4	Erythema nodosum, pyoderma, severe stomatitis, uveitis
Nutrition		
Height	10	> 2″/year
	5	< optimal %
	1	No growth
X-rays	15	Normal
	10	Ileitis, colitis to splenic flexure
	5	Total colon or ileocaecal involvement
	1	Toxic megacolon or obstruction
Laboratory		
HCT	5	> 40
	3	25–35
	1	< 25
ESR	5	Normal
	3	20–40
	1	> 40
WBC	5	Normal
	3	< 20,000
	1	> 20,000
Albumin	10	Normal
	5	3.0 g/dl
	1	< 2.5 g/dl

- Zinc picolinate, 50 mg a day.
- Vitamin A, 50,000 iu a day.
- Vitamin E, 200 iu a day.

Botanical medicines

- Mixed flavonoids, 500 mg 20 minutes before meals.
- Bastyr's Formula, two to three '00' capsules with each meal.

31

Cystitis

- Burning pain on urination.
- Frequent need to urinate; excessive urge to urinate at night.
- Turbid, foul-smelling or dark urine.
- Lower abdominal pain.

General considerations

Bladder infections in women are surprisingly common: 21 per cent of all women have urinary tract discomfort at least once a year; 37.5 per cent of women with no history of urinary tract infection will have one within 10 years; and 2 to 4 per cent of apparently healthy women have elevated levels of bacteria in their urine, indicative of an unrecognised urinary tract infection. Women with a history of recurrent urinary tract infections will typically have an episode at least once every year.[1] Recurrent bladder infections can be a significant problem for some women since 55 per cent will eventually involve the upper urinary tract, i.e. the kidneys. Recurrent kidney infection can cause progressive damage resulting in scarring and, for some, kidney failure.

Urinary tract infections in males are much less common and in general indicate an anatomical abnormality or a prostate infection. Urinary tract infections are rare in boys (0.05 per cent), while 2 per cent of girls have excessive bacteria in their urine.[2]

Causes

Urine, as it is secreted by the kidneys, is sterile until it reaches the urethra which transports the urine from the bladder to the urethral opening. Bacteria can reach the urinary tract by ascending from the urethra or, much less commonly, through the bloodstream. Bacteria are introduced into the urethra from faecal contamination or, in women, vaginal secretions. Important factors in aiding or perpetuating an ascending infection are anatomical or functional obstructions to flow (allowing pooling of urine) and immune system dysfunction. Free flow, large urine volume, complete emptying of the bladder and optimal immune function are important antibacterial defences.

The body has many defences against bacterial growth in the urinary tract: urine flow tends to wash away bacteria; the surface of the bladder has antimicrobial properties; the pH (acidity or, in this case, alkalinity) of the urine inhibits the growth of many bacteria; the prostatic fluid has many antimicrobial substances; and the body quickly secretes white cells to control the bacteria.[3]

Many factors are associated with increased risk of bladder infections – pregnancy (twice as frequent), sexual intercourse (nuns have 1/10 the incidence), homosexual activity (in males), mechanical trauma or irritation and, perhaps most important, structural abnormalities of the urinary tract which block the free flow of urine. Reflux of infected urine from the bladder into the upper urinary tract is important in the development of kidney infections and the establishment of recurrent infections. Table 31.1 lists the types and frequencies of abnormalities associated with chronic urinary tract infections.

Table 31.1 Results of urologic evaluation of women with persistent bacteria in their urine, recurrent urinary infections or kidney infections[1]

Abnormality	Per cent
Normal	60
Abnormalities of unknown significance	15
Kidney structural abnormalities or scarring	10–20
Kidney stones	2–8
Reflux of urine	20 (children)
	5 (adults)
Hydronephrosis	< 1
Bladder outlet obstruction	< 1
Miscellaneous urinary tract lesions	< 1

Diagnosis

The diagnosis of bladder infection is imprecise since clinical symptoms and the presence of significant amounts of bacteria in the urine do not correlate well. As can be seen from Table 31.2, only 60 per cent of women with the typical symptoms of urinary tract infection actually have significant levels of bacteria in their urine. Equally important, however, is the fact that 20 per cent have the more potentially serious involvement of the upper tract.

In general, the diagnosis is made according to signs and symptoms and urinary findings. Microscopic examination of the infected urine will show high levels of white blood cells and bacteria. Culturing the urine will determine the quantity and type of bacteria involved. As shown in Table 31.3, *E. coli* (from the colon) are by far the most common. The presence of fever, chills and low back pain can indicate involvement of the kidneys. Those with recurrent infections should have specialised X-rays (intravenous urogram) to determine if there is a structural abnormality.

Table 31.2 Results of women presenting with typical urinary tract infection symptoms and no fever, vaginal symptoms or toxicity[4]

Diagnosis	Per cent
Upper urinary tract infection	20
Bladder infection	40
Low levels of bacteria in urethra	16
Urethral chlamydia	8
Unsuspected vaginitis	4
Other (herpes, gonorrhoea, pelvic inflammatory disease, etc.)	12

Therapy

The recommendations given in Chapter 6, Immune support, are appropriate to employ during a bladder infection. Additional and specific botanical medicines are given below.

Botanical medicines

Many herbs have been used through the centuries in the treatment of urinary tract infections. The following are several which have both folk and scientific support for their use.

Cranberry juice Cranberries and cranberry juice have been used to treat bladder infections and have been shown to be quite effective in several clinical studies.[5-7] In one study, 16 ounces (450 g) of cranberry juice per day was shown to produce beneficial effects in 73 per cent of the subjects (44 females and 16 males) with active urinary tract infections.[5] Furthermore, withdrawal of the cranberry juice in the people who benefited resulted in recurrence of bladder infection in 61 per cent.

Table 31.3 Bacteriologic findings in outpatients with urinary tract infections[3]

Bacteria species	Per cent of patients
Escherichia coli	89.2
Proteus miribilis	3.2
Klebsiella pneumonia	2.4
Enterococci	2.0
Staphylococcus saprophyticus	1.6*
Enterobacter aerogenes	0.8
Pseudomonas aeruginosa	0.4

*Recent evidence suggests that this may be more prevalent than currently thought – in sexually active college-age women it may account for as much as 20 per cent of asymptomatic urinary tract infections.

Although many people believe the action of cranberry juice is due to acidifying the urine and the antibacterial effects of a cranberry component hippuric acid,[8,9] these are probably not the major mechanisms of action. In order to acidify the urine at least 1½ pints (1 litre) of cranberry juice would have to be consumed.[8] In addition, the concentration of hippuric acid in the urine as a result of drinking cranberry juice is not sufficient to inhibit bacteria.[8,9]

Recent studies have shown components in cranberry juice to reduce the ability of bacteria to adhere, or stick, to the lining of the bladder and urethra.[10] In order for bacteria to infect they must first adhere to the mucosa. By interfering with adherence, cranberry juice greatly reduces the likelihood of infection and helps the body fight off infection. This is the most likely explanation of cranberry juice's positive effects in bladder infections.

It must be pointed out that most cranberry juices on the market contain one-third cranberry juice mixed with water and sugar. Since sugar has such a detrimental effect on the immune system,[11-13] use of sweetened cranberry juice cannot be recommended.

Bearberry (Uva ursi)   Most research has focused on *Uva ursi*'s (bearberry or upland cranberry) urinary antiseptic component, arbutin, which typically composes 7 to 9 per cent of the leaves. However, crude plant extracts are much more effective medicinally than isolated arbutin.[14] *Uva ursi* is reported to be especially active against *E. coli* and also has diuretic properties.[15-17]

Care must be taken to avoid excessive dosages of *Uva ursi*; as little as 15 grams (½ an ounce) of the dried leaves has been shown to produce toxicity in susceptible individuals. Toxic signs include ringing in the ears, nausea, vomiting, sense of suffocation, shortness of breath, convulsions, delirium and collapse.[14]

Garlic (Allium sativum)   Garlic has been shown to have antimicrobial activity against many disease causing organisms, including those associated with urinary tract infections – *Escherichia coli*, *Proteus spp.*, *Klebsiella pneumonia* and *Staphylococcus spp.*[18-20]

Goldenseal (Hydrastis canadensis)   Goldenseal is one of the most effective of the herbal antimicrobial agents. Its long history of use by herbalists and naturopathic physicians for the treatment of infections is well documented in the scientific literature.[21] Of particular importance here is its efficacy against *Escherichia coli*, *Proteus spp.*, *Klebsiella spp.*, *Staphylococcus spp.*, *Enterobacter aerogenes* (requires large dosage) and *Pseudomonas spp.*[22,23] Hydrastis also works better in an alkaline urine.

Sandalwood oil (Santalum album)   Sandalwood oil is an effective diuretic and urinary tract antiseptic.[16] However, large dosages can be quite toxic.

Treatment

If inadequately treated, bladder infections can become chronic or lead to kidney infections. The care of a physician is strongly encouraged.

General measures

- Drink large amounts of fluids (at least 5 pints, 3 litres, per day) including at least 16 ounces (450 g) of unsweetened cranberry juice per day.
- Urinate after intercourse. Women who develop bladder infections after intercourse should wash their labia and urethra with a strong tea of hydrastis (two tsp per cup) both before and after.

Diet

Avoid all simple sugars, refined carbohydrates, full-strength fruit juice (dilute fruit juice is acceptable) and food allergens. Restrict calories and eat liberal amounts of garlic and onions.

Nutritional supplements

- Vitamin C, 500 mg every two hours.
- Bioflavonoids, 1 g per day.
- Vitamin A, 25,000 iu per day.
- Beta-carotene, 200,000 iu per day.
- Zinc (picolinate), 30 mg per day.

Botanical medicines

Doses three times a day.
- *Uva ursi*
    Dried leaves or as a tea, 1.5 to 4.0 g (approximately 1–2 tsp).
    Freeze-dried leaves, 500 to 1,000 mg.
    Tincture (1:5), 4 to 6 ml (1 to 1.5 tsp).
    Fluid extract (1:1), 0.5 to 2.0 ml (¼ to ½ tsp).
    Powdered solid extract (4:1), 250–500 mg.
- *Hydrastis canadensis* (goldenseal)
    Dried root (or as tea), 1 to 2 g.
    Freeze-dried root, 500 to 1,000 mg.
    Tincture (1:5), 4 to 6 ml (1 to 1.5 tsp).
    Fluid extract (1:1), 0.5 to 2.0 ml (¼ to ½ tsp).
    Powdered solid extract (4:1), 250–500 mg.
- Sandalwood oil, 1–2 drops.

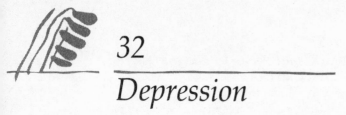

32

Depression

Depression, as defined by the American Psychiatric Association in its *Diagnostic and Statistical Manual of Mental Disorders* (*DSM*-III), is diagnosed according to eight primary criteria:

- Poor appetite with weight loss, or increased appetite with weight gain.
- Insomnia or hypersomnia.
- Physical hyperactivity or inactivity.
- Loss of interest or pleasure in usual activities, or decrease in sexual drive.
- Loss of energy and feelings of fatigue.
- Feelings of worthlessness, self-reproach or inappropriate guilt.
- Diminished ability to think or concentrate.
- Recurrent thoughts of death or suicide.

The presence of five of these eight symptoms definitely indicates depression; the individual with four is probably depressed. According to the *DSM*-III, the depressed state must be present for at least one month to be called depression. In many cases, depression is appropriate to a life event and specific medical treatment is not needed.

General considerations

Many nutritional, environmental and lifestyle factors are discussed in this chapter, and it is important to recognise that they have a much broader scope of therapeutic application than just to depression. This chapter is really a compilation of many chapters that address factors associated with mood disturbance.

As the biochemistry of mood and behaviour have become better understood, many conditions once thought of as having a psychological or sociological cause are now being shown to have a physiological or biochemical basis as well.

Causes

Nearly one in four individuals experiences some degree of clinical depression or mood disorder in their lifetime. The rates are slightly higher in women than men. Currently there are four basic theoretical models of depression[1]:

- The aggression-turned-inward construct which, although apparent in many clinical cases, has no substantial proof.
- The loss model, which postulates that depression is a reaction to the loss of a person, thing, status, self-esteem or even a habit pattern.
- The interpersonal relationship approach, which utilises behavioural concepts, i.e. the person who is depressed uses depression as a way of controlling other people (including doctors). It can be an extension and outgrowth of such simple behaviour as pouting, silence, or ignoring something or someone. It fails to serve the need and the problem worsens.
- The biogenic amine hypothesis, which stresses biochemical derangements characterised by imbalances of amino acids which form neurotransmitters (compounds which transmit information to and from nerve cells).

When an individual's depression is thought to be best defined by one of the first three theories presented above, counselling should be the primary therapy. These individuals will, however, also greatly benefit from supportive nutritional therapy.

The biogenic amine hypothesis has become the primary treatment approach for many practitioners – psychiatrists, allopaths and naturopaths alike. Many of the anti-depressant drugs and the nutritional treatments employed by physicians are designed to correct or lessen suspected imbalances in the biogenic amines (serotonin, melatonin, dopamine, adrenaline and noradrenaline). These compounds are also known as mono-amines. The amino acid tryptophan serves as the precursor to serotonin and melatonin while phenylalanine and tyrosine are precursors to dopamine, adrenaline and noradrenaline.

Therapy

As with most diseases, a general approach to the whole individual must be undertaken before specific therapy is utilised. The approach to a person suffering from any chronic illness is to determine what nutritional, environmental, social and psychological factors are involved in the disease. After the diagnosis of depression has been made by a physician, it is important to rule out the simple organic factors which are known to contribute to the depression, i.e. nutrient deficiency or excess, drugs (prescribed, illicit, alcohol, caffeine, nicotine, etc.), hypoglycaemia, hormonal derangement, allergy, environmental and microbial factors. Each of these is briefly discussed below.

Nutrient deficiency

Virtually any nutrient deficiency can result in depression. Table 32.1 provides a summary of the behavioural changes typically associated with specific vitamin deficiency states.[2] The table is followed by a discussion of tetrahydrobiopterin (a vitamin-like compound found in reduced levels in patients with depression), and some of the vitamins particularly indicated in depression.

Table 32.1 Behavioural effects of some vitamin deficiencies

Deficient vitamin	Behavioural effects
Ascorbic acid	Lassitude, hypochondriasis, depression, hysteria
Biotin	Depression, extreme lassitude, somnolence
Cyanocobalamin	Psychotic states, depression, irritability, confusion, memory loss, hallucinations, delusions, paranoia
Folic acid	Forgetfulness, insomnia, apathy, irritability, depression, psychosis, delirium, dementia
Niacin	Apathy, anxiety, depression, hyperirritability, mania, memory deficits, delirium, organic dementia, emotional lability
Pantothenic acid	Restlessness, irritability, depression, fatigue
Pyridoxine	Depression, irritability, hyperacousia (extremely acute hearing)
Thiamin	Korsakoff's psychosis, mental depression, apathy, anxiety, irritability

Tetrahydrobiopterin   This vitamin-like compound functions as an essential coenzyme in the synthesis of several neurotransmitters.[3] Although not considered a vitamin, functional deficiency states do exist. Patients with depression have been shown to have low levels of tetrahydrobiopterin (BH_4) in their brains.[4-6] These patients typically respond to BH_4 supplementation.[4-6] Although, to the authors' knowledge, BH_4 is not currently available commercially, BH_4 synthesis is stimulated by folic acid, vitamin B12 and ascorbic acid.[4,7]

Folic acid and vitamin B12   As stated above, these vitamins stimulate BH_4 formation and supplementation has been suggested for this reason.[4,7] Furthermore, serum folate and B12 levels are low in a substantial number of patients suffering from various psychiatric syndromes, especially depression.[8-11]

Folic acid deficiency is the most common nutrient deficiency in the world. In studies of psychiatric patients, as many as 30 per cent have been shown to be deficient in folic acid, and in one study 67 per cent of geriatric patients admitted to a psychiatric ward were folate-deficient.[8]

Folate-treated patients with organic psychosis, endogenous depression and schizophrenia fare much better than control subjects not receiving folate. Correction of folate deficiency may result in complete resolution of mental symptoms in some individuals.[8] At the very least, folate supplementation in psychiatric patients has led to a considerable decrease in hospital stays.[8]

The prevalence of B12 deficiency in psychiatric patients is less than that of folic acid.[8-11] Measuring B12 levels in the blood is considered a useful screening measure for psychiatric patients.[8,10] Patients with severe mania and psychosis secondary to B12 deficiency have had complete remission upon B12 supplementation.[11-13]

Folate and B12 are closely associated with methionine metabolism.[14-19] A popular biochemical model of depression concerns decreased brain levels of the methionine derivative S-adenosylmethionine (SAM).[16] Supplemental SAM has been demonstrated to possess significant antidepressant activity in double-blind placebo controlled studies.[18,19] An improvement is usually noted within four to seven days and virtually no side effects have been reported. Supplementing the diet with the amino acid methionine may offer the same benefit as SAM.

SAM, folate and B12 have been shown to influence monoamine metabolism, particularly serotonin metabolism.[14-19] These serotonin-elevating effects are not fully understood, but are undoubtedly responsible for the antidepressive effects of these nutrients. The most common psychological symptoms of B12 and folic acid deficiency are listed in Table 32.1.

Thiamin A vitamin B1 deficiency results in metabolic acidosis and altered brain chemistry.[8] Newly admitted psychiatric patients typically have low levels of vitamin B1 activity, although it is unclear whether this is secondary to malnutrition or an actual feature of disease.[20]

Niacin A niacin deficiency will result in a significant decrease in energy metabolism within the brain. Supplementing niacin could lead to a rise in tryptophan, as niacin is synthesised from tryptophan in the body.[8]

Pyridoxine Vitamin B6 is an important coenzyme in the synthesis of all monoamines.[1] Pyridoxine levels are typically quite low in depressed patients, especially those using oral contraceptives.[8,20-2] Patients with low pyridoxine status usually respond very well to supplementation.[8,20,21,23] Improvement in tryptophan metabolism is generally the mechanism used to explain this effect, although pyridoxine is involved in the synthesis and metabolism of all monoamines.[8]

Drug-induced depression

Depression is often a side effect of drug usage, particularly of substances not often considered drugs, i.e. oral contraceptives, caffeine and cigarettes. Other common drugs associated with depression include corticosteroids, beta-blockers and other blood pressure medications. All these drugs disrupt the normal balance between the monoamines in the brain.

Oral contraceptives The use of oral contraceptives has historically been associated with inducing several nutrient deficiencies, particularly folate, B12, riboflavin, pyridoxine, ascorbic acid and zinc, while iron, copper and vitamin A levels are typically increased.[2] These findings suggest decreased liver metabolism of these substances. (The many effects of oestrogen on mood are discussed extensively in Chapter 62, Premenstrual syndrome.)

Oestrogens further affect mood by disturbing vitamin B6 and tryptophan metabolism, and blood sugar metabolism.[2,8,20,21,23] Many of the side effects of oral contraceptive use can be corrected or reversed by vitamin B6 supplementation,[2,8,24,25]

Caffeine Caffeine is the most widely used drug in our society. Caffeine is everywhere – in coffee, tea and colas, and in over-the-counter drugs such as stimulants and analgesics. The average American consumes 150–225 mg of caffeine per day, 75 per cent of which comes from coffee.[26] A typical cup of coffee contains between 50 and 150 mg, while a cup of tea contains 50 mg and a 12-ounce cola contains about 35 mg.

Even though the average consumption is only 150–225 mg per day, some people consume an excess of 7,500 mg per day.[26] This has led to the term 'caffeinism' to describe a clinical syndrome similar to generalised anxiety and panic disorders, including such symptoms as depression, nervousness, heart palpitations, irritability, recurrent headache, twitching and the so-called 'restless leg syndrome'.[27-30] The intake of caffeine has also been positively correlated with the degree of mental illness in psychiatric patients.

Smoking Smoking affects behaviour through the actions of carbon monoxide (a known toxin to the brain) and nicotine and the induction of low vitamin C levels.[31-5] A low level of vitamin C contributes to the classical 'neurotic triad' of hypochondriasis, depression and hysteria.[33]

Nicotine stimulates adrenal hormone secretion, including increased adrenaline and cortisol secretion.[34] This is compounded by the fact that cigarette smoking is positively associated with increased sugar and caffeine consumption.[35] The effects of reactive hypoglycaemia and caffeine are discussed below. The adrenal hormone cortisol inhibits the uptake of tryptophan by the brain (this is discussed below) resulting in decreased serotonin activity in the brain.

Many strategies have been adopted to aid the individual in his/her attempt to quit smoking. Both psychological techniques and nicotine chewing gum replacement yield similar success rates, about 38 per cent.[36,37] Hypnosis may be effective in some instances.[38] The withdrawal symptoms of irritability, hunger, inability to concentrate and craving for cigarettes usually appear within 24 hours after cessation of smoking and continue for two weeks or more. Chewing gum that provides 2 mg of nicotine has been shown to be effective in alleviating these symptoms.[36] It is assumed that lobeline, as supplied from *Lobelia inflata*, would have similar effects on withdrawal symptoms, due to its similarity to nicotine. *Avena sativa* (oats) has also been reported to be of great value in helping the patient kick the habit.[39]

Hypoglycaemia

The brain is highly dependent on glucose (blood sugar) as an energy source. A drop in blood glucose levels results in the release of hormones which increase blood sugar levels, i.e. adrenaline, glucagon, cortisol and growth hormone. It appears that only adrenaline produces the physical symptoms of hypoglycaemia – sweating, tremor, increased heart rate, anxiety and hunger. If the onset of hypoglycaemia is sudden, these symptoms predominate. If, however, the onset is gradual, this physical phase may not be recognised. Instead symptoms such as dizziness, headache, clouding of vision, blunted mental acuity, emotional instability, confusion and abnormal behaviour predominate.[40]

There has been much controversy over the prevalence of hypoglycaemia in the United States. This is due largely to the inadequacies of the 5-hour glucose tolerance test (GTT), the standard laboratory test used in the diagnosis of hypoglycaemia.[41,42] It has been suggested that this somewhat stressful ordeal for the patient be abandoned as a diagnostic tool.[41] However, despite the inadequacy of GTT, psychiatric patients do have a higher incidence of hypoglycaemia as determined by GTT.[42-5] Correction of any underlying disturbance in glucose metabolism is the first step in treating psychiatric patients.

Hormonal factors in depression

Many hormones are known to influence mood; however, it is beyond the scope of this text to address all of them. Instead, the focus will be on the effects of the thyroid and adrenal hormones.

Thyroid function Low thyroid function and depression are closely tied, but whether the low thyroid function is a result of depression or the depression a result of low thyroid function remains to be definitively determined. It is probably a combination. Depressive illness is often a first or early manifestation of thyroid disease, as even subtle decreases in available thyroid hormone are suspected of producing symptoms of depression.[46,47] Depressed patients should be screened for hypothyroidism, particularly if they complain of fatigue as well.[49] (See Chapter 49, Hypothyroidism, for further discussion.)

Adrenal function Like the thyroid gland, dysfunction of the adrenal gland is closely associated with depression. Defects in adrenal function observed in depressed subjects include excessive cortisol secretion, abnormal nocturnal release of cortisol and inadequate suppression of the secretion of cortisone by the drug dexamethasone.[48]

The psychological effects of increased adrenal release of cortisol mirror the effects of orally administered corticosteroid drugs – depression, mania, nervousness, insomnia and schizophrenia.[30] The effects of corticosteroids on mood are related to their shunting of tryptophan away from serotonin synthesis.[49]

For information on the ways to improve adrenal gland function see Chapter 10, Stress.

Allergy

The idea that food and environmental allergy can produce psychological symptoms is not a new one. However, it is an idea not generally well accepted by orthodox medical practitioners and is discussed more extensively in lay publications. The evidence, although largely based on personal testimonials, is documented by a few controlled studies.[50] For more detail on food allergies see Chapter 38, Food allergy.

Environmental factors

Many environmental factors can produce psychological symptoms, particularly chronic exposure to solvents and heavy metals.[51-5] Hair mineral analysis is an accurate and cost-effective method of detecting these toxic substances and should be employed to aid diagnosis.

Exposure to numerous solvents, such as those used in paints, furniture making and boat building, has been reported to produce psychological symptoms, including depression.[53,54] Virtually any toxic chemical or environmental exposure is capable of producing psychological symptoms.[51] The diagnosis of an environmentally induced depression rests largely on a detailed medical history.

Candidiasis

Much attention has been focused on intestinal overgrowth of the yeast *Candida albicans*.[56] Virtually every symptom imaginable has been purported to be a result of candidiasis, although at the time of writing, the reports are largely anecdotal. It may be the causative factor in a wide variety of illnesses, or it may be representative of a deeper disorder, possibly of the immune system or liver.

Candida is believed to induce a wide variety of mental and neurological manifestations.[56] These may be due to disturbed intestinal flora or reduced hepatic clearance of candidal antigens and/or byproducts. (See Chapter 21, Candidiasis, for further discussion.)

Monoamine metabolism and precursor therapy in depression

The use of monoamine precursors has offered a more natural way of influencing monoamine metabolism than prescribed antidepressant drugs like monoamine oxidase inhibitors and tricyclic antidepressants. The amino acid tryptophan serves as the precursor to serotonin and melatonin while phenylalanine and tyrosine are precursors to dopamine, adrenaline and noradrenaline.

Clinical double-blind studies have demonstrated that precursor therapy is as effective as imipramine and far superior to unilateral electroconvulsive therapy.[57–62] Other studies have, however, demonstrated that there is an inconsistency of therapeutic effect in using monoamine precursors and that these substances offer little more than a placebo response.[58–60] This is apparently the result of inappropriate dosage, the use of the wrong precursor, interfering metabolic factors or factors other than an imbalance in monoamine activity being responsible for the depression. Tryptophan, phenylalanine and tyrosine are discussed briefly below.

Tryptophan The basic premise of tryptophan supplementation in depression is that there is a deficiency of serotonin within the brain of depressed individuals. The synthesis of central nervous system (brain and spinal cord) serotonin is entirely dependent on blood tryptophan levels, particularly unbound or free tryptophan levels.[58–62] Low serum tryptophan levels lead to reduced brain serotonin and melatonin synthesis.

Tryptophan transport into the brain may also be inhibited in depressed patients.[58–63] Tryptophan shares the transport system with the other large neutral amino acids, i.e. leucine, isoleucine, valine, tyrosine and phenylalanine. The quantity of these other amino acids in food is usually much greater than the amount of tryptophan. Therefore, a protein-rich meal will result in decreased brain tryptophan uptake. In contrast, a carbohydrate rich meal will result in increased tryptophan uptake via the lack of competing amino acids and the effects of insulin.

Supplementation with tryptophan has resulted in mixed results.[60] There are many variables to be considered when evaluating controlled studies of tryptophan supplementation, such as study size, duration and dosage. At this time the inconsistent results from studies utilising tryptophan appear to be due to a failure to address important considerations related to the nature of the depression and the factors affecting brain uptake of tryptophan. The use of tryptophan alone as the sole therapy is not as effective as when used in conjunction with other critical nutrients; in some cases tryptophan used by itself may worsen the condition. Tryptophan may also offer considerable benefit to depressed patients with sleep disorders, as it has been shown to be an effective sleep promoter (see Chapter 50, Insomnia).

Phenylalanine and tyrosine   Although the number of clinical studies utilising phenylalanine or tyrosine for depression does not approach the number using tryptophan, there is evidence that these monoamine precursors may be effective in some individuals.[57,64,65]

Phenylalanine can be converted to phenylethylamine (PEA).[64] This compound has amphetamine-like stimulant properties and is suggested to be an endogenous stimulatory or antidepressive substance in humans.[64] PEA is found in high concentrations in chocolate and is associated with the feeling of love, which might explain chocolate's addictiveness and association with romance.

Low PEA levels are found in depressed patients, while high levels are found in schizophrenia.[64,65] Phenylalanine, both D- and L- forms, has been demonstrated to increase urinary PEA output and CNS (central nervous system) PEA concentrations.[64]

The pharmacological activity of supplemental tyrosine in depressives may also be related to its increasing of trace amine levels (octopamine, tyramine and PEA), rather than just its enhancing of monoamine synthesis or possibly stimulating thyroid hormone synthesis.[64] Low blood tyrosine levels are seen in some depressed individuals.[57,65] Clinical studies using phenylalanine and/or tyrosine for depression indicate that phenylalanine and tyrosine supplementation offer encouraging alternatives to prescribed antidepressants.[64-5]

Exercise

The value of an exercise programme in the therapy of depression cannot be overstated. Exercise alone has been demonstrated to have a tremendous impact on improving mood and the ability to handle stress.[66] In a recent study it was found that increased participation in exercise, sports and physical activities is strongly associated with decreased symptoms of depression (feelings that life is not worthwhile, low spirits, etc.), anxiety (restlessness, tension, etc.) and malaise (rundown feeling, insomnia, etc.).[67]

It appears exercise is a critical component of a happy as well as a healthy life.

Treatment

As is obvious from the above discussion, full understanding of the causes of depression has not yet been achieved. However, many important potentially controllable factors have now been identified, and most individuals can be helped. Treatment is largely dependent upon accurate determination of which factors are contributing to the patient's depression, balancing of errant neurotransmitter levels and optimising the patient's nutrition, lifestyle and psychological health.

Diet

Eliminate or rotate allergic foods (see Chapter 38, Food allergy), prevent hypoglycaemia and eliminate all sources of caffeine and aspartame.

Lifestyle

Adopt a regular exercise programme (at least 30 minutes of physical activity sufficient to elevate the heart rate by 50 per cent three times a week). Eliminate smoking, oral contraceptives and caffeine.

Supplements

In general, dependent upon needs.
- B-vitamin complex, 50 times the recommended dietary allowance.
- Vitamin C, 1 gram three times daily.
- Folic acid, 400 μg a day.
- Vitamin B12, 250–1,000 μg a day.
- Magnesium, 500 mg daily.
- Amino acids – best if dosage is determined by a physician:
    Tryptophan, 6 grams per day.
    DLPA (D,L-phenylalanine), 400 mg a day.

Botanical Medicines

- St John's Wort   *(Hypericum perforatum)*

One of St John's Wort's most popular historical uses was as a mood elevator in cases of depression and other psychiatric illness. Researchers have discovered that components in St John's Wort do, in fact, alter brain chemistry in a way which improves mood.

A clinical study of 15 women with depression demonstrated that a standardised extract of St John's Wort led to significant improvement in symptoms of anxiety, depression, and feelings, of worthlessness.[*] In addition, the extract greatly improved the quality of sleep as it was effective in relieving both insomnia and hypersomnia (excessive sleep).

Take in doses three times a day:
    Dried herb, 2–4 g, or as tea tincture (1:5), 8–12 ml.
    Fluid extract (1:1), 2–4 ml.
    Solid (dry powdered) extract (4:1), 500–1,000 mg.

---

[*]Muldner, V. H. and Zoller, M. 'Antidepressive wirkung eines auf den wirkstoffkomplex hyperican standardisierten', *Arzneim Forsch*, 1984, 34, p.918.

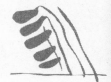

33

Diabetes mellitus

The National Diabetes Data Group of the US National Institutes of Health recommends the following criteria in diagnosing diabetes:

- Fasting (overnight) blood glucose concentration greater than or equal to 140 mg/dl on at least two separate occasions.
- Following ingestion of 75 g of glucose, blood glucose concentration greater than or equal to 200 mg/dl at two hours post ingestion and at least one other sample during the two hour test.
- Classic symptoms of frequent urination, excessive thirst and appetite.

General considerations

Diabetes mellitus, perhaps more than any other disease, is strongly associated with western culture and diet.[1] Diabetes is the most common of the serious metabolic diseases of humans. It is a chronic disorder of carbohydrate, fat and protein metabolism, characterised by fasting elevations of blood glucose levels and a greatly increased risk of atherosclerosis, kidney disease and loss of nerve function.[1]

The National Diabetes Data Group (NDDG) of the US National Institutes of Health distinguishes the following subclasses of diabetes:

- Insulin-dependent diabetes mellitus (IDDM or type 1) – this type of diabetes is associated with juvenile onset and complete destruction of the beta-cells of the pancreas which manufacture insulin.
- Non-insulin dependent diabetes mellitus (NIDDM or type 2) – NIDDM usually has an adult onset. It is subdivided into two subgroups, obese NIDDM and non-obese NIDDM.
- Secondary diabetes – this is associated with certain conditions and syndromes such as pancreatic disease, hormone disturbances, insulin receptor abnormalities, drug-induced diabetes, genetic syndromes and malnourished populations.
- Gestational diabetes, due to the glucose intolerance of some women during pregnancy.

- Impaired glucose tolerance (IGT) – this group includes such terms as prediabetic, chemical, latent, borderline, subclinical and asymptomatic, used to describe individuals whose plasma glucose levels and responses to glucose are intermediate, between normal and those that are clearly abnormal.

The percentage of individuals with diabetes in the United States is estimated at 4 per cent, of which 90 per cent are type 2 and the rest type 1. The prevalence of diabetes is rising and is now the seventh leading cause of death in the US. At the current rate of increase (6 per cent per year) the number of diabetics will double every 15 years.[2,3]

Diabetes has been linked to the western lifestyle as it is uncommon in cultures consuming a more 'primitive' diet.[1] As cultures switch from their native diets to the foods of commerce, their rate of diabetes increases, eventually reaching the same proportions seen in western societies.[1]

Although genetics appears important in susceptibility to diabetes, environmental and dietary factors are important in its development. Many have been identified. A diet high in refined fibre-depleted carbohydrate is believed to be the culprit in many individuals, while a high intake of high-fibre complex carbohydrate-rich foods is protective against diabetes.[1,4]

Obesity is another significant environmental factor, particularly considering the fact that 90 per cent of NIDDM type 2 sufferers are obese.[2] Even in normal individuals, significant weight gain results in carbohydrate intolerance, higher insulin levels and insulin insensitivity in fat and muscle tissue. The progressive development of insulin insensitivity (which will be discussed in more detail later) is believed to be the underlying factor in the genesis of type 2 diabetes. Weight loss corrects all of these abnormalities and significantly improves the metabolic disturbances of diabetes.[2,5]

Insulin-dependent diabetes

Type 1 diabetes is generally acknowledged to be due to an insulin deficiency.[2,3] Although the exact cause is unknown, current theory suggests it is due to a hereditary predisposition to injury to the pancreatic beta cells coupled with some defect in tissue regeneration capacity. The beta cells are responsible for producing and secreting insulin. Causes of injury are most likely due to free radicals, viral infection and auto-immune reactions. Alloxan, a uric acid derivative, is a potent beta-cell toxin and is used to induce experimental diabetes in animals.[6]

Streptozotocin This N-nitroso compound has now replaced alloxan as the preferred agent for destruction of beta cells in the induction of diabetes in experimental animals.[6] Circumstantial evidence suggests that dietary intake of the N-nitroso compounds found in smoked/cured meats can cause diabetes in susceptible individuals, producing beta-cell damage by the same mechanism as streptozocin.[7] Many other chemicals have also been implicated in beta-cell damage.[8]

Viral infection Recent evidence has strengthened the hypothesis of a viral cause of type 1 diabetes in some cases.[2,3] A viral cause was first suspected due to the seasonal variation in the onset of the disease (October to March). During these months, viral diseases such as mumps, hepatitis, infectious mononucleosis, congenital rubella and coxsackie virus are much more prevalent. Viruses are capable of infecting pancreatic beta cells and inducing diabetes.

Autoimmunity   Autoimmune factors may also be causative in many cases.[2,3] Antibodies to pancreatic cells are present in 75 per cent of all cases of type 1 diabetes, compared to 0.5 to 2.0 per cent of normals. The antibody levels decline progressively after the first few weeks of the disease, suggesting complete beta cell destruction.

It is probable that the antibodies to the beta cells develop in response to cell destruction due to other mechanisms (chemical, viral, etc.). It appears that normal individuals either do not develop as severe an antibody reaction, or are better able to repair the damage once it occurs.

In summary, type 1 diabetes is characterised by decreased insulin synthesis and/or secretion as a result of beta cell destruction caused by chemical, viral or antibody damage in susceptible individuals.

Non-insulin-dependent diabetes

Central to the development of type 2 diabetes is insulin insensitivity. This is evidenced by typically high levels of circulating insulin and the reversibility of blood sugar elevation by dietary changes and/or weight loss sufficient to restore insulin sensitivity.[2,3,5]

Chromium   Considerable evidence now indicates that chromium levels are a major determinant of insulin sensitivity.[9-14] Chromium, an essential micronutrient, functions as a cofactor in all insulin-regulating activities.[11,13] Its deficiency is widespread in the US.

Trivalent chromium (C^{3+}) is the only form of chromium that exhibits biological activity.[11] It is an integral component of the so-called glucose tolerance factor (GTF). This compound also contains two molecules of nicotinic acid, cysteine, glutamine and glycine.[14] Supplemental chromium, in the form of brewer's yeast (9 g daily) or chromium chloride (200 μg daily), significantly improve glucose tolerance, decreases fasting glucose, cholesterol and triglyceride levels and increases the HDL-cholesterol level by increasing insulin sensitivity in normal, elderly and type 2 diabetic patients.[9-14] It is not, however, a panacea for type 2 diabetic patients, since double blind studies of chromium alone have yielded conflicting results.[15]

Obesity   One factor in the origin of diabetes that is without dispute is the effect of obsesity on the condition.[1-3,5,16,17] As stated earlier, obesity is associated with insulin insensitivity, and the amount of fat and its distribution also seem to be important.[16,17]

Using cellular criteria, two types of obesity have been identified, hypertrophic obesity (enlarged fat cells) and hyperplastic obesity (increased number of fat cells). The hypertrophic form is more closely associated with the metabolic complications associated with obesity, i.e. diabetes, glucose intolerance, hypertension, hyperlipidaemia, etc.

Another system of categorising obesity is based on fat distribution and also results in two subgroups, android type (deposition in the upper body, i.e. abdomen, typical in the obese male) and gynaecoid type (with distribution in the lower body, i.e. gluteal and femoral, most common in the obese female). The abdominal fat cell activity is affected by plasma insulin and triglyceride levels, while the gluteal and femoral adipocytes are more sensitive to certain steroidal hormones such as corticosteroids and oestrogen. The incidence of diabetes is higher in both men and women with the hypertrophic, android-type obesity.[16,17]

Weight loss, in particular a significant decrease in body fat percentage, is a prime objective in treating the majority of type 2 diabetic patients since it improves all aspects of diabetes and may result in 'cure'.[18,19]

Prenatal factors   Recent evidence supports the concept that prenatal nutrition, in particular hyperglycaemia, may be a promoter of diabetes later in life. Studies done in Berlin have shown that adults born during the 'hypocaloric war and post-war period (1941–48)' have significantly less diabetes than those born during the relatively hyper-caloric years before and after. This is not a minor correlation, as the data show a greater than 50 per cent drop in the incidence of diabetes.[20]

Another study shows a significantly lower incidence of childhood diabetes during periods in which maternal elevations in blood glucose were carefully controlled and the foetus protected from elevations in insulin.[20] Although the data in this study is based on a number of suppositions, they again indicate a greater than 50 per cent drop in the incidence of childhood diabetes when the mother's blood glucose levels are controlled.

Monitoring the diabetic individual

There appears to be a causal relationship between the degree of blood glucose elevation (hyperglycaemia) and the development of the complications of diabetes (discussed below). Therefore monitoring and controlling the degree of hyperglycaemia is critical to the prevention of the major diabetic complications. The adequacy of control can be determined by several simple techniques.

Home glucose monitoring   The advent of home glucose monitoring, using reagent strips and capillary blood, has brought about major improvements in the care of diabetes. A sample can be obtained by the use of a simple spring-triggered device equipped with a disposable lancet, the best sites being the outsides of the fingers (taking care to avoid the nailbeds). Glucose levels are then determined by placing the sample on a reagent strip and measuring the colour change using a commercially available reflectance meter. There are also reagent strips that give satisfactory values by visual inspection using a dual-colour scale.

Glucose tolerance test   The GTT is a very sensitive test for diabetes. However, it is also very stressful to the patient. The National Diabetes Data Group recommends giving a 75 gram glucose dose, dissolved in 300 ml of water, for adults (1.75 g/kg ideal body weight for children) after an overnight fast in subjects who have been consuming at least 150 grams of carbohydrate daily for three days prior to the test. The patient is considered normal if the two-hour blood glucose is less than 140 mg/dl and no value exceeds 200 mg/dl. A confirmatory diagnosis of diabetes requires that blood levels be above 200 mg/dl at both two hours and at least once between zero time and two hours.[8]

Medications that impair glucose tolerance (diuretics, glucocorticoids, nicotinic acid and phenytoin) may invalidate the results. Because of difficulties in interpreting the results of the GTT and the lack of standards relating to age (glucose tolerance decreases with age, with a two-hour value of 150 mg/dl being considered normal between 70 and 80 years), the GTT is being replaced by other methods.[8]

HbAl$_c$ Proteins that have glucose molecules attached to them (glycosylated peptides) are elevated several-fold in diabetics.[2,18,19,21,22] The use of the glycosylated haemoglobin (HbAl$_c$) assay for long-term diabetic monitoring of diabetic control is gaining much wider use and acceptance.

Since the average lifespan of a red blood cell is 120 days, this assay is believed to represent time-averaged values for blood glucose over the preceding two to four months, thus providing a simple, useful method for assessing treatment and patient compliance. The clinical usefulness of the HbAl$_c$ assay has been validated by comparison with long-term fasting blood glucose levels.[21]

Although the oral glucose tolerance test is more sensitive than the HbAl$_c$ assay, it is also more stressful to the patient and less specific. An elevated HbAl$_c$ level almost always indicates diabetes.[21] It has been recommended that an HbAl$_c$ level be determined before subjecting patients, particularly pregnant women, to the stress of a GTT.

Normally about 5 to 7 per cent of haemoglobin is combined with carbohydrate (mostly glucose). Mild hyperglycaemia results in an HbAl$_c$ concentration of 8 to 10 per cent, while severe hyperglycaemia may result in concentrations up to 20 per cent. Measuring glycosylated haemoglobin (and possibly other glycosylated proteins such as albumin) is thus an important and useful test for diabetic control and the prevention of complications.

Post-hypoglycaemic hyperglycaemia (the Somogyi phenomenon)   The problem of hypoglycaemia is common in type 1 diabetes. This can be caused by missing a meal, overexercising or excessive insulin. Daytime hypoglycaemic episodes are usually recognised by adrenergic symptoms – sweating, nervousness, tremor and hunger. Night-time hypoglycaemia may be without symptoms or manifest itself as night sweats, unpleasant dreams or an early morning headache. In response to the hypoglycaemia, there is an increase in circulating levels of hormones which increase blood glucose levels (e.g. adrenaline, noradrenaline, growth hormone and cortisol). Often this results in rebound elevations in blood glucose.[2,23]

This phenomenon was first hypothesised by Somogyi in the late 1930s and is commonly referred to as the Somogyi phenomenon. It is very important to recognise this response when monitoring an individual's insulin needs. Therefore it is imperative that a good relationship exists between the physician prescribing the insulin and the individual using the therapies recommended here. As these therapies start improving the individual's insulin response and sensitivity, the patient may experience the Somogyi phenomenon. Even mild hypoglycaemia, which may be without symptoms, can cause substantial deterioration in glucose control,[1,23] so if the Somogyi effect is suspected the insulin dose should be decreased under careful supervision.

The Somogyi phenomenon should be suspected whenever there are wide swings in blood glucose over short periods of time during the day. For example, a blood glucose of 70 mg/dl before breakfast and 400 mg/dl before lunch suggests early morning hypoglycaemia with post-breakfast hyperglycaemia due to increased counter-regulatory hormone activity.[2] The advent of the insulin pump and continuous insulin infusion has lead to a decreased frequency of the Somogyi phenomenon.

Complications of diabetes

Acute complications of diabetes

Diabetics are susceptible to two major acute metabolic complications. In the type 1 patient this is usually diabetic acidosis, while in the type 2 patient it is usually hyperosmolar nonketogenic coma.[2,8]

Diabetic ketoacidosis   This condition primarily occurs in the type 1 diabetic and, if progressive, can result in coma and numerous metabolic derangements.[2,8] Since ketoacidosis is potentially a medical emergency, prompt recognition is imperative. The coma is usually preceded by a day or more of frequent urination and severe thirst along with severe fatigue, nausea and vomiting, and mental confusion.

Evidence of excessive ketone bodies in the blood necessitates hospitalisation. The individual must be adequately educated in recognising the early symptoms and signs of ketoacidosis.

Hyperosmolar nonketogenic coma   With a death rate of over 50 per cent, this condition constitutes a true medical emergency. It is usually the result of profound dehydration secondary to deficient fluid intake or precipitating events such as pneumonia, burns, stroke, a recent operation, or certain drugs such as phenytoin, diazoxide, glucocorticoids and diuretics.[2]

Onset may be insidious over a period of days or weeks, with symptoms of weakness, frequent urination and severe thirst and progressively worse signs of dehydration (weight loss, loss of skin elasticity, dry mucous membranes, racing heart beat and low blood pressure).

Complications of chronic diabetes

The diabetic patient's condition is worsened by the appearance of six major complications of diabetes – diabetic retinopathy, diabetic neuropathy, diabetic nephropathy and diabetic foot ulcers, as well as the probable causative roles of glycosylated proteins and sorbitol.

Diabetic retinopathy   Damage to the retina due to diabetes (diabetic retinopathy) is the leading cause of blindness in the US. One in 20 type 1 and one in 15 type 2 patients develop retinopathy, half of whom (32,000 in 1978) become legally blind.

The development of laser therapy will probably reduce the prevalence of diabetes-induced blindness. Laser therapy, however, is not indicated in milder forms of retinopathy since the occasional side effects (vitreous haemorrhage, vitreous contraction with retinal detachment, macular oedema and visual field loss) may outweigh the benefits.[2]

Diabetic neuropathy   Damage to the nervous system due to diabetes (diabetic neuropathy) is usually limited to the peripheral nerves.[2,3,8] This condition is characterised by feelings of numbness (paraesthesias) and pain. The neurological examination by a physician usually reveals dulled perception of vibration, pain and temperature, particularly in the lower extremities. Nerve conduction is delayed and there may be a delayed response of the Achilles reflex similar to that seen in hypothyroidism.[2]

Diabetic nephropathy   Damage to the kidneys as a result of diabetes (diabetic nephropathy) is a common complication and a leading cause of death in diabetics.[2] Periodic monitoring of a diabetic patient's kidney function (BUN, uric acid, creatinine and creatinine clearance) is important. Although studies are inconclusive, it appears that controlling blood sugar levels reduces the risks of these complications.

Diabetic foot ulcers   Lack of oxygen supply and peripheral nerve damage are the key factors in the development of diabetic foot ulcers. The foot ulcers are largely preventable through proper foot care, the avoidance of injury and tobacco in any form, and employing methods to improve the circulation in the area.

Proper foot care includes keeping the feet clean, dry and warm and wearing only well fitted shoes. Tobacco constricts the peripheral blood vessels and should be strictly avoided. Circulation can be improved by avoiding sitting with the legs crossed or in other positions that compromise circulation, and by massaging the feet lightly upwards.

Glycosylated proteins and diabetic complications   It appears that the glycosylation of albumin, of low-density lipoprotein (LDL) and of the proteins of the red blood cell, lens of the eye and nerve cells, causes abnormal structure and function of the involved cells and tissues and may contribute to the complications of diabetes.[19] For example, glycosylated LDL molecules (found in high levels in diabetics) do not bind to LDL-receptors or shut off cholesterol synthesis.[2] This results in the overproduction of cholesterol and elevated blood levels of cholesterol.

Aldose reductase and diabetic complications   The study of diabetic cataracts has led to the elucidation of the role of aldose reductase (AR) in the development of diabetic complications. AR is the enzyme involved in the formation of polyols, some of which (sorbitol and galactitol) are implicated in the development of diabetic complications.[24-6]

The mechanism by which aldose reductase is involved in the development of diabetic complications is best understood by considering its involvement in diabetic cataract formation. Elevated glucose levels in the lens results in the shunting of glucose to the sorbitol biochemical pathway or chain of reactions. Since the lens membranes are virtually impermeable to polyols, sorbitol accumulates in high concentrations that persist even if glucose levels return to normal. This creates an osmotic gradient that results in water being drawn into the cells to maintain osmotic balance. The cells also lose amino acids, inositol, magnesium, potassium, vitamins, glutathione and other important molecules; since these compounds function to protect the lens from damage, their loss results in an increased susceptibility to damage.

Diabetic neuropathy, the most frequent complication of long-term diabetes, is also believed to be the result of polyol accumulation.[2,24,25] The earliest and best measured signs of diabetic neuropathy are decreased sensory and nerve conduction velocities. In rats, increasing sorbitol concentrations in the sciatic nerve are directly related to decreasing nerve conduction velocities, possibly as a result of decreased myoinositol concentrations.[25] Sorbitol accumulation and myoinositol reduction have usually been regarded as independent phenomena; however, recent evidence now points to polyol accumulation being directly related to myoinositol loss.[25] Inositol supplementation improves nerve conduction velocities in both diabetic rats and humans.[6,23]

The use of drugs which inhibit aldose reductase, such as sorbinil, has led to improvement in some individuals with diabetes. Flavonoids, such as quercetin, are potent inhibitors of polyol accumulation[24,26] and, since they are widely distributed in the plant kingdom, may help explain the favourable effects of many botanical medicines, many of which are high in flavonoids, traditionally used in the treatment of diabetes.

Therapy

Diet

Dietary modification and treatment is fundamental to the successful treatment of diabetes. Since diabetics have a higher incidence of death from cardiovascular disease (60–70 per cent versus 20–25 per cent in matched non-diabetic controls)[3] most of the dietary recommendations given in Chapter 18, Atherosclerosis, are equally appropriate here. The rate of diabetes is highly correlated with the fibre-depleted high-refined carbohydrate diet of 'civilised' man.[1] Re-establishing the traditional diet and lifestyle reverses the carbohydrate and fat metabolism abnormalities associated with the foods of commerce and eventually results in a lower rate of occurrence of diabetes. The evidence indicating the western diet and lifestyle as the ultimate etiological factor in diabetes is overwhelming.[1]

Clinical trials of dietary treatment with a more primitive diet, high in plant cell-wall materials and complex carbohydrates and low in fat and animal products, have consistently demonstrated superior therapeutic effects over oral hypoglycaemic agents, insulin (when less than 30 units per day) and other previously recommended dietary regimes (carbohydrate restriction, high protein and the ADA diet).[4,27–30]

The ADA diet   The diet recommended by the American Diabetes Association and the American Dietetic Association is clearly inferior to the HCF diet (presented below). None the less, it is mentioned here for historical purposes; the exchange system is a useful concept and the diet is in common use by the typical physician. It offers some

Table 33.1 Composition of food exchanges (carbohydrate, fat and protein, in grams)

Exchange	Calories	Carbohydrate	Fat	Protein
Milk	170	12	10	8
Vegetables	35	7	—	2
Fruit	40	10	—	—
Bread	70	15	—	2
Meat	75	—	5	7
Fat	45	—	5	—

support to many, especially if supplemented with dietary fibre (guar, 15–30 g daily, or pectin, 30–45 g daily).[4,31]

A resurgence of interest in diet therapy resulted from the Universal Group Diabetes Program (UGDP) report which, in 1970, cast serious doubt on the efficacy and safety of oral hypoglycaemic drugs.[8] Prior to the report, the ADA diet consisted of high-protein, high-cholesterol and high-fat foods. This diet obviously increased the already high risk of atherosclerosis in diabetics. In 1971, a revised ADA diet was developed based on the exchange system, a very useful concept for diabetic diets.[2,8]

In the exchange system there are six groups of foods – milk, vegetables, fruit, bread, meat and fat. The composition of the typical exchange is listed in Table 33.1. Exchange lists for meal planning have been developed and are available through national diabetic associations. However Chapter 2, Basic principles of health, offers a healthier exchange list.

The current ADA diet stresses the major goal of calorie restriction as a means of achieving and maintaining ideal weight, a factor known to benefit diabetics. The major changes include the restriction of fat intake to 35 per cent or less of total calorie intake; the reduction of saturated fats to one-third of the fat intake by substituting poultry, veal and fish for red meats; and the reduction of cholesterol to less than 300 mg a day. The carbohydrate content is 40–50 per cent of total calories, and unrefined carbohydrates are recommended (supplying 15–20 g a day of fibre), to the exclusion of refined and simple carbohydrates.

Although easy to use, the diet suffers from significant limitations: it is not as effective as the other diets presented here; a large percentage of the recommended calories are still derived from fat; and the fibre content is much too low.

The HCF diet   The high-carbohydrate high plant-fibre (HCF) diet popularised by James Anderson has substantial support and validation in the scientific literature as the diet of choice in the treatment of diabetes.[4,27–30] It is high in cereal grains, legumes and root vegetables and restricts simple sugar and fat intake. The calorie intake consists of 70–75 per cent complex carbohydrates, 15–20 per cent protein and only 5–10 per cent fat, and the total fibre content is almost 100 grams per day. The positive metabolic effects of the HCF diet are many: reduced after-mealtime hyperglycaemia and delayed hypo-glycaemia; increased tissue sensitivity to insulin; reduced cholesterol and triglyceride levels with increased HDL-cholesterol levels; and progressive weight reduction. If

Table 33.2 Representative menus for the HCF and MHCF diets

Meal	HCF diet	MHCF diet
Breakfast	Whole oats, 1 cup Wholewheat bread, 2 slices Skimmed milk, 1 cup Grapefruit Margarine, 2 pats	Oat bran cereal, 1 cup Yogurt, plain low fat, 1 cup Bilberries, 1 cup
Snack, morning or afternoon	Yogurt, 1 cup Fresh strawberries, 1 cup	Wholegrain flat-bread cracker, 2 Apple, 1 medium

Lunch	Wholewheat bread, 2 slices
	Kidney bean and rice casserole, 1 cup
	Kale, cooked, 1 cup
	Cucumber and onion salad
	Potatoes, boiled, 1 cup
	Margarine, 4 pats
		Brown rice, cooked, 1 cup
		Lentil soup, 1 cup
		  carrot, 1 large
		  celery, large
		  onion, 1 cup
		  garlic, 1 clove

Evening meal	Wholewheat bread, 2 slices Lima beans, 1 cup Peas, ¾ cup Blackberries, ¾ cup Tomato, 1 small Asparagus, steamed, 1 cup Squash, winter, 1 cup Beef, roast, 100 g Margarine, 4 pats	Wholegrain bread, 1 slice Green beans, ¾ cup Tossed salad, 2 cups Broccoli, ¾ cup Salmon, 100 g Butter, 1 pat

patients resume a conventional ADA diet, their insulin requirements return to prior levels.

Anderson basically promotes two HCF diets: one for the initial treatment of the hospitalised patient which provides 70 per cent of total calories from carbohydrate, 19 per cent from protein and 11 per cent from fat, 50 mg a day of cholesterol and 35–49 g a day of dietary fibre per 1,000 Cal; and a home use, or maintenance, diet that provides 55–60 per cent of total calories from carbohydrate, 20 per cent from protein and 20–25 per cent from fat, 75–200 mg a day of cholesterol and 50 g a day of dietary fibre (approximately 25 g/1,000 Cal).[4] Anderson claims fair to good compliance in 90 per cent of patients.

On the home HCF diet, available carbohydrate calories come from grain products (50 per cent), fruits and vegetables (48 per cent) and skim milk (2 per cent). Protein is provided by fruits and vegetables (50 per cent), grain products (36 per cent) and skim milk and lean meat (14 per cent). The fat is derived from grain products (60 per cent), fruits and vegetables (20 per cent), and skim milk and meat (12 per cent). The HCF diet is also based on the exchange system. A representative menu for the maintenance HCF diet is shown in Table 33.2.

Some researchers have shown that despite liberal instructions to increase carbohydrate intake from unrefined sources, patients still only manage to average 36 per cent of their energy intake from carbohydrates, even lower than the ADA recommendation.[4,32] One study found that when patients on a complex carbohydrate diet were allowed free selection in their choice of carbohydrate-rich foods, even though their fibre intake was the recommended 50 g a day, their selections resulted in a disappointing 51 per cent simple and 49 per cent complex carbohydrates.[32] Serum triglyceride concentrations appear to be the most sensitive indicators of dietary compliance; as the individual deviates, serum triglyceride levels rise.[4] Average serum cholesterol levels while following the HCF diet are 180 mg/dl.

Type 1 diabetic patients have also benefited from the HCF diet.[4] In one representative study, when 16 type 1 patients were treated with HCF diets, their average insulin requirements dropped by 38 per cent and they demonstrated significantly lower fasting, after meal and urinary glucose levels than matched patients on control diets.[4]

Modified high fibre content diet (MHCF)   In general, the HCF diet and/or the Pritikin Diet[33,34] are adequate for the treatment of diabetes. However, improvements can be made, primarily by substituting more natural (i.e. primitive) foods wherever possible in the HCF diet and avoiding some foods that have deleterious effects. The MHCF diet recommends a higher intake of legumes, along with restriction of several foods allowed on the HCF diet, namely processed grains, and excludes fruit juices, low fibre fruits, skim milk and margarine.

There is a substantial rationale for these modifications. Legumes are low in fat and high in complex carbohydrates and fibre and are proved to be effective in treating diabetes. Fruit juices, low fibre fruits and processed grains (i.e. flour) induce a rapid

Table 33.3 Composition of the ADA, HCF and MHCF diets (all values in grams except ratios)

	ADA	HCF	MHCF
Protein	98	96	90
Carbohydrate	215	351	370
Simple (S)	100	94	70
Complex (C)	115	257	300
S/C ratio	0.87	0.37	0.23
Fat	83	23.5	20
Saturated (S)	19	4.7	4.0
Monounsaturated (M)	43	9.5	7
Polyunsaturated (P)	15	6.9	8
P/S ratio	0.79	1.47	2.0
Cholesterol	0.47	0.04	0.05
Fibre	27	82	100
Soluble (S)	15	67	80
Insoluble (I)	12	15	20
S/I ratio	1.25	4.47	5.0

elevation of serum glucose and insulin levels, and the casein in skim milk appears to raise cholesterol levels. The trans-fatty acids in margarine (and other synthetically saturated fats) also have significant injurious effects.

A comparison of the ADA, HCF and MHCF diets is shown in Table 33.3.

Dietary fibre

Guar and pectin   Supplementation with the plant fibres guar (5 g/meal) and pectin (10 g/meal) has demonstrated a positive impact on diabetic control. These fibre supplements are now being used, along with the standard ADA diet, by many physicians specialising in the treatment of diabetes.[4] Jenkins and colleagues developed a palatable crispbread containing guar gum.[4,31] When diabetic patients ate between 14 and 26 grams of guar per day they required less insulin and had less glycosuria.[4,31] These beneficial effects are most noticeable in patients on a diet containing at least 40 per cent complex carbohydrates.

Legumes   Consumption of legumes (beans) should be encouraged since a high carbohydrate legume-rich high-fibre diet has been shown to improve all aspects of diabetic control.[30] The beneficial effects of legumes are primarily due to their water-soluble gel-forming fibre components which have effects similar to those of guar and pectin.

Fibre supplementation vs high fibre diet   Although fibre-supplemented diets are beneficial, they are not as effective as the HCF diet and are therefore reserved for the type 2 diabetic patient who is unwilling to implement the more difficult dietary change and will settle for palliative results. Insulin dosages on fibre supplemented diets can usually be reduced to one-third those used on control (ADA) diets, while the HCF diet has led to discontinuation of insulin therapy in approximately 60 per cent of type 2 patients, and significantly reduces doses in the other 40 per cent.[4,27,28]

For a more complete discussion of the effects of fibre, see Chapter 4, Dietary fibre.

Exercise

An appropriate exercise training programme is vitally important in a diabetes treatment plan.[33-7] Exercise improves many parameters and is indicated in both type 1 and type 2 diabetes. Physically trained diabetics experience many benefits: enhanced insulin sensitivity with a consequent diminished need for insulin injections; improved glucose tolerance; reduced total serum cholesterol and triglycerides with increased HDL levels; and in obese diabetics, improved weight loss.[33-6] However, a physical fitness programme does present some risk to the diabetic and must be carefully adapted to the fitness of the patient. Exercise should be avoided during periods of hypoglycaemia.

Besides its well-known and documented value, exercise may have a more specific beneficial effect for diabetics; exercise increases tissue levels of chromium (in rats)[37] and increases the number of insulin receptors in type 1 diabetics.[38] It is possible, then, that many of the beneficial effects of exercise are directly related to improved chromium metabolism.

Botanical medicines

Since antiquity, diabetes has been treated with plant medicines. Recent scientific investigation has confirmed the efficacy of many of these preparations, some of which are remarkably effective. This discussion will, of necessity, be limited to a few plants – those which appear most effective, are relatively non-toxic and have substantial documentation of efficacy.[39]

Pterocarpus marsupium   This botanical medicine has a long history of use in India as a treatment for diabetes.[40] The flavonoid, (-)-epicatechin, extracted from the bark of this plant has been shown to prevent alloxan-induced beta cell damage in rats.[40-3] Further, both epicatechin and a crude alcohol extract of *Pterocarpus marsupium* have actually been shown to regenerate functional pancreatic beta cells. No other drug or natural agent has been shown to generate this activity.

*Bitter melon (*Momordica charantia*)*   Bitter melon, also known as balsam pear, is a tropical vegetable widely cultivated in Asia, Africa and South America, and has been used extensively in folk medicine as a remedy for diabetes.[39] The blood sugar lowering action of the fresh juice or extract of the unripe fruit has been clearly established in both experimental and clinical studies.[39,44-6]

Bitter melon is composed of several compounds with confirmed anti-diabetic properties. Charantin, extracted by alcohol, is a hypoglycaemic agent composed of mixed steroids that is more potent than the drug tolbutamide which is often used in the treatment of diabetes.[39] Momordica also contains an insulin-like polypeptide, polypeptide-P, which lowers blood sugar levels when injected subcutaneously into type 1 diabetic patients.[44] Since it appears to have fewer side effects than insulin, it has been suggested as a replacement for some patients. The oral administration of 50–60 ml of the juice has shown good results in clinical trials.[39]

*Onion and garlic (*Allium cepa *and* Allium sativum*)*   The common bulbs, onion and garlic, have significant blood sugar lowering action.[39,47] The active principles are believed to be allyl propyl disulphide (APDS) and diallyl disulphide oxide (allicin), although other constitutents such as flavonoids may play a role as well.

Experimental and clinical evidence suggests that APDS lowers glucose levels by competing with insulin (also a disulphide protein) for insulin-inactivating sites in the liver. This results in an increase of free insulin. APDS administered in doses of 125 mg/kg to fasting humans causes a marked fall in blood glucose levels and an increase in serum insulin.[39] Allicin doses of 100 mg/kg produce a similar effect.

Graded doses of onion extracts (1 ml of extract = 1 g of whole onion) at levels sometimes found in the diet, i.e. 25 to 200 grams, reduce blood sugar levels during oral and intravenous glucose tolerance in a dose-dependent manner, i.e. the higher the dose the greater the effect. The effects are similar in both raw and boiled onion extracts. The inhibition of adrenalin-induced hyperglycaemia suggests that onions affect the hepatic metabolism of glucose and/or increases the release of insulin, and/or prevent insulin's destruction.[47]

The cardiovascular effects of garlic and onions, i.e. lipid lowering, platelet aggregation inhibition, antihypertensive, etc. (see Chapter 48, Hypertension), further substantiate the liberal use of these common foods by the diabetic patient.[48,49]

Fenugreek (Trigonella foenum-graecum)   Fenugreek seeds have demonstrated anti-diabetic effects in experimental and clinical studies.[39,50] The active principle is in the defatted portion of the seed and contains the alkaloid trogonelline, nicotinic acid and coumarin.[50]

Administration of the defatted seed (in daily doses of 1.5–2 g/kg) to both normal and diabetic dogs reduces fasting and after-meal blood levels of glucose, glucagon, somatostatin, insulin, total cholesterol and triglycerides, while increasing HDL-cholesterol levels.[50]

Bilberry leaves (Vaccinium myrtillus)   A decoction of the leaves of the bilberry has a long history of folk use in the treatment of diabetes. Oral administration reduces levels in normal and depancreatised dogs, even when glucose is concurrently injected intravenously.[39,51]

The compound myrtillin (an anthocyanoside) is apparently the most active ingredient. Upon injection it is somewhat weaker than insulin, but is less toxic, even at 50 times the 1 g per day therapeutic dose. It is of great interest to note that a single dose can produce beneficial effects lasting for several weeks.

Bilberry anthocyanosides also increase capillary integrity, inhibit free-radical damage and improve the tone of the vascular system.[39] In Europe, hundreds of tons of bilberries are processed annually for use as an anti-haemorrhagic agent in the treatment of eye diseases including diabetic retinopathy.[39]

Single nutrients

Although the following discussion of specific nutrients documents their usefulness, they are not a panacea: as noted above, proper and adequate treatment of the diabetic patient requires much more than a bottle of supplements. In general, diabetics should be on a heavy supplementation programme to help prevent many of the major diabetic complications, particularly atherosclerosis and diabetic neuropathy.

Many of these nutrients, although only briefly discussed here, are considered in more detail in the chapters covering the diseases commonly associated with diabetes – atherosclerosis, obesity and hypertension. These conditions (and the nutritional abnormalities associated with them), in addition to the increased platelet adhesiveness seen in diabetes, help account for the threefold risk of cardiovascular mortality seen in the diabetic patient.

Sucrose   The first nutrient is actually an anti-nutrient for diabetics. Sucrose must be eliminated, as its consumption produces elevated plasma cholesterol, triglyceride and uric acid levels, diminished glucose tolerance and increased platelet adhesiveness, all of which are associated with diabetes and atherogenesis.[5,51]

Chromium   As a key constituent of the 'glucose tolerance factor', chromium is a critical nutrient in diabetes. Supplementation in the form of chromium chloride (200 µg daily) or high-chromium-containing brewer's yeast (9 g a day) has been demonstrated to decrease fasting glucose levels, improve glucose tolerance, lower insulin levels and decrease total cholesterol and triglyceride levels, while increasing HDL-cholesterol levels.[9–14] Niacin administered at relatively low levels (100 mg) along with 200 µg of chromium has been shown to be more effective than chromium alone.[53] Exercise increases tissue chromium concentrations[37] while the consumption of simple carbo-hydrates increases chromium excretion.[13] All these effects appear due to increased insulin sensitivity.

Pyridoxine Diabetics with neuropathy have been shown to be deficient in vitamin B6 and benefit from supplementation.[54–6] Peripheral neuropathy is a known result of pyridoxine deficiency and is indistinguishable from diabetic neuropathy.

Pyridoxine is also important in preventing other diabetic complications because it is an important coenzyme in the cross-linking of collagen and inhibits platelet aggre-gation.[57]

Vitamin C The transport of vitamin C into cells is facilitated by insulin.[58] It has been postulated that, due to impaired transport or dietary insufficiency, a relative vitamin C deficiency exists in the diabetic and that this may be responsible for the increased capillary permeability and other vascular disturbances seen in diabetics.[58] A chronic, latent vitamin deficiency will lead to a number of problems for the diabetic, including elevations in cholesterol levels, decreased membrane integrity and a depressed immune system. (See also Chapter 18, Atherosclerosis.)

Vitamin E Diabetic patients appear to have an increased requirement for vitamin E.[59] A vitamin E deficiency results in increased free-radical-induced damage, particularly of the lining of the vascular system.[60] Supplemental vitamin E may help prevent diabetic complications through its antioxidant activity, the inhibition of the platelet-releasing reaction and platelet aggregation, increasing HDL-cholesterol levels and its role in fatty acid metabolism.[59] (See also Chapter 18, Atherosclerosis.) The trace mineral selenium functions synergistically with vitamin E.

Manganese Manganese is an important cofactor in the key enzymes of glucose metabolism.[54,61] A deficiency results in diabetes in guinea pigs and the frequent birth of offspring who develop pancreatic abnormalities or no pancreas at all.[62] Diabetics have been shown to have only one-half the manganese of normal individuals.

Magnesium Magnesium levels are significantly lowered in diabetics, and lowest in those with severe retinopathy.[63] The degree of diabetic control affects serum magnesium levels; poorly controlled diabetics have significantly lowered magnesium levels. Low magnesium levels appears to be a significant risk factor in the development of cardiovascular disease, particularly coronary artery spasm.

Magnesium supplementation appears warranted in diabetics since it is a common deficiency, possibly prevents retinopathy and reduces the risk of atherosclerosis.[54] (See also Chapter 18, Atherosclerosis.)

Vitamin B12   Vitamin B12 supplementation has been used with some success in treating diabetic neuropathy.[64,65] It is not clear if this is due to the correcting of a deficiency state or normalising vitamin B12 metabolism.[66]

Clinically, diabetic neuropathy is very similar to that of classical vitamin B12 deficiency. Absence of anaemia is not an adequate criteria for ruling out a deficiency; blood levels of vitamin B12 are more reliable. Oral supplementation may be sufficient, but intramuscular vitamin B12 may be necessary in many cases.

Carnitine   Carnitine supplementation of diabetic patients has resulted in significantly decreased total serum cholesterol and triglyceride levels.[67] In addition, carnitine improves the breakdown of fatty acids, possibly playing a role in preventing diabetic ketoacidosis.

Zinc   Zinc deficiency has been suggested to play a role in the development of diabetes in humans.[54] Zinc is involved in virtually all aspects of insulin metabolism – synthesis, secretion and utilisation. Zinc also has a protective effect against beta cell destruction,[68] and has well-known anti-viral effects. Diabetics typically excrete too much zinc in the urine and therefore require supplementation.[69] Supplementation to diabetic mice has improved all aspects of glucose tolerance. Presumably zinc supplementation in humans may have similar effects.

Inositol   As mentioned above, inositol supplementation has shown some success in the treatment of experimental animal diabetic neuropathy since it helps re-establish normal myoinositol levels in the deficient nerve cell.[6] The myoinositol deficiency in nerves is believed to be due to the accumulation of sorbitol within the cell, which results in the loss of intracellular myoinositol.[25] Oral supplementation to human diabetics has not resulted in significant improvement.[70]

Potassium   Potassium supplementation yields improved insulin sensitivity, responsiveness and secretion in diabetics.[54,71] Insulin administration often causes a potassium deficiency.[72]

Biotin   This B vitamin has been shown to work synergistically with insulin and independently in increasing the activity of glucokinase.[73,74] This enzyme is responsible for the first step in glucose utilisation. Glucokinase is present only in the liver, where, in diabetics, its concentration is very low.[75]

Supplementation with large quantities of biotin may significantly enhance glucokinase activity, thereby improving glucose metabolism in diabetics. In one study, 16 mg of biotin per day resulted in significant improvements in blood glucose control in diabetics.[76]

Treatment

Proper and effective treatment of the diabetic patient requires the careful integration of a wide range of therapies and patients who are willing to alter their lifestyles substantially. Adult onset diabetes (type 2) is usually the end result of many years of chronic metabolic insult and, although treatable with the natural metabolic approach presented here, its ultimate resolution will take persistence. Although this programme is primarily designed for the type 2 patient, it is equally appropriate for the type 1 patient. The ultimate goal is to re-establish normal glycaemia and prevent the development (or ameliorate) the complications of diabetes.

The diabetic individual must be monitored carefully, particularly if he/she is on insulin or has relatively uncontrolled diabetes. Careful attention to symptoms, home glucose monitoring and the HbAI$_c$ test are, at this time, the best way to monitor the progress of the diabetic individual. It is important to recognise that as the diabetic individual employs some of the suggestions here, drug dosages will have to be altered and that a good working relationship with the prescribing doctor will greatly aid the healing process.

Diabetes is a serious condition that requires strict medical supervision. Please consult a physician before employing any of the recommendations below.

Diet

The HCF diet, modified to incorporate more natural foods, is clearly the diet of choice. All simple, processed and concentrated carbohydrates must be avoided, complex-carbohydrate high-fibre foods should be stressed, and fats should be kept to a minimum. Legumes, onions and garlic are particularly useful, and should be encouraged.

Supplements

The following are daily doses.
- Vitamin C, 1 g.
- Vitamin E, 200 mg.
- Magnesium, 400 mg.
- Selenium, 200 μg.
- Zinc, 25 mg.
- Brewer's yeast, 3 tblsp.
- Chromium (GTF), 200 μg.
- Fibre – guar, pectin or oat bran, 20–30 g.

Botanical medicines

Liberal consumption of garlic, onions and fenugreek. Additional herbal medications may include the fresh juice of unripe *Momordica charantia* (1–2 oz, 25–50 g, three times daily), bilberry leaf tea or anthocyanoside extracts of *Vaccinium myrtillus*, and *Pterocarpus marsupium*.

Exercise

A graded exercise programme should be developed, related to the individual's fitness level and interest, yet which elevates heart rate by at least 60 per cent of maximum for half an hour three times a week.

34

Diarrhoea

- Increase in frequency, fluidity and volume of bowel movements.

General considerations

Diarrhoea is a common symptom whose presence usually indicates a mild functional disorder. However, it may also be the first suggestion of a serious underlying disease. Diarrhoea lasting more than a few days should not be taken lightly; its cause must be determined and treated appropriately. The accompanying box lists the various types of diarrhoea.

- Osmotic diarrhoea is caused by an excess of water-soluble molecules in the stool which results in an increased retention of fluids in the bowel.
- Secretory diarrhoea is due to excessive secretion of ions into the bowel, with the same results of excessive water retention in the stools.
- Inadequate contact between the intestinal contents and the absorbing surfaces resulting in inadequate absorption.
- Exudative diarrhoea is usually due to infections and inflammatory bowel diseases, resulting in abnormal intestinal permeability, with intestinal loss of serum proteins, blood, mucus and pus.
- Frequent small, painful evacuations are usually a result of disease in the rectum or at the end of the colon.

Table 34.1 on page 288 lists the most common causes of diarrhoea.

Diagnosis

Diagnosis of the cause of diarrhoea can be difficult and usually requires the assistance of a physician. It may require microscopic examination and culturing of the stools for infectious agents, special tests such as the breath hydrogen test to discover missing enzymes, intestinal biopsy and X-rays. In general, acute diarrhoea is usually due to dietary problems such as excessive fruit consumption, eating allergic food, or an

286

Types of diarrhoea[1]

- Osmotic
  Saline laxatives containing magnesium, phosphate or sulphate
  Carbohydrate malabsorption
  Antacids containing magnesium salts
  General nutrient malabsorption
  Excess consumption of non-metabolisable low-calorie sweets
  Excessive vitamin C intake
- Secretory
  Toxigenic bacteria
  Hormone-producing tumours
  Fat malabsorption
  Laxative abuse
  Ileal resection
- Exudative
  Inflammatory bowel disease
  Pseudomembranous colitis
  Invasive bacteria
- Impaired mixing or contact
  Short bowel syndrome
  Intestinal resection

intestinal viral infection. Table 34.2 on page 289 lists the key diagnostic criteria for common causes of diarrhoea.

Therapy

One of the most common causes of osmotic diarrhoea is the ingestion of carbohydrates in excess of the individual's ability to digest them. This can be due to the lack of needed enzymes (see Lactose intolerance and Disaccharide deficiency below), excessive consumption (see Artificial sweeteners below) or the consumption of large amounts of legumes. This type of vegetable contains oligosaccharides, such as stachyose and raffinose, which can cause abdominal distension, gas and osmotic diarrhoea.

Dietary considerations

Food allergy   Chronic diarrhoea is one of the most common symptoms of food allergy.[3] It can be diagnosed by either laboratory or challenge testing. After the food allergens have been diagnosed, significant allergens should be avoided and milder allergens

Table 34.1 Causes of diarrhoea[2]

Cause	Most common examples
Psychogenic disorders	Nervous diarrhoea
Intestinal infections	
Viral infections	Enterovirus, rotavirus
Bacterial infections	*Campylobacter jejuni*, shigella, salmonella, *Yersinia enterocolitica*
Bacterial toxins	*Clostridium difficile*, pathogenic *Escherichia coli*, staphylococcus, *Vibrio parahaemolytica*, *Vibrio cholerae*
Parasitic infections	*Giardia lamblia*, *Entamoeba histolytica*, cryptosporium, isospora
Inflammatory bowel disease	Crohn's disease, ulcerative colitis, diverticulitis
Antibiotic therapy	Tetracycline
Inadequate bile secretion	Hepatitis, bile duct obstruction
Malabsorption states	Coeliac sprue (severe wheat allergy), short small bowel, lactose intolerance
Pancreatic disease	Pancreatic insufficiency, pancreatic tumour
Reflex from other areas	Pelvic inflammatory disease
Neurologic disease	Tabes dorsalis (syphilis of the spinal cord), diabetic neuropathy
Metabolic disease	Hyperthyroidism
Malnutrition	Marasmus, kwashiorkor
Food allergy	
Dietary factors	Excessive fresh fruit intake, excessive low-calorie sweeteners
Laxative abuse	
Heavy metal poisoning	
Miscellaneous	Foecal impaction, cancer, vagotomy

should be rotated on a four-day cycle. (This topic is fully discussed in Chapter 38, Food allergy.)

Lactose intolerance   Deficiency in the enzyme lactase, responsible for digesting the lactose-form dairy products, is common worldwide. It has been estimated that 70 to 90 per cent of oriental, black, Native American and Mediterranean adults lack this enzyme. The incidence of deficiency is 10 to 15 per cent in northern and western Europeans.[2] While almost all infants are able to digest milk and other dairy products, most children lose their lactase enzyme by three to seven years of age.[4] Symptoms range from minor abdominal discomfort and bloating to severe diarrhoea in response to even small amounts of lactose. The deficiency is confirmed by the lactose challenge test.

Disaccharidase deficiency   Acute illnesses, such as viral and bacterial intestinal infections, will frequency injure the mucosal cells of the small intestine resulting in a temporary deficiency of the lactase and other disaccharide enzymes.[1,2] This is one reason why many physicians of natural medicine recommend fasting during acute infections.

Excessive consumption of vitamin C   Dosages of vitamin C in excess of bowel tolerance (typically over 6 grams) will cause diarrhoea. This is usually intentional as doses of

Table 34.2 Diagnostic criteria for common causes of diarrhoea

Cause	Key diagnostic criteria
Lactase deficiency	Bloated feeling, flatulence, cramps, belching, watery explosive diarrhoea relieved by stopping dairy products
Infectious diarrhoea	Acute diarrhoea in most members of the family, fever, debility
Food allergy	Eczema, asthma, chronic infections, dark circles and puffiness under the eyes
Low-calorie sweets	Explosive, watery diarrhoea after consumption of large amounts of undigestible, low-calorie sweets (e.g. mannitol)

vitamin C up to bowel tolerance levels are a common recommendation for boosting infection resistance.

Artificial sweeteners Unlike cyclamates or saccharin, sugar alcohols (mannitol and sorbitol) must be used in large quantities to provide a sweet taste. In these large amounts they are likely to produce osmotic diarrhoea.[1]

Herbal therapies

Hydrastis canadensis Berberine, a major alkaloid in goldenseal, has been shown in several clinical studies to be highly successful in the treatment of acute diarrhoeas caused by *E. coli*, *Shigella dysenteriae*, *Salmonella paratyphi B*, klebsiella, *Giardia lamblia* and *Vibrio cholerae*.[5–8] Both *in vivo* and *in vitro* studies in hamsters and rats[9] have shown that berberine also has significant antibiotic activity against *Entamoeba histolytica*.

In addition to its direct antimicrobial activity, experimental results indicate that berberine-containing plants are particularly appropriate in diarrhoeas caused by enterotoxins (e.g. *Vibrio cholerae* and *E. coli*).[10–12] The mechanisms of action in these diseases are due to berberine's anti-secretory activity, metabolic inhibition of infective organisms, inhibition of toxin formation by the organisms and direct antagonism of the formed toxin at the site of target organs.[11,12]

For those planning to travel to an underdeveloped country or an area of poor water quality or sanitation, the prophylactic use of berberine-containing herbs during and one week prior to and after visiting may be useful.

Robert's Formula Although no research has been done to document its efficacy, an old naturopathic remedy, Robert's Formula, has a long history of use in inflammatory bowel disease and other causes of diarrhoea.[13,14] It is composed of several botanical medicines:

- *Althaea officinalis*, marshmallow root, a demulcent with soothing properties on the mucous membranes.
- *Baptisia tinctora*, wild indigo, for gastrointestinal infections.
- *Echinacea angustifolia*, purple coneflower, antibacterial and used to promote normalisation of the immune system.

- *Geranium maculatum,* a gastrointestinal haemostatic.
- *Hydrastis canadensis,* goldenseal, inhibits the growth of many enteropathic bacteria – see above.
- *Phytolacca americana,* poke root, used for healing ulcerations of the intestinal mucosa.
- *Symphytum officinale,* comfrey, anti-inflammatory and promotes tissue growth and wound healing.
- *Ulmus fulva,* slippery elm, a demulcent.

Other considerations

Pectin   Pectin is a polysaccharide present in the cell walls of virtually all plants. It forms a gel when mixed with water, and has long been used in the symptomatic treatment of diarrhoea (often in combination with kaolin).[14,15] Pectin is found in high concentrations in the peel of citrus fruits, apples, carrots, potatoes, sugar beet and tomatoes. (For more discussion, see Chapter 4, Dietary fibre.)

Lactobacillus acidophilus   Re-establishment of proper bowel microbial flora is crucial in the treatment of diarrhoea. Lactobacilli are important for many reasons; they are antibacterial (against salmonella, streptococci, *Escherichia coli,* shigella and staphylococci), antiviral, antifungal, produce several vitamins and make up a significant portion of the dry weight of the stool.[16,17]

Treatment

Since most acute diarrhoeal states are self-limited and are due to dietary indiscretions or mild gastrointestinal infections, simple dietary and herbal approaches should be used first. If there is no response, then more detailed diagnostic procedures should be used. If significant illness (e.g. fever or debility) accompanies the diarrhoea or it lasts for more than a few days, a physician should be consulted. (See Chapter 27, Coeliac disease, Chapter 30, Crohn's disease and ulcerative colitis, Chapter 38, Food allergy, Chapter 44, Hepatitis, Chapter 51, Irritable bowel syndrome, for the specific therapies for these diseases.)

Diet

During the acute phase of diarrhoea, no food should be eaten. Instead fluids should be freely consumed, particularly dilute fruit and vegetable juices to help maintain electrolyte balance. An old naturopathic remedy is to sip a drink made of equal parts sauerkraut and tomato juice. It is high in electrolytes, and cabbage juice has been shown to help heal intestinal lesions.[18]

After the acute phase, start with easily digested low-allergen foods (e.g. soups, yogurt, cooked fruits, grated apples, etc.). For chronic diarrhoea, allergic foods must be determined and avoided. A four-day rotation diet may be necessary.

Dairy products should be avoided if deficient in lactase; mannitol and sorbitol consumption should be limited; and bean consumption curtailed.

Botanical medicines

Hydrastis canadensis (goldenseal), the following doses three times a day:

- Dried root (or as tea), 1 to 2 g.
- Freeze-dried root, 500 to 1,000 mg.
- Tincture (1:5), 4 to 6 ml (1 to 1.5 tsp).
- Fluid extract (1:1), 0.5 to 2.0 ml (¼ to ½ tsp).
- Powdered solid extract (4:1), 250–500 mg.

Modified Robert's formula   The dosage for the formula given below would be ¼ to ½ tsp, or 1 to 2 '00' capsules between meals, three times a day. Equal amounts of: marshmallow (*Althae officinalis*), wild indigo (*Baptisia tinctora*), purple coneflower (*Echinacea angustifolia*), American cranesbill (*Geranium maculatum*), goldenseal (*Hydrastis canadensis*), American poke root (*Phytolacca americana*), comfrey (*Symphytum officinale*), slippery elm (*Ulmus fulva*).

Other therapies

- Pectin, 1 tblsp three times a day.
- *Lactobacillus acidophilus* and *L. bulgaricus*, ½ tsp three times a day.

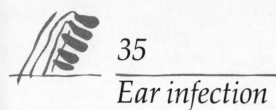

35
Ear infection

- Chronic ear inflammation of the middle ear (serous otitis media):
    Painless hearing loss.
    Dull immobile ear-drum (tympanic membrane).
- Acute middle ear infection (acute otitis media):
    Earache or irritability.
    History of recent upper respiratory tract infection or allergy.
    Red, opaque, bulging ear-drum with loss of the normal features.
    Fever and chills.
- Infection or inflammation of the external ear canal (otitis externa):
    Itching, discharge or burning pain.
    Proper diagnosis by a physician is necessary before otitis externa can be treated.

General considerations

A middle ear infection (otitis media) is characterised by a sharp, stabbing, dull and/or throbbing pain in the ear. The pain is due to inflammation, swelling or infection of the middle ear and is a common affliction of childhood. There are basically two types of earache, chronic and acute.

- Chronic otitis media (also known as serous, secretory or non-suppurative otitis media, chronic otitis media with effusion and 'glue ear') refers to a constant swelling of the middle ear.[1]
- Acute otitis media (also known as bacterial otitis media) is an acute infection of the middle ear and is usually preceded by an upper respiratory infection or allergy. The organisms most commonly cultured from middle ear fluid during acute otitis media include *Streptococcus pneumoniae* (40 per cent) and *Haemophilus influenzae* (25 per cent).[1]

Chronic otitis media affects 20 to 40 per cent of children under the age of six, and acute otitis media is the most frequent diagnosis of children in a clinical practice. The unnecessary surgery of yesterday, the tonsillectomy, has been replaced by a different procedure during the 1980s, known as a myringotomy. It involves the placement of a tiny plastic tube or grommet through the ear-drum to assist drainage of fluid into the throat via the Eustachian tube. It is not a curative procedure, as children with tubes in their ears are in fact more likely to have further problems with ear infections.

A number of studies have demonstrated that there are no significant differences in the clinical course of acute otitis media when conventional treatments are compared with placebo. Specifically, no differences are found between non-antibiotic treatment, ear tubes, ear tubes with antibiotics, and antibiotics alone.[2–4] Children not receiving antibiotics, however, did have fewer recurrences than those receiving antibiotics.[2] These results, when coupled with the high rate of recurrent ear infections following insertion of ear tubes, suggest that conservative treatment alone would reduce the rate and decrease the yearly financial costs of otitis media.

The risk of the infection spreading to the mastoid and brain is of major concern, and is the most common justification given for conventional medical therapy. Again, there is no evidence to document that the rate (0.2 to 2.0 per cent) is any different with or without antibiotics, with or without myringotomy.[2]

Although standard antibiotic and surgical procedures may not be statistically effective, each individual patient should be evaluated by a physician before a decision to not use these procedures is considered. As with all potentially dangerous diseases, otitis media should be treated under the supervision of a physician.

Causes

Abnormal eustachian tube function is the underlying cause in virtually all cases of otitis media. The eustachian tube regulates gas pressure in the middle ear, protects the middle ear from nose and throat secretions and bacteria, and clears fluids from the middle ear. Swallowing causes active opening of the eustachian tube due to the action of the surrounding muscles. Infants and small children are particularly susceptible to eustachian tube dysfunction since it is smaller in diameter, and closer to the horizontal.

Obstruction of the eustachian tube leads first to serous (fluid from the blood) build-up and then, if bacteria start to grow, bacterial infection. Obstruction results from collapse of the tube (due to weak tissues holding the tube in place and/or an abnormal opening mechanism), allergic blockage with mucous, or infection.[1]

Therapy

Since an ear infection can be quite serious, it is necessary that any individual with symptoms of an acute ear infection be seen by a physician. The recommendations given below are to be used along with those recommendations given in Chapter 6, Immune support.

Bottle feeding

Recurrent ear infection is strongly associated with early bottle feeding, while prolonged breastfeeding (minimum of six months) has a protective effect.[5] Whether this is due to cow's milk intolerance or the protective effect of human milk against infection has not yet been conclusively ascertained. It is probably a combination of both. In addition, bottle feeding while a child is lying on his or her back (bottle propping) leads to regurgitation of the bottle's contents into the middle ear and should be avoided.

Whatever the 'causative' organism in otitis media, viral (respiratory syncitial virus or influenza A) or bacterial (*Streptococcus pneumonia* or *Haemophilus influenzae*), human milk offers protection due to its high antibody content which helps inhibit infectious agents.[6]

Another way in which breastmilk helps decrease ear problems is possibly due to its anti-inflammatory properties. Mother's milk is rich in the fatty acids gamma-linolenic acid and dihomo-gamma-linolenic acid, which elevate the anti-inflammatory prosta-glandins (hormone-like compounds).[7]

Food allergy

Prolonged breastfeeding prevents food allergies, particularly if the mother avoids sensi-tising foods (i.e. those to which she is allergic) during pregnancy and lactation. Also of value is excluding the foods to which children are most commonly allergic – wheat, egg, fowl and dairy produce, particularly during the first nine months.

Since a child's digestive tract is quite permeable to food antigens, especially during the first three months, careful control of eating patterns (no frequent repetitions of any food, avoiding the common allergenic foods, and introduction of foods in a controlled manner, that is, introduction of one food at a time and carefully watching for a reaction) will reduce and prevent the development of food allergies.

The role of allergy as the major cause of chronic otitis media has been firmly estab-lished in the medical literature.[8-11] Most studies show that 85 to 93 per cent of these children have allergies, 16 per cent to inhalants, 14 per cent to food and 70 per cent to both.

The allergic reaction causes blockage of the Eustachian tube by two mechanisms; inflammatory swelling of the tube and inflammatory swelling of the nose causing the Toynbee phenomenon (swallowing when both mouth and nose are closed, forcing air and secretions into the middle ear).[8] In chronic earaches, an allergic cause should always be considered, and the offending allergens determined and avoided.

One illustrative study of 153 children with earaches demonstrated that 93.3 per cent of the children (using the RAST test for diagnosis) were allergic to foods, inhalants, or both. The 12-month success rate for 119 of the children, when treated with serial dilution titration therapy for inhalant sensitivities and an elimination diet for food allergens, showed that 92 per cent improved. This compares favourably with the surgically-treated control group (ear tubes and, as indicated, tonsillectomy and adenoidectomy), which showed only a 52 per cent response.[8]

Thymus gland extract

The thymus gland secretes a family of hormones which act on white cells to ensure their proper development and function. Studies with calf thymus extracts given orally have demonstrated impressive clinical results in a variety of clinical conditions.[12-14] These extracts have been shown to improve immune function, decrease children's food allergies and improve a child's resistance to chronic respiratory infections. Thymus extracts may be of particular benefit in chronic otitis media.

Treatment

The key dietary consideration is the recognition and elimination of the foods to which a child is allergic. Many methods are available for this determination, with the RAST test being perhaps the best (see Chapter 38, Food allergy, for description).

Since it is usually not possible to determine the exact allergen during an acute attack, the most common allergic foods should be eliminated from the diet, i.e. milk and dairy products, eggs, wheat, corn, oranges and peanut butter. The diet should also eliminate concentrated simple carbohydrates (sugar, honey, dried fruit, concentrated fruit juice, etc.) since they inhibit the immune system.

If many food allergens are detected, a four-day rotation diet is necessary. In general, the most common food allergens, i.e. dairy products and wheat, should be limited.

Nutritional supplements

- Beta-carotene, (age × 20,000) iu a day (200,000 iu max.).
- Vitamin C, (age × 500) mg a day.
- Zinc picolinate, (age × 2.5) mg a day (15 mg max.).
- Bioflavonoids, (age × 50) mg a day (250 mg max.).
- Evening primrose oil, (age × 1) capsule a day.
- Thymus extract, (age × 50) mg a day.

Botanical medicines

Echinacea angustifolia, *Hydrastis canadensis* (goldenseal) and *Glycyrrhiza glabra* (liquorice) can be taken at the following doses during an infectious processes (three times a day doses):
- Dried root (or as tea), 1 to 2 g.
- Freeze-dried root, 500 to 1,000 mg.
- Tincture (1:5), 4 to 6 ml (1 to 1.5 tsp).
- Fluid extract (1:1), 0.5 to 2.0 ml (¼ to ½ tsp).
- Powdered solid extract (4:1), 250–500 mg.

Other therapies

Locally applied heat is often very helpful in reducing discomfort. It can be applied as a hot pack, with warm oil (especially mullein oil), by blowing hot air into the ear, etc. Also of value is putting hygroscopic anhydrous glycerine into the ear. This helps pull fluids out and reduces the pressure in the middle ear.

36
Eczema

- Chronic, itching, inflammatory skin condition.
- Skin is dry and thickened.
- Lesions include scratches, papules, patches of redness, weeping fluid and scaling with small blisters formed within the skin, and hyperpigmented plaques of thickened skin with accentuated furrows.
- Personal or family history of eczema and/or asthma.

General considerations

Eczema (atopic dermatitis) is an intensely itchy, inflammatory disease of the skin. It is commonly found on the face, wrists and insides of the elbows and knees. Although it may occur at any age, it is most common in infants and completely clears in half the cases by 18 months of age.

Eczema is a very common condition affecting 2.4 to 7 per cent of the population. It is often associated with asthma, and when associated with a heredity tendency to develop immediate allergic reactions is referred to as atopy.

Causes

Current research indicates that eczema is, at least partially, an allergic disease:

- Serum IgE (one of the classes of antibodies) is elevated in 80 per cent of patients.
- All patients have positive allergy (skin and RAST, see Chapter 38, Food allergy) tests.
- Two-thirds of eczema patients have family members who also have eczema.
- Many eventually develop hayfever (allergic rhinitis) and/or asthma.
- Most improve on a diet which eliminates common allergenic foods.[1]

Abnormalities of the skin

Eczema is characterised by a variety of physiological and anatomical abnormalities of the skin. The type of abnormality determines the manner in which it manifests itself. The major abnormalities are:

- A higher than normal tendency to itch.
- Dry thickened skin, which has decreased water-holding capacity.
- An increased tendency to thickening of the skin in response to rubbing and scratching.
- A tendency of the skin to be overgrown by bacteria, especially *Staphylococcus aureus*.[2]

Immunological abnormalities

White blood cells from patients with eczema show decreased levels of prostaglandins, increased histamine release and decreased ability to kill bacteria.[3,4]

These defects, coupled with scratching and the large amounts of the bacteria *Staphylococcus aureus* in the skin in 90 per cent of these patients, leads to the increased susceptibility to staph infections.[3] There are also other immune system defects which lead to increased susceptibility to viral skin diseases such as *Herpes simplex*, vaccina, *Molluscum contagiosum* and warts. It is interesting to note that these immune system abnormalities normalise when the eczema improves and become abnormal again during recurrences of the dermatitis.[3]

Low stomach acid

Low stomach acid (hypochlorhydria) is very common in patients with eczema and other inflammatory conditions of the skin such as hives.[5,6] This is perhaps not surprising considering the association of hypochlorhydria with food allergies, a major cause of eczema.[7]

Several methods exist to test for stomach acid. The most accurate and useful are gastric intubation (inserting a small tube through the throat into the stomach to remove a sample of the stomach fluids) and the Heidelberg gastric analysis (a vitamin pill-sized capsule with a pH meter and small radio transmitter inside it is swallowed and measures the pH throughout the intestinal tract).[8]

Stress

Emotional tension can provoke and aggravate itching. And, according to a number of studies, people with eczema show higher levels of anxiety, hostility and neurosis than matched controls.[9]

Therapy

Food allergy

Many studies have documented that food allergy is a very important cause in eczema.[1,10,11] In infants, milk appears to be the most common allergic food.[12] Control of eczema is critically dependent on finding and eliminating all, or at least most, of the food allergens.

A food allergy screening test, such as the RAST test (see Chapter 38, Food allergy), is used to identify the major food allergy families. Then other foods in the offending food families are also eliminated. For example, if a person is found to be allergic to wheat, then not only wheat, but also barley, rye, rice, oats and millet should be eliminated. (See Chapter 38 for complete discussion.)

Nutrients

Essential fatty acids Patients with eczema appear to have an essential fatty acid deficiency or a defect in a zinc-dependent enzyme involved in essential fatty acid metabolism. This results in decreased synthesis of the anti-inflammatory prostaglandins.[13,14] Treatment with evening primrose oil both normalises the essential fatty acid abnormalities and relieves the symptoms of eczema.[13–15]

It is also important to increase the dietary intake of fish oils (eicosapentaenoic acid, EPA), either by eating more fatty fish (e.g. mackerel, herring and salmon) or supplementation. Fish oils have significant anti-inflammatory and anti-allergy effects by inhibiting arachidonic acid metabolism.[16–18]

Arachidonic acid (from animal fats) is the necessary fatty acid source of inflammatory agents produced by the body, known as leukotrienes. In contrast, fish oils as well as vegetable oils (linolenic, linoleic and dihomo-gamma-linolenic acid) possess anti-inflammatory effects. By decreasing animal fat intake and increasing the intake of fish and vegetable oils a significant reduction in the inflammatory and allergic process can be achieved.

Therapeutic doses of fish oils, flaxseed oil and/or evening primrose oil are typically 3–4 grams as a loading dose for 1 month, which is then reduced to 1 gram a day and fish twice a week.

Bioflavonoids Bioflavonoids are indicated in virtually all inflammatory and allergic conditions, as they appear to control directly the factors involved in inflammation and allergy. They do this by inhibiting the inflammatory process, decreasing the release of mediators of inflammation, stabilising cell membranes and decreasing the contraction of smooth muscle.[19–23] They also increase the effectiveness and levels of vitamin C.

Vitamin A Vitamin A is critical to the proper development and maintenance of the skin. When deficient, the skin is particularly vulnerable to hyperkeratinisation (thickening of the skin), as is commonly found in eczema.[24]

Zinc Clinical experience has shown that zinc supplementation is particularly helpful for those with eczema. Its efficacy is probably due to the fact that it is a common deficiency, necessary for the enzyme that produces hydrochloric acid in the stomach and necessary (as discussed above) for the conversion of fatty acids to anti-inflammatory prostaglandins.

Botanical medicines

A number of herbs reduce histamine production and secretion, particularly those containing flavonoids such as quercetin.[25,26] Flavonoid extracts from *Vaccinium myrtillus* (bilberry leaf), *Rosa damascena* (Turkish attar of rose), *Ruta graveolens* (rue), *Prunus spinosa* (blackthorn) and *Crataegus monogyna* (hawthorn berry) were the most potent inhibitors of inflammation, according to one study.[25] These flavonoids are also potent inhibitors of mast cell degranulation (the process by which histamine is released).[27] *Coleus forskolii, Inula britannica* and *Glycyrrhiza glabra* (liquorice root) also help reduce the excessive histamine production common in the patient with eczema.[28,29]

*Burdock root (*Arctium lappa*)* Burdock root has a long history of use in the treatment of eczema.[30,31] There is good scientific support for this use, since its primary active component, inulin, tends to correct the underlying defects in the inflammatory mechanisms and immune system commonly found in patients with eczema.[7] Burdock also has direct antimicrobial activity which helps control the staph infections so common in eczema.[30]

Topical botanical preparations A number of botanicals have demonstrated an effect equal to or superior to cortisone when applied topically. *Glycyrrhiza glabra* (liquorice) and *Matricaria chamomilla* (German chamomile) are the most active.[32,33] Proprietary formulas containing these botanicals may be quite beneficial for the temporary relief of eczema.

Treatment

Since food allergy is such an important factor in eczema, all major allergens, and other foods in their food family, must be identified and eliminated. In addition, at the start, a four-day diversified rotation diet should be used. As the condition improves, the allergic foods can be slowly reintroduced. Animal products should be greatly reduced until symptoms have improved, and fatty fish should be consumed regularly.

Nutritional supplements

These are all adult doses; reduce for children in proportion to body weight.
- Vitamin A, 25,000 iu a day.
- Vitamin E, 400 iu a day (mixed tocopherols).
- Vitamin C, 500 mg a day.

- Zinc, 50 mg a day picolinate (decrease as condition clears).
- Bioflavonoids, 500 mg a day.
- Evening primrose oil, 2–4 capsules three times a day.
- Flaxseed oil, 1 tsp three times a day.

Botanical medicines

Doses three times a day.
- *Glycyrrhiza glabra* (liquorice):
   Dried root (or as tea), 1 to 2 g.
   Tincture (1:5), 4 to 6 ml (1 to 1.5 tsp).
   Fluid extract (1:1), 0.5 to 2.0 ml (¼ to ½ tsp).
   Powdered solid extract (4:1), 250–500 mg.
- *Arctium lappa* (burdock):
   Dried root (or as tea), 3 to 6 g.
   Fluid extract (1:1), 2 to 4 ml (½ to 1 tsp).
   Powdered solid extract (4:1), 500–750 mg.

Other therapies

Local pain and itching is a significant problem for those with eczema. Many therapies have been tried. The authors have found a non-oily zinc ointment to be useful. Only the mildest of soaps should be used, the affected tissues should be kept dry and clean, and all irritants, such as wool, should be assiduously avoided.

If the lesions become infected, goldenseal packs are often useful. However, severe infections should be treated with antibiotics.

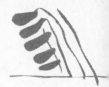

37

Fibrocystic breast disease

- Recurrent, typically premenstrual, breast swelling, pain and tenderness, although often without symptoms.
- Characterisically affects both breasts, with multiple cysts of varying sizes giving each breast a nodular consistency.
- The size of the cysts typically fluctuate.
- Noninvasive procedures such as ultrasonography and thermography aid in diagnosis, but definitive diagnosis depends upon biopsy.
- Most common age is 30–50.

General considerations

Fibrocystic breast disease (FBD), also known as cystic mastitis, is a mildly uncomfortable to severely painful benign cystic swelling of the breasts. It is typically cyclic, and usually precedes a woman's period. It is the most frequent disease of the breast.

Fibrocystic breast disease is very common, affecting 20–40 per cent of premenopausal women. It is usually a component of the premenstrual syndrome (PMS) and is considered a risk factor for breast cancer. It is not, however, as significant a factor as the classical breast cancer risk factors, i.e. family history, early menarche and late or no first pregnancy.

Causes

The development of fibrocystic breast disease is apparently due to an increased oestrogen-to-progesterone ratio. During each menstrual cycle there is a recurring hormonal stimulation of the breast. As the hormone levels fall after a few days the breasts normally return to their prestimulation size and function. In many women these changes are so slight that clinical signs or symptoms do not appear. In others, however, significant inflammatory processes occur.

The cells of a fibrocystic breast are characterised by overgrowth and enlargement, increased secretory activity, dilation of the milk ducts and scarring. These effects may be due to increased levels of the hormone prolactin which is secreted by the pituitary.[1,2] Oestrogen, both internally produced and in birth control pills, causes an increase in prolactin secretion.

Several lifestyle and nutritional abnormalities appear to cause the hormonal imbalances seen in FBD.

Therapy

Chapter 62, Premenstrual syndrome, contains a much more comprehensive discussion of the many factors involved in FBD; the reader is encouraged to read it first. The factors discussed here were chosen since they are not covered in depth in the PMS chapter and are particularly relevant to fibrocystic breast disease.

Methylxanthines

There is very strong evidence supporting an association between consumption of caffeine, theophylline and theobromine, as found in coffee, tea, cola, chocolate and caffeinated medications, and fibrocystic breast disease.[3-6] Caffeine, theophylline and theobromine are all known to stimulate overproduction of cellular products, such as fibrous tissue and cyst fluid.[4-6]

In one study, limiting methylxanthines (caffeine, theophylline and theobromine) in the diet resulted in improvement in 97.5 per cent of the 45 women who completely abstained and in 75 per cent of the 28 who limited their consumption of coffee, tea, cola, chocolate and caffeinated medications. Those who continued with little change in their methylxanthine consumption showed little improvement.[4] According to this study, women may have varying thresholds of response to methylxanthines.

Vitamin E

Several double-blind clinical studies have shown vitamin E (alpha-tocopherol) to relieve many premenstrual symptoms, particularly FBD.[7,8] The mode of action remains obscure, although vitamin E has been shown to normalise circulating hormones in PMS and FBD patients.[7-9] Vitamin E supplementation (600 iu a day) also lowers the elevated follicle stimulating and luteinising hormone levels commonly seen in FBD patients.[9]

Vitamin A

After three months of 150,000 iu a day supplementation with vitamin A, five of the nine patients who completed the study had complete or partial remission of their fibrocystic breast disease.[10] However, some patients developed mild side effects, resulting in two of the original 12 withdrawing due to headaches (an early sign of vitamin A toxicity), and one patient having her dosage reduced. Beta-carotene would appear to be more appropriate due to its greatly decreased toxicity and similar activity.

Thyroid and iodine

Hypothyroidism and/or iodine deficiency are associated with a higher incidence of breast cancer. There is evidence of an association between low thyroid function and FBD as well.

Thyroid hormone replacement therapy in hypothyroid, and some normal thyroid, individuals may result in improvement.[11,12] Research has shown that thyroid supplementation decreases breast pain, serum prolactin levels and breast nodules in, supposedly, normal thyroid patients. These results suggest that unrecognised hypothyroidism and/or iodine deficiency may be a causative factor in FBD.

Experimental iodine deficiency in rats results in mammary changes similar on the cellular level to human FBD. This indicates that iodine may be very important in the treatment and prevention of FBD. Iodine supplementation is known to have significant anti-inflammatory and anti-scarring effects.[13]

Liver function

Since the liver is the primary site for oestrogen clearance, any factor (e.g. cholestasis, 'toxic liver syndrome', environmental pollution) that interferes with proper liver function may lead to oestrogen excess. Adequate levels of lipotropic factors and B vitamins are necessary for oestrogen detoxification. (See Chapter 8, Liver support for full description.)

Colon function

Breast disease has been linked to the western diet and bowel dysfunction. There is an association between cellular abnormalities in breast fluid and the frequency of bowel movements.[14] Women having fewer than three bowel movements per week have a risk of fibrocystic breast disease 4.5 times greater than women having at least one a day.

This association is probably due to the bacterial flora in the large intestine transforming colon contents into a variety of toxic metabolites, including carcinogens and mutagens.[15] Faecal microorganisms are capable of resynthesising oestrogen from previously excreted and detoxified oestrogen. Diet plays a major role in the colon microflora, transit time and the concentration of absorbable bowel toxins and metabolites.[16]

Women on a vegetarian diet excrete two to three times more detoxified oestrogens than women on an omnivorous diet who also reabsorb more oestrogens.[16] Furthermore, omnivorous women have 50 per cent higher mean levels of undetoxified oestrogens. *Lactobacillus acidophilus* supplementation has been shown to lower the faecal enzymes which result in resynthesis of oestrogen.[16]

Treatment

Unless a woman has pure fibrocystic breast disease, the therapeutic approach outlined in Chapter 62, Premenstrual syndrome, will meet her individual needs more definitively. The therapy recommended here includes key factors discussed in that chapter.

Diet

The diet should be primarily vegetarian, with large amounts of dietary fibre. All methylxanthine-containing foods (coffee, tea, cola and chocolate) should be eliminated until symptoms are alleviated. They can then be reintroduced in small amounts. Oestrogens from drugs and contaminated food should be avoided (oral contraceptives, high oestrogen-containing animal products, etc.).

Supplements

- B-complex, 10 times the recommended dietary allowance.
- Choline, 1 g a day.
- Methionine, 1 g a day.
- Vitamin B6, 200 mg a day.
- Vitamin C, 500 mg a day.
- Vitamin E, 600 iu a day of d-alpha tocopherol.
- Beta-carotene, 50,000–300,000 iu a day.
- Iodine, 0.25 mg a day.
- Zinc, 15 mg a day (picolinate preferred).
- Flaxseed oil, 300 ml a day.
- *Lactobacillus acidophilus*, 1 tsp three times a day.

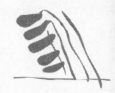

38
Food allergy[1]

- Immediate or delayed adverse reactions to the ingestion of specific foods.
- Chronic symptoms for which no satisfactory explanation can be found.
- Common signs and symptoms of food allergy are dark circles and puffiness under the eyes, chronic diarrhoea, malabsorption, chronic infections, chronic inflammation.

General considerations

Although there is as yet no agreed definition for food allergy, for the purposes of this chapter it is considered to exist when there is an inappropriate adverse reaction to the ingestion of a food. The reaction may or may not be mediated by the immune system. The reaction may be caused by a food protein, starch or other food component, or by a contaminant found in the food (colourings, preservatives, etc.). There is considerable debate among physicians and researchers as to whether food sensitivity without immune system involvement exists, and there is even disagreement concerning which elements of the immune system are involved.

Reactions express themselves in many different ways and in diverse body systems. Common synonyms for food allergy are food hypersensitivity, food anaphylaxis, food idiosyncrasy, food intolerance, pharmacologic reaction to food, metabolic reaction to food and food sensitivity.

The recognition of food sensitivity was first recorded by Hippocrates, who observed that milk could cause gastric upset and urticaria. He wrote 'to many this has been the commencement of a serious disease when they have merely taken twice in a day the same food which they have been in the custom of taking once'.[2]

The incidence of food allergies and the number of allergic (atopic) individuals has increased dramatically since the early 1970s. Some physicians claim that food allergies are the leading cause of most undiagnosed symptoms. Others maintain that at least 60 per cent of the US population suffers from symptoms associated with food reactions. Theories of why the incidence has increased include increased stresses on the immune system (such as greater chemical pollution in the air, water and food), earlier weaning and earlier introduction of solid foods to infants, genetic manipulation of plants resulting in food components which cross-react with normal tissues, and increased ingestion of fewer foods. Probably all of these and more have contributed to the increased frequency and severity of symptoms.

Definition

The accompanying box lists the definitions accepted by the US Academy of Allergy and Immunology. From a clinical perspective, clinical ecologists and preventive- and nutrition-oriented physicians recognise two basic types of food allergies:

- Cyclic: this form accounts for 80–90 per cent of food allergies. The sensitivity is slowly developed by repetitive eating of a food. If the allergic food is avoided for a period of time (typically over four months), it may be reintroduced and tolerated unless it is again eaten too frequently.
- Fixed allergies: these are sensitivities that occur whenever a food is eaten, no

---

Definitions accepted by the Academy of Allergy and Immunology[3]

- Adverse reaction (sensitivity) to a food
  A general term that can be applied to a clinically-recognisable abnormal response attributed to an ingested food or food additive.
- Food hypersensitivity (allergy)
  An immunological reaction resulting from the ingestion of a food or food additive. This reaction occurs only in some patients, may occur after only a small amount of the substance is ingested and is unrelated to any physiological effect of the food or additive. To many, it is a term which would be restricted to those hypersensitivity reactions that involve an IgE immunological mechanism of which anaphylaxis is the classic example. To others it is a term which may include any food reaction which is known to involve an immune mechanism. This term is one which is overused and one which has been incorrectly applied to any and all adverse reactions to a food or food additive.
- Food anaphylaxis
  A classic allergic hypersensitivity food or food additive reaction which involves the immunologic activity of IgE homocytotrophic antibody and release of chemical mediators.
- Food intolerance
  A general term describing abnormal physiological response to an ingested food or food additive which is not proven to be immunological in nature. This response could include idiosyncratic, metabolic, pharmacological or toxic food or food additive reactions. This term is often overused and, like the term food 'allergy', is one which has been applied incorrectly to any or all adverse reactions to foods.

---

matter what the length of time between ingestion. Long-term avoidance may re-establish tolerance.

Cause

Genetic predisposition It is well-documented that food allergy is often an expression of an inherited genetic predisposition.[4] Allergic histories can often be found in parents and siblings. When both parents are allergic, 67 per cent of the children are allergic. Where only one parent is allergic, 33 per cent of the children are allergic.[5] The actual expression can be triggered by a variety of stressors – physical and emotional trauma, excessive use of drugs, immunisation reactions, excessive frequency of consumption of a specific food, and/or environmental toxins.

Immune mediated The clinical expression of immune-system-mediated food allergy is the result of interactions between ingested food antigens, the digestive tract, histamine-

- Food toxicity (poisoning)
  A term used to imply an adverse effect as a result of a direct action of a food or food additive upon the host recipient without involving immune mechanisms. This type of reaction may involve non-immune release of chemical mediators. 'Toxins' may either be contained within food or released by microorganisms or parasites contaminating food products. On some occasions this term may be synonymous with idiosyncratic adverse reaction. When the reaction is anaphylaxis-like, it may be called anaphylactoid.
- Food idiosyncrasy
  A quantitatively abnormal response to a food substance or food additive that differs from its physiological or pharmacological effect. The reaction resembles hypersensitivity but does not involve immune mechanisms. Food idiosyncratic reactions include those which occur in specific groups of individuals who may be genetically predisposed. When the reaction is anaphylaxis-like, it may be called anaphylactoid.
- Anaphylactoid reaction to a food
  An anaphylaxis-like food or food additive reaction as a result of non-immune release of chemical mediators which mimic the signs and symptoms of food hypersensitivity (allergy).
- Pharmacological food reaction
  An adverse reaction to a food or food additive as a result of a naturally derived or added chemical which produces a drug-like or pharmaceutical effect in the host.
- Metabolic food reaction
  An adverse reaction to a food or food additive as a result of the effect of the food substance upon the metabolism of the host recipient.

containing tissue mast cells and circulating basophils, and food-specific immuno-globulins such as IgE and IgG.

Food represents the largest antigenic challenge confronting the human immune system.[6] The immune system controls most food allergy reactions. When the immune system is activated, cells and antibodies cooperate in an immune response which, under

---

Mechanisms of immune-mediated tissue injury[7]

- Type I – immediate hypersensitivity (reactions occurring in less than 2 hours)
  Antigens bind to preformed IgE antibodies attached to the surface of the mast cell or the basophil and cause release of mediators – histamine, leukotrienes, etc. A variety of allergic symptoms may result, depending on the location of the mast cell: in the nasal passages it cause sinus conges-tion; in the bronchioles, constriction (asthma); in the skin, hives and eczema; in the synovial cells that line the joints, arthritis; in the intestinal mucosa, inflammation with resulting malabsorption; and in the brain, headaches, loss of memory and 'spaciness'. It has been estimated that Type I reactions account for only 10 to 15 per cent of food allergy reactions.[8]

- Type II – cytotoxic reactions
  Cytotoxic reactions involve the binding of either IgG or IgM antibody to cell-bound antigen. Antigen-antibody binding activates factors which result in the destruction of the cell to which the antigen is bound. Examples of tissue injury include immune haemolytic anaemia. It has been estimated that at least 75 per cent of all food allergy reactions are accom-panied by cell destruction.[9]

- Type III – immune complex-mediated reactions
  Immune complexes are formed when antigens bind to antibodies. They are usually cleared from the circulation by the phagocytic system. However, if these complexes are deposited in tissues they can produce tissue injury. Two important factors which promote tissue injury are increased quantities of circulating complexes and the presence of vasoactive amines (which increase vascular permeability and favour tissue deposition of immune complexes). These responses are of the delayed type, often occurring two hours after exposure. This type of hypersensitivity has been shown to involve IgG and IgG immune complexes.[10,11] It is estimated that 80 per cent of food allergy reactions involve IgG and IgG complex mediators.[8]

- Type IV – T-cell dependent
  This delayed type reaction is mediated primarily by T-lymphoctyes. It results when an allergen contacts a mucosal surface. Within 36 to 72 hours of contact it can cause inflammation by stimulating sensitised T-cells. Type IV does not involve any antibodies. Examples include contact dermatitis, allergic colitis and regional ileitis.

certain circumstances, can have negative effects.

There are five major families of immunoglobulins – IgE, IgD, IgG, IgM and IgA. IgE is involved primarily in the classic immediate reaction, while the others seem to be involved in delayed reactions such as those seen in the cyclic type of food allergy. Although the function of the immune system is protection of the host from infections and malignancies, abnormal immune responses can lead to tissue injury and disease (food allergy reactions being but one expression). Gell and Coombs have classified the mechanisms of immune tissue injury into four distinct types, as shown in the accompanying box.

Immune system disorders   There are several immune disorders which can play a major role in food allergy reactivity.[12] Some studies have shown atopic individuals (i.e. those with a tendency to develop asthma and eczema) to have abnormalities in T-cell number and ratios. Atopic individuals have nearly 50 per cent more helper T-cells than non-allergenic persons.[13]

An emerging theory suggests that atopics have a lower immunological set point. With more helper T-cells in circulation, the level of attack required to trigger an immune response is lowered. Suppressor T-cell dysfunction has also been noted in patients with migraines[14] and asthmatic children,[15] both groups which commonly suffer from food allergies. Because T-cells regulate important immune system functions, it is not surprising that abnormalities in other immune system parameters have also been noted.

Food-sensitive people have been observed to have unusually low levels of serum IgA.[16] IgA plays an important role on the mucosal membrane surfaces of the intestinal tract, where it helps protect against the entrance of foreign substances into the body. It has been suggested that a relative short-term IgA deficiency predisposes to the development of allergy during the first months of life.[17]

There is also evidence that psychosocial stress is sometimes correlated with impaired T-cell function,[18] and stress is known to lead to decreased secretory IgA.[19] These findings might explain the relationship that many observers report between food allergy and severe mental stress.

Non-immunological mechanisms   Many adverse reactions to foods are triggered by non-immunological mechanisms in which antibody formation is not involved. Instead, the reaction is mediated and triggered by inflammatory mediators (prostaglandins, leukotrienes, SRS-A, serotonin, platelet-activating factor, histamine, kinins, etc.).

Foods may also produce a pseudo-allergic reaction due to histamine content or histamine releasing effects and reactions to biogenic amines in the foods. The box on the next page describes mechanisms responsible for non-immunological allergic (or pseudo-allergic) reactions.

Maldigestion   Repetitive exposure, improper digestion and poor integrity of the intestinal barrier are all factors in the development and maintenance of food allergy.

It has been well documented that partially digested dietary protein can cross the intestinal barrier and be absorbed into the bloodstream. It then causes a food-allergic

> **Mechanisms responsible for 'pseudo-allergic' reactions to non-steroidal anti-inflammatory drugs, food additives and foods[20]**
>
> - Inhibition of the anti-inflammatory (cyclo-oxygenase) pathway in arachidonic acid metabolism resulting in increased prostaglandin products from the inflammatory (lipoxygenase) pathway.
> - Activation of platelets resulting in serotonin release.
> - Enhanced reactivity of mast cells and/or basophils to various triggering stimuli.
> - Activation of the alternative complement pathway.
> - Excessive intake of histamine-containing foods – sausage, sauerkraut, tuna, wine, preserves, spinach, tomato.
> - Excessive intake of histamine-releasing foods – ovomucoid, crustaceans, strawberry, tomato, chocolate, protease-containing fruits (bananas, papaya), lecithin-containing nuts, peptones, alcohol.
> - Intolerance to foods containing vasoactive amines – tyramine (cabbage, cheese, citrus, seafood, potato), serotonin (banana), phenylethylamine (chocolate).

response which can occur directly at the intestinal barrier, at distant sites or throughout the body.[21] Factors which can increase intestinal macromolecular absorption include immaturity of the gastrointestinal system, abnormal bacteria in the gut, vitamin A deficiency, decreased stomach acid, insufficient pancreatic digestive enzyme secretion, inflammation of the intestinal tract, intestinal ulceration and diarrhoea.

Gastric acidity limits the passage of organisms into the intestinal tract and is important in the digestion of protein. Low stomach hydrochloric acid levels are associated with an increased incidence of intestinal infections and increased circulating antibodies to foods. When properly chewed and digested, 98 per cent of ingested proteins are absorbed as amino acids and small peptides.

Research has shown that incompletely digested proteins may reduce the reponsiveness of the immune system, leading to long-term allergic reactions by producing a state of low tolerance.[22] An irritated and inflamed intestine could adversely affect the immunologic defence mechanism of the gut.

Proper functioning of the liver is very important, due to its role in removing foreign proteins. The normal bacterial and viral populations that inhabit the intestinal tract are important in maintaining normal intestinal function and proper immune system function of the intestinal tract.[23]

Premature newborn infants absorb much larger quantities of ingested food proteins than do older children.[24] This suggests that the weaning of infants to solid foods should be done slowly and carefully in order to lessen their exposure to potential allergic foods. The development of the mucosal barrier during the neonatal period is an important mechanism against allergic reactions. Animal experiments show that diseases affecting the gut may interfere with intestinal protection against food allergens.[25]

Diagnosis

Food allergies have been implicated as a causative factor in a wide range of conditions; no part of the human body is immune from being a target cell or organ. The actual symptoms produced during an allergic response depend on the location of the immune system activation, the mediators of inflammation involved, migraine[26] and the sensitivity of the tissues to specific mediators.

Diseases caused by or associated with food allergy

Food allergies have been shown to cause migraine,[26] eczema,[27] thrombophlebitis,[28] arthritis, colitis,[29] enuresis, ear infections, gall bladder disease,[30] childhood hyperactivity,[31] asthma,[32] glaucoma,[33] and many other pathological conditions. Common symptoms and diseases that should make the clinician suspicious of food allergies are listed in Table 38.1, while some common physical signs of food allergy are listed in the accompanying box.

Table 38.1 Symptoms and diseases commonly associated with food allergy[34]

System	Symptoms and diseases
Gastrointestinal	Canker sores, coeliac disease, chronic diarrhoea, stomach ulcer, gas, gastritis, irritable colon, malaborption, ulcerative colitis
Genitourinary	Bed-wetting, chronic bladder infections, kidney disease
Immune	Chronic infections, frequent ear infections
Mental/emotional	Anxiety, depression, hyeractivity, inability to concentrate, insomnia, irritability, mental confusion, personality change, seizures
Musculoskeletal	Bursitis, joint pain, low back pain
Respiratory	Asthma, chronic bronchitis, wheezing
Skin	Acne, eczema, hives, itching, skin rash
Miscellaneous	Arrhythmia, oedema, fainting, fatigue, headache, hypoglycaemia, itchy nose or throat, migraines, sinusitis

---

Common physical signs of food allergy

- Dark circles under the eyes.
- Puffiness under the eyes.
- Horizontal creases in the lower lid.
- Chronic non-cyclic fluid retention.
- Chronic swollen glands.

The symptom process may involve the following three stages, as shown in the next box.[35]

The three stages of cyclic food allergy development

- Hypersensitivity (pre-adapted)

  Clinically apparent, acute symptomatic response following each antigen exposure.
- Adaptive

  Less recognisable response after eating the allergic food, and an increase in chronic symptoms. This can be considered an addictive phase, since ingestion of the allergic food(s) may actually temporarily relieve symptoms. This stage typically involves food cravings and withdrawal responses. It is also known as 'masked allergy'.
- Maladaptive

  The body is in a constant state of biochemical dysfunction. The allergic person is totally unaware of sensitivities as a cause of their ill health.

Laboratory diagnosis of food allergy

The diagnosis of food allergy/intolerance is still controversial. There are two basic categories of tests commonly used:

- Laboratory methods that attempt to measure immune complex formation in a variety of ways.
- Clinical tests which challenge the patient with suspected allergens while carefully monitoring for reactions.

Listed in Table 38.2 are the advantages and disadvantages of the laboratory-based food allergy testing methodologies. The RAST (radio-allergo-sorbent test) test is perhaps the best laboratory method currently available.

Table 38.2 Advantages and disadvantages of the food allergy testing methodologies[36]

Procedure	Advantages	Disadvantages
RAST	Patient convenience	Low accuracy
	Good for inhalants and foods	Expensive
	Office kits available	
FICA	Patient convenience	Expensive
	Good accuracy	Not widely available
	Detects IgG and IgE	Few clinical studies
Cytotoxic	Patient convenience	Poor reproducibility
	Moderate cost	Limited availability
	Many foods tested	
Skin prick	Widely available	Poor accuracy
	Good for inhalants	Inconvenient
EAV acupuncture	Inexpensive	No scientific basis
	Easily applied	Few clinical studies
Kinesiologic	Inexpensive	No scientific basis
	Easily applied	Few clinical studies

Radio-allergo-sorbent test (RAST)

This test is performed on blood drawn from an individual. Suspected allergens are bound to a solid matrix, followed by the application of a sample of the individual's serum. If the serum contains an antibody specific to the antigen, it will bind with the antigen, thus becoming attached to the solid matrix. A minute amount of radioactive material which binds to antibodies is then added. After incubation and subsequent washing, the residual radiation is measured to determine what percentage of the radio-active material became bound to the antibodies on the solid matrix. The higher the radioactive bond, the greater the amount of antibody specific to the allergen tested is present in the individual's blood.

The underlying assumption in this test is that a person without food sensitivity will have little or no food-antigen-specific antibodies in their blood. For the patient, the procedure is comfortable, although expensive.

Food immune complex assay (FICA)

The FICA, like the RAST, is performed on a blood sample. The FICA test measures the level of circulating food immune complexes, in other words, food molecules which are bound to antibodies. Like the RAST, the FICA is a very good test, in terms of patient convenience and accuracy.

Cytotoxic test

The cytotoxic blood test is based on the principle that extracts of foods to which a patient is sensitive will induce visible damage when in contact with the individual's white blood cells. The white blood cells are separated from the blood and are mixed on a slide with an allergen and observed for two hours under a microscope. A positive reaction is marked by changes in the shape of the white cells.

While the cytotoxic test is in widespread clinical use, there is much controversy over its validity and reproducibility. The most common criticism is that the technique is susceptible to the subjective judgments of technicians and that the methods used by different labs produce widely varying results. The cost is considerably less than that of the RAST and FICA, but it is not as reliable.

Skin testing

Skin testing with food extracts is usually done by either the prick or scratch methods. Interaction of the test antigen and IgE skin-sensitising antibody bound to local tissue mast cells produces an immediate visible reaction. The test procedure delivers antigens beneath the skin. When the antigen interacts with allergic antibodies, mast cells release mediator substances, most notably histamine. These mediators cause local vasodilation and increase capillary permeability, resulting in the immediate (15-minute) wheal-and-flare or hive reaction.

The most commonly used skin test is the prick test, in which the tester places a drop of antigen solution on the skin and inserts a needle through the external surface of the skin, but not deep enough to draw blood. The accuracy of the skin test depends on the experience of the interpreter.

The skin tests measure only IgE mediated reactions. While there is general agreement on their value for determining inhalant allergies, there is broad disagreement on their merits in diagnosing food sensitivities. While the skin tests are economical, they can cause great patient discomfort and are contraindicated in various types of patients.

Electroacupuncture (EAV) techniques

Electroacupuncture, according to Voll, has been used in Europe for many years to determine the abnormalities or energy imbalances of the body. Proponents claim that food allergies can be measured using this technique.

The patient holds a negative electrode in one hand, and the positive electrode probe is used to press selected acupuncture points. When a suspected food is placed on an aluminium tray which is connected into the circuit, certain galvanometer reading changes indicate sensitivity. If the appropriately diluted form of the extract is then placed on the tray, equilibrium of the reading should occur.

In order for this technique to gain wider acceptance, more research and clinical trials will have to be conducted, and a scientifically satisfactory explanation of its mode of operation will have to be developed.

Kinesiologic

Practitioners of applied kinesiology (AK) claim that muscle testing can diagnose food allergies. After either the patient has ingested a small amount of the antigen, or the antigen has been placed on the surface of the patient's body, certain muscles are tested for strength and weakness. This technique is widely used by AK practitioners (particularly chiropractors), and, if it is effective, does have the advantage of being inexpensive and fast.

More research needs to be done in order to confirm the limited clinical claims, and, as with the EAV technique, a satisfactory explanation of its mode of action must be developed.

Experiential testing   Many physicians believe that oral food challenge is the best way of diagnosing food sensitivities. Orthodox practitioners, clinical ecologists and naturopathic physicians agree that food challenge is an accurate and useful procedure when used with an appropriate patient. There is, however, a wide variety of protocols and indications among the physicians using these methods.

There are two broad categories of food provocation challenge testing:
- Elimination (also known as oligoantigenic) diet, followed by food reintroduction.
- Pure water fast, followed by food challenge.

In the elimination diet method the person is placed on a limited diet; commonly eaten foods are eliminated and replaced with either hypoallergenic and foods rarely eaten, or special hypoallergenic formulas.[37,38] The fewer the allergic foods the greater the ease of establishing a diagnosis with an elimination diet. The standard elimination diet consists of lamb, chicken, potatoes, rice, banana, apple and a brassica family vegetable (cabbage, Brussels sprouts, broccoli, etc.).

The individual stays on this limited diet for at least one week and up to one month. If the symptoms are related to food sensitivity, they will typically disappear by the fifth or sixth day of the diet. If the symptoms do not disappear it is possible that a reaction to a food in the elimination diet is responsible, in which case an even more restricted diet must be utilised.

After one week, individual foods are reintroduced according to some plan whereby a particular food is reintroduced every two days. Methods range from reintroducing only a single food every two days, to one every one or two meals. Usually after the one week 'cleansing' period the patient will develop an increased sensitivity to offending foods.

Reintroduction of sensitive foods will typically produce a more severe or recognisable symptom than before. A careful detailed record must be maintained describing when foods were reintroduced and what symptoms appeared upon reintroduction.[39] It can be very useful to track the wrist pulse during reintroduction, as pulse changes may occur when an allergic food is consumed.[40]

For those with limited financial resources, as well as those with less severe health problems, elimination diets offer a viable means of detection. Because one can sometimes dramatically experience the effects of food reactions, motivation to eliminate the food can be high. The procedure is time consuming and requires discipline.

A refinement which yields more results than the simple elimination diet is the five day water fast with subsequent challenge. Proponents of this approach believe that it is necessary for the patient to fast for at least five days in order to clear the body of allergic responses.[41] This procedure can be performed at home, or in a special clinical ecology unit.[41] During the fast, 'withdrawal' symptoms will likely be experienced. These symptoms will usually subside by the fourth day. As in the elimination diet, symptoms caused by food allergy will diminish or be eliminated after the fourth day.

After the five day fast, individual foods are singly reintroduced, with the monitoring of symptoms and pulse. Due to the hyper-reactive state, symptoms tend to be more acute and pronounced than before the fast. This method can produce dramatic results, greatly motivating avoidance of the offending foods.

This method is only advisable for people who are physically and mentally capable of a five day water fast. Close monitoring by a physician with experience in fasting is highly recommended. At times, careful interpretation of results is needed, due to the occurrence of delayed reactions.

Food challenge testing should not be used in people with symptoms that are potentially life threatening (such as airway constriction or severe allergic reactions).

Therapy

Avoidance and elimination

The simplest and most effective method of treating food allergies is through avoidance of allergic foods. Elimination of the offending antigens from the diet will begin to alleviate associated symptoms after the body has cleared itself of the antigen/antibody complexes and after the intestinal tract has got rid of any remaining food (usually three to five days). Avoidance means not only avoiding the food in its most identifiable state (e.g. eggs in an omelette), but also in its hidden state (e.g. eggs in cake). For severe reactions, closely related foods with similar antigenic components may also need to be eliminated (e.g. rice and millet in patients with severe wheat allergy).

Avoiding allergic foods may not be simple or practical, for several reasons:

- Common allergic foods such as wheat, corn and soy are found as components of many processed foods.

- When eating away from home it is often difficult to determine what ingredients are used in purchased foods and prepared meals.

- There has been a dramatic increase in the number of foods that single individuals are allergic to. This condition represents a 'syndrome' that is possibly indicative of broad immune system dysfunction. It may be difficult (psychologically, socially and nutritionally) to eliminate a large number of common foods from a person's diet.

Rotary diversified diet

Many experts believe the key to the dietary control of food allergies is the rotary diversified diet. The diet was first developed by Dr Herbert J. Rinkel in 1934, and is made up of a highly varied selection of foods which are eaten in a definite rotation in order to prevent the formation of new allergies and to control pre-existing ones.

Tolerated foods are eaten at regularly spaced intervals of four to seven days.[42] For example, if a person has wheat on Monday, they will have to wait until Friday to have anything with wheat in it again. This approach is based on the principle that infrequent consumption of tolerated foods is not likely to induce new allergies or increase any mild allergies, even in highly sensitised and immune-compromised individuals. As tolerance for eliminated foods returns, they may be added back into the rotation schedule without reactivation of the allergy (this of course applies only to cyclic food allergies – fixed allergenic foods may never be eaten again).

However, it is not simply a matter of rotating tolerated foods. Food families must also be rotated. Foods, whether animal or vegetable, come in families. The reason it is important to rotate food families is that foods in one family can cross-react with allergic foods. Steady consumption of foods which are members of the same family can lead to allergies. Food families need not be as strictly rotated as individual foods, but it is usually recommended to avoid eating members of the same food family two days in a row.

A simplified four day rotation diet plan is given in the accompanying box. However, in order to insure proper nutritional intake and classification of foods by related family groupings, professional nutritional counselling can be utilised. There are several excellent books and aids available which go into rotation diets to a much greater extent (e.g. *An Alternative Approach to Allergies* by T.G. Randolph and R.W. Moss, Bantam Books, New York, NY, 1980, and *Coping with Your Allergies* by N. Golos and F.G. Golos, Simon and Schuster, New York, NY, 1986).

Four day rotation diet

Food family   *Food*

Day 1

Citrus   Lemon, orange, grapefruit, lime, tangerine, kumquat, citron
Banana   Banana, plantain, arrowroot (musa)
Palm   Coconut, date, date sugar
Parsley   Carrots, parsnips, celery, celery seed, celeriac, anise, dill, fennel, cumin, parsley, coriander, caraway
Pepper   Black and white pepper, peppercorn
Herbs   Nutmeg, mace
Subucaya   Brazil nut
Bird   All fowl and game birds including chicken, turkey, duck, goose, guinea, pigeon, quail, pheasant, eggs
Tea   Comfrey tea (borage family), fennel tea
Oil   Coconut oil, fats from any bird listed above
Sweetener (use sparingly) Date sugar, orange honey if honey not used on another day of rotation
Juices   Juices may be made and used without adding sweeteners from the following

	Fruits	Any listed above in any combination desired
	Vegetables	Any listed above in any combination desired, including fresh comfrey

Day 2

Grape   All varieties of grapes, raisins
Pineapple   Juice pack, water pack or fresh
Rose   Strawberry, raspberry, blackberry, loganberry, rose hips
Melon   Watermelon, cucumber, cantaloupe, pumpkin, squash, other melons, zucchini, pumpkin or squash seeds
Mallow   Okra, cottonseed
Beet   Beet, spinach, chard
Pea (legume)   Pea, black-eyed pea, dry beans, green beans, carob, soybeans, lentils, liquorice, peanut, alfalfa
Cashew   Cashew, pistachio, mango
Birch   Filberts, hazelnuts
Flaxseed   Flaxseed

Swine	All pork products
Molluscs	Abalone, snail, squid, clam, mussel, oyster, scallop
Crustaceans	Crab, crayfish, lobster, prawn, shrimp
Tea	Alfalfa tea, fenugreek
Oil	Soybean oil, peanut oil, cottonseed oil
Sweeteners (use sparingly)	Carob syrup or beet syrup
Clover honey	If honey not used on another day
Juices	Juices may be made and used without added sweeteners from the following
	Fruits or berries — Any listed above in any combination desired
	Vegetables — Any listed above in any combination desired including fresh alfalfa and some legumes

Day 3

Apple	Apple, pear, quince
Mulberry	Mulberry, figs
Honeysuckle	Elderberry
Olive	Black or green or stuffed with pimento
Gooseberry	Currant, gooseberry
Buckwheat	Buckwheat, rhubarb
Aster	Lettuce, chicory, endive, escarole, globe artichoke, dandelion, sunflower seeds, tarragon
Potato	Potato, tomato, eggplant, peppers (red and green), chili pepper, paprika, cayenne, ground cherries
Lily (onion)	Onion, garlic, asparagus, chives, leeks
Spurge	Tapioca
Herb	Basil, savory, sage, oregano, horehound, catnip, spearmint, peppermint, thyme, marjoram, lemon balm
Walnut	English walnut, black walnut, pecan, hickory nut, butternut
Pedalium	Sesame
Beech	Chestnut
Saltwater fish	Herring, anchovy, cod, sea bass, sea trout, mackerel, tuna, swordfish, flounder, sole
Freshwater fish	Sturgeon, salmon, whitefish, bass, perch
Tea	Kaffir tea
Oil	Safflower oil
Honey (use sparingly)	Buckwheat, safflower or sage honey if not used on another day
Juices	Juices may be made and used without added sweeteners from the following

Fruits	Any listed above in any combination desired
Vegetables and herbs	Any listed above in any combination desired

Day 4

Plum	Plum, cherry, peach, apricot, nectarine, almond, wild cherry
Bilberry	Bilberry, huckleberry, cranberry, wintergreen
Pawpaws	Pawpaw, papaya, papain
Mustard	Mustard, turnip, radish, horseradish, watercress, cabbage, chinese cabbage, broccoli, cauliflower, Brussels sprouts, kale, kohlrabi, rutabaga
Laurel	Avocado, cinnamon, bay leaf, sasafras, cassia buds or bark
Sweet potato or yam	
Grass	Wheat, corn, rice, oats, barley, rye, wild rice, cane, millet, sorghum, bamboo sprouts
Orchid	Vanilla
Protea	Macadamia nut
Conifer	Pine nut
Fungus	Mushrooms and yeast (brewer's yeast, etc.)
Bovid	Milk products – butter, cheese, yogurt, beef and milk products, oleomargarine, lamb
Tea	Sassafras tea or papaya leaf tea, maté tea, lemon verbena tea
Oil	Corn oil, butter
Sweetener (use sparingly)	Cane sugar, sorghum, corn syrup, glucose, dextrose, avocado honey if honey is not used on another day
Juices	Juices may be made and used without added sweeteners, from the following
Fruits	Any listed above in any combination desired
Vegetables	Any listed above in any combination desired, including any of the tea herbs obtained fresh

Desensitisation

The intradermal/sublingual provocation and neutralisation (P-N) technique is used both to diagnose and treat food allergies.[43-45] The P-N procedure assesses the ability of a test dose (under the skin or under the tongue) to provoke symptoms and induce a weal, and then attempts to discover which dosage will neutralise the symptoms and change the weal according to a specific pattern. Intradermal injections or sublingual drops of 0.05 ml of a particular dilution of antigen in glycerine are given in sequential serial dilutions. It has been found that certain dilutions of food antigens will invoke, while other dilutions will block, the characteristic allergy symptoms.[35]

Based on the neutralising dilution, a sublingual vaccine is prepared and taken one drop sublingually per day for a period usually ranging from five to 12 months. During this time the person eats a fixed-frequency diet which specifies the number of times an allergic (yet treated) food shall be eaten (usually two or three times per week). The vaccine appears to block and relieve most symptoms, even when ingesting allergic foods. Many patients report that after six months to a year of therapy they can stop therapy and continue to eat formerly symptom-provoking foods.

Immune system support

Due to the association of food allergy with immune system dysfunction, immune support can be very beneficial. Selenium,[46] zinc,[47] B-complex and thymus extract all help normalise the immune system. Vitamin A may increase IgA levels at the mucosal surfaces.

Minimising systemic reactions

Quercetin (a bioflavonoid) has been shown to stabilise mast cells (thereby reducing histamine release) and lessen production of mediators of inflammation.[48] Flavonoids also reduce permeability of the capillary cell wall. Vitamin C and bromelain have strong antihistaminic properties, and bromelain interferes with the release of inflammatory particles.

Essential fatty acid deficiency has been shown to decrease anti-inflammatory prostaglandin (PGE1) production, favouring arachidonic acid shunting to inflammatory prostaglandins (PGE2) and lower levels of T-cell suppressor cells.[49] Vegetable oils, evening primrose oil and fish oils help reverse this process.

Underlying and associated conditions

It is necessary to identify and treat any underlying conditions which may contribute to the allergic process. Improper digestion of food and malabsorption should be tested for (see Chapter 5, Digestion).

Due to the association of chronic candidiasis with imbalanced bowel flora and intestinal mucosal inflammation, candida infection should be identified and treated (see Chapter 21, Candidiasis).

Treatment

While there is no known simple 'cure' for food allergies, there are a number of measures that will help avoid and lessen symptoms and correct the underlying causes.

Eventually the damaged tissues will heal, and in most cases one will become progressively less sensitive to the environment.

First, all allergenic foods should be identified using one of the methods discussed above. Then, all possible causes of food allergy (inadequate stomach acid, inadequate pancreatic enzyme secretion, bowel toxicity or bacterial imbalance, impaired liver function, chronic candida infection, and excessive frequency of consumption of specific foods) should be identified and controlled. Finally, the significantly allergic foods should be avoided.

Diet

The best approach is clearly avoidance of all major allergens, and rotation of all other foods for at least the first few months. As one improves, the dietary restrictions can be relaxed after four months, although some individuals may always require a rotation diet. For strongly allergic foods, all members of the food family should be avoided.

Supplements

- Vitamin C, 1 g four times a day.
- Selenium, 100 µg two times a day.
- Quercetin, 250 mg 20 minutes before meals.
- Bromelain, 125 mg 20 minutes before meals.
- Pancreatin (8× USP, i.e., eight times the United States Pharmacopea standard for pancreatin), one to two tablets with meals.
- Zinc, 15 mg a day.
- Vitamin A, 15,000 iu two times a day
- Linseed oil, 1 tblsp two times a day.
- Thymus extract, dosage will vary with product, follow label instructions.
- B-complex, 50 mg per day.

39

Gallstones

- May be without symptoms or may cause intense abdominal pain with irregular pain-free intervals of days or months.
- Bloating, gas, nausea and discomfort after a heavy meal of rich, fatty food.
- Definitive diagnosis is made using diagnostic ultrasound.

General considerations

Gallstones are another example of a western-diet induced disease. In the United States autopsy studies have shown that gallstones exist in about 20 per cent of the women and 8 per cent of the men over age 40.[1-4]

Gallstones arise when a normally solubilised component of bile becomes super-saturated and precipitates to begin the formation of a stone. Gallstones can be divided into four major categories:
- Pure cholesterol.
- Pure pigment (calcium bilirubinate).
- Mixed, containing cholesterol and its derivatives along with varying amounts of bile salts, bile pigments and inorganic salts of calcium.
- Stones composed entirely of minerals.[1-3]

Pure stones, either cholesterol or calcium bilirubinate, are extremely rare in the US. Recent studies indicate that in the US, approximately 80 per cent of the stones are of the mixed variety, the remaining 20 per cent of the stones being composed entirely of minerals, principly calcium salts, although some stones contain oxides of silicon and aluminium.[1-3]

What causes gallstones

The formation of gallstones has been divided into three steps:
- Bile supersaturation
- Nucleation and initiation of stone formation
- Enlargement of the gallstone

Cholesterol and mixed stones   The required step in cholesterol and mixed stones is cholesterol becoming insoluble (supersaturation of bile) within the gallbladder. The solubility of bile is based on the relative concentrations of cholesterol, bile acids, phosphatidylcholine (lecithin) and water. Since free cholesterol is water insoluble, it must be incorporated into a lecithin-bile salt mixture. Either an increase in cholesterol or a decrease in bile acids, lecithin or water within the bile will result in cholesterol becoming insoluble within the bile.

Risk factors for the development of cholesterol and mixed gallstones include diet, sex, race, obesity, certain drugs, various gastrointestinal diseases (especially Crohn's disease and cystic fibrosis) and age.[1–3]

The role of a low fibre, high-fat diet in the development of gallstones is discussed below. Women are thought to be predisposed to gallstones because of either an increased cholesterol content in the bile or suppression of bile acid synthesis by oestrogens. The rate of occurrence of gallstones is highest in women of American Indian and northern European origin over the age of 30. Age is also an important risk factor, especially among men.[1–3]

Risk factors for pigmented gallstones are not related to diet as much as they are to geography and severe diseases. Pigmented gallstones are more common in the orient due to the higher incidence of parasitic infection of the liver and gallbladder by a variety of organisms including the liver fluke *Clonorchis sinensis*. Bacteria and protozoa can cause stagnation of bile or act as nucleating agents. In the United States, pigmented stones are usually due to chronic haemolysis (bursting of red blood cells) or alcoholic cirrhosis of the liver.[1–3]

Therapy

Gallstones are easier to prevent than reverse. Primary treatment, therefore, involves reducing those risk factors listed above, involved in developing gallstones. Once gallstones have formed, it is important to avoid aggravating foods and to employ measures which increase the solubility of cholesterol in bile.

A number of dietary factors are important in the prevention and treatment of gallstones. Foremost is the elimination of foods which can produce symptoms. In addition to this general recommendation, it is also important to increase dietary fibre, eliminate food allergies and reduce intake of animal protein.

Other treatment measures involve the use of nutritional lipotropic compounds, herbal choleretics and other natural compounds in an attempt to increase the solubility of bile.

Dietary fibre

The hypothesis that the main cause of gallstones is the consumption of fibre-depleted refined foods has a great deal of support.[3,4] As mentioned earlier, gallstones are associated with the western diet in population studies. Such a diet, high in refined carbohydrate (sugar) and fat and low in fibre, leads to a reduction in the synthesis of bile acids by the liver and a lower bile acid pool in the gallbladder. Since the solubility of cholesterol is dependent upon the bile acid content of bile, when bile acid levels are reduced, cholesterol-rich gallstones form.

Another way in which fibre may prevent gallstone formation is by reducing the absorption of deoxycholic acid.[3,4] This compound is produced from bile acids by bacteria in the intestine. Deoxycholic acid greatly reduces the solubility of cholesterol in bile. In other words a high level of deoxycholic acid in the gallbladder leads to cholesterol-rich gallstones.

Dietary fibre has been shown to decrease the formation of deoxycholic acid as well as to bind to deoxycholic acid and promote its excretion in the faeces. This greatly increases the solubility of cholesterol in the bile. A diet high in fibre, especially those fibres capable of binding to deoxycholic acid (predominantly water-soluble fibres found in vegetables and fruits, pectin, oat bran and guar gum), is extremely important in the prevention as well as reversal of most gallstones.[4]

Vegetarian diet

A vegetarian diet has been shown to be protective against gallstone formation.[4,5] In a study of a large group of healthy non-vegetarian women and a comparable group of vegetarian women, it was shown that gallstones (using ultrasound techniques) occurred significantly less frequently in the vegetarian group.

This may simply be a result of the increased fibre content of the vegetarian diet, although other factors may be equally important. Animal proteins, like casein from dairy products, have been shown to increase the formation of gallstones in animals, while vegetable proteins, like soy, were shown to be preventive against gallstone formation.[3,4,6]

Food allergies

Since 1948 Dr J.C. Breneman, author of *Basics of Food Allergy*, has used a very successful therapeutic regime to prevent gallbladder attacks – allergy elimination diets. There is support for food allergies causing gallbladder pain in the scientific literature.[7-10] A 1968 study revealed that 100 per cent of a group of patients were free from symptoms while they were on a basic elimination diet (beef, rye, soybean, rice, cherry, peach, apricot, beet and spinach).[7]

Foods inducing symptoms in decreasing order of their occurrence were egg, pork, onion, fowl, milk, coffee, citrus, corn, beans and nuts. Adding eggs to the diet caused gallbladder attacks in 93 per cent of the patients.

Several mechanisms have been proposed to explain the association of food allergy and gallbladder attacks. Dr Breneman believes the ingestion of allergy-causing substances causes swelling of the bile ducts, resulting in impairment of bile flow from the gallbladder.

Lecithin (phosphatidylcholine)

A low lecithin concentration in the bile may be a causative factor for many individuals with gallstones. Studies have shown that as little as 100 mg of lecithin three times per day will increase the concentration of lecithin in the bile; larger doses (up to 10 grams) produce even greater increases.[11,12] This is extremely significant as an increased lecithin content of bile usually increases the solubility of cholesterol. However, no significant effects on gallstone dissolution have been obtained using lecithin alone.

Nutrient deficiencies

Deficiencies of vitamins E and C have been shown to cause gallstones in experimental studies in animals.[13,14]

Olive oil

A very popular lay remedy for gallstones is the so-called olive oil liver flush. There are several variations. The most popular is drinking one cup of unrefined olive oil plus the juice of two lemons in the morning for several days. Many people tell tales of passing huges stones while on the liver flush. However, what they think are gallstones are actually a complex of minerals, olive oil and lemon juice produced within the gastrointestinal tract.

  The olive oil liver flush is not a good idea for a couple of reasons. First of all, consuming a large quantity of any oil will result in contraction of the gallbladder. It is quite possible that violent contraction of the gallbladder would increase the likelihood of a stone blocking the bile duct. This is a very serious condition that often requires immediate surgery to prevent death. In addition, oleic acid, the main component of olive oil has been shown to increase the development of gallstones in rabbits and rats by increasing the content of cholesterol within the gallbladder.[15,16] Although this effect has not yet been observed in humans,[17] the animal research suggests it to be unwise to use an olive oil liver flush as a treatment of gallbladder disease.

Lipotropic factors and herbal choleretics

The naturopathic approach to the treatment of gallstones has typically involved the use of lipotropic and choleretic formulas (see Chapter 8, Liver support, for complete discussion). Lipotropic factors are, by definition, substances that hasten the removal or decrease the deposit of fat in the liver through their interaction with fat metabolism. Compounds commonly employed as lipotropic agents include choline, methionine, betaine, folic acid and vitamin B12. Often these nutritional factors are used along with herbal cholagogues and choleretics. Cholagogues are agents that stimulate gallbladder contraction to promote bile flow, while choleretics are agents that stimulate bile secretion by the liver, as opposed to the expulsion of bile by the gallbladder.

  Many of the herbal choleretics have a favourable effect on the solubility of bile. Those choleretics discussed in Chapter 8, Liver support, are appropriate to use in the treatment of gallstones, including dandelion root (*Taraxacum officinale*), silymarin (from *Silybum marianum*), artichoke leaves (*Cynara scolymus*) and turmeric (*Curcuma longa*). In addition, boldo (*Peumus boldo*) contains substances quite useful in the treatment of gallstones.

Chemical dissolution of gallstones

There appears to be a successful non-surgical alternative to the treatment of gallstones by using a complex of plant terpenes (i.e. menthol, menthone, pinene, borneol, cineol and camphene) alone or preferably in combination with oral bile acids. This approach is available only through a physician's prescription.

As the formation of the stone is dependent on either increased accumulation of cholesterol or reduced levels of bile acids or lecithin, decreasing gallbladder cholesterol levels and/or increasing bile acid or lecithin levels should result in dissolution of the stone. Oral bile acid therapy (chenodeoxycholic acid or ursodeoxycholic acid) has resulted in dissolution of the gallstone in a number of patients by promoting increased cholesterol solubility. However, this therapy often takes several years and is associated with mild diarrhoea and liver damage.

Gallstone dissolution by a natural terpene combination (Rowachol, Rowa Ltd, UK) has been demonstrated in several studies.[18-22] This non-surgical approach to gallstone removal offers an effective alternative to surgery and has been demonstrated to be safe even when it has been consumed for prolonged periods of time (up to four years). Although effective alone, best results appear to be achieved when plant terpene complexes are used in combination with bile acid therapy.[22-25]

This combined approach offers better results than when either bile acids or plant terpenes were used alone.[23-25] Furthermore, since a lower dose of bile acid can be used, there is a significant reduction in the risk of complications or side effects, and in the cost of bile acid therapy. Chemical dissolution of gallstones is especially indicated in the treatment of gallstones in the elderly who cannot withstand the stress of surgery and in other cases where surgery is quite risky.

Treatment

Prevention is easier to attain than reversal of gallstones. The risk factors and causes of gallstones are well known. In most cases, it is simply a matter of adopting a healthier diet rich in dietary fibre.

If gallstones are already developed it is necessary to take stronger measures to avoid gallbladder attacks, as well as increase the solubility of the bile. Food allergies and fatty foods can aggravate the symptoms of gallstones. To increase the solubility of the bile it is necessary to follow the dietary guidelines given below, as well as supplement the diet with the nutritional and herbal factors listed below.

Diet

Increase intake of vegetables and fruits. Increase intake of dietary fibre, especially the gel-forming or mucilaginous fibres (flax seed, oat bran, guar gum, pectin, etc.), while reducing the consumption of saturated fats, cholesterol, sugar and animal proteins. All fried foods should be avoided.

An allergy elimination diet can be used to reduce gallbladder attacks (see Chapter 38, Food allergy, for a description of an elimination diet).

Water

It is extremely important that six to eight glasses of water be consumed each day to maintain the water content of bile.

Nutritional supplements

- Vitamin C, 1 to 3 grams a day.
- Vitamin E, 200 to 400 iu a day.
- Phosphatidylcholine, 500 milligrams a day.
- Choline, 1 gram a day.
- L-methionine, 1 gram a day.
- Fibre supplement (guar gum, pectin, psyllium or oat bran), minimum of 5 grams a day.

Botanical medicines

- *Taraxacum officinale*
    Dried root, 4 grams three times a day.
    Fluid extract (1:1), 4–8 ml three times a day.
    Solid extract (4:1), 250–500 mg three times a day.
- *Peumus boldo*
    Dried leaves (or by infusion), 250–500 mg three times a day.
    Tincture (1:10), 2–4 ml three times a day.
    Fluid extract (1:1), 05.–1.0 ml.
- *Silybum marianum* – the standard dose of *Silybum marianum* is based on its silymarin content, 70–210 mg of silymarin three times daily.
- *Cynara scolymus* – extract (15 per cent cynarin), 500 mg three times a day.
- *Curcuma longa* can be used liberally as spice.
    Curcumin, 300 mg three times a day.

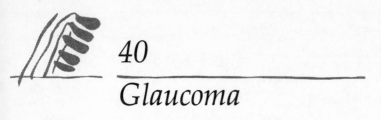

40

Glaucoma

Acute (closed-angle) glaucoma:

- Severe throbbing pain in eye with markedly blurred vision.
- Pupil moderately dilated and fixed.
- Pupil does not respond to light appropriately.
- Nausea and vomiting is common.
- Increased pressure in the inner eye, usually on one side.

Chronic (open angle) glaucoma:

- Usually asymptomatic until later stages.
- Gradual loss of peripheral vision resulting in tunnel vision.
- Extreme pain, blurring of vision, conjunctivitis, and fixed and dilated pupil in later, emergency stage.
- Persistent elevation of inner eye pressure associated with pathological cupping of the optic discs, i.e. the portion of the eye where the optic nerve enters the eyeball.

General considerations

In the United States there are approximately 2 million people with glaucoma, 25 per cent of which is undetected.[1] Ten per cent have the acute closed-angle type and 90 per cent is of the chronic open-angle type.[1]

Glaucoma refers to increased pressure within the eye as a result of an imbalance between production and outflow of the fluid in the eye. Obstruction to outflow is the main factor responsible for this imbalance in acute glaucoma. While there appears to be no anatomical basis for the chronic form, there is a strong correlation between the content and composition of collagen and the glaucomatous eye.[2]

Collagen is the most abundant protein in the body, including the eye. In the eye it gives strength and integrity to the tissues. Errors of collagen metabolism (e.g. osteogenesis imperfecta, Ehlers–Danlos syndrome and Marfan's syndrome) are often associated with eye complications – glaucoma, myopia (near sightedness), retinal detachment, ectopia lentis (dislocated lens) and blue sclera.[3]

Abnormalities in the tissue at the back of the eye, through which pass the optic

Table 40.1 Differential diagnosis of the inflamed eye[1]

	Acute conjunctivitis	Acute iritis	Acute glaucoma	Corneal trauma or infection
Incidence	Very common	Common	Uncommon	Common
Discharge	Moderate to copious	None	None	Watery or purulent
Vision	No effect	Slightly blurred	Markedly blurred	Usually blurred
Pain	None	Moderate	Severe	Moderate to severe
Conjunctival injection	Diffuse, mostly fornices	Circumcorneal	Diffuse	Diffuse
Cornea	Clear	Usually clear	Steamy	Clarity may change
Pupil size	Normal	Small	Dilated and fixed	Normal
Pupil light and response	Normal	Poor	None	Normal
Intraocular pressure	Normal	Normal	Elevated	Normal
Anterior chamber	Normal depth	Normal depth	Very shallow	Normal depth
Iris	Normal	Dull, swollen	Congested and bulging	Normal unless infected
Smear	Causative organisms	No organisms	No organisms	Causative organisms if infection

nerve fibres and blood vessels, the connective tissue network the eye fluid must pass through to leave the eye and the blood vessels in the eye, have all been observed in glaucomatous eyes.[2,4–6] These changes may result in elevated inner eye pressure or lead to progressive loss of peripheral vision. Table 40.1 summarises the conditions associated with an inflamed eye.

Therapy

Treatment and prevention of glaucoma is dependent upon:
- Reduction of the elevated inner eye pressure.
- Improvement of collagen metabolism, particularly at the back of the eye where the optic nerve exits and in the tissues that drain the eye fluids.

Acute glaucoma

Acute glaucoma represents a medical emergency. A person with suspected acute glaucoma should go immediately to an ophthalmologist or hospital accident and emergency department. Effective therapy must be started within 12 to 48 hours or permanent loss of vision will occur within three to five days.

The standard medical approach is immediately to reduce the eye pressure through the use of an osmotic agent, followed by surgery. Although the osmotic agent (such as glycerin, 1–2 g/kg body weight mixed with an equal amount of water) will usually quickly improve the symptoms, surgery is still necessary since each acute attack diminishes vision and contracts the visual field, and an apparently improving eye may worsen rapidly. Agents (e.g. belladonna and ephedra) which dilate the pupils must be strictly avoided.

Chronic glaucoma

Vitamin C   Of foremost importance in achieving collagen integrity is optimal tissue concentrations of vitamin C. Furthermore, vitamin C supplementation has been demonstrated to lower inner eye pressure levels in many clinical studies.[7-11] A daily dose of 0.5 grams per kilogram body weight, whether in single or divided doses, reduces inner eye pressure by an average of 16 mm Hg.[11] Almost normal tension levels have been achieved in some patients unresponsive to standard medical therapies (acetazolamide and pilocarpine).[11]

This pressure-lowering action of vitamin C is long lasting if supplementation is continued, and intravenous administration results in an even greater initial reduction.[7,9-11] Careful monitoring by a physician is required to determine the appropriate dose, as some people will respond to as little as 2 grams per day while others will respond only to extremely high doses, e.g. 35 grams per day.[7-11] Abdominal discomfort when using high doses is common, but usually resolves after three to four days.[11]

The proposed mechanisms by which vitamin C lowers inner eye pressure include increased blood osmolarity, diminished production of eye fluid, and improved fluid outflow. In the light of recent research, however, its role in collagen formation may be the key to its action.

Bioflavonoids   To aid normal collagen metabolism further, bioflavonoid supplements, particularly the anthocyanosides (the blue-red pigments found in berries), are very useful. These compounds prevent the breakdown of vitamin C, improve capillary integrity and stabilise the collagen matrix by preventing free radical damage, inhibiting enzymatic breakdown of the collagen matrix and cross linking with collagen fibres to form a more stable collagen matrix.[12-14] *Vaccinium myrtillus* (bilberry) extract is particularly rich in these flavonoid and anthocyanidin compounds and has been used with good results in reducing near-sightedness, improving night vision and reversing diabetic retinopathy.[15] Rutin has also been demonstrated to lower inner eye pressure when used in conjunction with standard drugs.[16]

Allergy   The successful treatment of chronic glaucoma by anti-allergic measures has been reported in the literature.[17] In one study, many of the 113 patients demonstrated an immediate rise in intraocular pressure of up to 20 mm Hg (in addition to other typical allergic symptoms) when challenged with the appropriate allergen, whether food borne or environmental. The author speculated that the known allergic responses of altered vascular permeability and vasospasm could result in the congestion and oedema characteristic of glaucoma.

Other considerations

Corticosteroids induce glaucoma by destroying collagen structures in the eye.[1,2] Corticosteroid use should therefore be discouraged in the patient with glaucoma.[1,2]

Treatment

Acute glaucoma is a medical emergency. Go to the nearest accident and emergency department immediately. Effective therapy must be started within 12 to 48 hours or permanent loss of vision will occur within three to five days. The following are only meant to prevent further attacks in the other eye and for the treatment of chronic glaucoma under the care of a physician. An asymptomatic eye may convert spontaneously to acute glaucoma. The process can be precipitated by anything that dilates the pupil, such as atropine and epinephrine-like drugs. Typical signs and symptoms include extreme pain, blurring of vision, inflammation of the eye and a fixed, dilated pupil.

Supplement

- Vitamin C, 2–5 g a day in divided doses.
- Bioflavonoids (mixed), 1 gram a day.

Botanical medicines

Vaccinium myrtillus (bilberries):
- Fresh berries, 2–4 oz (50–100 grams) three times a day.
- Extracts containing 25 per cent anthocyanoside, 80–160 mg three times a day.

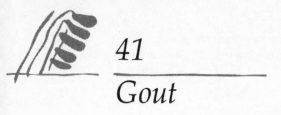

41
Gout

- Acute onset of intense joint pain, typically involving the first joint of the big toe (about 50 per cent of cases).
- Elevated serum uric acid level.
- Periods without symptoms between acute attacks.
- Identification of urate crystals in joint fluid.
- Aggregated deposits of monosodium urate monohydrate (tophi) chiefly in and around the joints of the extremities, but also in subcutaneous tissue, bone, cartilage and other tissues.
- Uric acid kidney stones.
- Familial disease; 95 per cent males.

General considerations

Gout is a common type of arthritis caused by an increased concentration of uric acid (the final breakdown product of purine metabolism) in biological fluids. In gout, uric acid, crystals (monosodium urate) are deposited in joints, tendons, kidneys, and other tissues, where they cause considerable inflammation and damage.[1,2]

Gout is associated with affluence and is often called the rich man's disease. Throughout history, the sufferer of gout has been depicted as a portly, middle-aged man sitting in a comfortable chair with one foot resting painfully on a soft cushion as he consumes great quantities of meat and wine. In fact, the traditional picture does have some basis in reality, as meats, particularly organ meats, are high purine foods, while alcohol inhibits uric acid secretion by the kidneys. Furthermore, even today, gout is primarily a disease of adult men; over 95 per cent of sufferers of gout are men over the age of 30.[1,2] The incidence of gout is approximately three adults in 1,000, although as many as 10–20 per cent of the adult population have hyperuricaemia.[3]

Causes of gout

Gout is classified into two major categories, primary and secondary. Primary gout accounts for about 90 per cent of all cases, while secondary gout accounts for only 10 per cent. The cause of primary gout is usually unknown. There are, however, several genetic defects in which the exact cause of the elevated uric acid is known.[1,2]

Causes of gout[3,4]

- Metabolic
  - Increased production of purine (primary)
    - Idiopathic (unknown).
    - Specific enzyme defects, e.g. Lesch-Nyhan syndrome, glycogen storage disease.
    - Decreased enzyme activity, e.g. hypoxanthine-guanine phosphoribosyl-transferase is decreased in 1–2 per cent of adult gouty individuals.
    - Increased enzyme activity, e.g. phosphoribosylpyrophosphate synthetase.
  - Increased production of purine (secondary)
    - Increased turnover of purines
      - Cancer.
      - Chronic haemolytic anaemia.
      - Cytotoxic drugs.
      - Psoriasis.
    - Increased synthesis, e.g. glucose-6-phosphatase deficiency.
    - Increased catabolism of purines
      - Fructose ingestion or infusion.
      - Exercise.
- Renal
  - Decreased renal clearance of uric acid (primary)
    - Intrinsic kidney disease.
  - Decreased renal clearance of uric acid (secondary)
    - Functional impairment of tubular secretion
      - Drug-induced, e.g. thiazides, probenecid, salicylates, ethambutol, pyrazinamide.
      - Hyperlacticaemia, e.g. lactic acidosis, alcoholism, toxaemia of pregnancy, chronic beryllium disease.
      - Hyperketoacidaemia, e.g. diabetic ketoacidosis, diabetes insipidus.
      - Bartter's syndrome.
      - Chronic lead intoxication.
      - Glucose-6-phosphatase deficiency.

The increased serum uric acid level observed in primary gout can be divided into three categories:

- Increased synthesis of uric acid, found in a majority of individuals.
- Reduced ability to excrete uric acid, typical of a smaller group (about 30 per cent).
- Overproduction of uric acid as well as under-excretion of uric acid – a small minority.

Although the exact metabolic defect in gout is not known in the majority of cases, gout is one of the most controllable metabolic diseases.[1,2] The causes of gout are summarised in the box on the preceding page.

Secondary gout refers to those cases in which the elevated uric acid level is secondary to some other disorder, such as excessive breakdown of cells or some form of kidney disease. Diuretic therapy for hypertension and low dose aspirin therapy are also important causes of secondary gout since they cause decreased uric acid excretion.[1,2]

About 200 to 600 mg of uric acid are excreted daily in the urine of an adult male. This is two-thirds of the amount produced, the rest being excreted in the bile and other gastrointestinal tract secretions. The dietary component of the uric acid in the blood is usually only 10–20 per cent of the total, but in an individual with significant uric acid in the blood enough uric acid through the diet can increase crystal formation in tissues.[3]

Almost all of the uric acid in the blood is filtered in the kidney: only the small amount bound to protein is not filtered. Excretion into the urine is peculiar in that about 80 per cent of the filtered uric acid is reabsorbed.[3]

Uric acid is a highly insoluble molecule, and at pH 7.4 and body temperature the serum is saturated at 6.4–7.0 mg/100 ml. Although higher concentrations do not necessarily result in deposition of uric acid crystals (some unknown factor in serum appears to inhibit crystal precipitation), the chance of an acute attack is greater than 90 per cent when the level is above 9 mg/100 ml (see Table 41.1). Lower temperatures decrease the saturation point of uric acid, which may explain why urate deposits tend to form in areas such as the top of the ear, where the temperature is lower than the mean body temperature (see Table 41.2). Uric acid is insoluble below pH 6.0 and can precipitate as the urine is concentrated in the collecting ducts and passed to the bladder.

Diagnosis

The first attack of gout is characterised by intense pain, usually involving only one joint. The first joint of the big toe is affected in nearly half of the first attacks and is at some time involved in over 90 per cent of individuals with gout. If the attack progresses, fever and chills will appear. The first attacks usually occur at night and are usually preceded by a specific event such as dietary excess, alcohol ingestion, trauma, certain drugs or surgery.[2]

The classic description of gout was by an English physician, Sydenham, who suffered from gout in 1683. Little has changed in the clinical picture of gout in over 300 years.

The victim goes to bed and sleeps in good health. About two o'clock in the morning he is awakened by a severe pain in the great toe; more rarely in the heel, ankle, or

Table 41.1 Prevalence of gouty arthritis by maximum urate level[5]

Serum urate (mg/100 ml)	Men (%)	Women (%)
<6	0.6	0.08
6.0–6.9	1.9	3.3
7.0–7.9	16.7	17.4
8.0–8.9	25.0	0
9+	90.0	0

Table 41.2 Solubility of urate ion as a function of temperature in 140 mmol Na^{+5}

Temperature (°C)	Maximum solubility (mg/100 ml)
37	6.8
35	6.0
30	4.5
25	3.3
20	2.5
15	1.8
10	1.2

instep. The pain is like that of a dislocation, and yet parts feel as if cold water were poured over them. Then follows chills and shivers, and a little fever. The pain which at first was moderate, becomes more intense. With its intensity the chills and fever increase. After a time this comes to a height, accommodating itself to the bones and ligaments of the tarsus and metatarsus. Now it is a violent stretching and tearing of the ligaments – now it is a gnawing pain and now a pressure and tightening. So exquisite and lively meanwhile is the feeling of the part affected, that it cannot bear the weight of bedclothes nor the jar of a person walking in the room. The night is passed in torture, sleeplessness, turning the part affected, and perpetual change of posture; the tossing about of the body being as incessant as the pain of the tortured joint, and being worse as the fit comes on. Hence the vain effort by change of posture, both in the body and the limb affected, to obtain an abatement of pain.

Subsequent attacks are common, with the majority having another attack within one year. However, nearly 7 per cent never have a second attack. Chronic gout is extremely rare, due to the advent of dietary therapy and drugs that lower uric acid levels. Some degree of kidney dysfunction occurs in nearly 90 per cent of subjects with gout, and there is a higher risk of kidney stones.[2]

Therapy

The current standard medical treatment of acute gout is administration of colchicine, the anti-inflammatory drug originally isolated from the plant *Colchicum autumnale* (autumn crocus, meadow saffron).[2] Colchicine has no effect on uric acid levels; rather it stops the inflammatory process by inhibiting the migration of white blood cells into areas of inflammation.

Over 75 per cent of patients with gout show major improvement in symptoms within the first 12 hours after receiving colchicine. However, as many as 80 per cent of patients are unable to tolerate an optimal dose because of gastrointestinal side effects, which may precede or coincide with clinical improvement.[2]

Colchicine may also cause bone marrow depression, hair loss, liver damage, depression, seizures, respiratory depression and even death. Other anti-inflammatory agents are also used in acute gout, including indomethacin, phenylbutazone, naproxen and fenoprofen.[2]

Once the acute episode has resolved, a number of measures are taken to reduce the likelihood of recurrence:

- Drugs to keep uric acid levels within a normal range.
- Controlled weight loss in obese individuals.
- Avoidance of known precipitating factors, such as heavy alcohol consumption or a diet rich in purines.
- Low doses of colchicine to prevent further acute attacks.[2]

Several dietary factors are known to be causes of gout – consumption of alcohol, high purine containing foods (organ meats, meat, yeast, poultry, etc.), fats and refined carbohydrates, and overconsumption of calories.[6,7] Individuals with gout are typically obese, prone to hypertension and diabetes, and at a greater risk for cardiovascular disease. Obesity is probably the most important dietary factor.[6,7]

In concept, the naturopathic approach for chronic gout does not differ substantially from the standard medical approach:

- Dietary and herbal measures are employed instead of drugs to keep uric acid levels within the normal range.
- Obese individuals are put on a careful weight loss programme.
- Known precipitating factors, such as heavy alcohol consumption and numerous dietary factors are controlled.
- Nutritional substances are used to prevent further acute attacks.

Lead toxicity An additional item of concern relates to lead toxicity. A secondary type of gout, sometimes called saturnine gout, can result from lead toxicity.[7,8,9] Historically, saturnine gout was due to the consumption of alcoholic beverages stored in containers containing lead.[9] However, chronic lead intoxication can lead to gout regardless of source. The mechanism of action is related to a decrease in renal urate excretion.

Dietary considerations

The dietary treatment of gout involves the following guidelines:

- Elimination of alcohol intake.

- Low purine diet.
- Achievement of ideal body weight.
- Liberal consumption of complex carbohydrates.
- Low fat intake.
- Low protein intake.
- Liberal fluid intake.

Alcohol   Alcohol (ethanol) increases uric acid production by accelerating purine nucleotide degradation and reduces uric acid excretion by increasing lactate production (a result of ethanol oxidation) which impairs kidney function. The net effect is a significant increase in serum uric acid levels. This explains why alcohol consumption is often a precipitating factor in acute attacks of gout. Elimination of alcohol is all that is needed to reduce uric acid levels and prevent gouty arthritis in many individuals.[6,7,10]

Low-purine diet   A low-purine diet has been the mainstay of the dietary therapy of gout for many years. However, with the advent of potent drugs that lower uric acid levels, many physicians 'lower the serum urate levels without subjecting the patient to the inconvenience and deprivation associated with a purine-free diet'. Dietary restriction of purines is, however, recommended to reduce metabolic stress. Foods with high purine levels should be entirely omitted. These include organ meats, meats, shellfish, yeast (brewer's and baker's), herring, sardines, mackerel and anchovies. Foods with moderate levels of protein should be curtailed as well. These include dried legumes, spinach, asparagus, fish, poultry and mushrooms.[6,7]

Weight reduction   Weight reduction in obese individuals significantly reduces serum uric acid levels. Weight reduction should involve the use of a high-fibre, low-fat diet, as this type of diet will help manage the elevated cholesterol and triglycerides which are also common in obesity. This diet is also an alkaline ash diet, recommended in the dietary treatment of gout, since a more alkaline pH increases uric acid solubility.

Carbohydrates, fats and protein   Refined carbohydrates and saturated fats should be kept to a minimum, as the former increase uric acid production while the latter increase uric acid retention.[6,7,11,12]

Protein intake should not be excessive (i.e. greater than 0.8 g/kg body weight per day), as it has been shown that uric acid synthesis may be accelerated in both normal and gouty patients by a high protein intake.[6] Adequate protein is necessary (0.8 g/kg body weight), however, as amino acids decrease resorption of uric acid in the renal tubules, thus increasing uric acid excretion and reducing serum uric acid concentrations.[7,13]

Fluid intake   Liberal fluid intake keeps the urine dilute and promotes the excretion of uric acid. Furthermore, dilution of the urine reduces the risk of kidney stones.[6]

Nutritional supplements

Eicosapentaenoic acid   Eicosapentaenoic acid (EPA) supplementation is very useful in the treatment of gout. EPA limits the production of the pro-inflammatory leukotrienes, which are the mediators of much of the inflammation and tissue damage observed in gout.[14,15]

Vitamin E   Vitamin E is indicated in the treatment of gout since it also (mildly) inhibits the production of leukotrienes and acts as an antioxidant.[16] Selenium functions synergistically with vitamin E.

Folic acid   Folic acid has been shown to inhibit xanthine oxidase, the enzyme responsible for producing uric acid.[17] The drug allopurinol, used in the medical treatment of gout, is a potent inhibitor of this enzyme. Research has demonstrated that a derivative of folic acid is an even greater inhibitor of xanthine oxidase than allopurinol, suggesting that folic acid at pharmacological doses may be an effective treatment in gout.[18] Positive results in the treatment of gout have been reported, but the data is incomplete and uncontrolled.[19]

Bromelain   The proteolytic enzyme of pineapple has been demonstrated to be an effective anti-inflammatory agent in both clinical human studies and experimental animal models.[20] It is a suitable alternative to stronger prescription anti-inflammatory agents used in the treatment of gout. For best results, bromelain should be taken between meals.

Quercetin   The bioflavonoid quercetin has demonstrated several effects in experimental studies that indicate its possible benefit to individuals with gout.[21-24] Quercetin may offer significant protection by inhibiting:
- xanthine oxidase, in a similar fashion to the drug allopurinol[21];
- leukotriene synthesis and release[23];
- neutrophil accumulation and enzyme release.[22]

For best results, quercetin should be taken with bromelain between meals (bromelain is believed to enhance the absorption of quercetin and other medications[24]).

Alanine, aspartic acid, glutamic acid and glycine   These amino acids have been shown to lower serum uric acid levels, presumably as a result of decreasing uric acid resorption in the renal tubule. This results in an increase in uric acid excretion.[7,13]

Vitamin C   Megadoses of vitamin C are probably contraindicated in individuals with gout as vitamin C may increase uric acid levels in a small number of individuals.[25]

Niacin   High doses of niacin, i.e. above 50 mg per day, are probably contraindicated in the treatment of gout, as niacin competes with uric acid for excretion.[26]

Botanical medicines

Cherries   Consuming half a pound (225 g) of fresh or canned cherries per day has been shown to be very effective in lowering uric acid levels and preventing attacks of gout.[27] Cherries, hawthorn berries, bilberries and other dark red-blue berries are rich sources of anthocyanidins and proanthocyanidins. These compounds are flavonoid molecules that give these fruits their deep red-blue colour, and are remarkable in their ability to prevent collagen destruction.[28,29]

Anthocyanidins and other flavonoids affect collagen metabolism in many ways:

- They have the unique ability actually to crosslink collagen fibres, resulting in reinforcement of the natural crosslinking of collagen that forms the collagen matrix of connective tissue (ground substance, cartilage, tendon, etc.).[28–30]
- They prevent free radical damage through their potent antioxidant and free radical scavenging action.[28–31]
- They inhibit enzymatic cleavage of collagen by enzymes secreted by leucocytes during inflammation.[30,31]
- They prevent the release and synthesis of compounds that promote inflammation, such as histamine, serine proteases, prostaglandins and leukotrienes.[31]

These effects on collagen structures make flavonoids extremely useful in the treatment of a wide variety of inflammatory conditions, including gout, rheumatoid arthritis and periodontal disease.

Harpagophytum procumbens (devil's claw)   Devil's claw has been used in folk medicine for the treatment of a variety of diseases, including gout and rheumatoid arthritis. Clinical research appears to indicate devil's claw may be of benefit in the treatment of gout; in addition to relieving joint pain, clinical trials found devil's claw also reduced serum cholesterol and uric acid levels.[32]

Several pharmacological studies utilising experimental models of inflammation in animals have reported that devil's claw possesses an anti-inflammatory and analgesic effect comparable to the potent drug phenylbutazone.[33] However, other studies have indicated that devil's claw has little, if any, anti-inflammatory activity.[34,35]

The equivocal research results found in experimental models may reflect a mechanism of action that is inconsistent with current anti-inflammatory drugs or a lack of quality control (standardisation) of the preparations used. Further clinical research is needed to clarify these inconsistencies.

At this time it can be stated that devil's claw may be useful in the short-term management of gout. However, since gout can be successfully prevented and treated by following simple dietary changes in most instances, the use of devil's claw in long-term management of gout is probably unnecessary.

Treatment

As stated earlier, the naturopathic approach to the prevention and treatment of gout does not differ substantially from the standard medical approach. The basic approach involves dietary and herbal measures which maintain uric acid levels within the normal range, controlled weight loss in obese individuals, avoidance of known precipitating factors (such as heavy alcohol consumption and a high-purine diet), the use of nutritional substances to prevent further acute attacks and the use of herbal and nutritional substances to inhibit the inflammatory process.

Diet

Eliminate alcohol intake, maintain a low-purine diet, increase consumption of complex carbohydrates and decrease consumption of simple carbohydrates, maintain a low fat intake, optimise protein intake (0.8 g/kg body weight) and consume liberal quantities of fluid. Urinary 24-hour uric acid levels can be used to monitor compliance with purine-free diet (maintain below 0.8 g per day.)

In addition, liberal amounts (0.5–1.0 pounds, 0.25–0.5 kg, per day) of cherries, bilberries and other anthocyanoside-rich, i.e. red-blue, berries (or extracts) should be consumed.

Nutritional supplements

- EPA, 1.8 g a day.
- Vitamin E, 400–800 iu a day.
- Folic acid, 10–40 mg a day.
- Bromelain, 125–250 mg three times a day between meals.
- Quercetin, 125–250 mg, three times a day between meals.

Botanical medicines

- *Harpagophytum procumbens*
  Dried powdered root, 1–2 grams three times a day.
  Tincture (1:5), 4–5 ml three times a day.
  Dry solid extract (3:1), 400 mg three times a day.
- Anthocyanoside extracts (e.g. *Vaccinium myrtillus*, *Ribes nigrum*), equivalent to 80 mg anthocyanoside content daily.

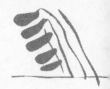

42

Haemorrhoids

- Abnormally large or painful conglomerates of blood vessels, supporting tissues and overlying mucous membrane or skin of the anorectal area.
- Bright red bleeding on the surface of the stool, on the toilet tissue and/or in the toilet bowl.

General considerations

In the industrialised countries, haemorrhoidal disease is extremely common. Although most individuals may begin to develop haemorrhoids in their 20s, haemorrhoidal symptoms usually do not become evident until the 30s.[1,2] Estimates have indicated that 50 per cent of persons over 50 years of age have symptomatic haemorrhoidal disease and up to one-third of the total US population have haemorrhoids to some degree.[3]

Cause

The causes of haemorrhoidal disease are similar to those which cause varicose veins (see Chapter 73, Varicose veins), i.e. genetic weakness of the veins, excessive venous pressure, pregnancy, long periods of standing or sitting and heavy lifting are considered the major factors.

Because the venous system supplying the rectal area contains no valves, factors which increase venous congestion in the region can precipitate haemorrhoid formation. This includes increasing intra-abdominal pressure (e.g. defaecation, pregnancy, coughing, sneezing, vomiting, physical exertion and portal hypertension due to cirrhosis), a low-fibre-diet-induced increase in straining during defaecation and standing or sitting for prolonged periods of time.

Classification of haemorrhoids

Haemorrhoids are typically classified according to location and degree of severity.

External haemorrhoids   External haemorrhoids occur below the anorectal line, the point in the 3-cm-long anal canal at which the skin lining changes to mucous membrane (see Figure 42.1). They may be either full blood clots (thrombotic haemorrhoid) or connective tissue (cutaneous haemorrhoid). A thrombotic haemorrhoid is produced when a haemorrhoidal vessel has ruptured and formed a blood clot (thrombus), while a cutaneous haemorrhoid consists of fibrous connective tissue covered by anal skin. Cutaneous haemorrhoids can be located at any point on the circumference of the anus. Typically, they are caused by the resolution of a thrombotic haemorrhoid, i.e. the thrombus becomes organised and replaced by connective tissue.

Internal haemorrhoids   Internal haemorrhoids occur above the anorectal line. Occasionally an internal haemorrhoid will enlarge to such a degree that it will prolapse and descend below the anal sphincter.

Internal-external haemorrhoids   Internal-external, or mixed, haemorrhoids are a combination of contiguous external and internal haemorrhoids that appear as baggy swellings. The following type occur:
- Without prolapse – bleeding may be present, but there is no pain.
- Prolapsed – characterised by pain and possibly bleeding.
- Strangulated – the haemorrhoid has prolapsed to such a degree and for so long that its blood supply is occluded by the anal sphincter's constricting action. Strangulated haemorrhoids are very painful and usually become thrombosed.

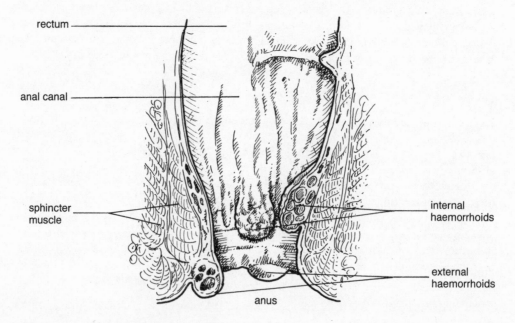

Figure 42.1   Haemorrhoids

Diagnosis

The symptoms most often associated with haemorrhoids include itching, burning, pain, inflammation, irritation, swelling, bleeding and seepage. Itching is rarely due to haemorrhoids except when there is mucous discharge from prolapsing internal haemorrhoids. The common causes of anal itching include tissue trauma secondary to excessive use of harsh toilet paper, *Candida albicans*, parasitic infections and allergies. Pain does not usually occur unless there is acute inflammation of external haemorrhoids. As there are no sensory nerves ending above the anorectal line, uncomplicated internal haemorrhoids rarely cause pain. Bleeding is almost always associated with internal haemorrhoids and may occur before, during or after defaecation. When bleeding occurs from an external haemorrhoid, it is due to rupture of an acute thrombotic haemorrhoid. Bleeding haemorrhoids can produce severe anaemia due to chronic blood loss.

Therapy

Dietary factors

In contrast to the westernised countries, haemorrhoids are rarely seen in parts of the world where high-fibre, unrefined diets are consumed.[3] A low-fibre diet, high in refined foods, contributes greatly to the development of haemorrhoids.

Individuals consuming a low-fibre diet tend to strain more during bowel movements, since their smaller and harder stools are more difficult to pass. This straining increases the pressure in the abdomen, which obstructs venous return. The increased pressure will increase pelvic congestion and may significantly weaken the veins, causing haemorrhoids to form.

A high-fibre diet is perhaps the most important component in the prevention of haemorrhoids. A diet rich in vegetables, fruits, legumes and grains promotes peristalsis; and many fibre components attract water and form a gelatinous mass which keeps the faeces soft, bulky and easy to pass. The net effect of a high-fibre diet is significantly less straining during defaecation. (The importance of fibre is discussed in more detail in Chapter 4, Dietary fibre, and Chapter 73, Varicose veins.)

Bulking agents

Natural bulking compounds can also be used to reduce faecal straining. These fibrous substances, particularly psyllium seed and guar gum, possess mild laxative action due to their ability to attract water and form a gelatinous mass. They are generally less irritating than wheat bran and other cellulose fibre products. Several double-blind clinical trials have demonstrated that supplementing the diet with bulk-forming fibres can significantly reduce the symptoms of haemorrhoids (bleeding, pain, pruritis and prolapse) and improve bowel habits.[4,5]

Hydrotherapy

The warm Sitz bath is an effective non-invasive treatment for uncomplicated haemorrhoids.[2] A Sitz bath is a partial immersion bath of the pelvic region. The temperature of the water in the warm Sitz bath should be between 100–105 °F (37.7–40.5 °C).

Topical therapy

Topical therapy, in most circumstances, will only provide temporary relief. Topical treatment involve the use of suppositories, ointments and anorectal pads. Many over-the-counter products for haemorrhoids contain primarily natural ingredients, such as witch hazel (Hamamelis water), shark liver oil, cod liver oil, cocoa butter, Peruvian balsam, zinc oxide, live yeast cell derivative and allantoin.

Botanical medicines

The botanicals described in Chapter 73, Varicose veins (particularly *Ruscus aculeatus* or butcher's broom), and flavonoids are useful for enhancing the integrity of the venous structures of the rectum.

Monopolar direct current therapy

The monopolar direct current technique is purely an outpatient procedure. No anaesthetic is needed, except local anaesthetic for the occasional hypersensitive or nervous patient (in such instances, a 2 per cent procaine solution is injected directly into the haemorrhoid). To date, there have been no reported cases of adverse effects, which speaks well for the procedure's safety.

The monopolar direct current technique for haemorrhoid management is fast becoming the treatment of choice in the United States. According to an article in *Gastrointestinal Endoscopy*,[6] 'This painless outpatient treatment of all grades of haemorrhoids is effective and safe. This methodology warrants consideration as the treatment of choice of haemorrhoidal disease.'

The first published work on monopolar direct current (also called inverse galvanism) was *Obliteration of Haemorrhoids with Negative Galvanism* by Wilbur E. Keesey MD of Chicago.[7] Dr. Keesey dated the first use of this approach to 1897, although the technical problems (producing a smooth uninterrupted galvanic current source) were not worked out until approximately 1925. The technique then began to be used in general practice.

Treatment

As with all diseases, the primary treatment of haemorrhoids is prevention. This involves reducing those factors which may be responsible for increasing pelvic congestion – straining during defaecation, sitting or standing for prolonged periods of time, or underlying liver disease. A high-fibre diet is crucial for the maintenance of proper bowel activity, and nutrients and botanical substances which enhance the integrity of venous structures may also be of benefit.

Warm Sitz baths and topical preparations are useful to ameliorate the discomfort, but have only transient results.

When indicated, the monopolar direct current method, specifically designed for haemorrhoid treatment, will give permanent results. This technique is especially useful in advanced haemorrhoidal disease.

Diet

A high-complex carbohydrate diet rich in dietary fibre is indicated. The diet should contain liberal amounts of proanthocyanidin- and anthocyanidin-rich foods such as blackberries, cherries, bilberries, etc., to strengthen vein structures.

Supplements

- Vitamin A, 10,000 iu a day.
- Vitamin B-complex, 10–100 mg a day.
- Vitamin C, 500–3,000 mg a day.
- Vitamin E, 200–600 iu a day.
- Bioflavonoids, 100–1,000 mg a day.
- Zinc, 15–30 mg a day.

Botanical medicines

- *Ruscus aculeatus*, butcher's broom, extract (9–11 per cent ruscogenin content), 100 mg three times daily.

Physical medicine

- Hydrotherapy – warm Sitz baths to relieve uncomplicated haemorrhoids.
- Monopolar direct current therapy, as performed by a trained physician.

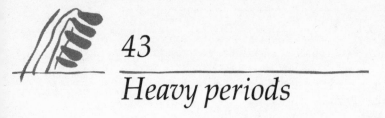

43

Heavy periods

- Excessive menstrual bleeding refers to a blood loss greater than 80 ml, occurring at regular menstrual cycles (cycles are usually, but not necessarily, of normal length).
- Often caused by local lesions, e.g. uterine fibroids, endometrial polyps, endometrial hyperplasia and endometriosis.

General considerations

Excessive menstrual bleeding or menorrhagia is a common female complaint that may be entirely prevented by taking proper nutritional measures. As with any disease, proper determination of the cause is essential for effective treatment.

The cause of functional menorrhagia is currently believed to involve abnormalities in the biochemical processes of the endometrium which control the supply of arachidonic acid, a fatty acid, for prostaglandin synthesis.[1,2] Prostaglandins are hormone-like molecules manufactured from fatty acids. The endometrium (lining of the uterus) of women with menorrhagia concentrates arachidonic acid to a much greater extent than normal. The increased arachidonic acid released during menstruation results in increased production of series 2 prostaglandins, which are thought to be the major factor both in the excessive bleeding seen at menstruation, as well as menstrual cramps.

Other factors believed to contribute to menorrhagia are iron deficiency, hypo-thyroidism, vitamin A deficiency, intrauterine devices and various local factors (e.g. uterine myomas, endometrial polyps, adenomyosis, endometrial hyperplasia, salpingitis and endometriosis).

Therapy

Iron deficiency

A menstrual blood loss above 60 ml per period is associated with negative iron balance in most cases.[3] Although menstrual blood loss is well recognised as a major cause of iron deficiency anaemia in fertile women, it is not as well known that chronic iron deficiency can be a cause of menorrhagia. This has been suggested, based on several observations:

- Response to iron supplementation alone in 74 of 83 patients (in whom organic pathology had been excluded).
- High rate of organic pathology (fibroids, polyps, adenomyosis, etc.) in the patients who failed to respond to iron supplementation.
- Associated rise in serum iron levels in 44 of 57 patients.
- Decreased response to iron therapy when initial serum iron levels were high.
- Correlation of menorrhagia with depleted tissue iron stores (bone marrow) irrespective of serum iron level.
- A significant double-blind placebo-controlled study displaying improvement in 75 per cent of those on iron supplementation, compared with 32.5 per cent for the placebo group.[4]

Iron supplementation, at a daily dose of 100 mg elemental iron, has been recommended as a preventive therapy by several researchers, since it appears that chronic iron deficiency may promote menorrhagia, and iron-containing enzymes are depleted before haematological changes are observed.[3,4]

Vitamin A

In one study, serum vitamin A levels were found to be significantly lower in 71 women with menorrhagia than in healthy controls. After 40 of these were given 25,000 iu of vitamin A twice a day for 15 days, blood loss returned to normal in 23 and was reduced in 14, i.e. 92.5 per cent of these women had either complete relief or significant improvement.[5]

Vitamin C and bioflavonoids

Capillary fragility is believed to play a role in many cases of menorrhagia. Supplementation with vitamin C (200 mg three times a day) and bioflavonoids has been shown to reduce menorrhagia in 14 out of 16 patients.[6] One of the patients failing to respond had endometriosis and the other had metrorrhagia (bleeding from the uterus not associated with the menstrual cycle).

As vitamin C is known to increase iron absorption significantly, its therapeutic effect could be also due to enhanced iron absorption.

Vitamin E

One group of investigators has suggested that free radicals have a causative role in endometrial bleeding, particularly in the presence of an intrauterine device.[7] Vitamin E supplementation (100 iu every two days) resulted in improvement in all patients by the end of 10 weeks.[7] Although vitamin E may have produced its effects via its antioxidant activity, it is equally plausible that it affected prostaglandin metabolism in a manner that would reduce bleeding.

Vitamin K and chlorophyll

Although bleeding time and prothrombin levels in women with menorrhagia are typically normal, the use of vitamin K (historically in the form of crude preparations of chlorophyll) has clinical and limited research support.[8] Also, some women will be found to have an inherited or acquired bleeding disorder.

Thyroid abnormalities

The association of overt hypothyroidism or hyperthyroidism with menstrual disturbances is well known. However, even minimal thyroid dysfunction, particularly minimal subclinical insufficiency (as determined by basal body temperature or the thyroid stimulation (TRH) test), may be responsible for menorrhagia and other menstrual disturbances.[9] Patients with even mild hypothyroidism and menorrhagia have responded dramatically to thyroid hormone.[9]

Essential fatty acids

Since it now appears that the majority of arachidonic acid in tissues is derived from the diet,[10] it is possible that reducing the intake of animal products and/or increasing the intake of the vegetable oils like linoleic, linolenic and di-homo-gamma-linolenic acid could curtail blood loss by decreasing the availability of arachidonic acid.

Botanical medicines

Numerous botanicals have been used in the treatment of menorrhagia, including spotted cranesbill (*Geranium maculatum*), birthroot (*Trillium pendulum*), blue cohosh (*Caulophyllum thalictroides*), witch hazel (*Hamamelis virginiana*) and shepherd's purse (*Capsella bursa-pastoris*). The latter, shepherd's purse, has a long history of use in the management of obstetric and gynaecological haemorrhage. Clinical studies have shown it to be effective in menorrhagia.[11,12]

Treatment

The first step in treating a woman with menorrhagia is to rule out serious causes. As excessive menstrual blood can reflect a serious condition, it is essential that any woman experiencing excessive menstrual blood loss consult a physician. When the excessive bleeding has been determined to be functional, i.e. not due to any disease state, the following guidelines will usually be of great value.

Diet

The diet should be relatively low in sources of arachidonic acid (animal fats) and high in linolenic and linoleic acids (vegetable oil sources). Green leafy vegetables and other sources of vitamin K should be eaten freely.

Supplements

- Vitamin C, 1 g a day.
- Bioflavonoids, 250 mg a day.
- Vitamin A, 25,000 iu a day.
- Vitamin E, 200 iu a day.
- Chlorophyll (fat soluble), 25 mg a day.
- Iron, 100 mg a day.

Botanical medicine

- *Capsella bursa-pastoris:*
      Dried herb or as tea, 2–4 grams.
      Fluid extract, 2–4 ml.
      Solid (dry, powdered) extract, 500–1,000 mg.

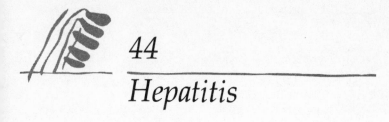

44

Hepatitis

- Loss of appetite, nausea, vomiting, fatigue, flu-like symptoms.
- Fever, enlarged tender liver, jaundice (yellowing of skin due to the increased level of bilirubin in the blood).
- Dark urine.
- Elevated liver enzymes in the blood.

General considerations

There are several types of viral hepatitis, with types A, B and non-A, non-B being the most common. Hepatitis A occurs sporadically or in epidemics, and is transmitted primarily through faecal contamination. Its incubation period is two to six weeks, carrier states are unknown and mortality rate is low (0.0–0.2 per cent). Hepatitis B is transmitted through infected blood or blood products, although it is occasionally transmitted through saliva and sexual secretions. It is very common in homosexuals and intravenous drug users. About 5 to 10 per cent become carriers. Its incubation period is six weeks to six months and fatality rate is moderate (0.3–1.5 per cent). Hepatitis non-A, non-B is much less common, but is seen in about 90 per cent of post-transfusion cases (about 10 per cent of people receiving blood transfusions develop hepatitis). Its incubation period is two to 20 weeks and mortality rate is unclear, but higher than for the other forms (1–12 per cent).[1,2] Hepatitis is also caused by type D virus, Epstein-Barr virus and cytomegalovirus.[2]

For as yet unknown reasons, 10 per cent of hepatitis B and 10 to 40 per cent of hepatitis non-A, non-B cases develop into chronic forms. The symptomatology varies from an asymptomatic state to chronic fatigue, serious liver damage and even death.[1]

The rate of hepatitis A in the general population of the United States is surprisingly high. Antibodies to the heptatitis A virus are detected in 10 to 20 per cent of children below 10 years of age and increases to 50 to 60 per cent of adults by age 50.[3] Antibodies to the hepatitis B virus are found in 5 to 10 per cent of adults. Only 3 to 5 per cent of adults were aware that they had had hepatitis A, indicating that the majority of cases are mild or asymptomatic.[3]

Diagnosis

Diagnosis is suspected when the typical signs and symptoms (see Table 44.1) are present, and confirmed by blood tests for elevated liver enzymes. The type of virus involved is determined by measuring antibodies to specific viruses in the blood. The typical blood tests are listed in Table 44.2.

Table 44.1 Incidence of symptoms in viral hepatitis[2]

Symptom	% of patients
Dark urine	94
Fatigue	91
Loss of appetite	90
Nausea	87
Fever	76
Vomiting	71
Headache	70
Abdominal discomfort	65
Light stools	52
Muscle pain	52
Drowsiness	49
Irritability	43
Itching	42
Diarrhoea	25
Joint pain	21

Table 44.2 Laboratory tests for the diagnosis of viral hepatitis[2]

Test	Use	Timing
Alanine aminotransferase	Acute hepatitis A	1–3 months
	Acute hepatitis B	2–5 months
Anti-HAV antibody	Acute hepatitis A	1 month to several years
Anti-HBc antibody	Acute hepatitis B	2 months to 2 years
Anti-HBs antibody	Chronic hepatitis B	5 months to several years

Therapy

Hepatitis is a disease which greatly benefits from the use of natural therapies. Several nutrients and herbs have been shown to inhibit viral reproduction, improve immune system function and greatly stimulate regeneration of the damaged liver cells. Therapies to protect the liver are discussed in more detail in the Chapter 8, Liver support.

Dietary considerations

Although a diet high in saturated fat increases the risk of developing fatty infiltration and/or stasis of bile in the liver and gall bladder, research on the effects of various diets on the rate of recovery from hepatitis is inconclusive.[2] However, clinical experience indicates the value of a natural diet, low in saturated fats, simple carbohydrates (sugar, white flour, fruit juice, honey, etc.), oxidised fatty acids (fried oils) and animal fat. A high fibre diet has been shown to increase the elimination of bile acids, drugs and toxic bile substances from the system.[4]

Nutritional considerations

Vitamin C   Large doses of vitamin C (40–100 grams orally or intravenous) were found to improve viral hepatitis greatly in two to four days, with clearing of jaundice within six days.[5] While several other studies found similar results,[6,7,8] one controlled study[9] failed to confirm this work. However, Linus Pauling claims that systematic errors invalidated the study.[10] Another controlled study found that 2 grams or more of vitamin C per day were dramatically able to prevent hepatitis B in hospitalised patients. While 7 per cent of the control patients (receiving less than 1.5 grams of vitamin C per day) developed hepatitis, none of the treated patients did.[11]

Vitamin B12 and folic acid   Intravenous and oral supplementation with vitamin B12 and folic acid have been found to shorten recovery time moderately.

Liver extracts   The oral administration of concentrated liver extracts has been used in the treatment of many chronic liver diseases since 1896.[12] Numerous scientific investigations into the therapeutic efficacy of liver hydrolysates have demonstrated that these extracts promote hepatic regeneration[13] and are quite effective in the treatment of chronic liver disease, including chronic active hepatitis.[14,15]

Botanical medicines

Catechin   An international workshop in 1981 on the use of catechin in diseases of the liver concluded that this flavonoid (isolated from *Uncaria gambier*) has much promise for the treatment of many types of liver disease, particularly both acute and chronic viral hepatitis.[16] Catechin has been shown, in numerous double-blind clinical studies, to decrease serum bilirubin levels in patients with all types of acute viral hepatitis (i.e. types A, B and non-A, non-B).[16–23] Furthermore, there is also more rapid relief of clinical symptoms (i.e. loss of appetite, nausea, weakness, itching and abdominal discomfort), more accelerated clearance of hepatitis virus antibodies from the blood and greater reduction of liver enzyme levels than in control groups. One study of patients with chronic liver disease found that catechin improved liver blood tests about twice as fast as compared to untreated controls.[17]

The liver-protecting effect of catechin is related to its free radical and antioxidant properties, its anti-toxin effects in stimulation of immune system function and its ability to stabilise membranes.[16,24,25]

Alcohol and other toxic-substance-induced liver damage (as evidenced by fatty infiltration) is usually unresponsive to commonly used lipotropic agents (choline, cysteine, inositol, niacin, etc.), but catechin as well as silymarin, due to its wide range of actions, appears to prevent this hepatic damage.[24,25]

Dandelion (Taraxacum officinale) The common dandelion is recognised by herbalists all over the world as an excellent liver remedy. It is a very rich source of many nutrients, being particularly high in vitamins, minerals, proteins, choline, inulin and pectins. Its carotenoid content is extremely high, even higher than carrots (14,000 iu of vitamin A per 100 grams compared with 11,000 iu for carrots).

Studies in humans and laboratory animals have shown that dandelion enhances the flow of bile, improving such conditions as liver congestion, bile duct inflammation, hepatitis, gallstones and jaundice.[26,27] Dandelion's beneficial effect on such a wide variety of conditions is probably closely related to its ability to improve the functional capacity of the liver.

Milk thistle (Silybum marianum) The common milk thistle contains silymarin, one of the most potent liver medicines known. Silymarin's effect in preventing liver destruction relates to its ability, in many instances, to inhibit the factors that are responsible for the damage, i.e. free radicals and leukotrienes.[17–23,28,29] Equally important is its ability to stimulate protein synthesis, which results in an increase in the production of new liver cells to replace the damaged ones.[28]

In human studies, silymarin has been shown to have positive effects in treating several types of liver disease, including cirrhosis, chronic hepatitis, fatty infiltration of the liver (chemical and alcohol induced), subclinical cholestasis of pregnancy and gallbladder inflammation.[4,12,30–8] The therapeutic effect of silymarin in these disorders has been confirmed by microscopic examination of the cells (biopsy), clinical and laboratory data.

Artichoke (Cynara scolymus) The globe artichoke has a long folk history of use in the treatment of many liver diseases. Recent evidence supports this use. The active ingredient in artichoke is cynarin, which is found in highest concentrations in the leaves. Like silymarin, cynara extract has demonstrated significant liver protecting and regenerating effects.[17,22]

It also stimulates the elimination of bile from the liver. This is a very important property; if the bile is not being eliminated from the liver, the liver is at increased risk of damage. Clearing bile from the liver is very important in the treatment of hepatitis and other liver diseases since it helps decongest the liver.

Liquorice (Glycyrrhiza glabra) Double-blind studies have shown a liquorice component to be effective in treating viral hepatitis, particularly chronic active hepatitis.[39] This activity is probably due to its well documented antiviral activity.[40,41] A glycyrrhizin-containing product (Stronger Neo-minophagen C), consisting of 0.2 per cent glycyrrhizin, 0.1 per cent cysteine and 2.0 per cent glycine in physiological saline solution, is widely used intravenously in Japan for the treatment of hepatitis. The other components, glycine and cysteine, appear to modulate glycyrrhizin's actions. Glycine has been shown to prevent the sodium- and water-retaining effects of glycyrrhizin, while cysteine aids in detoxification via increased glutathione synthesis and cystine conjugation.

Treatment

Remember, hepatitis is a serious disease requiring the care of a physician.

Bed rest is important during the acute phase of viral hepatitis, with slow resumption of activities as health improves. Strenuous exertion, alcohol and other liver-toxic drugs and chemicals should be avoided. During the contagious phase (two to three weeks before symptoms appear to three weeks after) careful hygiene and avoiding close contact with others is important. In particular, once diagnosis is made, work in a day care centre, restaurant and similar occupations is not recommended.

Diet

A natural diet, low in natural and synthetically saturated fats, simple carbohydrates (sugar, white flour, fruit juice, honey, etc.), oxidised fatty acids (fried oils) and animal fat, and high in fibre is recommended.

Nutritional supplements

- B complex, five times the recommended dietary allowance per day.
- Vitamin C, to bowel tolerance (10–50 g a day).
- Choline, 1 g three times a day.
- Methionine, 1 g three times a day.
- Liver hydrolysate, 500 mg three times a day.
- Free form amino acids, 2 g three times a day.

Botanical medicines

Doses three times a day, unless otherwise stated.
- *Taraxacum officinale*, dandelion:
    Dried root, 4 grams.
    Fluid extract (1:1), 4–8 ml.
    Solid extract (4:1), 250–500 mg.
- *Silybum marianum*, milk thistle – the standard dose of *Silybum marianum* is based on its silymarin content, 70–210 mg of silymarin three times daily.
- *Cynara scolymus*, globe artichoke:
    Crude dried leaves, 4–6 grams.
    Solid extract (15 per cent cynarin), 500 mg.
    Cynarin, 500 mg a day.

- *Glycyrrhiza glabra*, liquorice:
    Dried root (or as tea), 1 to 2 g.
    Tincture (1:5), 4–6 ml (1 to 1.5 tsp).
    Fluid extract (1:1), 0.5–2.0 ml (¼ to ½ tsp).
    Powdered solid extract (4:1), 250–500 mg.

If liquorice is to be used over a long time it is necessary to increase the intake of potassium rich foods.

- Catechin or uncaria gambier extract, 1 gram.

- Multiple, small fluid-filled blisters on an inflamed base.
- Local burning or stinging pain.
- Fatigue and mild fever.
- Regional lymph nodes may be tender and swollen.

General considerations

Herpes simplex is a recurrent viral infection of the skin or mucous membranes character-ised by the appearance of single or multiple clusters of small vesicles (blisters) filled with a clear fluid on an inflamed base. It typically occurs about the mouth (herpes gingivostomatitis), lips (herpes labialis), genitals (herpes genitalis) and eye (herpes keratoconjunctivitis). After the initial infection, the virus becomes dormant in the nerve ganglia, and recurs following minor infections, trauma, stress (emotional, dietary and environmental) and sun exposure. Its incubation period is two to 12 days (averaging six to 12) and the typical infection lasts one to two weeks.

The incidence of herpes infections is somewhat difficult to determine. Studies show that 30 to 100 per cent of the adults in the United States have had oral herpes, while genital herpes is found in 3 per cent of nuns to 70 per cent of prostitutes.[1] Current estimates indicate that 20–40 per cent of the US population have recurrent herpes infections.

Causes

More than 70 viruses compose the herpes family. Of these, four are important in human disease – *Herpes simplex* (HSV), *Varicella zoster* (VZV), Epstein-Barr (EBV) and cyto-megalovirus (CMV). Blood studies have distinguished two types of HSV, which have been designated HSV-1 and HSV-2. Serum studies have shown that 30–100 per cent of adults have been infected with one or both HSV, with the greatest incidence among the lower socioeconomic groups. HSV-1 is primarily isolated from extragenital sites, while genital infections are primarily by HSV-2 (10–40 per cent are due to HSV-1). Transmission is by direct contact with contaminated tissues and fluids – saliva, skin discharge, sexual fluids, etc.

Recurrence rate

HSV-1 genital lesions have a recurrence rate of 14 per cent while the HSV-2 recurrence rate is 60 per cent. Men seem more susceptible to recurrences. After resolution of the primary infection, HSV apparently becomes a dormant inhabitant within the nerve ganglia. Recurrences develop at or near the sites of primary infection and may be precipitated by many different stimuli – sunburn, sexual activity, menses, stress, food allergy, drugs and certain foods. The risk of clinical herpes infection after sexual contact with an individual with active lesions is estimated to be 75 per cent.

Immunological aspects

Since not everyone exposed to HSV develops clinical infection, it appears that the host defence mechanisms are important in protecting against HSV infection. Chronic, persistent infections are seen in immunosuppressed individuals. The cell-mediated immune system is undoubtedly the major factor in determining the outcome of herpes exposure – resistance, latent infection or clinical disease.

Therapy

Carotenes

Beta-carotene potentiates the immune system and inhibits viruses.[2,3] Beta-carotene supplementation in humans can enhance the action of interferon,[4] stimulate white cell antiviral activity and increase the number of circulating T-helper cells.[5]

Zinc and vitamin C

Oral supplementation with zinc[6] and a bioflavonoid-ascorbate complex[7] has been shown to be effective in clinical studies. Although zinc is an effective inhibitor of *Herpes simplex* virus replication in vitro,[8] its effect in vivo is probably more related to its enhancing cell-mediated immunity. The topical application of 0.01–0.025 per cent zinc sulphate solutions has also been shown to be effective in both reducing symptoms and inhibiting recurrences.[8,9]

Vitamin E

Vitamin E has been shown effective in decreasing the pain and shortening the healing time of herpes lesions.[10]

Thymus extract

Enhancement of the person's immunological status is the key to the control of herpes infection. There is some evidence that a defect in specific cell-mediated immunity is present even in apparently normal subjects with recurrent *Herpes simplex* virus infection.[11] Thymus extracts have been shown to be effective in preventing both the number and the severity of recurrent infections in immune-suppressed individuals. The thymus extract appears to increase the white cell response to the *Herpes simplex* virus, natural killer cell activity and interferon production. The extract, therefore, appears to prevent viral activation by potentiating cell-mediated responses.[12]

Lithium

A topical treatment for herpes is a lithium ointment. Lithium interferes with replication of DNA-type viruses, such as herpes virus, without affecting host cells. Lithium succinate (8 per cent solution) may be combined with zinc in a topical ointment, or it may be used alone.[13,14]

Dietary considerations

A lysine-rich/arginine-poor diet has become a popular treatment for herpes infections. This approach came from research showing that lysine has antiviral activity in vitro due to antagonism of the metabolism of the amino acid arginine.[15,16] A preponderance of lysine over arginine is believed either to inhibit the synthesis of the arginine-rich proteins necessary for viral replication or to repress the activation of the control genes.

Double-blind placebo-controlled studies on the effectiveness of lysine supplementation with uncontrolled avoidance of arginine-rich foods have shown inconsistent results.[16,17] These results may be due to the relatively low levels of lysine used (1,200 mg per day), the lack of control of the amounts of arginine-rich foods or the severity of the cases (both placebo and treated groups had lesions for a remarkable 40 per cent of the time in one negative study).

From a theoretical perspective this approach should be effective, since studies in test tubes have shown that HSV is dependent on adequate levels of arginine and low levels of lysine.[17] They compete with each other for intestinal transport, and rats fed a lysine-rich diet displayed a 60 per cent decrease in brain tissue arginine levels, although there was no change in serum levels.[16] Since HSV is believed to reside in the nerve ganglia, lysine supplementation and arginine avoidance seem appropriate. However, this approach is not curative – it only inhibits recurrences. In some patients, withdrawal from lysine is followed by relapse within 1–4 weeks.[17]

Some care should be taken, however, not to use excessive doses of lysine. There is inconsistent animal data suggesting that large doses of lysine may increase serum cholesterol levels.[9,18] Table 45.1 shows the lysine and arginine content of selected foods. Notice that most vegetable proteins have large amounts of arginine, while animal proteins have balanced levels.

Considering the importance of the immune system in preventing recurrent herpes infections, optimisation of its function is of primary importance. This requires the

Table 45.1 Arginine and lysine content of selected foods (100 g)

Food	Arginine	Lysine
Almonds	2,730	580
Bacon	2,100	2,000
Beans, green	80	80
Beans, lima	1,170	1,470
Beans, red	340	420
Beans, mung	1,320	1,930
Beef	1,600	2,200
Brazil nut	2,250	470
Bread, wholewheat	510	290
Buckwheat	1,200	460
Carob	710	340
Cashews	1,950	740
Cheese, Cheddar	850	1,700
Chicken	1,930	2,700
Chocolate	4,500	2,000
Clams	830	840
Coconut	470	148
Crustaceans	1,330	1,260
Eggs	840	820
Fish fingers	940	1,460
Halibut	140	2,220
Hazel nut	3,510	690
Lentil	2,100	1,740
Linseed	2,030	810
Liver, beef	1,590	1,950
Milk, whole	130	280
Millet	410	260
Oatmeal, cooked	130	70
Oysters	310	280
Peanuts, w/o skins*	3,240	1,090
Peas, green	420	220
Peas, chick	1,900	1,380
Pecan	2,030	810
Pork, lean	1,510	1,850
Rice, brown	120	100
Salmon	1,530	2,350
Sardines	1,190	1,850
Sesame	2,590	580
Shrimp	1,360	2,130
Soybeans, boiled	620	620
Sunflower	1,190	540
Tuna	1,530	2,530
Turkey	1,700	2,450
Walnuts	2,250	490
Yeast	1,940	3,510

*The US literature lists 7,500 g lysine per 3.5 oz

avoidance of concentrated and simple carbohydrates and of all significant food allergens, since sugar consumption and allergic reactions seriously impair immune function.[19]

Herbal therapy

Glycyrrhizic acid, a component of liquorice root (*Glycyrrhiza glabra*), inhibits both the growth and cell-damaging effects of herpes simplex. At high concentration in vitro, glycyrrhizic acid produces irreversible inactivation of HSV,[20] suggesting its usefulness as a topical treatment.

Treatment

Every care should be taken to maintain optimal immune system function (i.e. avoid allergenic foods, limit stress, optimise diet, etc.). The diet should be low in refined carbohydrates and arginine-rich foods. Those guidelines and recommendations discussed in Chapter 6, Immune support, are appropriate in the prevention and treatment of herpes infections.

Supplements

- Beta-carotene, 100,000 iu a day.
- Vitamin C, 2 g a day.
- Bioflavonoids, 1 g a day.
- Vitamin E, 400 iu a day.
- Zinc picolinate, 15 mg a day.
- Lysine, 2 g a day (increase if arginine-rich foods are consumed).
- Thymus extract, two tablets three times a day.

Topical treatment

- Ice, 10 minutes on, 5 minutes off, during early stages.
- Zinc sulphate solution, 0.025 per cent solution three times a day.
- Glycyrrhizinic acid ointment, three times a day.
- Lithium succinate, 8 per cent solution, three times a day.

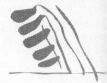

46

Hives

- Hives (urticaria) – raised and swollen welts with blanched centres (weals) which may coalesce to become giant welts. Limited to the superficial portion of the skin.
- Angioedema – similar eruptions to hives, but with larger swollen areas that involve structures beneath the skin.
- Chronic versus acute – recurrent episodes of hives and/or angioedema of less than six weeks duration are considered acute, while attacks persisting beyond this period are designated chronic.

General considerations

Hives or urticaria is a localised swelling of the skin which usually itches intensely. The medical term for a hive is a weal. Weals are caused by the release of histamine within the skin. About 50 per cent of patients with urticaria develop angioedema, a deeper, less-defined swelling that involves tissues beneath the skin as well as the skin.

Urticaria and angioedema are relatively common conditions; it is estimated that 15–20 per cent of the general population has had hives at some time. Although persons in any age group may experience acute or chronic urticaria and/or angioedema, young adults (post-adolescence through to the third decade of life) are most often affected.[1,2]

Causes

The basic development of a weal involves the release of inflammatory mediators from mast cells or basophilic leucocytes. Although classically this occurs as a result of allergy complexes (IgE-antigen complexes) causing these cells to release histamine, other mechanisms are probably more important in the majority of patients. The true incidence of classic IgE-mediated urticaria is probably quite low when compared to other mechanisms.[1,3]

The signs and symptoms of acute and chronic urticaria show consistent patterns, despite the many diverse causes and initiating factors (see below) that have been found, yet the development of urticaria cannot be entirely ascribed to any one mechanism. However, at present, it appears that mast cells and mast cell-dependent mediators play the most prominent role.[3]

Mast cells are widely distributed throughout the body and are found primarily near small blood vessels, particularly in the skin. The mast cell is a secretory cell capable of releasing both preformed and newly synthesised molecules, termed mediators. These mediators (listed in the box) play key roles in the development of inflammatory reactions. The actual events initiated by the mediators depend on the tissues into which they are released. For example, the release of histamine into the skin primarily produces itching and swelling, while histamine released into the lung may induce asthma (bronchospasm) and released into joint spaces causes arthritis.

Mast cell-derived mediators[3]

- Preformed, rapidly released
    Histamine
    Eosinophil chemotactic factors of anaphylaxis (ECF-A)
    Eosinophil chemotactic oligopeptides
    Neutrophil chemotactic factor
    Superoxide anions
    Exoglycosidases (beta-hexosaminidase, beta-delta-galactosidase,* beta-glucuronidase)
    Serotonin*
    Arylsulphatase A
- Secondary or newly generated
    Slow-reacting substances (SRS-A) – LTC, LTD, LTE
    Prostaglandins
    Monohydroxyeicosatetraenoic acids (HETEs)
    Hydroperoxyeicosatetraenoic acids (HPETEs)
    Thromboxanes
    Platelet activating factor (PAF)*
    Prostaglandin generating factor of anaphylaxis (PGF-A)
- Preformed, granule-associated
    Heparin
    Proteases (chymotrypsin/trypsin)
    Peroxidase*
    Superoxide dismutase*
    Arylsulphatase B
    Inflammatory factors of anaphylaxis (IFA)*

*Found in mast cells of species other than human

Physical causes of urticaria

Urticaria can be produced as a result of reactions to various physical stimuli. The most common forms of physical urticarias are dermographic, cholinergic and cold urticarias. These are briefly described below. Less common types of physical urticarias or angioedema are contact, solar, pressure, heat contact, aquagenic, vibratory and exercise-induced.[1]

Table 46.1 Clinical aspects of physical urticarias[1]

Type	Eliciting stimulus	Time of onset	Duration of lesion	Diagnostic test	Associated symptoms
Dermographic urticaria (tarda)	Stroking, scratching (rubbing for red dermographism)	2–5 min (0.5–5 hr)	1–5 hr (48 hr)	Firm stroking of skin	Headache, malaise
Cholinergic urticaria	Physical exercise + Overheating = Mental stress	2–20 min	30–60 min	Bicycling, running, sauna	Headache, GI upset, wheezing, salivation, lachrimation, syncope
Cold urticaria	Cold contact	2–5 min	1–2 hr	Ice cube, cold arm bath, cold air	Wheezing, syncope
Solar urticaria	Light of varying wavelengths	2–15 min	0.25–3 hr	Phototest	Wheezing, dizziness, syncope
Pressure urticaria	Pressure	3–8 hr	8–24 hr	Locally applied weights	Flu-like syndrome, fever, leucocytosis, arthralgias
Heat contact urticaria	Contact with heat	2–15 min	30–60 min	Hot arm bath	Gastrointestinal upset, dizziness, fatigue, wheezing, dyspnoea
Aquagenic urticaria	Contact with water	2–30 min	30–60 min	Bath, compresses	
Vibratory angioedema	Vibration	0.5–4 min	1 hr	Vibrating motor	Faintness, headache
Exercise-induced anaphylaxis	Exercise after a heavy meal	2–5 min	10–30 min	Exercise	Flushing, headache, disorientation, glottis oedema, dyspnoea, collapse
Familial cold urticaria	Cold wind, change from cold to warm air	0.5–3 hr	48 hr	Cold wind and subsequent rewarming	Tremor, headache, arthralgias, fever

Dermographism

Dermographism or dermographic urticaria is a readily elicited welting of the skin which evolves rapidly when moderate amounts of pressure are applied. This may occur as a result of simple contact with furniture, garters, bracelets, watch bands, towels or bedding.

The rate of dermographic urticaria has been estimated at 1.5–5 per cent in the general population. It is the most frequent type of physical urticaria and is found twice as frequently in women as in men, with the average age of onset in the third decade. The rate is much greater among the obese, especially those who wear tight clothing.

Dermographism may be associated with other diseases including parasite infections, insect bites, psychiatric disorders, hormonal changes, thyroid disorders, pregnancy, menopause, diabetes, other urticarias, during or following drug therapy, and *Candida albicans*.[1]

Cholinergic urticaria

Cholinergic, or heat reflex urticaria, is the second most frequent physical urticaria. These lesions, which depend upon the stimulation of the sweat gland, consist of pinpoint weals surrounded by reddened skin. The weals arise at or between hair follicles and develop preferentially on the upper trunk and arms.

The three basic types of stimuli that may produce cholinergic urticaria include:
- passive overheating;
- physical exercise; and
- emotional stress.

Typical eliciting activities, besides physical exercise, may include taking a warm bath or sauna, eating hot spices, or drinking alcoholic beverages. The weals usually arise within two to ten minutes after provocation and last for 30–50 minutes.

A variety of systemic symptoms may also occur, suggesting a more generalised mast cell release of the mediators than in the skin. Headache and burning of the eyes are common symptoms. Less frequent symptoms include nausea, vomiting, abdominal cramps, diarrhoea, dizziness, hypotension and asthmatic attacks.[1]

Cold urticaria

Cold urticaria is a urticarial reaction of the skin when it comes in contact with cold objects, water or air. Weal formation is usually restricted to the area of exposure, and develops within a few seconds to minutes after the removal of the cold object and rewarming of the skin. The lower the object's or element's temperature, the faster the reaction.

Widespread local exposure and generalised urticaria can be accompanied by flushing, headaches, chills, dizziness, increased heart rate, abdominal pain, nausea, vomiting, muscle pain, shortness of breath, wheezing or unconsciousness.

Cold urticaria has been observed to accompany a variety of clinical conditions including viral infections, parasitic infestations, syphilis, multiple insect bites, penicillin injections, dietary changes and stress.[1] The association of cold urticaria with infectious mononucleosis is well established.[1]

Non-physical causes of urticaria

Drugs are the leading cause of urticarial reactions in adults. In children, hives are usually due to foods, food additives or infections.[1]

Drugs

Most drugs are composed of small molecules incapable of inducing antigenic/allergenic activity on their own. Typically, they act by binding to larger molecules in the body. This results in the development of allergic antibodies to the altered human protein. Alternatively, drugs can interact directly with mast cells to induce degranulation. Many drugs have been shown to produce urticaria. The two most common hive-inducing drugs, penicillin and aspirin, are briefly discussed below.

Drugs which can cause urticaria

Acetylsalicylic acid	Griseofulvin (cold urticaria)	Phenobarbitol
Allopurinol	Insulin	Pilocarpine
Antimony	Iodines	Poliomyelitis vaccine
Antipyrines	Liver extract	Potassium sulphocyanate
Barbiturates	Menthol	Procaine
Bismuth	Meprobamate	Promethazine
Chlorhydrate	Mercury	Quinine
Chlorpromazine	Morphine, opium	Reserpine
Corticotropin (ACTH)	Para-aminosalicylic acid	Saccharin
Eucalyptus	Penicillin	Thiamine chloride
Fluorides	Phenacetin	Thiouracil
Gold		

Penicillin Antibiotics, including penicillin and related compounds, are the most common cause of drug-induced urticaria. The rate of allergy to penicillin in the general population is thought to be at least 10 per cent. Nearly 25 per cent of these individuals will display urticaria, angioedema or anaphylaxis upon ingestion of penicillin.[1,4] An important characteristic of penicillin is that it cannot be destroyed by boiling or steam distillation. This is a problem since penicillin and related contaminants can exist undetected in foods.

It is not known to what degree penicillin in our food supply contributes to urticarial reactions. However, urticaria and allergic symptoms have been traced to penicillin in milk,[5] soft drinks[6] and frozen dinners.[7] In one study of 245 patients with chronic urticaria, 24 per cent had positive skin tests and 12 per cent positive allergy tests for penicillin sensitivity.[8] Of those 42 patients sensitive to penicillin, 22 improved clinically on a dairy product-free diet while only two out of 40 patients with negative skin tests improved on the same diet. This study would seem to provide indirect evidence of the importance of penicillin in the food supply in urticaria.

In an attempt to provide direct evidence, penicillin-contaminated pork was given to penicillin-allergic volunteers. No significant reactions were noted other than transient pruritis in two volunteers.[9] Penicillin in milk appears to be more allergenic than penicillin in meat.[5] Presumably this is due to the fact that penicillin can be degraded into more allergenic compounds in the presence of carbohydrate and metals, suggesting that penicillin in milk may be more allergenic than artificially contaminated meat.[5]

Aspirin   Urticaria is a more common indicator of aspirin sensitivity than is asthma (see Chapter 17, Asthma and hayfever). The incidence of aspirin sensitivity in patients with chronic urticaria is at least 20 times greater than in normal controls.[10] Studies have demonstrated that 6.5–54 per cent of patients with chronic urticaria are sensitive to aspirin.

Aspirin and other anti-inflammatory drugs have been shown to increase gut permeability dramatically and may alter the normal handling of antigens.[11,12]

The daily administration of 650 mg of aspirin for three weeks has been shown to desensitise patients with urticaria and aspirin sensitivity. While taking the aspirin, patients also become nonresponsive to foods to which they usually reacted (pineapple, milk, egg, cheese, fish, chocolate, pork, strawberries and plums).[13] Others have noted this effect in patients with asthma, but they have also found that the effect disappears within nine days after stopping the treatment, suggesting the loss of effect or a possible placebo response.[14]

Food allergy

Classic allergic (IgE-mediated) urticaria can occur upon the ingestion of a specific allergic antigen. Although any food can cause an allergic reaction, the most common offenders are milk, fish, meat, eggs, beans and nuts.[1,4,15–19]

A basic requirement for the development of a food allergy is the absorption of the allergen through the intestinal barrier. Several factors are known to increase gut permeability significantly, including vasoactive amines ingested in foods or produced by bacterial action on essential amino acids, alcohol, aspirin and possibly many food additives. In addition, several investigators have reported alterations in gastric acidity, intestinal motility and the function of the small intestine and biliary tract in up to 85 per cent of patients with chronic urticaria.[20–4] Lack of hydrochloric acid or other digestive factors, intestinal infection and other disruptive factors reported in patients with chronic urticaria may temporarily or permanently alter the barrier and immune function of the gut wall and predispose an individual to allergies.

In one study with 77 patients having chronic urticaria, 24 (31 per cent) were diagnosed as lacking stomach acid entirely (achlorhydric) and 41 (53 per cent) were shown to be deficient in hydrochloric acid (hypochlorhydric).[22] Treatment with hydrochloric acid and a vitamin B complex gave impressive clinical results, highlighting the importance of correcting any underlying factor in the treatment of chronic urticaria.

Although classic allergic (IgE-mediated) reactions are thought to predominate in urticaria, it has been suggested that IgG-mediated reactions are probably responsible for the majority of adverse reactions to foods seen in general practice (see Chapter 38, Food allergy). IgG antigen-antibody complexes are capable of promoting events which cause mast cell degranulation. This could be a significant factor in some cases of urticaria.

Food colourants

Food additives appear to be a major factor in many cases of chronic urticaria in children. Colourings (azo dyes), flavourings (salicylates, aspartame), preservatives (benzoates, nitrates, sorbic acid), antioxidants (hydroxytoluene, sulphite, gallate) and emulsifiers/stabilisers (polysorbates, vegetable gums) have all been shown to produce hives in sensitive individuals.

Tartrazine In 1959 the azo dye tartrazine was the first food dye reported to induce urticaria.[25] Tartrazine is one of the most widely used colourants; it is added to almost every packaged food as well as many drugs, including some antihistamines, antibiotics, steroids and sedatives.[26] In the United States the average daily per capita consumption of certified dyes is 15 mg, of which 85 per cent is tartrazine. Among children, consumption is usually much higher. Tartrazine sensitivity has been calculated as occurring in 0.1 per cent of the population.[26]

Tartrazine sensitivity is extremely common (20–50 per cent) in individuals sensitive to aspirin.[4,26] Like aspirin, tartrazine is a known inducer of asthma, urticaria and other allergic conditions, particularly in children.[26] In addition, tartrazine, as well as benzoate and aspirin, increases the production of a compound which increases the number of mast cells in the body.[27] This is of considerable significance as tissue examination of patients with urticaria shows that greater than 95 per cent have an increase in mast cells.[28]

Food flavourings

Salicylates A broad range of salicylic acid esters (aspirin-like compounds) are used to flavour foods such as cake mixes, puddings, ice cream, chewing gum and soft drinks. The mechanism of action of these agents is thought to be similar to that of aspirin.[4]

Salicylates are also found naturally in many foodstuffs. It is estimated that daily salicylate intake from foods is in the range of 10–200 mg/day. As this is very close to the level of salicylate used in clinical testing (usually 300 mg), dietary salicylate may be a significant factor in aspirin-sensitive individuals.

Most fruit, especially berries and dried fruits, contain salicylates. Raisins and prunes have the highest amounts. Salicylates are also found in appreciable amounts in sweets made of liquorice and peppermint. Moderate levels of salicylate are found in nuts and seeds. Vegetables, legumes, grains, meat, poultry, fish, eggs and dairy products typically contain insignificant levels of salicylates. Salicylate levels are especially high in some herbs and spices including curry powder, paprika, thyme, dill, oregano and turmeric. Although the intake of these herbs and spices is relatively small, they can make a significant contribution to dietary salicylate.[29]

Other flavouring agents   Other flavouring agents such as cinnamon, vanilla, menthol and other volatile compounds may produce urticaria in some individuals.[4] Recently the artificial sweetener aspartame has been shown to induce urticaria.[30]

Food preservatives

Benzoates   Benzoic acid and benzoates are the most commonly used food preservatives. Although for the general population the incidence of adverse reactions to these compounds is thought to be less than 1 per cent, the frequency of positive challenges in patients with chronic urticaria varies from 4–44 per cent. Fish and shrimp frequently contain extremely high quantities of benzoates. This may be one reason why adverse reactions to these foods is so common in patients with urticaria.

BHT and BHA   Butylated hydroxytoluene (BHT) and butylated hydroxyanisol (BHA) are the primary antioxidants used in prepared and packaged foods. Typically, 15 per cent of patients with chronic urticaria test positive to oral challenge with BHT.[31-34] The use of chewing gum containing BHT was enough to induce urticaria in one patient.[35]

Sulphites   Sulphites, like tartrazine, have been shown to induce asthma, urticaria and angioedema in sensitive individuals.[36] The source may be varied as these compounds are ubiquitous in foods and drugs. They are typically added to processed foods to prevent microbial spoilage and to keep them from browning or changing colour. The earliest known use of sulphites was in the treatment of wines with sulphur dioxide by the Romans. Sulphites are typically sprayed on fresh foods such as shrimps, fruits and vegetables. They are also used as antioxidants and preservatives in many pharmaceuticals.

The average person consumes an average of 2 to 3 mg of sulphites per day. Wine and beer drinkers typically consume up to 10 mg a day and individuals who rely on restaurants for meals may ingest up to 150 mg a day.[36]

Food emulsifiers and stabilisers

A variety of compounds is used to emulsify and stabilise many commercial foods to ensure that the solids, oils and liquids do not separate out. Most of the foods containing these compounds are heterogeneous as they usually contain antioxidants, preservatives and dyes as well. Polysorbate in ice cream has been reported to induce urticaria, and vegetable gums such as acacia, gum arabic, tragacanth, quince and carrageenan may also induce urticaria in susceptible individuals.[4]

Infections

Infections are a major cause of urticaria in children.[1] Apparently in adults immuno-logical tolerance occurs to many microorganisms due to repeated massive antigen exposure. The role of bacteria, viruses and yeast (*Candida albicans*) in urticaria is briefly reviewed below. Chronic trichomonas infections have also been found to cause urticaria.

Bacteria   Bacterial infections contribute to urticaria in two major settings: in acute streptococcal tonsillitis (strep throat) in children; and in chronic dental infections in adults. In the first setting acute urticaria predominates while in the second, chronic urticaria predominates.[1]

Viruses   Hepatitis B is the most frequent cause of viral-induced urticaria; in one study 15.3 per cent of the patients with chronic urticaria had anti-hepatitis B surface anti-bodies.[37]

Urticaria has also been strongly linked to infectious mononucleosis and may develop several weeks before clinical manifestation. The incidence of urticaria during infectious mononucleosis is 5 per cent.[1]

Candida albicans   The association between *Candida albicans* and chronic urticaria has been suggested in several clinical studies. The number of patients with chronic urticaria who react positively to an immediate skin test with candida antigens is 19–81 per cent, compared to 10–15 per cent of normals.[38–45] It appears that sensitivity to *Candida albicans* is an important factor in at least 25 per cent of patients with chronic urticaria.[42] Approx-imately 70 per cent of patients with positive allergy tests also react to foods prepared with yeasts.

Treatment with nystatin and diet have proved that elimination of the organism can achieve a cure in a number of individuals with positive skin tests, although a placebo response cannot be ruled out. More patients responded to a yeast-free diet than to simple elimination of the organism. The yeast-free diet employed excluded bread, buns, sausage, wine, beer, cider, grapes, sultanas, Marmite, Bovril, vinegar, tomato, ketchup, pickles and prepared foods containing food yeasts.

In one study of 49 patients with positive sensitivity to candida, nine responded to a three-week course of nystatin while 18 became symptom-free only after adopting the yeast-free diet.[40] This would seem to support the importance of diet along with elimin-ating the yeast. Further support for the importance of diet can be found in another study of 36 patients with a positive allergy test to candida. Only three patients became symptom-free from nystatin alone, compared with 23 on diet therapy following the nystatin therapy.

Desensitising patients to *Candida albicans* with the use of a candida cell wall extract has also demonstrated encouraging results in some patients, although the treatment of these individuals also included supportive therapies.[44,45]

Other considerations

Psychological aspects

In one study involving 236 cases of chronic urticaria, psychological factors, i.e. stress, were reported to be the most frequent primary cause.[46] Stress appears to play an important role by increasing the susceptibility to allergies.

In one study of 15 patients with chronic urticaria, relaxation therapy and hypnosis was shown to provide significant benefit.[47] Patients were given an audio tape and asked to use the relaxation techniques described on the tape at home. At a follow-up examination five to 14 months after the initial session, six patients were free of hives and an additional seven reported improvement.

Ultraviolet light therapy

Ultraviolet light has been shown to be of some benefit to patients with chronic urticaria.[48,49] Both ultraviolet A (UVA) and ultraviolet B (UVB) have been used. Patients with cold, cholinergic and dermographic urticaria display the greatest therapeutic response.

Vitamin B12

Vitamin B12 has been reported to be of value in the treatment of acute and chronic urticaria.[50,51] Although serum B12 levels are normal in most patients, additional B12 appears to be of value. However, since injectable B12 was used, the placebo effect cannot be ruled out.

Treatment

The basic therapeutic approach is identification and control of all factors which promote the patient's urticarial response. Your physician can be invaluable in this process. Acute urticaria is usually a self-limiting disease, especially once the eliciting agent has been removed or reduced. Chronic urticaria also responds to the removal of the eliciting agent(s). In severe allergic reactions (anaphylaxis) emergency care is necessary.

Diet

An elimination or oligoantigenic diet is of utmost importance in the treatment of chronic non-physical urticaria (see Chapter 38, Food allergy). The diet should not only eliminate suspected allergens, but also all food additives.

The strictest elimination diets allow only water, lamb, rice, pears and vegetables. Those foods most commonly associated with inducing urticaria (milk, eggs, chicken, fruits, nuts and additives) should definitely be avoided.[19] Foods containing vasoactive amines should be eliminated, even if no direct allergy to them is noted. The primary foods to eliminate are cured meat, alcoholic beverages, cheese, chocolate, citrus fruits and shellfish.

The importance of eliminating food additives cannot be overstated. If food additives do in fact increase the number of mast cells in the skin, they may also do the same in the small intestine thereby greatly increasing the risk of developing a 'leaky' gut. Measures to support digestive function, such as hydrochloric acid or pancreatic enzyme supplementation, are often extremely important (see Chapter 5, Digestion).

Supplements

- Vitamin C, 1 g three times a day.
- Vitamin B12, 1 mg daily.

Psychological

Daily performance of relaxation techniques. Listening to audio-tape relaxation programmes may be an appropriate way to induce the desired state.

Physical medicine

Daily sunbathing for 15–20 minutes or the use of a UVA solarium, especially in chronic physical urticaria.

47

Hyperactivity and learning disorders

- Hyperactivity (attention deficit disorder with hyperactivity) – the child displays signs of inattention, impulsiveness and hyperactivity inappropriate for mental and chronological age.
- Learning disability – the child displays developmentally inappropriate short attention span and poor concentration for mental and chronological age.

General considerations

Attention deficit disorder is the current term that encompasses a wide variety of names used in the past to describe similar disorders, e.g. hyperkinetic reaction of childhood, hyperkinetic syndrome, hyperactive child syndrome, minimal brain damage, minimal brain dysfunction, minimal cerebral dysfunction and minor cerebral dysfunction.

Currently three separate disorders are described:
- Attention deficit disorder without hyperactivity.
- Attention deficit disorder with hyperactivity.
- Attention deficit disorder – residual type.

The first two disorders are considered individually below. The discussion of hyperactivity is concerned largely with the role of food additives, food allergies and sucrose, while the discussion of attention deficit disorder without hyperactivity focuses on heavy metals. Residual attention deficit disorder (individual 18 years or older) is viewed primarily as a continuation of the process.

Although these two syndromes are discussed separately, it is important to recognise that the factors discussed under one may be equally relevant to the other.

Hyperactivity

The rate of this disorder has been reported to be from 4 to 20 per cent of school-age children. A more widely accepted conservative figure of 3 per cent is currently acknowledged, due to improved diagnostic criteria.[1] Clinical observation and population surveys report a substantially greater incidence in boys than girls (10:1). Onset is usually by the age of three, although diagnosis is not generally made until later when the child is in school. The characteristics of this disorder are listed in the box.

Characteristics of hyperactivity disorder

- Hyperactivity.
- Perceptual motor impairment.
- Emotional instability.
- General coordination deficit.
- Disorders of attention (short attention span, distractibility, lack of perseverance, failure to finish thing off, not listening, poor concentration).
- Impulsiveness (action before thought, abrupt shifts in activity, poor organising, jumping up in class).
- Disorders of memory and thinking.
- Specific learning disabilities.
- Disorders of speech and hearing.
- Neurological signs and electroencephalographic irregularities.

These characteristics are frequently associated with difficulties in school, both in learning and behaviour. Although other factors may be involved in the cause, considerable evidence points towards food additives, food sensitivities and sucrose consumption as being responsible for the majority of hyperactivity.

Food additives

The term food additives covers a wide range of chemicals (5,000 additives are used in the USA), such as anticaking agents (e.g. calcium silicate), antioxidants (e.g. common food additives such as butylated hydroxytoluene, BHT, and butylated hydroxyanisole, BHA), bleaching agents (e.g. benzoyl peroxide), colourings (e.g. artificial azo dye derivatives), flavourings, emulsifiers, mineral salts, preservatives (e.g. benzoates, nitrates, sulphites), thickeners and vegetable gums. The 1985 per capita daily consumption of food additives in the US was approximately 13–15 g. The hypothesis that food additives induce hyperactivity, commonly referred to as the Feingold hypothesis, stemmed from the research of Benjamin Feingold. According to Feingold, many hyperactive children, perhaps 40–50 per cent, are sensitive to artificial food colours, flavours and preservatives and to naturally occurring salicylates and phenolic compounds.[2]

Feingold's claims were based on his experience with over 1,200 cases in which food additives were linked to learning and behaviour disorders. Since Feingold's presentation to the American Medical Association in 1973, the role of food additives in the cause of hyperactivity has been hotly debated in the scientific literature.[3-15] However, these researchers have focused on only ten food dyes versus the 3,000 food additives with which Feingold was concerned.

At first glance, it appears that the majority of the double-blind studies designed to test the hypothesis have shown essentially negative results.[3–8] On closer examination of these studies, though, and further investigation into the literature, it becomes evident that food additives do, in fact, play a major role in hyperactivity.[9–15] This is somewhat in opposition to the final report filed by the National Advisory Committee on Hyperkinesis and Food Additives to the USA Nutrition Foundation in 1980. However, the US National Institutes of Health, Consensus Conference on Defined Diets and Childhood Hyperactivity agreed to reconsider the Feingold diet in the amelioration of hyperkinesis.[16,17] The reason for this reconsideration is largely due to the overwhelming evidence produced in several studies [7–9,12,13] and the fact that, despite major inadequacies in the negative studies, about 50 per cent of those who tried the Feingold diet in these studies displayed a decrease in symptoms of hyperactivity.[3,6]

Schauss[10] and Rippere[11] have reviewed much of the literature concerning food additives and hyperactive children and have formulated guidelines and recommendations for future research designs that we hope will be utilised. Rippere's review is primarily a critique of C. Keith Conners' studies and book, *Food Additives and Hyperactive Children.* (Conners has been the primary researcher refuting the Feingold hypothesis.[3–5]) Rippere's major criticisms of Conners' work focused on six areas:

- Type of placebo. In Conners' studies the placebo used was a chocolate cookie. In Table 47.1 below it can be seen that in double-blind studies of reactions to foods in hyperactive children, chocolate has produced a reaction in 33 per cent in one study and 59 per cent in another. Conners himself acknowledges that reaction to the placebo was not uncommon. Furthermore, Conners reports that at a two-year follow-up 21 per cent of the mothers whose children took part in the diet trials mentioned that chocolate is a food that appeared to affect behaviour adversely. When the other constituents of the cookie are also taken into consideration, e.g. cow's milk, sugar, wheat, corn, yeast and other additives besides artificial colours, this placebo can hardly be termed inert.
- Adequacy of challenge dosages. The dose of mixed food dyes in these challenge trials was based on erroneous information, being far below the average daily intake based on FDA (US Food and Drug Agency) data. The dose given in Conners' studies was 13 mg twice daily, compared with a daily dose of 150 mg estimated to be at the 90th percentile for children from 5 to 12 years of age (average daily dose for children between 5 and 12 years of age is estimated at 76.5 mg).
- Length of dose interval. The doses of food dyes were given at relatively long intervals. This, combined with the inadequate dosage, indicates that the model fell far short of real-life exposure experienced by these victims of the technicolour breakfast cereal generation.
- Type of blood test for allergy determination. Conners' use of the cytotoxic test for allergy is irrelevant. The test is very unreliable, and Feingold's hypothesis does not require an allergic basis for the reactions to the various additives.
- Outcome measures. Conners' main outcome measures, a standardised rating procedure using subjective judgments and administered at less than daily intervals in the majority of studies, is potentially insensitive to true effects.
- Bias in the presentation of other investigators' data. Conners consistently

minimises and discounts findings which support Feingold's hypothesis, including even his own findings. The fact that teacher ratings failed to improve may indicate that other environmental factors were having an effect; in particular, it has been demonstrated that standard cool-white fluorescent lighting increases hyperactive behaviour, while full-spectrum light with radiation shields decreases hyper-activity.[18]

It is interesting to note that, while the US studies have been largely negative, the reports from Australia and Canada have been more supportive.[7,9,13,19,20] Feingold contended that there is a conflict of interest on the part of the Nutrition Foundation, a US organisation supported by the major food manufacturers – Coca Cola, Nabisco, General Foods, etc. It appears significant that the Nutrition Foundation has financed most of the negative studies.[18,21] Feingold contends that the conflict of interest arises because these companies would suffer economically if food additives were found to be harmful. Other countries have significantly restricted the use of artificial food additives because of the possible harmful effects.[22]

Sucrose

There appears to be a strong association between sucrose consumption and artificial food dyes.[23] In addition to this incriminating evidence connecting sucrose with negative effects on behaviour, there are the Langseth and Dowd findings. These researchers performed 5-hour oral glucose tolerance tests on 261 hyperactive children, with the result that 74 per cent displayed abnormal glucose tolerance curves.[24] The predominant abnormality was a low, flat curve. Hypoglycaemia eventually results in hyperactivity as adrenaline and other stimulants are released by the adrenal glands in response to the low blood sugar level. Refined carbohydrate appears to be the major factor in pro-moting reactive hypoglycaemia.[25]

Food allergies (sensitivities)

The contention that food allergies provoke hyperactivity in children is another popular notion in lay publications. There are, however, much more consistent results in double-blind studies that examined the relationship between food and food additive allergies and behaviour.[26-9] While artificial colourings and preservatives are the most common provoking substances in two of these studies, no child was sensitive to these substances alone.[26,27] This suggests that, since food sensitivities provoke psychological symptoms, mere elimination of food additives from the diet is inadequate.

One large controlled trial treated 76 severely handicapped children with an oligo-antigenic diet (lamb, chicken, potatoes, rice, bananas, apple, brassica family vegetable, calcium gluconate 3 g/day and a multiple vitamin).[26] After a four-week trial, 82 per cent improved and a normal range of behaviour was achieved in 21 of these. Other symptoms, such as headaches, abdominal pains and fits, also improved.[26] Reintro-duction of the foods to which the child was sensitive led to reappearance of symptoms and hyperactive behaviour. No mention was made of the possibility that non-responders were reacting to foods on the oligoantigenic diet or perhaps the vitamins,

Table 47.1 Food allergy reactions in hyperactive children – results from two studies

Item	% Reacting[27]	% Reacting[26]
Red dye	88	NT
Yellow dye	80	NT
Blue dye	80	NT
Colouring and preserv.		79
Cow's milk	73	64
Soya	NT	73
Chocolate	33	64
Grape	40	50
Orange	40	45
Peanuts	47	32
Wheat	30	49
Corn	40	29
Tomato	47	20
Egg	20	40
Cane sugar	40	16
Apple	40	13
Fish	NT	23
Oats	NT	23

NT Not tested

although it was noted that physical complaints were reduced in the non-responders as well. Table 47.1 summarises the results of two studies on food sensitivities and hyperactivity.

Treatment

Considering the importance of food allergy, recognition and control of the offending allergens is critical. The elimination diet (see Chapter 38, Food allergy) for a period of four weeks, followed by reintroduction/challenge of suspected foods (full servings at least once a day, one food introduced per week), is the most sensible and economical approach. If symptoms recur or worsen upon reintroduction/challenge, the food should be withdrawn. If there is no improvement on the elimination diet, it is possible that the child is reacting to something in the diet or environment. Further testing may be indicated in these patients.

All refined sugars should be eliminated from the diet, and a general multivitamin and mineral supplement should be used (with special care to insure that the child is not allergic to the product used).

Also, the factors discussed below under Learning disability should be considered. For example, hyperactive children have been shown to have increased lead levels.[30,31]

Learning disability

Three factors are considered by the authors to be particularly relevant to learning disabilities:
- Chronic fluid retention in the ear (otitis media).
- Nutrient deficiency.
- Heavy metals.

Otitis media

Children with moderate to severe hearing loss tend to have impaired speech and language development, lowered general intelligence scores and learning difficulties.[32,33] Current and early incidence of otitis media have been reported to be twice as common in learning-disabled children as non-learning-disabled children.[33] This reconfirms the necessity of dealing with otitis media from a preventive standpoint (see Chapter 35, Ear infection), since many of the factors associated with hyperactivity are also associated with otitis media.

Nutrient deficiency

Virtually any nutrient deficiency can result in impaired brain function.[34-6] Iron deficiency is the most common nutrient deficiency in American children.[34,36] Iron deficiency is associated with markedly decreased attentiveness, less complex or purposeful, narrower attention span, decreased persistence and decreased voluntary activity that is usually responsive to supplementation.[34,36-8]

Several investigators have demonstrated that correction of even subtle nutritional variables exerts a substantial influence on learning and behaviour. [35,39-41]

Heavy metals

Numerous studies have demonstrated a strong relationship between childhood learning disabilities (and other disorders including criminal behaviour) and body stores of heavy metals, particularly lead.[30,31,42-5]

Learning disabilities seem to be characterised by a general pattern of high hair levels of mercury, cadmium, lead, copper and manganese.[39,40] Poor nutrition and elevation of heavy metals usually go hand in hand, due to decreased consumption of food factors known to chelate these heavy metals or decrease their absorption (see Chapter 3, Detoxification).

Treatment

The treatment plan involves the elimination of any ear infection, detection and elimination of any heavy metal toxicity, and establishment of optimum nutrition for these children. Counselling is also indicated in most cases and, for the best results, should involve the whole family.

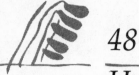

48

Hypertension

- A repeatable blood pressure (BP) reading of greater than 150/90 mm Hg.

General considerations

Hypertension or high blood pressure is one of the major medical problems of the 20th century. Hypertension is divided into two main categories – primary or essential hypertension and secondary hypertension. Currently 92–4 per cent of all diagnosed hypertension is termed essential, i.e. the underlying mechanism is unknown. However, there is considerable research showing that a variety of genetic, nutritional and environmental factors are responsible for the condition. In the other 6–8 per cent the hypertension is secondary to another disease.

The number of individuals with hypertension (blood pressure over 160/95 mm Hg) in the US is estimated at 20 per cent in the adult white population and 30 per cent in black adults. These values are nearly doubled if the blood pressure reading of 140/90 mm Hg is considered the upper limit of normal.[1]

Since hypertension is associated with an increase in cardiovascular illness and death, monitoring blood pressure offers an invaluable non-invasive diagnostic and prognostic aid. Some factors associated with an unfavourable outcome in hypertension are:

- Black racial background.
- Youth.
- Male.
- Persistent diastolic blood pressure (i.e. pressure between the pulses, when the heart is relaxed) of greater than 115 mm Hg.
- Smoking.
- Diabetes mellitus.
- Elevated blood cholesterol levels.
- Obesity.
- Evidence of end-organ damage, e.g. cardiac enlargement, ECG abnormalities and congestive heart failure.

Although physicians are primarily concerned with diastolic blood pressure (the second number in the blood pressure reading), systolic pressure (i.e. the reading when the heart is contracting and pumping) is also an important factor. Males with a normal diastolic pressure (less than 82 mm Hg) but elevated systolic pressure (over 158 mm Hg) have a two-fold increase in their cardiovascular death rates when compared to individuals with normal systolic pressures (less than 130 mm Hg).

Most cases of hypertension can be brought under control through changes in diet and life-style.[1] Although recent long-term clinical studies have found that people with hypertension not taking blood-pressure lowering medicines actually fare much better than those taking the prescription drugs,[2,3] antihypertensive medications are among the most widely prescribed drugs. Drug therapy usually involves the use of diuretics and/or beta-adrenergic blocking drugs. These drugs are associated with many side effects. There are other classes of hypotensive drugs which also may be used, including vaso-dilators and reserpine alkaloids.

Causes

Although behaviour patterns and stress play an important part, hypertension is most closely related to dietary factors. Hypertension is another of the many diseases or syndromes associated with the western diet, and is found almost entirely in developed countries. People living in remote areas of China, the Solomon Islands, New Guinea, Panama, Brazil and Africa show virtually no evidence of essential hypertension, nor do they experience a rise in blood pressure with advancing age.[4,5] Furthermore, when racially identical members of these societies migrate to less remote areas and adopt a more 'civilised' diet the incidence of hypertension increases dramatically.[4,5]

Weight   Population as well as clinical studies have repeatedly demonstrated that obesity is a major factor in hypertension.[6] Possible mechanisms include:
- Elevated cardiac output.
- Increased body sodium due to increased insulin levels or abnormal aldosterone/renin relationships.
- Alterations in hormonal/nervous system control mechanisms.

Weight reduction reduces blood pressure in normotensive, hypotensive and hyper-tensive individuals. Weight reduction should be a primary therapeutic goal for decreasing hypertension in obese patients, and may contribute to the management of moderately overweight hypertensives as well.

Lifestyle   Lifestyle factors are also very important causes of elevated blood pressure. Coffee consumption, alcohol intake, lack of exercise and smoking are all things that may contribute to an elevated blood pressure reading.

Caffeine   The effects of long-term caffeine consumption on blood pressure have not yet been clearly determined. Short-term studies consistently show elevation in blood pressure in both normotensive and hypertensive individuals which usually normalise after a few days. One large study (6,321 adults) demonstrated a small but statistically significant elevation in blood pressure when comparing those who drank five or more cups a day to non-coffee drinkers.[7]

Alcohol   Even moderate amounts of alcohol produce acute hypertension in some patients via increased adrenaline secretion.[8,9] Chronic alcohol consumption is one of the strongest predictors (sodium consumption being the other) of blood pressure.[8,10]

Smoking   It is a well documented fact that cigarette smoking is a contributing factor to hypertension. Smokeless tobacco, i.e. snuff, chewing tobacco and plug, also induces hypertension via its nicotine and sodium content.[11,12] Smoking is also positively associated with increased sugar, alcohol and caffeine consumption.[13] The hypertensive response to nicotine is due to its adrenal stimulation, which results in increased adrenaline secretion.[14] Furthermore, cigarette smokers are known to have higher concentrations of lead and cadmium and lower concentrations of ascorbic acid than non-smokers.[15]

Stress   Stress can be the causative factor of high blood pressure in many instances. Relaxation techniques such as biofeedback, autogenics, transcendental meditation, yoga, progressive muscle relaxation and hypnosis have all been shown to have some value in lowering blood pressure.[10]

Exercise   Exercise is strongly indicated since it reduces both stress and blood pressure.[20] The exercise programme should, of course, be carefully designed, taking into consideration the patient's needs and cardiovascular condition.

Heavy metals   Chronic exposure to lead from environmental sources, including drinking water, is associated with increased cardiovascular mortality. Elevated blood lead levels have been found in a significant number of hypertensives.[16,17] Areas with a soft water supply have an increased lead concentration in drinking water due to the acidity of the water, and people living in these areas may be predisposed to hypertension. It should be noted that soft water is also, of course, low in calcium and magnesium.[16]

Cadmium has also been shown to induce hypertension, with untreated hypertensives showing blood cadmium levels three to four times those in matched normotensives.[18] Cigarette smokers typically have much higher body cadmium levels due to cadmium's presence in cigarette smoke.

Therapy

Diet

Many dietary factors have been shown to correlate with blood pressure, including sodium to potassium ratio, percentage of polyunsaturated fatty acids, fibre and magnesium content, and levels of simple carbohydrates, total fats and cholesterol.

Sodium and potassium   The role of a high sodium–low potassium intake in the development of essential hypertension has been considered extensively and conclusively.[4,5,21]

Excessive consumption of dietary sodium chloride (salt), coupled with diminished dietary potassium, induces an increase in fluid volume and an impairment of blood pressure regulating mechanisms. This results in hypertension in susceptible individuals.

A high potassium–low sodium diet reduces the rise in blood pressure during mental stress by reducing the blood vessel constricting effect of adrenaline.[22] Sodium restriction alone does not improve blood pressure control; it must be accompanied by a high potassium intake.[22] This combined approach also improves patient compliance, since it includes many foods that do not warrant salting. (A list of high potassium foods is given in Chapter 10, Stress.)

In general, individuals with hypertension consume higher levels of salt than normotensives. This results in an elevated salt taste threshold, which means it takes more salt on the food before the individual senses the saltiness. This abnormal salt threshold returns to normal after long-term sodium restriction.[23] As public consciousness of the harmful effects of excess sodium has risen, consumer purchases of table salt have decreased.[4] Unfortunately, the salt content of processed and prepared foods has also risen.[4] It is therefore important to look closely for 'hidden salt' in prepared food and condiments.

Substituting potassium chloride for sodium chloride may have a useful effect. However, many of the salt substitutes still contain up to 50 per cent sodium chloride; and there is experimental evidence suggesting that chloride consumed concomitantly with sodium is the necessary factor in salt sensitive individuals' hypertensive response.[24]

Vegetarian diet When compared with non-vegetarians, vegetarians generally have lower blood pressure levels and a lower incidence of hypertension and other cardiovascular diseases. Dietary levels of sodium do not differ significantly between these two groups. However, a typical vegetarian's diet contains more potassium, complex carbohydrates, polyunsaturated fat, fibre, calcium, magnesium, vitamin C and vitamin A, which may have a favourable influence on blood pressure.[25]

Fibre The lack of dietary fibre is a common underlying factor in many diseases of western 'civilisation'. The high-fibre diet has been shown to be effective in preventing and treating many forms of cardiovascular disease, including hypertension. As even mild hypertension is associated with an increased risk of cardiovascular disease, the dietary plan outlined for the prevention of atherosclerosis is indicated in treating hypertension (see Chapter 18, Atherosclerosis).

The types of dietary fibre that are of the greatest benefit are the water soluble gel-forming fibres such as oat bran, apple pectin, psyllium seeds, guar gum and gum karaya. A fibre source containing these fibres should be taken by individuals with hypertension for a variety of reasons (e.g. to reduce cholesterol levels, promote weight loss, chelate out heavy metals, etc.).

Sugar Sucrose, common table sugar, elevates blood pressure. Mechanisms which have been proposed to explain this include:

- Increased sodium retention.
- Increased aldosterone secretion.
- Elevated insulin levels.
- Increased catecholamine (adrenaline) secretion.[26]

The most plausible of these appears to involve increased adrenaline production resulting in increased blood vessel constriction and increased sodium retention.

Nutritional considerations

Calcium and magnesium Population studies indicate that hypertensive individuals consume less daily calcium than normotensives and may benefit from calcium supplementation.[27,28] Several clinical studies have demonstrated that calcium supplementation does indeed have a blood pressure lowering effect.[29,30,31] It is generally agreed that daily administration of 1 gram elemental calcium, along with other non-drug approaches, should be given a trial of at least three to six months in patients with mild to moderate hypertension.

Magnesium may be shown to be an even more important factor in lowering blood pressure than calcium.[32] Magnesium was first recommended as a therapy for malignant hypertension as early as 1925.[33] An intracellular deficiency of free magnesium is a major etiological factor in hypertension, as its levels are consistently low in hypertensives as compared with normotensives, and they show an inverse correlation with blood pressure.[33] In one double-blind clinical study, magnesium supplementation lowered blood pressure by 12/8 mm Hg in 19 of 20 subjects in the experimental group, compared to 0/4 in the placebo group.[34]

Essential fatty acids Increasing dietary linoleic acid as found in vegetable oils has a profound hypotensive action in man.[35,36] This is due to normalisation of the E series prostaglandins which are known to be decreased in hypertensive patients.[35,36] This simple dietary effect is prevented by aspirin and other inhibitors of prostaglandin synthesis, implying that use of these types of agents should be avoided in hypertensive individuals.[36]

Coenzyme Q10 Coenzyme Q10 (CoQ10) is an essential component of the metabolic processes involved in energy (ATP) production. Individuals with cardiovascular disease (including hypertension, angina and congestive heart failure) often are deficient in CoQ10 and require increased tissue levels of CoQ10. Clinical studies have indicated that CoQ10 is of considerable benefit in the treatment of hypertension and other cardiovascular disease.[37,38]

Vitamin C There is an inverse relationship between serum vitamin C levels and blood pressure in hypertensive men, i.e. the lower the vitamin C level the higher the blood pressure.[39] Whether this is due to dietary habits or a blood pressure lowering effect of vitamin C has yet to be determined.

Zinc Zinc has been shown to reverse cadmium induced hypertension effectively in rats and presumably has a similar effect in humans.[40]

Bovine renal extract Bovine renal extract has also been shown to possess blood pressure lowering effects in animals and hypertensive human subjects.[41]

Botanical medicines

Garlic and onion Although most recent research has focused on its blood lipid lowering effects, garlic has been shown to have hypotensive qualities.[42-4] In humans, garlic has been shown to decrease the systolic pressure by 20–30 mm Hg and the diastolic by 10–20 mm Hg.[42] The pharmaceutical mechanism of garlic's hypotensive effect is related to its effect on the autonomic nervous system, hypolipidaemic properties and perhaps its high content of sulphur-containing compounds.[42] It has been shown that there are decreased levels of sulphur-containing amino acids in the plasma of patients with essential hypertension.[45] Like garlic, onion has also been shown to possess lipid lowering and blood pressure lowering activity.[42]

Hawthorn berry (Crataegus monogyna) The leaves, berries and blossoms of hawthorn contain many biologically active flavonoid compounds. Hawthorn berries and flowers are a particularly good source of anthocyanidins and proanthocyanidins (polymers of anthocyanidins). These flavonoids are responsible for the red to blue colours not only of hawthorn berries but also of blackberries, cherries, bilberries, grapes and many flowers as well.

In addition to their roles as plant pigments, these flavonoids have very strong 'vitamin P' activity. Included in their effects are an ability to increase intracellular vitamin C levels and decrease capillary permeability and fragility. In hawthorn berry and flower extracts, these compounds are highly concentrated.

Hawthorn berry and flower extracts are effective in reducing blood pressure and angina attacks, as well as in lowering serum cholesterol levels and preventing the deposition of cholesterol in arterial walls.[42,46] Hawthorn extracts are widely used in Europe for their blood pressure lowering and cardiotonic activity. The beneficial and pharmocological effects of hawthorn extracts in the treatment of high blood pressure appear to be a result of dilating the larger blood vessels.

Mistletoe (Viscum album) The mechanism underlying the long known anti-hypertensive action of mistletoe has not yet been clarified.[42] Although mistletoe contains a large number of biologically active substances, it appears that the healing effect is produced not by one or another of its components. Rather it is produced by the whole complex of biologically active substances contained in the plant. Mistletoe is believed to function as a regulator of blood pressure, exerting a healing effect in both hypertension and hypotension.[42] In Europe, mistletoe has often been combined with crataegus in treating hypertension. Potentially toxic, this herb should not be used at high doses (i.e. greater than the equivalent of 4 grams crude herb) or extended periods of time except under the supervision of a naturopathic physician.

Treatment

This chapter outlines many factors which can reduce elevated blood pressures. Although hypertension can be treated effectively without prescribed medications, or for that matter the aid of a physician, a physician's assistance in composing a non-drug treatment plan can be invaluable. Furthermore, this chapter represents only a fraction of possible natural treatments of hypertension. Most individuals will see a reduction in blood pressure by adhering to the following guidelines.

Diet

Attaining an ideal weight is imperative. The diet should be rich in high potassium foods (vegetables and fruits) and essential fatty acids. Daily intake of potassium should total 7 grams per day. The diet should be low in saturated fat, sugar and salt. In general, a wholefood diet emphasising vegetables and members of the garlic/onion family should be consumed.

Fibre

Typically, we recommend one to three tablespoons of herbal bulking formula containing such things as oat fibre, guar gum, apple pectin, gum karaya, psyllium seed, dandelion root powder, ginger root powder, fenugreek seed powder and fennel seed powder.

Lifestyle

Caffeine, alcohol and tobacco use should be eliminated. Stress reduction techniques such as biofeedback, autogenics, meditation, yoga, hypnosis and progressive muscle relaxation may offer some benefit. Regular aerobic exercise is also strongly recommended.

Supplements

In addition to a general multiple vitamin-mineral supplement the following recommendations are given.
- Calcium, 1–1.5 g per day.
- Magnesium, 500 mg per day.

An ionised source of calcium and magnesium is most beneficial, e.g. citrates, orotates, aspartates or Kreb's cycle chelates.
- Coenzyme Q10, 20 mg three times daily.
- Vitamin C, 1 to 3 grams per day.
- Zinc (picolinate), 15–30 mg per day.
- Renal extract, 500 mg per day.

Herbal medicines

- *Crataegus monogyna*:
    Berries or flowers (dried), 3–5 grams or as a tea.
    Tincture (1:5), 4–6 ml (1–1.5 tsp).
    Fluid extract (1:1), 1–2 ml (0.25–0.5 tsp).
    Solid extract (10 per cent procyanidins), 100–250 mg.
- *Viscum album*:
    Dried leaves, 2–4 grams.
    Tincture (1:5), 1–3 ml (0.25–0.75 tsp).
    Fluid extract (1:1), 0.5 ml.
    Solid extract (4:1), 100–250 mg.

High blood pressure should not be taken lightly. If, after following the above recommendations for a period of three months, blood pressure has not returned to normal, please consult your general practitioner.

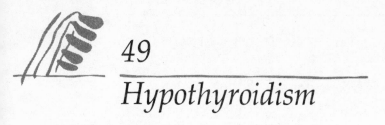

49

Hypothyroidism

- Hypothyroidism in children – delayed growth and mental development, along with the signs and symptoms listed below.
- Hypothyroidism in adults – common signs and symptoms of hypothyroidism are low basal body temperature, depression, difficulty in losing weight, dry skin, headaches, lethargy or fatigue, menstrual problems, recurrent infections, constipation and sensitivity to cold.

General considerations

Since the hormones of the thyroid gland regulate metabolism in every cell of the body, a deficiency of thyroid hormones can affect virtually all body functions. The degree of severity of symptoms in the adult range from extremely mild deficiency states which are barely detectable (subclinical hypothyroidism) to severe deficiency states which are life-threatening (myxoedema).[1-4]

Deficiency of thyroid hormone may be due to defective hormone synthesis or lack of stimulation by the pituitary gland which secretes thyroid stimulating hormone (TSH). When thyroid hormone levels in the blood are low, the pituitary secretes TSH. If thyroid hormone levels are decreased and TSH levels are elevated in the blood, it usually indicates defective thyroid hormone synthesis. This is termed primary hypothyroidism. If TSH levels are low and thyroid hormone levels are also low this indicates that the pituitary gland is responsible for the low thyroid function. This is termed secondary hypothyroidism.

There is much controversy over the diagnosis of hypothyroidism. Before the use of blood measurements, it was common to diagnose hypothyroidism based on basal body temperature (the temperature of the body at rest) and Achilles reflex time (reflexes are slowed in hypothyroidism). With the advent of sophisticated laboratory measurement of thyroid hormones in the blood, these 'functional' tests of thyroid activity fell by the wayside. However, it is now known that the blood tests are not sensitive enough to diagnose milder forms of hypothyroidism. As mild hypothyroidism is the most common form of hypothyroidism, the majority of people with hypothyroidism are going undiagnosed.[3,4,5]

This is a serious concern as failure to treat an underlying condition like hypo-thyroidism will reduce the effectiveness of nutritional therapies. For example, in most cases zinc, vitamin A and essential fatty acids are effective in relieving dry, scaly skin. However, if a person had hypothyroidism, no improvement would occur. It is critical that thyroid function be evaluated, as hypothyroidism is thought to be an underlying factor in a large number of diseases.

The basal body temperature is perhaps the most sensitive functional test of thyroid function.[3,4] A simple method for taking your basal body temperature is detailed below.

Most estimates on the rate of hypothyroidism are based on using low levels of thyroid hormone levels in the blood. As already mentioned, this may mean a large number of people with mild hypothyroidism go undetected. None the less, using blood levels of thyroid hormones as the criteria, it is estimated that between 1 per cent and 4 per cent of the adult population have moderate to severe hypothyroidism, and another 10 per cent to 12 per cent have mild hypothyroidism.[2,6,7,8] The rate of hypothyroidism increases steadily with advancing age.

Some writers of popular books using medical history, physical examination and basal body temperatures, along with the blood thyroid levels, as the diagnostic criteria estimate the rate of hypothyroidism in the general adult population to be approximately 40 per cent.[2,3] It is likely that the true rate of hypothyroidism using this criteria is some-where near 25 per cent of the population.

Taking your basal body temperature

Your body temperature reflects your metabolic rate, which is largely determined by hormones secreted by the thyroid gland. The function of the thyroid gland can be determined simply by measuring your basal body temperature. All that is needed is a thermometer.

- Shake down the thermometer to below 95 °F (35 °C) and place it by your bed before going to sleep at night.
- On waking, place the thermometer in your armpit for a full 10 minutes. It is important to make as little movement as possible. Lying and resting with your eyes closed is best. Do not get up until the 10-minute test is completed.
- After 10 minutes, read and record the temperature and date.
- Record the temperature for at least three mornings (preferably at the same time of day) and give the information to your physician. Menstruating women must perform the test on the second, third and fourth days of menstruation. Men and postmenopausal women can perform the test at any time.

Your basal body temperature should be between 97.6 °F (36.4 °C) and 98.2 °F (36.7 °C). Low basal body temperatures are quite common and may reflect hypothyroidism. High basal body temperatures (above 98.6 °F, 37.0 °C) are less common, but may be evidence of hyperthyroidism. Common signs and symptoms of hyperthyroidism include bulging eyeballs, fast pulse, hyperactivity, inability to gain weight, insomnia, irritability, menstrual problems and nervousness.

Manifestations of adult hypothyroidism

Since thyroid hormone affects every cell of the body, a deficiency will usually result in a large number of signs and symptoms. A brief review of the common manifestations of hypothyroidism on several body systems is given below.

Metabolic   The metabolic manifestations of hypothyroidism reflect a general decrease in the rate of utilisation of fat, protein and carbohydrate. Moderate weight gain combined with cold intolerance is a common finding.[2]

Cholesterol and triglyceride levels are increased in even the mildest forms of hypothyroidism.[2,9] This greatly increases the risk of serious cardiovascular disease. Studies have shown an increased rate of heart disease due to atherosclerosis in individuals with hypothyroidism.[10,11]

Hypothyroidism also leads to increased capillary permeability and slow lymphatic drainage.[2] Often this will result in swelling of tissue (oedema).

Endocrine   A variety of hormonal symptoms can exist in hypothyroidism. Perhaps the most common is a loss of libido (sexual drive) in men and menstrual abnormalities in women.[2]

Women with mild hypothyroidism have prolonged and heavy menstrual bleeding, with a shorter menstrual cycle (time from the start of one period to the next). Infertility may also be a problem. If the hypothyroid woman does become pregnant, miscarriages, premature deliveries and stillbirths are common. Rarely does a pregnancy terminate in normal labour and delivery in the hypothyroid woman.

Skin, hair and nails   Dry, rough skin covered with fine superficial scales is seen in most hypothyroid individuals while the hair is coarse, dry and brittle. Hair loss can be quite severe. The nails become thin and brittle and typically show transverse grooves.[2]

Psychological   The brain appears to be quite sensitive to low levels of thyroid hormone. Depression along with weakness and fatigue are usually the first symptoms of hypothyroidism.[2,5,12] Later the hypothyroid individual will have difficulty concentrating and be extremely forgetful.

Muscular and skeletal   Muscle weakness and joint stiffness is a predominant feature of hypothyroidism.[2,13] Some individuals with hypothyroidism may also experience muscle and joint pain, and tenderness.[14]

Cardiovascular   Hypothyroidism is thought to predispose to atherosclerosis due to the increase in cholesterol and triglycerides.[9,10,11] Hypothyroidism can also cause hypertension, reduce the function of the heart and reduce heart rate.[2]

Other manifestations   Shortness of breath, constipation and impaired kidney function are some of the other common features of hypothyroidism.[2]

Therapy

The manufacture of thyroid hormones within the thyroid gland is dependent on several important nutrients. Deficiency of any one of the nutritional factors described below, or ingestion of foods rich in goitrogens, could result in hypothyroidism.

Iodine and tyrosine

Thyroid hormones are made from iodine and the amino acid tyrosine. A deficiency of iodine results in the development of a goitre, an enlarged thyroid gland. When the level of the iodine is low in the diet and blood, it causes the cells of the thyroid gland to become quite large due to pituitary stimulation (TSH).[1]

Goitre is estimated to affect over 200 million people the world over.[1,15] In all but 4 per cent of these cases the goitre is caused by an iodine deficiency. Iodine deficiency is now quite rare in the US and other industrialised countries due to the addition of iodine to table salt. Adding iodine to table salt began in Michigan, where in 1924 the goitre rate was an incredible 47 per cent.

Few people in the US are now considered iodine deficient, yet the rate of goitre is still relatively high (5 to 6 per cent) in certain high risk areas. The goitre in these people is probably a result of the ingestion of certain foods which block iodine utilisation. These foods are known as goitrogens and are discussed below.

The recommended dietary allowance (RDA) for iodine in adults is quite small, 150 micrograms.[15] Seafoods, including seaweeds like kelp, clams, lobsters, oysters and sardines and other saltwater fish, are nature's richest sources of iodine. However, the majority of iodine is derived from the use of iodised salt (70 micrograms of iodine per gram of salt). Sea salt has little iodine. The average intake of iodine in the US is estimated to be over 600 micrograms per day.

Too much iodine can actually inhibit thyroid gland synthesis. For this reason, and because the only function of iodine in the body is for thyroid hormone synthesis, it is recommended that dietary levels or supplementation of iodine not exceed 1 milligram per day for any length of time.

Goitrogens

Some foods contain substances which prevent the utilisation of iodine. These are termed goitrogens and include such foods as turnips, cabbage, mustard, cassava root, soybean, peanuts, pine nuts and millet. Cooking usually inactivates goitrogens.[15]

Vitamins and minerals

Zinc, vitamin E and vitamin A function together in many body processes, including the manufacture of thyroid hormone.[16] A deficiency of any of these nutrients would result in lower levels of active thyroid hormone being produced. Low zinc levels are common in the elderly, as is hypothyroidism.[17] There may be a correlation.

The B vitamins riboflavin (B2), niacin (B3) and pyridoxine (B6), and vitamin C are also necessary for normal thyroid hormone manufacture.[16]

Exercise

Exercise stimulates thyroid gland secretion and increases tissue sensitivity to thyroid hormone. Many of the health benefits of exercise may be a result of improved thyroid function. Exercise is particularly important in a treatment programme for hypo-thyroidism.

This is especially true in overweight hypothyroid individuals who are dieting (restricting food intake). A consistent effect of dieting is a decrease in the metabolic rate as the body strives to conserve fuel. Exercise has been shown to prevent the decline in metabolic rate in response to dieting.[18]

Treatment

The medical treatment of hypothyroidism, in all but its mildest forms, involves the use of dessicated thyroid or synthetic thyroid hormone. Naturopathic physicians prefer the use of dessicated natural thyroid complete with all thyroid hormones. At this time it appears that thyroid hormone replacement is necessary in the majority of people with hypothyroidism.

It is important to support the thyroid gland nutritionally by ensuring adequate intake of key nutrients required in the manufacture of thyroid hormone, and avoiding goitrogens.

Diet

The diet should be free of goitrogens like turnips, cabbage, mustard, cassava root, soybean, peanuts, pine nuts and millet. Otherwise the diet should follow those guide-lines in Chapter 2, Basic principles of health.

Nutritional supplements

- Iodine, 300 micrograms.
- Tyrosine, 250 mg.
- Vitamin A, 25,000 iu.
- Zinc (picolinate), 30 mg.
- Vitamin E, 400 iu.
- Riboflavin, 15 mg.
- Niacin, 25–50 mg.
- Pyridoxine, 25–50 mg.
- Vitamin C, 1 gram.

Exercise

Daily aerobic exercise for 15 to 20 minutes.

50

Insomnia

- Difficulty falling asleep (sleep onset insomnia).
- Frequent or early awakening (maintenance insomnia).

General considerations

Insomnia is an extremely common complaint. Within the course of a year, up to 30 per cent of the population suffers from insomnia.[1] Many use over-the-counter medications to combat the problem, while others seek stronger sedatives. Each year 4 to 6 million people in the US receive prescriptions for sedative hypnotics.[2] Psychological factors account for 50 per cent of all insomnias evaluated in sleep laboratories.[1] Insomnia is closely associated with depression.[2]

Various compounds in food and drink can interfere with normal sleep, including stimulants, thyroid preparations, oral contraceptives, beta-blockers, marijuana, alcohol, tea and chocolate. Insomnia is definitely a symptom that can have many causes. Table 50.1 summarises some of the more common causes.

Table 50.1 Causes of insomnia

Sleep onset insomnia	Sleep maintenance insomnia
Anxiety or tension	Depression
Environmental change	Environmental change
Emotional arousal	Sleep apnoea
Fear of insomnia	Nocturnal myoclonus
Phobia of sleep	Hypoglycaemia
Disruptive environment	Parasomnias
Pain or discomfort	Pain or discomfort
Caffeine	Drugs
Alcohol	Alcohol

Therapy

Since insomnia is largely due to psychological factors, these should be considered and handled before simply inducing sleep pharmacologically. Counselling and/or stress reduction techniques (including biofeedback and hypnosis) may be very effective (see Chapter 10, Stress).

The following topics are discussed as they relate to promoting sleep: nocturnal glucose levels; serotonin precursor and cofactor therapy; exercise; restless legs syndrome; and botanicals with sedative properties.

Night-time glucose levels

Low night-time blood glucose levels are an important cause of maintenance insomnia. The brain is highly dependent on glucose as an energy substrate, and a drop in blood glucose level promotes awakening via the release of glucose regulatory hormones, i.e. adrenaline, glucagon, cortisol and growth hormone. Hypoglycaemia must be ruled out in maintenance type insomnia (see Chapter 33, Diabetes mellitus).

Serotonin precursor and cofactor therapy

Serotonin is a transmitting compound in the brain that is an important initiator of sleep. The synthesis of serotonin within the brain is dependent on the availability of the amino acid tryptophan (this subject is discussed in more detail in Chapter 32, Depression). Tryptophan administration is indicated more for cases of sleep-onset insomnia, since its greatest effect is shortening sleep latency (the time required to go to sleep).[3-5] However, tryptophan administration (5 g at bedtime) has also been reported to increase total sleep time and decrease awakenings in numerous double-blind clinical studies.[3-5]

The important cofactors vitamin B6 and magnesium should be administered along with the tryptophan to ensure its conversion to serotonin. Also, since other amino acids compete with tryptophan for transport into the CNS (central nervous system – the brain and spinal cord) across the blood–brain barrier and insulin increases tryptophan uptake by the CNS, protein consumption should be avoided near administration and a carbohydrate source such as fruit or fruit juice should accompany tryptophan administration.[3]

Niacin has been reported to have a sedative effect due to its peripheral dilating action and shunting of tryptophan metabolism towards serotonin synthesis.

Exercise

Regular physical exercise is known to improve general well-being as well as promote improvement in sleep quality.[1,6] Exercise should be performed in the morning or early evening, not before bedtime, and should be of moderate intensity.[1,6] Usually 20 minutes of aerobic exercise at a heart rate between 60–75 per cent of maximum (approximately 220 − age in years) is sufficient.

Restless legs syndrome and nocturnal myoclonus

These disorders are significant causes of insomnia. The restless legs syndrome is characterised during waking by an irresistible urge to move the legs. Almost all patients with restless legs syndrome have nocturnal myoclonus.[1] It has been demonstrated that some patients with restless legs syndrome respond well to high doses of folic acid (35–60 mg daily).[7] This syndrome is believed to be a result of folate deficiency or perhaps a folate dependency in some individuals. It is a common finding in people with malabsorption syndromes and caffeine sensitivity.[7]

Nocturnal myoclonus is a nerve and muscular disorder characterised by repeated contractions of one or more muscle groups, typically of the leg, during sleep. Each jerk usually lasts less than ten seconds. The patient is normally unaware of the myoclonus and only complains of either frequent nocturnal awakenings or excessive daytime sleepiness, but questioning the sleep partner often reveals the myoclonus. Vitamin E has been used successfully in nocturnal myoclonus.[1]

Botanicals with sedative properties

Numerous plants have sedative action. Plants commonly prescribed as aids in promoting sleep include passion flower (*Passiflora incarnata*), hops (*Humulus lupulus*), valerian (*Valeriana officinalis*), skullcap (*Scutellarea latriflora*) and chamomille (*Matricaria chamomilla*).[8–10] Only passiflora and valerian will be discussed here.

Passion flower (Passiflora incarnata)   Passion flower was widely used by the Aztecs as a diaphoretic, a sedative and an analgesic. Its constituents include harmol, harman, harmine, harmalol, harmaline and passicol.[9,10] Harmine was originally known as telepathine for reason of its peculiar ability to induce a contemplative state and mild euphoria.[10] It was later used by the Germans in World War II as 'truth serum'.[10] Harma alkaloids are monoamine oxidase inhibitors,[11] and therefore their use with tryptophan would have an additive effect.

Valerian (Valeriana officinalis)   Valerian has been widely used in folk medicine as a sedative. Recent scientific studies have substantiated valerian's ability to improve sleep quality and relieve insomnia.[12,13] In a large double-blind study involving 128 subjects it was shown that an aqueous extract of valerian root improved the subjective ratings for sleep quality and sleep latency (the time required to get to sleep) but left no 'hangover' the next morning.[12]

In a follow-up study, valerian extract was shown to reduce sleep latency significantly and improve sleep quality in sufferers of insomnia under laboratory conditions and was suggested to be as effective in reducing sleep latency as small doses of barbiturate or benzodiazepans.[13] The difference, however, arises in the fact that these compounds also result in increased morning sleepiness. Valerian, on the other hand, actually reduces morning sleepiness.

Treatment

The treatment should be as conservative as possible and should include some means of dealing with psychological factors contributing to the insomnia. Foremost is the elimination of those factors known to disrupt normal sleep patterns, such as coffee (be sure to consider less obvious caffeine sources such as chocolate, coffee-flavoured ice cream, etc.), tea, alcohol, hypoglycaemia, stimulant containing herbs, marijuana and other recreational drugs, numerous over-the-counter medications and prescription drugs. If this approach produces no response, more aggressive measures can be taken. Once a normal sleep pattern has been established, the recommended supplements and botanicals should be slowly decreased.

Supplements

Forty-five minutes before bedtime:
- Niacin, 100 mg (decrease dose if uncomfortable flushing interferes with sleep induction).
- Vitamin B6, 50 mg.
- Magnesium, 250 mg.
- Tryptophan, 3–5 grams.

Botanical medicines

Forty-five minutes before bedtime:
- *Valeriana officinalis*:
    Dried root or as tea, 1–2 grams.
    Fluid extract, 1–2 ml (0.5–1.0 tsp).
    Solid extract (1.0–1.5 per cent valtrate or 0.5 per cent valeric acid), 150–300 mg.
- *Passiflora incarnata*:
    Dried herb or as tea, 1–2 grams.
    Fluid extract, 1–2 ml (0.5–1.0 tsp).
    Solid extract, 150–300 mg.

Lifestyle

Institute a regular exercise programme that elevates heart rate by 50–75 per cent for at least 20 minutes a day.

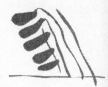

51

Irritable bowel syndrome

A syndrome characterised by some combination of:

- Abdominal pain.
- Altered bowel function, constipation or diarrhoea.
- Hypersecretion of colonic mucus.
- Dyspeptic symptoms (flatulence, nausea, anorexia).
- Varying degrees of anxiety or depression.

General considerations

The irritable bowel syndrome (IBS) is a very common condition in which the large intestine, or colon, fails to function properly. It is also known as nervous indigestion, spastic colitis, mucus colitis and intestinal neurosis.

IBS has characteristic symptoms which can include a combination of any of the following: abdominal pain and distension; more frequent bowel movements with pain, or relief of pain with bowel movements; constipation; diarrhoea; excessive production of mucus in the colon; symptoms of indigestion such as flatulence, nausea or anorexia; and varying degrees of anxiety or depression.

The irritable bowel syndrome (IBS) is the most common gastrointestinal disorder reported to general practitioners; 30–50 per cent of all referrals to gastroenterologists suffer from the condition.[1,2] However, it is almost impossible to determine the exact number of sufferers as many do not seek medical attention. Some estimates suggest that approximately 15 per cent of the population have suffered from IBS, and that there are twice as many women sufferers as men. (Though it is more likely that the number are equal, but that men do not report the symptoms as often.)

Causes

The causes of IBS are not entirely clear. There is no evidence that any structural defects of the bowel are associated with IBS, but a variety of physiological, psychological and dietary factors have been identified as possible causes.

395

Diagnosis

Diagnosing IBS can be quite difficult, and is often achieved by a process of elimination. Your physician provides valuable assistance in diagnosis, as a detailed history and physical examination has been shown to eliminate much of the vagueness involved in diagnosing IBS.[3] Conditions which may mimic IBS are shown in the accompanying box.

Conditions which may mimic IBS[2]

- Miscellaneous dietary factors such as excessive tea, coffee, carbonated beverages and simple sugars.
- Infectious enteritis such as amoebiasis and giardiasis.
- Inflammatory bowel disease (Crohn's disease and ulcerative colitis).
- Lactose (milk-sugar) intolerance.
- Laxative abuse.
- Intestinal candidiasis.
- Disturbed bacterial microflora as a result of antibiotic or antacid use.
- Malabsorption diseases such as pancreatic insufficiency and coeliac disease.
- Metabolic disorders such as adrenal insufficiency, diabetes mellitus and hyperthyroidism.
- Mechanical causes such as faecal impaction.
- Diverticular disease.
- Cancer.

Therapy

From a therapeutic standpoint, once other conditions have been ruled out, there appear to be four major treatments to consider when formulating a treatment plan:
- Increasing dietary fibre.
- Eliminating allergic/intolerant foods.
- Controlling psychological components.
- Using herbal therapy when appropriate.

Dietary fibre

The treatment of irritable bowel syndrome by increasing the intake of dietary fibre has a long, although irregular, history.[1] In general, consuming a diet rich in complex carbo-hydrates and dietary fibre is often curative.

One problem that has not been addressed in studies on the therapeutic use of dietary fibre is the role of food allergy. The type of fibre often used in both research and clinical practice is wheat bran.[4] As wheat is among the most commonly implicated foods in malabsorptive and allergic conditions, the use of wheat bran is usually not indicated in individuals with symptoms of IBS since food allergy is a significant causative factor in this condition. In addition, while patients with constipation are much more likely to respond to wheat bran, those with diarrhoea may actually worsen their symptoms.

Individuals will usually respond better to fibre from sources other than cereals, particularly water-soluble fibre like that found in vegetables, fruits, oat bran, guar, psyllium and legumes (beans, peas, etc.).[5]

Food sensitivity

Recent research has further documented the connection, recognised since the early 1900s, between IBS and sensitivity to certain foods.[6-9] The type of food sensitivity most significant in IBS is not believed to be mediated by the immune system, so food intolerance rather than food allergy is the more appropriate term to describe the sensitivity. According to double-blind challenge methods, the majority of patients with IBS (approximately two-thirds) have at least one food intolerance, and some have multiple intolerances.[8]

Since in most cases the reaction appears not to be mediated by the immune system, many food allergy tests are inappropriate. Current food allergy tests are designed to determine only immune-system mediated food sensitivities. In addition, since the majority of food allergies are mediated by IgG rather than the classic allergic antibody IgE, traditional allergy tests like the skin scratch test and the IgE-RAST (radio-allergo-absorbent test) are usually poor indicators of food intolerance (although they are widely used for this purpose). The IgE/IgG-RAST may be a better indicator, although many sensitivities may still be undetectable by currently available laboratory procedures. The elimination/challenge method is the least expensive food sensitivity detector and appears to yield the best results in patients with IBS.

In an elimination diet, the individual is placed on a limited diet; common foods are eliminated and replaced with either hypoallergenic and foods rarely eaten, or special hypoallergenic formulas. Typically the low antigenic diet (oligoantigenic or elimination diet) consists of lamb, chicken, potatoes, rice, banana, apple and a brassica family vegetable. The individual stays on this limited diet for at least one week and up to one month. If the symptoms are related to food sensitivity, they will typically disappear by the fifth or sixth day of the diet. If the symptoms do not disappear it is possible that a reaction to a food in the oligoantigenic diet is responsible, in which case an even more restricted diet must be utilised. A large number of individuals feel a marked improvement when they are on this oligoantigenic diet.[8,9]

After one week, individual foods are reintroduced, according to some plan whereby a particular food is reintroduced every two days. Usually after the one week 'cleansing' period the patient will develop an increased sensitivity to offending foods. Reintroduction of sensitive foods will typically produce a more severe or recognisable symptom than before. Try and consume the food being reintroduced as an entire meal. It can be very useful to track the wrist pulse during reintroduction, as pulse changes may occur when an allergic food is consumed. A careful, detailed, record must be maintained describing when foods were reintroduced and what symptoms appeared upon reintroduction.

It is interesting to note that many IBS patients have other symptoms suggestive of food allergy (such as heart palpitation, hyperventilation, fatigue, excessive sweating, headaches, etc.). (Food allergy is discussed in greater detail in Chapter 38.)

Candida albicans

The presence of the yeast *Candida albicans* in the intestinal tract favours the development of allergic and pseudo-allergic reactions, and this often makes it a complicating factor in IBS. *Candida albicans*, commonly known as thrush (or monilia), is a type of yeast which is present in the gut and is normally kept under control by digestive secretions and friendly bacteria. If the secretion of digestive juices or if the balance of microflora in the gut is disturbed, following a course of antibiotics for example, the candida may multiply unchecked and cause candidiasis (see Chapter 21, Candidiasis), thereby increasing the risk of allergies developing.

In one interesting study, a small group of patients who did not respond to an allergy elimination diet nor to the anti-yeast drug nystatin (600,000 units per day for ten days) were found at the six-month follow-up visit still to have the candida yeast in their faeces.[9] It is quite possible that the dramatic clinical improvement noted in the other participants in this study was due to the elimination of *Candida albicans* as well as food allergens. For this reason those factors discussed in Chapter 21, Candidiasis, may be appropriate to employ in IBS as well.

Psychological factors

Almost all patients with IBS complain of mental/emotional problems such as anxiety, fatigue, hostile feelings, depression and sleep disturbances.[10] There are several theories that link psychological factors to the symptoms of IBS.[11] The 'learning model' holds that when exposed to stressful situations some children learn to develop gastrointestinal symptoms to cope with stress. Another theory holds that the IBS is a manifestation of depression or chronic anxiety, or both. Personality assessments of IBS sufferers have shown them to have higher than average anxiety levels and a greater feeling of depression.[12] However, these studies were based on personality assessments after the individual developed IBS. It has since been determined by pre-illness personality assessment that IBS sufferers have normal personality profiles before their illness. Therefore, many of the common psychological symptoms of IBS sufferers may be either a result of the bowel disturbances (particularly malabsorption) or be caused by a problem such as stress, food allergy, environmental illness or candidiasis.

Some researchers believe that IBS sufferers have difficulty in adapting to life events, although this has not been fully demonstrated in clinical studies. However, increased contractions of the colon during exposure to stressful situations has been shown to occur in both normal subjects and those suffering IBS.[13] This could account for the increased abdominal pain and irregular bowel functions experienced by most people during periods of emotional stress.

Various methods have been used to tackle these psychological factors as a part of the standard medical treatment of IBS. Psychotherapy in the form of biofeedback[14] or short-term individual counselling[15] has sometimes proved successful. An increase in physical exercise also appears helpful for IBS patients suffering from stress. Many people find that daily leisurely walks markedly reduce symptoms, probably due to the known stress reduction effects of exercise.[16]

Botanical medicines

Peppermint oil   Peppermint oil inhibits gastrointestinal contraction and relieves gas.[17,18] An enteric-coated peppermint oil capsule has been used in treating the irritable bowel syndrome in Europe.[18] Enteric coating prevents the oil from being released in the stomach. It is necessary to do this as menthol and other plant monoterpenes in peppermint oil are rapidly absorbed. In order for these compounds to be of benefit in treating IBS they must reach the colon. Without enteric coating, peppermint oil's effects are predominantly upper gastrointestinal, with common side effects such as oesophageal reflux and heartburn often accompanying administration.

The administration of an enteric-coated peppermint oil capsule prevents this from occurring. Instead of being absorbed in the stomach and upper intestine, peppermint oil in enteric-coated capsules is allowed to move into the small intestine and eventually the colon where it relaxes the spastic intestinal muscles.[18]

In one double-blind cross-over study, enteric-coated peppermint oil was shown to reduce significantly the abdominal symptoms of the irritable bowel syndrome.[19] The study concluded that 'Peppermint oil in enteric-coated capsules appears to be an effective and safe preparation for symptomatic treatment of the irritable bowel syndrome.' This is quite significant since many sufferers of the irritable bowel syndrome are told that it is a condition they will just have to live with.

Enteric-coated peppermint oil (0.2 ml) is available on the market. The standard dose is two to three capsules taken between meals. Some patients have noted a transient hot burning sensation in the rectum during defaecation due to unabsorbed menthol. If this occurs do not be alarmed, simply reduce the dose.

Ginger (Zingiber officinale)   Common ginger has a very long history of use in the treatment of a wide variety of intestinal ailments, among other things. A clue to ginger's usefulness in alleviating gastrointestinal distress was offered in a recent double-blind study which showed that ginger is very effective in preventing the symptoms of motion sickness.[20] In fact, in this study ginger was shown to be far superior to Dramamine, a commonly used over-the-counter and prescription drug for motion sickness.

Although ginger's mechanism of action in alleviating gastrointestinal distress is yet to be clearly understood, it has been regarded as a carminative or a compound that expels gas from the gastrointestinal tract for thousands of years.

Herbal antispasmodics

Many plants possess direct antispasmodic action on the gastrointestinal tract. Perhaps the most commonly used herbs with this activity are chamomile (*Matricaria chamomilla*), valerian (*Valeriana officinalis*), rosemary (*Rosmarinus officinalis*), peppermint (*Mentha piperita*) and balm (*Melissa officinalis*). The antispasmodic activities of these herbs has been demonstrated in experimental studies.[21,22] These herbs are referred to as:

- Intestinal antispasmodics or compounds which relieve intestinal spasms or cramps.
- Carminatives or compounds which relieve or expel gas.
- Stomachics or compounds which tone and strengthen the stomach.
- Anodynes or compounds that relieve or soothe pain.

The use of these herbs alone or in combination may be of great benefit in mild intestinal colic and the irritable bowel syndrome.

Treatment

Since the diagnosis of irritable bowel syndrome is typically made by exclusion, a careful diagnosis is always required. Your physician can provide valuable service if he/she is knowledgeable of the causes of IBS and conditions that may mimic IBS. As discussed in this chapter, IBS is a multifactorial condition, with a diet low in fibre, food sensitivities and psychological factors all playing major roles.

The treatment of IBS involves increasing the intake of dietary fibre (especially water soluble fibre), elimination of food allergies, reducing stress and getting some exercise. In addition, the use of gel-forming/mucilaginous fibre supplements (e.g. guar, pectin, psyllium seed, oat bran), enteric peppermint oil capsules, ginger, herbal antispasmodics and measures designed to reduce the overgrowth of the common yeast (*Candida albicans*) may offer further relief of symptoms.

- Diet – high fibre diet, rich in vegetables. Avoidance of aggravating foods and any food sensitivities.
- Nutritional supplements – fibre supplement (psyllium seed husks, guar gum, pectin or oat bran), 5 grams per day.
- Botanical medicine – Enteric-coated peppermint oil, one to two capsules between meals. Any of the above mentioned botanicals would also be appropriate to use in the form of teas.
- Psychological – stress reduction techniques like biofeedback and hypnosis are often quite helpful in reducing symptoms.

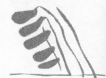

52

Kidney stones

- Usually no symptoms are apparent until the stone blocks the urinary tract, resulting in excruciating pain which originates in the flank and radiates.
- Nausea, vomiting, chills and fever may also be experienced.

General considerations

Stone formation in the urinary tract has been recognised for thousands of years but during the last few decades the pattern and rate of disease have changed markedly. In the past, stone formation was almost exclusively in the bladder, while today most stones form in the kidney or upper urinary tract. Over 10 per cent of all males and 5 per cent of all females experience a kidney stone during their lifetime. Each year nearly 6 per cent of the entire US population develops a kidney stone. In the US, one out of every 1,000 hospital admissions is for kidney stones. The rate of kidney stones has been steadily increasing, paralleling the rise in other diseases associated with the so-called western diet, i.e. atherosclerotic heart disease, gallstones, high blood pressure and diabetes.

In the western hemisphere, kidney stones are usually composed of calcium salts (75–85 per cent), uric acid (5–8 per cent) or struvite (10–15 per cent). The incidence varies geographically, reflecting differences in environmental factors, diet and components of drinking water. Males are affected more than females, and most patients are over 30 years of age.

Causes

Human urine is usually saturated to the limit with calcium oxalate, uric acid and phosphates. These compounds normally remain in solution, due to pH control and the secretion of various protective compounds. If these protective factors are overwhelmed, crystallisation will occur. In general, the majority of cases of kidney stones are entirely preventable. Occasionally a number of metabolic diseases cause kidney stones; these include such conditions as hyperparathyroidism, cystinuria, vitamin D excess, milk-alkali syndrome, destructive bone disease, primary oxaluria, Cushing's syndrome and sarcoidosis.

In general, conditions favouring stone formation can be divided into two groups:
- Factors increasing the concentration of stone crystalloids.
- Factors favouring stone formation at normal urinary concentrations of stone crystalloids.

The first group includes reduction in urine volume (dehydration) and an increased rate of excretion of stone constituents. The second group of factors is related to reduced urinary flow, pH changes, foreign bodies and reduction of normal substances which solubilise stone constituents.

Tables 52.1 and 52.2 outline possible causative factors involved in the development of kidney stones. Accurate determination of the type of stone and the cause of its development leads to a better designed prevention programme. If a stone is not available for chemical analysis, careful evaluation of a number of criteria (diet, underly-

Table 52.1 Causes of excessive excretion of relatively insoluble urinary constituents

Constituent	Cause of excess excretion
Calcium (> 250 mg/day excreted)	Absorptive hypercalciuria, 30–40% of all stone formers
	Renal hypercalciuria (renal tubular acidosis)
	Primary hyperparathyroidism, 5–7% of all stone formers
	Hyperthyroidism
	High vitamin D intake
	Excess intake of milk and alkali
	Aluminium salts
	Destructive bone disease
	Sarcoidosis
	Prolonged immobility
Oxalate	Familial oxaluria
	Ileal disease, resection, or bypass
	Steatorrhoea
	High oxalate intake
	Ethylene glycol poisoning
	Vitamin C excess
	Vitamin B6 deficiency
	Abnormal oxalate metabolism
	Methoxyflourane anaesthesia
Uric acid (> 750 mg/day excreted)	Gout
	Idiopathic hyperuricosuria
	Excess purine intake
	Anticancer drugs
	Myeloproliferative disease
Cystine	Hereditary cystinuria

Table 52.2 Physical changes in the urine and kidney

Condition	Possible cause
Increased concentration	Dehydration
	Stasis
	Obstruction
	Foreign body concretions
Urinary pH	Low – uric acid, cystine
	High – calcium oxalate and PO_4
Infection	Proteus – struvite
Uricosuria	Crystals of uric acid initiate precipitation of calcium oxalate from solution
Low urinary citrate	Acidosis, infection, idiopathic
Nuclei for stone formation	Cells, bacteria, blood clots, etc., initiate precipitation
Deformities of kidney	Sponge kidney, horseshoe kidney, caliceal obstruction or defect

ing metabolic or disease factors. serum and urinary calcium, uric acid, creatinine and electrolyte levels, urinalysis and urine culture) will usually determine the composition of the stone. Your physician is invaluable in this process.

Therapy

As calcium-containing stones are the most common type of kidney stones, the focus here will be on this type. Calcium-containing stones are composed of calcium oxalate, calcium oxalate mixed with calcium phosphate, or, very rarely, calcium phosphate alone.

The high rate of calcium-containing stones in affluent societies is directly associated with dietary patterns of low fibre,[1] highly refined carbohydrates,[2,3] high alcohol consumption,[4] large amounts of animal protein,[4,5] high fat,[6] high calcium-containing food, high salt and high vitamin-D enriched food.

The classification of most stones as either caused by idiopathic hypercalciuria (i.e. unknown reason as to why there is increased calcium in the urine) or just idiopathic by many physicians is a reflection of the ignorance of dietary factors that induce increased urinary calcium levels and stone formation. Although each one of the dietary factors listed above can increase calcium levels in the urine, the cumulative effect of these dietary factors is undoubtedly the reason for the rising incidence of kidney stones.

Vegetarian diet

As a group, vegetarians have a decreased risk of developing stones.[5] Studies have shown that even among meat eaters, those who ate higher amounts of fresh fruits and vegetables had a lower incidence of stones.[7] None the less, over-consumption of protein should be avoided. Bran supplementation, as well as the simple change from white to wholewheat bread, has resulted in lowering urinary calcium.[1]

These simple dietary factors of eating more fruits and vegetables, and switching from white bread to wholewheat would probably prevent kidney stone development in many individuals.

Weight and carbohydrate metabolism

Weight control and correction of carbohydrate metabolism are important, since excess weight and insulin insensitivity lead to hypercalciuria and are high risk factors for stone formation.[8,9] This is particularly relevant because, following sugar ingestion, there is a rise in urinary calcium along with a decreased phosphate reabsorption. This leads to a low plasma phosphate which stimulates active vitamin D (1,25 dihydroxycholecalciferol) production which results in increased intestinal absorption of calcium and, simultaneously, increased excretion of calcium.

Nutritional considerations

Magnesium and vitamin B6   A magnesium deficient diet in rats is one of the quickest ways to produce kidney stones.[10] Magnesium is of critical importance in the prevention of kidney stones in humans as well. Magnesium has been shown to increase the solubility of calcium oxalate and inhibit the precipitation of both calcium phosphate and calcium oxalate.[11,12,13] A low urinary magnesium:calcium ratio is an independent risk factor in stone formation[14] and supplemental magnesium alone has been shown to be effective in preventing recurrences of kidney stones.[12,13,14] However, when used in conjunction with vitamin B6 (pyridoxine) an even greater effect is noted.[15,16]

Pyridoxine is known to reduce the production and urinary excretion of oxalates.[17,18,19] Patients with recurrent oxalate stones show abnormal vitamin B6-dependent enzyme levels, indicating clinical insufficiency of vitamin B6 and impaired glutamic acid synthesis. These levels return to normal but usually only after at least three months of treatment.[19] Restoration of normal vitamin B6 and magnesium levels are of great importance in preventing further kidney stones.

Depressed levels of glutamic acid (due to vitamin B6 deficiency or other reasons) in individuals experiencing recurrent kidney stones is significant, since an increased concentration of glutamic acid in the urine reduces calcium oxalate precipitation. Glutamic acid supplementation in rats significantly reduces the incidence of calculi, and it may do so in humans as well.[20,21]

Vitamin K   The urinary glycoprotein that is a powerful inhibitor of calcium oxalate crystalline growth requires vitamin K for its synthesis.[22] Impairment of glutamic acid formation or a vitamin K deficiency will reduce the formation of this glycoprotein. The presence of vitamin K in green leafy vegetables may be one reason vegetarians have a lower incidence of kidney stones.[23]

Fat soluble, but not water soluble, chlorophyll is an excellent source of naturally occurring vitamin K.

Citrate   Decreased urinary citrate is found in 20 per cent to 60 per cent of patients with kidney stones.[24,25] This is extremely important since citrate reduces urinary saturation of stone-forming calcium salts by forming complexes with calcium. It also retards the nucleation and crystalline growth of the calcium salts. If citrate levels are low, this inhibitory activity is not present and stone formation is likely to occur. Low citrate levels can result from a variety of metabolic disturbances (acidosis, chronic diarrhoea, urinary tract infection, etc.), but in general the reason for low levels in many individuals who develop kidney stones remains unknown.[24,25]

Citrate supplementation has been shown to be quite successful in preventing recurrent kidney stones.[24,25] Potassium citrate or sodium citrate have been used in clinical studies. A more advantageous salt of citric acid in the prevention of kidney stones would appear to be magnesium citrate.[11,12,13]

Concern has arisen that increased calcium supplementation may result in increased calcium-containing kidney stones (see below discussion on milk-alkali syndrome). Calcium citrate appears to bypass this justifiable concern. In addition, calcium citrate has been shown to be much better absorbed than calcium carbonate. It has been demonstrated that mean calcium absorption in patients with deficient stomach acid output was 45 per cent for calcium citrate, compared to 4.2 per cent for calcium carbonate.[26] In individuals with normal secretion of stomach acid output, calcium citrate was also demonstrated to be the more optimum calcium form.[27] While urinary calcium will rise in patients consuming calcium citrate, some of the citrate's effects inhibit the formation of calcium oxalate stones. Generally, over 95 per cent of the citrate ingested is used as an energy substrate, with the remainder being excreted in the urine where it demonstrates its inhibitory action against stone formation.

Milk-alkali syndrome

The long-term over-consumption of milk or antacids often results in the development of kidney stones. This condition has been termed the milk-alkali syndrome. Recently, due to the increase in the incidence of osteoporosis, there has been a tremendous push from physicians and manufacturers of antacids to use calcium carbonate antacids as calcium supplements. This does not appear to be sound medical advice, due to the risk of developing kidney stones with the over-consumption of antacids.

Milk may not be suitable for people at risk for developing kidney stones, due to the fortification of some milk products, particularly in the US, with vitamin D. This results in increased absorption of calcium, but also increases the urinary calcium concentration. Increasing the amount of urinary calcium greatly increases the risk of stone formation. Compounding this negative effect is the fact that milk fortified with vitamin D results in lowered magnesium levels.[28]

Heavy metals

Hair mineral analysis may be of value in patients with recurrent kidney stones, since many heavy metals (mercury, aluminium, gold, uranium and cadmium) are toxic to the kidney. Cadmium, in particular, has been shown to increase the incidence of kidney stones greatly; cadmium is concentrated in the kidneys where it causes much damage. A study of coppersmiths showed a 40 per cent incidence of kidney stones, which correlated very strongly with elevated serum cadmium levels.[29] Cadmium levels are also much higher in the tissues of cigarette smokers and individuals who live in areas where the drinking water is soft. Hair mineral analysis will often (but not always) detect increased body-burden of cadmium and other heavy metals.

Botanical medicines

Compounds (anthraquinones) isolated from the rubia, cassia and aloe species bind calcium in the urinary tract and significantly reduce the growth rate of urinary calcium crystals when used in oral doses lower than their laxative dose.[30,31] Madder root (*Rubia tinctoria*) and *Aloe vera* are especially good sources of these anthraquinones and may be used to prevent stone formation and, during acute attacks, to reduce the size of the stone.[32,33]

Khella (*Ammi visnaga*) has been shown to be unusually effective in relaxing the ureter and allowing the stone to pass.[34,35] This plant was used by the Egyptians nearly 4,000 years ago in the treatment of kidney stones.

Treatment

Effective treatment requires accurate differentiation between the various stone types and the recognition and control of any underlying metabolic diseases or structural abnormalities of the urinary tract. Tables 52.1 and 52.2 list diagnosable causes of kidney stones.

Prevention of recurrence is the therapeutic aim in the treatment of kidney stones. Since dietary management is effective, inexpensive and free from side effects, it is the treatment of choice. For all types of stones increasing urine flow to dilute the urine is vital. Enough fluids should be consumed to produce a daily urinary volume of at least 2 litres.

The following suggestions are primarily for calcium oxalate stones, although they are also appropriate for the majority of other types of kidney stones.

Diets

- Increase intake of dietary fibre, complex carbohydrates and green leafy vegetables, and decrease simple carbohydrates and high purines (meat, fish, poultry, yeast).
- Increase intake of foods with a high magnesium:calcium ratio (barley, bran, corn, buckwheat, rye, soy, oats, brown rice, avocado, banana, lima beans, potato).
- Reduce intake of high oxalate containing foods (black tea, cocoa, spinach, beet leaves, rhubarb, parsley, cranberry, nuts).
- Limit dairy products, particularly those fortified with vitamin D.

Supplements

- Vitamin B6, 25 mg per day.
- Vitamin K, 200 micrograms a day.
- Glutamate, 300 mg per day.
- Magnesium (citrate), 450 mg per day.
- Potassium (citrate), 150 mg per day.

Botanical medicines

Aloe vera juice at levels below that which can cause a laxative effect may be useful as a preventive measure and to reduce the size of a stone during an acute attack.

Miscellaneous

Avoid aluminium compounds and alkalis (antacids).

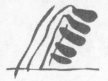

53

Macular degeneration of the eye

- Progressive visual loss due to degeneration of the macula.

General considerations

The macula is the portion of the retina of the eye responsible for fine vision; it is located at the centre of the retina. Degeneration of the macula is the leading cause of severe visual loss in the United States and Europe in persons aged 55 years or older. Presumably, the degeneration is a result of free radical damage similar to the type of damage that induces cataracts (see Chapter 23, Cataracts). The risk factors for macular degeneration include aging, atherosclerosis and hypertension.

There is no current medical treatment for macular degeneration. Laser surgery is used for those individuals who develop a less common type of macular degeneration.

Therapy

Clinical studies in humans have demonstrated that *Vaccinium myrtillus* (bilberry) extract (25 per cent anthocyanidin content), *Ginkgo biloba* extract (24 per cent ginkgo heteroside content) and zinc sulphate are capable of halting the progressive visual loss.[1-4] Presumably other natural compounds may also be of benefit, including the important antioxidants vitamin C, selenium and vitamin E.

The nutritional antioxidants are certainly important in the prevention and treatment of senile macular degeneration. However, in comparison the anthocyanosides from *Vaccinium myrtillus* and flavonoids from *Ginkgo biloba* address the problem to a much greater extent. Specifically, these plant extracts are many times more potent in their antioxidant and free radical scavenging activity than other nutritional antioxidants. Perhaps even more important is the fact that the anthocyanosides and ginkgo heterosides appear to have some degree of specificity for the eye.

Vaccinium myrtillus extracts (25 per cent anthocyanidin content) are widely used for ophthalmological applications, including poor day and night vision, glaucoma, diabetic retinopathy and macular degeneration.[1,2] The anthocyanosides of *Vaccinum myrtillus* have a very strong affinity for the pigmented epithelium of the retina which composes the optical or functional portion of the retina where they reinforce the collagen structures of the retina and prevent free radical damage.

Standardised *Ginkgo biloba* extracts (24 per cent ginkgo heteroside content) are used primarily for signs and symptoms of insufficient blood flow to the brain. Studies using this extract have also demonstrated impressive results in the treatment of macular degeneration.[3] The *Ginkgo biloba* extract possesses remarkable effects in preventing ischaemia and free radical damage to the retina and macula.

Treatment

As with most diseases, prevention or treatment at an early stage is most effective. Since free radical damage and lack of blood and oxygen supply to the macula appear to be the primary factors in macular degeneration, individuals with macular degeneration should greatly increase intake of antioxidant nutrients. Although nutritional antioxidants (e.g. vitamin C and E, zinc and selenium) are important in the treatment of macular degeneration, standardised *Ginkgo biloba* or *Vaccinium myrtillus* extracts offer even greater benefit.

Diet

Avoid rancid foods and other sources of free radicals. Increase consumption of legumes (high in sulphur-containing amino acids), yellow vegetables (carotenes), flavonoid rich berries (bilberries, blackberries, cherries, etc.) and vitamin E and C rich foods (fresh fruits and vegetables).

Supplements

- Vitamin C, 1 g three times a day.
- Vitamin E, 600 to 800 iu a day.
- Selenium, 400 micrograms per day.
- Beta-carotene, 200,000 iu a day.
- Zinc (picolinate), 45 mg a day.

Botanical medicines

Doses three times a day.
- *Ginkgo biloba* extract (24 per cent ginkgo heterosides), 40 mg.
- *Vaccinium myrtillus* (bilberry) extract (25 per cent anthocyanidin content), 80–160 mg.
- Fresh bilberries (blueberries), 4–8 oz (100–200 g).

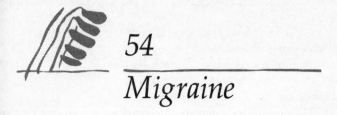

54

Migraine

Classic migraine:
- Severe throbbing pain, always beginning, and often remaining, on one side of the head.
- Head pain accompanied by nausea, with or without vomiting.
- Half have warning symptoms (auras) before the onset of pain. Typical auras last a few minutes and include blurring or bright spots in the vision, anxiety, fatigue, disturbed thinking, numbness or tingling on one side of the body.
- The attack typically starts in the morning, peaks within an hour, lasts 4 to 24 hours and happens several times a month.

Common migraine:
- The most common type.
- Severe throbbing pain on one or both sides of the head.
- Warning symptoms are rare.
- May last one to three days.

Cluster headache:
- Severe pain, usually localised around one eye.
- Tends to occur in clusters of one to three headaches a day over a few days, recurring every few months.
- No warning symptoms.
- May be associated with sensitivity to light, tearing, nasal stuffiness and agitated behaviour.

General considerations

Migraine headache is a surprisingly common disorder, affecting 15 to 20 per cent of men and 25 to 30 per cent of women.[1] Symptoms usually begin in childhood, but during this early period they often do not manifest as headache. Instead, such non-specific symptoms as colic, periodic abdominal pains and vomiting, dizziness or, unusually, severe motion sickness are the most common complaints.[1] The peak incidence is

Table 54.1 Migraine classification[2,3]

	Common	Classic	Complicated
Incidence	80%	10%	10%
Pain	Frontal, uni- or bilateral	Unilateral	Unpredictable, may be absent
Aura	Unusual	½ hr, striking	Neurological aura, dizziness, visual disturbance, loss of sensation on one side
Duration of headache	1–3 days	2–6 hr	Unpredictable
Physical signs	Unhappiness	Palor, vomiting	Mild neurological signs, speech disorder, loss of sensation, unsteadiness

between 20 and 35 years of age, then gradually declining. More than half of the patients have a family history of the illness.

Classification and diagnosis

Migraine headache has been subdivided into several types, based on the presence or absence of preceding or concomitant neurological manifestations and the nature of the manifestations. Although there are several subtypes, three (common, classic and complicated) comprise the vast majority of patients, and differentiation between them, while important, does not at this time have any therapeutic significance.

Cluster headache was once considered a migraine-type headache, since vasodilation is a key component, but it is now separately classified. Also referred to as histamine cephalgia, Horton's headache or atypical facial neuralgia, it is much less common than migraine.

Cause

Considerable evidence supports an association between migraine headache and vascular system instability, but the mechanisms are not yet known. Although most clinicians and researchers believe that the sequence of events is excessive intracranial arterial constriction (causing inadequate blood supply to the brain) followed by rebound dilation of the extracranial vessels (the headache phase), sophisticated studies of brain blood flow before, during and after are inconsistent in their support of this hypothesis.[4,5] The three leading hypotheses are discussed below.

Vascular system instability   It is a well-known clinical observation that the blood vessels over the temples are visibly dilated, and that the local compression of these vessels or the carotid artery temporarily relieves migraine pain.[6] However, other types of extracranial vasodilation (e.g. heat or exercise induced) are not associated with migraine. Despite the extracranial vasodilation, the patient appears pale during the headache, suggesting constriction of the small vessels. This is supported by the observation of lower skin temperature on the affected side.

The clinical manifestations of local or diffuse brain dysfunction have been attributed to intracranial vasoconstriction. A majority, but not all, of the studies measuring cerebral blood flow have confirmed a reduction of blood flow, sometimes to very low and critical levels, during the prodromal (warning) stage. This is followed by a stage of increased blood flow that can persist for more than 48 hours. The best current research shows that there is a significant decrease in regional cerebral blood flow in classic, but not common, migraine.[7] The abnormal blood flow appears confined to the cerebral cortex, while deeper structures have normal blood flow.

There is some evidence that migraine patients have an inherited abnormality of vascular system control. Migraine patients suffer from a tendency to faint when standing suddenly, more often than normal people, and they seem to be abnormally sensitive to the vasodilatory effects of physical and chemical agents.

Platelet disorder   The platelets in migraine sufferers show significant differences from the normal platelet, both during and between headaches.[8] These differences include a significant increase in spontaneous aggregation, highly significant differences in the manner of serotonin (a very potent vasoconstrictor neurotransmitter derived from tryptophan) release and significant differences in platelet composition.

The major proponent of the platelet hypothesis is Hanington, who starts with the observation that the most common precipitant of migraine is some type of stressor.[8] This results in a rise in plasma catecholamines (adrenaline and related neurotransmitters) levels which triggers the release of serotonin with resultant platelet aggregation and vasoconstriction.

The platelets of migraine sufferers aggregate more readily than normal platelets, both spontaneously and when exposed to serotonin and catecholamines. The increase in spontaneous aggregation is similar to that reported in patients suffering from transient cerebral ischaemic attacks. This is significant, considering the close resemblance of the symptomatology of such attacks and the prodromal (warning) phase of the migraine headache.

The onset of an attack is accompanied by a significant rise in plasma serotonin levels, followed by an increase in the urine of breakdown products of serotonin metabolism. All of the serotonin normally in the blood is stored in the platelets and is released by platelet aggregation and in response to various stimuli, such as catecholamines. There is no difference in total serotonin content between normal platelets and the platelets of migraine patients. However, the quantity of serotonin released by the platelets of the migraine patient in response to serotonin stimulation, while normal or even subnormal immediately after an attack, becomes progressively higher as the next attack approaches.[8]

The platelet hypothesis is strengthened by the observation that patients with classic migraine have a two-fold increase in incidence of prolapse of the mitral valve in the heart.[9] Using careful clinical and echocardiographic criteria and matched controls, the authors found in the migraine patients definite mitral valve prolapse in 16 per cent and possible prolapse in 15 per cent. The controls had 7 per cent and 8 per cent respectively.

This is of significance, since the prolapsing mitral valve is known to damage platelets and increase their aggregation. This work has been confirmed in several studies.[10,11]

Neuronal disorder   A third major hypothesis is that the nervous system plays a role in initiating the vascular events in migraine.[1] It has been suggested that the neurones which ennervate the arteries in the structures surrounding the brain release substance P (a neurotransmitter). This happens either in direct response to the various initiators or secondarily to changes in the central nervous system.[12] Substance P is an important mediator of pain, and its release into the arteries is associated with vasodilation, release of mediators of inflammation from mast cells and increased vascular permeability.

This theory suggests that functional changes within the sympathetic nervous system determine the threshold for migraine activation, and it is through its modulation that potentiators exert their effect.[12] Chronic stress is thought to be an important potentiator in this model.

A unified hypothesis   Although a definitive statement about the mechanism of migraine is not yet possible, particularly considering the unusually high level of contradictory information available, general observations may be made.

The mechanism of migraine can be described as a three-stage process – initiation, prodrome and headache. Although a particular stressor may be associated with the onset of a specific attack, it appears that initiation is dependent on the accumulation over time of several stressors. Once a critical point of susceptibility (or threshold) is reached, a cascade event is initiated. This susceptibility is probably a combination of changes in the platelet, alteration in the responsiveness of key cerebrovascular end-organs, increased sensitivity of the intrinsic sympathetic nervous system of the brain and the build-up of histamine, arachidonic acid metabolites or other mediators of inflammation. The platelet changes include increased adhesiveness, enhanced tendency to release serotonin and increased levels of arachidonic acid in the membranes. Once the platelet is stimulated to secrete serotonin, platelet aggregation, vasospasm and inflammatory processes result in local cerebral ischaemia. This is followed by rebound vasodilation and the release of substance P and other mediators of pain. These events are summarised in Figure 54.1 on the next page.

Therapy

Migraine headache is the result of a remarkably diverse range of causes. Although food intolerance/allergy is the most important, many other factors must be considered as either primary causes or contributors to the migraine process.

Dietary considerations

Food allergy/intolerance   There is little doubt that food allergy/intolerance is the major cause of migraine headache. Many careful double-blind placebo-controlled studies have demonstrated that the detection and removal of allergic/intolerant foods will eliminate

Figure 54.1 The mechanism of migraine

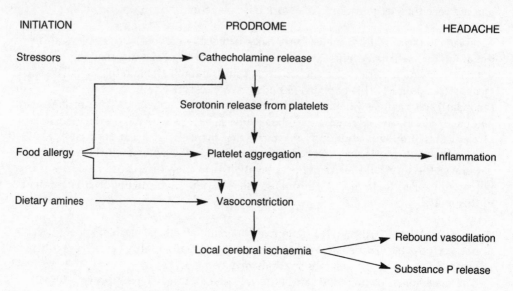

or greatly reduce migraine symptoms in the majority of sufferers. What is unclear is the percentage of migraine patients for whom food control is the most important factor; studies show a range from 30 to 93 per cent, with the majority showing a remarkably high degree of correlation.[13–19] These studies found the incidence of food allergy to be similar for the three major types of migraine. The foods most commonly found to induce migraine headaches are listed in Table 54.2.

The mechanism by which food allergy/intolerance induces a migraine attack is still unknown. Several theories have been proposed: abnormal response to pharmacologically active substances in the foods (such as tyramine); deficiency in the enzyme monoamine oxidase which normally eliminates such substances; food allergy; and platelet abnormalities.[16] One study suggests that migraine headache may result from chronic alternation of the non-specific responsiveness of a cerebrovascular end organ as a result of long-term stimulation by food allergens.[16] This mechanism would be similar to the response in asthma of the bronchioles to exercise or cold after antigen contact. Allergic reactions to foods are known to cause the platelets to release serotonin.[19]

There are several methods which can be used to detect food allergies, most of which are described in Chapter 38, Food allergy. Although the FICA (food immune complex assay) and RAST (radio-allergo-sorbent test) procedures are probably the most accurate and convenient, challenge testing is ultimately the most reliable. Unfortunately, however, challenge testing has limitations; some foods evoke a slow response, which may require several days of repeated challenge to elicit recognisable symptoms. Also, ingestion of large amounts of several foods may be necessary to detect those that are marginally reactive. The recommended procedure for the diagnosis and management of food allergy/intolerance is described below.

Table 54.2 Foods which most commonly induce migraine headaches[15-17]

Food	Egger et al.[16](%)	Hughes et al.[15](%)	Monro et al.[17](%)
Cows' milk	67	57	65
Wheat	52	43	57
Chocolate	55	57	26
Egg	60	24	22
Orange	52	—	13
Benzoic acid	35	—	—
Cheese	32	—	—
Tomato	32	14	—
Tartrazine	30	—	—
Rye	30	—	—
Rice	—	—	30
Fish	22	29 (shell)	17
Grapes	12	33	—
Onion	—	24	—
Soy	17	24	—
Pork	22	—	17
Peanut	12	29	—
Alcohol	—	29	9
Monosodium glutamate	—	19	—
Walnut	—	19	—
Beef	20	14	—
Tea	17	—	17
Coffee	15	19	17
Nuts	12	19 (cashew)	17
Goats milk	15	14	—
Corn	20	9	—
Oats	15	—	—
Cane sugar	7	19	—
Yeast	12	14	—
Apple	12	—	—
Peach	12	—	—
Potato	12	—	—
Chicken	7	14	—
Banana	7	—	4
Strawberry	7	—	—
Melon	7	—	—
Carrot	7	—	—

Dietary amines Foods such as chocolate, cheese and alcohol have been reported to precipitate migraine attacks. They contain vasoactive amines which cause vasoconstriction either directly or indirectly through the liberation of catecholamines. These vasoactive amines are normally broken down by the monoamine oxidase group of enzymes, the activity of which is reduced in the platelets of migraine patients, particularly during attacks, although this deficiency has not been found consistently.[8,20]

Patients with dietary migraine have been found to have significantly lower levels of a platelet enzyme (phenolsulphotransferase, which normally breaks down these dietary amines) than either migraine patients without a history of dietary provocation or normal controls.[20] Red wine contains substances (possibly flavonoids) which are potent inhibitors of this enzyme and can initiate a migraine attack.[21]

The vasoactive amine content of several foods can be found in Table 54.3. In general, tyramine is produced by the aging of protein-rich foods.

Table 54.3 Biogenic amine content of selected foods (microgram/gram)

Food	Serotonin	Tryptamine	Tyramine	Dopamine
Avocado	10	0	23	4–5
Banana (pulp)	28	0	7	8
Cabbage	—	—	440–800	—
Egg plant	2	0.5–3	3	0
Pineapple	2	—	—	—
Plum (red)	10	0.2	6	0
Potato	0	0	560–1,300	—
Tomato	10	—	4	0
Cheese	—	—	—	$\leqslant 2,170$
Canned fish	—	—	—	$\leqslant 3,303$
Wine	—	—	—	$\leqslant 24$
Beer	—	—	—	1.8–11.22
Aged meats	—	—	—	$\leqslant 1,237$
Yeast extracts	—	—	—	66–2,256

Essential fatty acids and arachidonic acid The role of essential fatty acids in the development of migraine may be quite important, but does not appear to have received much research attention. Considering the importance of platelet aggregation and arachidonic acid metabolites in the events leading to the cerebral ischaemia preceding migraine, manipulation of dietary fatty acids may be very useful. It has been well demonstrated that reducing the consumption of animal fats and increasing the consumption of fish will significantly change platelet and membrane fatty acid ratios and decrease platelet aggregation.[22-4]

Physical medicines

Many forms of physical medicine have been used in the treatment of migraine headache. Although most have been shown effective in shortening the duration and decreasing the intensity of an attack, they appear relatively ineffective in actually curing this disorder.

Cervical manipulation In a six-month trial in Australia, 85 patients were studied to determine the efficacy of manipulation of the cervical spine by a chiropractor in the treatment of migraine headache. The study was controlled by comparing chiropractic manipulation to manipulation by a medical doctor or physiotherapist and to cervical mobilisation. Although the study found no difference in frequency to recurrence, duration or disability, the chiropractic patients reported greater reduction in the pain associated with the attacks.[25]

Temporomandibular joint dysfunction syndrome   It has been claimed that a substantial portion of headaches diagnosed as classic or common migraine are in reality the symptoms of temporomandibular joint dysfunction syndrome (TMJ).[26] However, a recent careful study found that the incidence of migraine in patients with TMJ is similar to that in the general population, while the incidence of headache due to muscle tension is much higher.[27] These results suggest that, while correction of TMJ dysfunction may be of use in the treatment of migraine headaches, it is far more important in muscle tension headaches.

Relaxation training and biofeedback   Several investigations have shown that electro-thermal biofeedback can lead to a reduction in the frequency and intensity of attacks.[1,28] Temperature biofeedback is based on the assumption that when the patient increases his/her finger temperature there will be a normalisation of the vasomotor response of cranial blood vessels, and this will reduce the occurrence of headaches.

Transcutaneous electrical stimulation   Transcutaneous electrical stimulation (TENS) has been shown in a placebo-controlled trial to be effective in the treatment of patients with migraine and muscle tension headaches (55 per cent responded to treatment versus an 18 per cent placebo response).[29] However, the study also found that inappropriately applied TENS, i.e. TENS applied below perception threshold, was ineffective.

Acupuncture   The use of acupuncture in the treatment of migraine headache has received considerable research attention. However, assessing its efficacy is difficult since the studies have not been blind, migraine patients were seldom studied separately and most of the research has been reported in foreign languages, with only summaries available in English. Despite these limitations, sufficient evidence exists to support the use of acupuncture to relieve migraine pain.[30-2]

It is interesting to note that the mechanism of relief is apparently not endorphin-mediated. One study found that the injection of saline or naloxone (an endorphin blocker) did not affect the efficacy of the therapy,[33] and another found that, while acupuncture increased endorphin levels in controls, the low levels of serum endorphins found in migraine patients did not increase with treatment.[34] The mechanism of action may instead be through normalisation of serotonin levels. One study found that acupuncture was effective in relieving pain when it normalised serotonin levels, but was ineffective in relieving pain and in raising serotonin levels in those patients with very low levels of serotonin.[35]

Acupuncture appears to have some success in reducing the frequency of migraine attacks, although, as mentioned above, limitations in experimental design make interpretation difficult. One study found that 40 per cent of the subjects experienced a 50–100 per cent reduction in severity and frequency.[33] Although the authors used a double-blind cross-over design, the patients were only followed for two months. Another (uncontrolled) study found that five treatments (over a period of one month) decreased recurrence in 45 per cent of the patients over a period of six months.[36]

Botanical medicines

Botanical medicines have a long history of use as folk cures for migraine headache. Although many botanicals, e.g. *Gelsemium sempervirens* (yellow jasmine), *Helichrysum angustifolium* (everlasting), *Lavandula angustifolia*, *Valeriana officinalis* and *Galium odoratum* (sweet woodruff) have been used, few have received careful evaluation.[37] Discussed here are those with well-documented efficacy.

Ergotamine Ergotamine tartrate, with or without caffeine, belladonna or barbiturates, is the most widely used medical drug in the treatment of migraine. Although definitely effective when administered intramuscularly, a controlled clinical study has shown oral ergotamine tartrate (which is poorly absorbed by the gastrointestinal tract) to be no more effective than a placebo.[1]

Considering its widespread use for treatment and chronic application for prevention, recognition of the common signs and symptoms of acute and chronic toxicity is important. Symptoms of acute poisoning include vomiting, diarrhoea, dizziness, rise or fall of blood pressure, slow weak pulse, dyspnoea, convulsions and loss of consciousness. Symptoms of chronic poisoning include two types of manifestations: those resulting from blood vessel contraction and reduced circulation – numbness and coldness of the extremities, tingling, pain in the chest, heart valve lesions, hair loss, decreased urination and gangrene of the fingers and toes; and those resulting from nervous system disturbances – vomiting, diarrhoea, headache, tremors, contractions of the facial muscles and convulsions.[38]

Feverfew (Tanacetum parthenium) A recent survey found that 70 per cent of 270 migraine sufferers who had eaten feverfew daily for prolonged periods claimed that the herb decreased the frequency and/or intensity of their attacks.[39] Many of these patients had been unresponsive to orthodox medicines. This prompted the clinical investigation of the therapeutic and preventive effects of feverfew in the treatment of migraine. The double-blind study was done in a controlled setting at the London Migraine Clinic, using patients who reported being helped by feverfew.[39] Those patients who received the placebo (and as a result stopped using feverfew) had a significant increase in the frequency and severity of headache, nausea and vomiting during the six months of the study, while patients taking feverfew showed no change in the frequency or severity of their symptoms. Two patients in the placebo group who had been in complete remission during self-treatment with feverfew leaves developed recurrence of incapacitating migraine and had to withdraw from the study. The resumption of self-treatment led to renewed remission of symptoms in both patients.

The efficacy of feverfew in the prevention of migraine headaches is probably due to its ability to:
- Inhibit the secretion of serotonin from platelets.

- Decrease blood vessel response to vasoconstrictors (adrenaline, acetylcholine, bradykinin, prostaglandins, histamine and serotonin).
- Inhibit the production of inflammatory substances (prostaglandins, leukotrienes and thromboxanes).[40–2]

Cayenne pepper (Capsicum frutescens) Capsaicin is the major pungent ingredient of hot peppers.[37] Although capsicum does not appear to have been tested for efficacy in the treatment of migraine, there is sufficient theoretical basis, particularly if the neuronal model of migraine is accurate, to consider its use. Capsaicin depletes substance P in sensory nerves after an initial stimulation of substance P release,[43] acts as a potent inhibitor of platelet aggregation[44] and has a long history of use in the control of pain.[45] Considering the initial increased release of substance P induced by capsaicin, it is probably more useful in the prevention of migraine than in the treatment of an attack. The chemical structure of capsaicin is similar to that of eugenol, the active principle of clove oil, which also can induce long-lasting local anaesthesia of the trigeminal nerve.[43]

Valeriana officinalis Many herbs have been used in folk medicine in the treatment of migraine headaches. In general, the most common physiological characteristics they share are sedative and anti-spasmodic properties. Valerian has well documented sedative properties, which, although they would not cure the migraine headache, would help reduce the discomfort associated with them.[46]

Nutritional considerations

Quercetin The bioflavonoid quercetin has apparently not been clinically tested for efficacy in the treatment of migraine headache. However, its activity as a mast cell stabiliser and inhibitor of many of the pathways of inflammation suggests it may be useful. This possibility is strengthened by the observation that sodium cromoglycate (at 200–400 mg, four times a day), a molecule very similar to quercetin, confers excellent protection from challenges of foods known to induce an attack.[17]

Niacin Niacin, due to its obvious vasodilatory effects, has long been recommended in the popular literature for the treatment of migraine headache. This use was studied in the 1940s, and researchers found that intravenous injections of up to 50 mg resulted in relief of symptoms in 17 out of 21 patients.[47] These results were confirmed in one study[48] but unconfirmed in another.[49] Niacin should probably not be used in cluster headaches.

Magnesium As discussed above, mitral valve prolapse may be a significant factor in the development of the platelet abnormalities seen in migraine patients. Research has shown that 85 per cent of patients with mitral valve prolapse have chronic magnesium deficiency.[50] A magnesium deficiency hinders the mechanism by which the body repairs defective collagen (connective tissue abnormalities are common in mitral valve prolapse), increases circulating catecholamines (an important mediator in platelet aggregation) and predisposes to heart beat irregularities, blood clotting and poor regulation of the immune and autonomic nervous systems. Oral magnesium supplementation provides relief of mitral valve prolapse symptoms.[50,51]

Other considerations

Bowel toxaemia　Of possible significance in the development of migraine is the conversion of the amino acid tyrosine to tyramine by colon bacteria.[52] Although normally considered important only in patients with liver cirrhosis, the highly sensitive migraine patient might respond to the tyramine thus formed. This conversion by bacteria is blocked by berberine, the active alkaloid of *Hydrastis canadensis* (goldenseal).[53]

Initiators　The most common initiators of migraine headache are listed in the accompanying box.

Precipitating factors in migraine

- Alcohol, especially red wine.
- Nitrates, monosodium glutamate, nitroglycerin.
- Emotional changes, especially let-down after stress and intense emotions such as anger.
- Hormonal changes, e.g. menstruation, ovulation, birth control pills.
- Too little or excess sleep, exhaustion.
- Foods, e.g. allergic, chocolate, cheese, cured meats.
- Weather changes, e.g. barometric pressure changes, exposure to sun.
- Glare.
- Withdrawal from vasopressors, e.g. caffeine, sympathomimetic drugs, ergotamine.

Treatment

Migraine headache is a multifaceted disease, and indeed could be accurately described as a symptom rather than a disease. The challenge is determining which of the several factors discussed here are responsible for each patient's migraine process.

Identification of the precipitating factors (see box), and their avoidance, is important in reducing the frequency of headaches. Avoidance of initiators is particularly significant considering that they are cumulative in effect.

Due to the high incidence (80–90 per cent) of food allergy/intolerance in migraine sufferers, diagnosis and management begins with one week of careful avoidance of all foods to which one may be allergic or intolerant. This can be accomplished through either a pure water fast or the use of an elimination diet (which is much less desirable since allergenic foods may be inadvertently included). All other possible allergens, e.g. vitamins, unnecessary drugs, herbs, etc., should also be avoided. During this procedure, some people will exhibit a strong exacerbation of symptoms early in the week, followed by almost total relief by the end of the fast/modified diet.[15] (This sequence is due to the addictive characteristic of the reactive foods.) Once the person is symptom-free, one new food is reintroduced and eaten several times each day while symptoms are carefully recorded. (Some authors recommend reintroduction on a four-day cycle). Suspected foods (symptom onset ranges from 20 minutes to two weeks) are eliminated, and apparently safe foods are rotated through a four day cycle (see rotary diversified diet in Chapter 38, Food allergy, for further discussion). Once a symptom-free period of at least six months has been established, the four-day rotation diet should no longer be necessary.

Diet

As discussed above, all food allergens must be eliminated and a four-day rotation diet utilised until symptom free for at least six months. Foods containing vasoactive amines should initially be eliminated. After symptoms have been controlled they can be carefully reintroduced. The primary foods to eliminate are alcoholic beverages, cheese, chocolate, citrus fruits and shellfish. The diet should be low in sources of arachidonic acid (animal fats) and high in foods which inhibit platelet aggregation, e.g. vegetable oils, fish oils, garlic and onion.

Supplements

- Quercetin, 500 mg a day.
- Evening primrose oil, 2 g a day.
- Niacin, 50 mg a day.
- Magnesium, 500 mg a day.

Botanical medicines

- *Tanacetum parthenium*, 25 mg dried leaves two times a day as a preventive measure.
- *Capsicum frutescens*, 25 mg two times a day.
- *Hydrastis canadensis*, three times a day doses of one of the following:
    Dried root (or as tea), 1 to 2 g.
    Freeze-dried root, 500 to 1,000 mg.
    Tincture (1:5), 4 to 6 ml (1 to 1.5 tsp).
    Fluid extract (1:1), 0.5 to 2.0 ml (¼ to ½ tsp).
    Powdered solid extract (4:1), 250–500 mg.

Physical medicines

All require the services of a professional physician.
- Transcutaneous electrical stimulation to control secondary muscle spasm.
- Acupuncture to balance meridians.
- Cervical manipulation.
- Relaxation training.

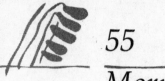

55

Morning sickness

- Morning or evening nausea and vomiting occurring during the first trimester of pregnancy.

General considerations

Many physiological and psychological factors have been proposed to explain the high frequency of nausea and vomiting during pregnancy (morning sickness). It has been estimated that 50 per cent of women complain of these symptoms at some time during pregnancy. Considering the multitude of hormonal and metabolic changes which occur during pregnancy, the existence of these symptoms is not surprising; none the less, emotional factors undoubtedly contribute to the perceived, and actual, severity of the nausea and vomiting. Effective psychological support is paramount to any effective therapy.

Therapy

The physiological factor largely responsible for nausea and vomiting of pregnancy appears to be impaired liver function.[1] The liver is responsible for detoxifying the hormones produced during pregnancy. If the liver is not functioning properly in detoxification processes (See Chapter 8, Liver support), toxic substances will circulate in the blood and eventually stimulate the nausea and vomiting centre located at the base of the brain.

Standard liver function tests are not usually sensitive enough to detect impaired liver function during pregnancy. One test that does appear to be sensitive enough is the measurement of serum bile acids. Studies have demonstrated a significant correlation between impaired liver function, as shown by an elevated serum bile acid level, and the symptoms of morning sickness.[1]

Those factors, particularly choline and methionine, discussed in Chapter 8, Liver support, are appropriate to employ in the treatment of nausea and vomiting of pregnancy, along with the additional recommendations given here.

Pyridoxine

Vitamin B6 has been used as a simple and somewhat effective treatment for the nausea and vomiting of pregnancy,[2,3] low serum pyridoxine levels being common among pregnant women.[2] A pyridoxine deficiency may be the causative factor in many cases.

Vitamin K and C

Vitamins K and C, when used together have shown considerable clinical efficacy, with 91 per cent of patients in one study showing complete remission within 72 hours.[4] The mechanism for this effect is unknown, and both vitamins administered alone show little effect.

Ginger (Zingiber officinale)

Historically, the majority of complaints for which common ginger was used concerned the gastrointestinal system. Ginger is generally regarded as an excellent carminative (a substance which promotes the elimination of intestinal gas) and intestinal spasmolytic (a substance which relaxes and soothes the intestinal tract).

A clue to ginger's effectiveness in eliminating gastrointestinal distress is offered by recent double-blind studies which demonstrated that ginger is very effective in preventing the symptoms of motion sickness, especially seasickness.[5-7] In fact, in one double-blind study ginger was shown to be far superior to Dramamine, a commonly used over-the-counter and prescription medication.[5]

Ginger has a long tradition of being very useful in alleviating the symptoms of gastrointestinal distress, including the nausea and vomiting typical of pregnancy. Although the mechanism of action has yet to be elucidated, current thought is that it is due to its aromatic and carminative effects on the gastrointestinal tract.

Psychological aspects

Many studies have been performed in an attempt to understand why 50 per cent of normal women experience no nausea and vomiting during pregnancy and why in some women this symptom continues beyond the first trimester.[8] Although many theories have been proposed, the lack of consistent data has hampered the development of a widely accepted viewpoint.

There appears to be general agreement that mild symptoms of nausea and vomiting during the first trimester have a strong physiological basis (linked to hormone changes during pregnancy) and are predictive of positive pregnancy adjustment and outcome. More serious or longer-lasting symptoms are thought more likely to have a psychological component.

A prospective study of 86 pregnant women showed a significant increase in both nausea and vomiting in the first trimester in women who reported more unplanned, undesired pregnancies and negative relationships with their own mothers. Those with problems continuing into the third trimester were also significantly more negative in their assessment of their relationships with their mothers.[9]

Treatment

A woman with nausea or vomiting during pregnancy must always consult her physician or midwife. Although it is usually a functional symptom, it can be a sign of serious disease, which must be ruled out.

Diet

- Small, frequent meals. Dry toast immediately after rising.

Supplements

- Choline, 1 gram per day.
- L-methionine, 1 gram per day.
- Vitamin B6, 50 mg two times a day.
- Vitamin C, 250 mg two times a day.
- Vitamin K, 5 micrograms a day.
- Methionine, 750 mg per day.

Botanical medicines

- Ginger root powder, 1 tsp decoction one to three times a day, or 1 gram in capsule.

Counselling

Women who are having an unplanned or undesired pregnancy or who report a poor relationship with their own mother should consult a qualified counsellor for assistance in resolving these conflicts.

56

Mouth ulcers

- Single or clustered shallow painful ulcers found anywhere in the oral cavity.
- Lesions are from 1 to 15 mm in diameter, have fairly even borders, are surrounded by a reddened border and are often covered by a white membrane.
- Lesions usually resolve in 7 to 21 days, but are recurrent in many people.

General considerations

Recurrent canker sores, mouth ulcers of aphthous stomatitis is an extremely common condition, estimated to affect 20 per cent of the population. The cause of recurrent canker sores, based on studies of initiating factors, appears to be related to food sensitivities,[1] stress[2] and/or nutrient deficiency.[3,4]

Therapy

Food and environmental allergens

The oral cavity is, obviously, the first site of contact for ingested, and many inhaled, allergens. The association of recurrent mouth ulcers with increased serum antibodies to food antigens suggests an allergic reaction is involved.[5,6] Furthermore, allergic antibody-bearing lymphocytes are significantly increased in mouth ulcers[7] and mast cells are increased in tissue sections from prodromal stages of recurrent ulcers.[8] Mast cell release of histamine and other inflammatory particles play an important role in the production of the mouth ulcer.[1] A diet eliminating allergens has been shown to have good therapeutic results.[9] (See Chapter 38, Food allergy for further discussion.)

Stress

Stress is often a precipitating factor in recurrent mouth ulcers, suggesting a breakdown in normal host protective factors.[2] Stress greatly increases the development of allergies.

Nutrient deficiency

A study of 330 patients with recurrent mouth ulcers found that 47 (14.2 per cent) were deficient in iron, folate or vitamin B12, or a combination of these nutrients.[4] When these patients' deficiencies were corrected by supplementation, the majority had complete remission. Other studies have shown similar deficiency rates for the same nutrients and equally good response to supplementation.[3]

Zinc supplementation has also been shown to be effective in some patients (particularly those with low serum zinc levels).

Gluten sensitivity

The incidence of recurrent mouth ulcers is increased in patients with coeliac disease, a condition caused by sensitivity to wheat gluten (See Chapter 27, Coeliac disease).[10–14] Biopsy of the small intestine in 33 patients with recurrent mouth ulcers showed eight to have the intestinal damage typical of coeliac disease, along with signs of allergic reactions to food antigens.[10] The remaining patients also exhibited these types of signs, but to a lesser degree.

An underlying gluten sensitivity would also contribute to nutritional deficiencies. Withdrawing gluten from the diet results in complete remission of recurrent mouth ulcers in patients with coeliac disease[10,11] and usually some improvement in the rest of the patients.[12,13]

Flavonoids

Several flavonoids are known to inhibit mast cell degranulation, basophil histamine release and the formation of other mediators of inflammation.[14,15] The anti-allergy drug di-sodium cromoglycate, a compound very similar in structure and function to the flavonoids,[14] has been shown to be effective in the treatment of recurrent mouth ulcers, resulting in an increase in the number of ulcer-free days and in mild symptomatic relief.[16] Several flavonoids, including quercetin, acacetin, apigenin, chrysin and phloretin have also shown anti-allergy effects similar to disodium cromoglycate.[14]

Treatment

The data described above suggests that no single factor is solely responsible for the initiation of mouth ulcers in any specific individual. The therapeutic approach to mouth ulcers is similar to that in other diseases with an allergic basis. Foremost is the recognition and control of allergens, particularly gluten (see Chapter 38, Food allergy). In addition, nutrient deficiencies need to be corrected and anti-inflammatory nutrients prescribed.

Diet

The diet should be low in animal products, high in complex carbohydrates and free of known allergens and all gluten sources (i.e. grains).

Supplements

- Vitamin C, 1 g per day.
- Zinc (picolinate), 25 mg per day.
- Multiple vitamin and mineral, one to five times the recommended dietary allowance.
- Mixed bioflavonoids, 1 g per day.

Multiple sclerosis

The early symptoms of multiple sclerosis may include:

- Muscular – feeling of heaviness, weakness, leg dragging, stiffness, tendency to drop things, clumsiness.
- Sensory – tingling, pins and needles sensation, numbness, dead feeling, band-like tightness, electrical sensations.
- Visual – blurring, fogginess, haziness, eyeball pain, blindness, double vision.
- Vestibular – light-headedness, feeling of spinning, sensation of drunkenness, nausea, vomiting.
- Genitourinary – incontinence, loss of bladder sensation, loss of sexual function.

General considerations

Multiple sclerosis is a syndrome of progressive nervous system disturbances occurring early in life, recognised since the description by Charcot in 1868. Despite considerable research, there are still many questions about MS. Mainstream medicine has become almost obsessed with finding a viral cause for this disease, although most current work suggests immune disturbances and autoimmunity.

In MS, the myelin sheath that surrounds nerves is destroyed. For this reason MS is classified as a 'demyelinating' disease. Zones of demyelination (plaques) vary in size and location within the spinal cord. Symptoms correspond in a general way to the distribution of the plaques.

In about two-thirds of the cases, onset is between ages 20 and 40 (rarely is the onset after 50) and women are affected slightly more often than males (60 per cent female: 40 per cent male). One of the more interesting features of MS is the geographic distribution of the disease. Areas with the highest rates of MS are all located in the higher latitudes, in both the northern and southern hemispheres (50–100 cases per 100,000 versus 10 per 100,000 in the tropics). These high-risk areas include the northern United States, Canada, Great Britain, Scandinavia, northern Europe, New Zealand and Tasmania. There are interesting exceptions to this geographic distribution, as the disease is uncommon in Japan at any latitude.[1,2]

It appears that the initial event in the development actually occurs in early life. This statement is based on the observation that people who move from a low-risk area to a high-risk area before age 15 acquire a high risk of developing MS, whereas those who make the same move after adolescence retain their low risk.

There are many possible reasons for the geographic distribution of MS. Obviously, such considerations as sun exposure, genetics, diet and other environmental factors quickly come to mind. There is reason to consider all of these as contributing to the development of MS, and they are discussed below.

Suspected causes of MS

The cause of MS remains to be definitively determined. A large number of causative factors have been proposed, but the data supporting many of these postulates are fragmentary and indirect. The following factors represent only a fraction of the possible explanations as to the cause of MS. It should be kept in mind that MS may be the epitome of a multifactorial disease.

Viruses   Viruses cause several demyelinating diseases in humans and animals that are quite similar to MS. Post-infectious encephalomyelitis is a demyelinating disease which starts 10 to 40 days after an acute viral infection or after an immunisation. Progressive multifocal leucoencephalopathy and subacute sclerosing panencephalitis are other human demyelinating diseases caused by the human papovavirus and the measles virus respectively. In animals, many viruses are capable of producing demyelination.[1-3] The studies, when looked at collectively, have clearly demonstrated that demyelination can occur as a result of viral infection. The demyelination may be direct viral destruction of the myelin-producing cells, or viral infection leading to immune system attack of the myelin.

This information has indicated to many that MS has a viral etiology. However, the viruses that have actually been isolated from cultures of material from patients with multiple sclerosis most likely have represented contaminants rather than causal agents.[1-3] Isolated viruses include rabies virus, *Herpes simplex* virus, scrapie virus, parainfluenza virus, subacute myelo-opticoneuropathy virus, measles virus and coronavirus.[1-3] Evidence has also pointed to several viruses, particularly the measles virus. In 1962 Adams and Imagawa reported that the blood of patients with multiple sclerosis had elevated levels of antibodies against measles. Subsequent studies confirmed this association and also demonstrated that patients with MS had CNS synthesis of measles antibody. Based on this data, MS was at one time believed to be due to an ongoing measles infection. This view has been modified by more recent studies indicating that a high percentage of patients with MS have elevated cerebrospinal fluid antibody levels to two or more viruses. More importantly, studies have shown that the measles-specific antibody in MS patients accounts for only a small percentage of the total antibody levels.[1-3]

The cerebrospinal fluid of most MS patients contains an elevated level of antibodies, which is characteristic of an infectious process. One hypothesis states that this is in fact due to an unrecognised infectious agent that causes MS. This hypothesis has been termed the 'sense antibody' hypothesis. An alternative hypothesis states that MS is not an infectious disease and that all the IgG in the CNS is nonspecific or 'nonsense antibody'.

At present, the data available does not appear to support a common infectious agent as the antigen for the increased antibodies. Increased activity of circulating antibody-producing cells during acute attacks is thought to be the factor responsible for the excessive antibody production within the CNS.[1–3]

Autoimmune factors　The lesions of MS are mimicked by those of experimental allergic encephalomyelitis (EAE), an autoimmune disease induced in animals by immunisation with myelin. However, in EAE immune sensitivity is to a single antigen, i.e. myelin basic protein, while in MS sensitivity to myelin basic protein cannot be demonstrated. This indicates that if MS is an autoimmune disease it is due to some other antigen. Attempts to find an antigen to which only MS patients react have failed.[1,2] However, a variety of immune system abnormalities have been reported in MS patients that would seem to support an autoimmune etiology.[1]

Diet　Many researchers have attempted to correlate various dietary patterns and the geographic distribution of MS. Diets high in gluten[5] and milk[6,7] are much more common in areas where there is a high rate of MS. As intriguing as these associations are, the majority of research concerning nutrition and MS has focused on the role that dietary fat plays in the epidemiology and etiology of MS.[8–11]

Some of the first investigations into diet and MS centred around trying to explain why inland farming communities in Norway had a higher incidence than areas near the coastline.[11] It was discovered that the diets of the farmers were much higher in animal and dairy products than the diets of the coastal dwellers, and the latter's diet had much higher levels of cold-water fishes. Since animal and dairy products are much higher in saturated fatty acids and lower in polyunsaturated fatty acids than fish, researchers explored this association in greater detail. Subsequent studies have upheld a strong association between a diet rich in animal and dairy products and the incidence of MS.[8,9]

It is interesting to note that the incidence of MS is quite low in Japan, where consumption of marine foods, seeds and fruit oil is quite high. These foods contain abundant polyunsaturated fatty acids, including the omega-3 oils (alpha-linolenic, eicosapentaenoic and docosahexanoic acids). Deficiencies of the omega-3 oils are thought to interfere with lipid elongation and permanently impair formation of normal myelin.[12]

Individuals with MS are thought to have a defect in essential fatty acid absorption and/or transport, which results in a functional deficiency state. In addition, consumption of saturated fats increases the requirements of essential fatty acids, creating a relative deficiency state in some individuals. This is probably significant in patients with MS. The role of diet in the cause and development of MS is discussed further below.

Excessive lipid peroxidation　Many studies have demonstrated reduced glutathione peroxidase (GSH-Px) activity in the erythrocytes and leucocytes (red and white blood cells) of patients affected by multiple sclerosis.[13–16] As GSH-Px is intricately involved in the protection of cells from free radical damage, decreased activity would leave the myelinated sheath particularly sensitive to lipid peroxidation.

GSH-Px is found in two forms, a selenium-dependent enzyme and a non-selenium-dependent enzyme. Since low-selenium areas often overlap high-prevalence areas for MS, it is natural to speculate that there may be a correlation between selenium levels, GSH-Px activity and MS. Initial studies seemed to support this correlation.[13,17] However, subsequent studies indicated that the reduced GSH-Px activity found in MS patients is independent of the selenium concentration and probably is due more to genetic factors.[14,15,16]

In patients with MS there appears to be an increased occurrence in individuals who inherently possess low GSH-Px activity (GSH-Px^L), compared with individuals who possess high GSH-Px activity (GSH-Px^H).[14] A decreased GSH-Px activity in the myelin-producing cells would render these cells extremely susceptible to lipid peroxidation and demyelination.

Therapy

From a natural therapeutic standpoint there appear to be three major approaches – dietary therapy, supplementation and physical therapy. Obviously, including all three provides the most comprehensive treatment plan.

Primary nutritional considerations

Dietary considerations   Dr Roy Swank, Professor of Neurology, University of Oregon Medical School, has provided convincing evidence that a diet low in saturated fats, maintained over a long time, tends to retard the disease process and reduce the number of attacks.[10,18] Swank began successfully treating patients with his low-fat diet in 1948. Swank's diet recommends:
- A saturated fat intake of no more than 10 grams per day.
- A daily intake of 40 to 50 grams of polyunsaturated oils (margarine, shortening and hydrogenated oils are not allowed).
- At least 1 tsp of cod liver oil daily.
- A normal allowance of protein.
- The consumption of fish three or more times a week.[10,18]

A diet low in saturated fats significantly restricts many animal sources of protein. The patient will have to derive protein from other sources, e.g. legumes, grains and vegetables. While meat consumption is contraindicated, fish appears to be particularly indicated due to its excellent protein content and, perhaps more importantly, its oil content. Cold-water fish such as mackerel, salmon and herring are rich in the beneficial oils eicosapentaenoic and docosaphexanoic acid (omega-3 oils). These oils are important in maintaining normal nerve cell function and myelin production.[12] They are incorporated into the myelin sheath where they may increase fluidity and improve neural transmission.

Swank's diet was originally thought to help patients with MS by overcoming an essential fatty acid deficiency. Currently, it is thought that the beneficial effects are probably a result of:

- Decreasing platelet aggregation.
- Decreasing an autonimmune response.
- Normalising the decreased essential fatty acid levels found in the serum, red blood cells, platelets and, perhaps most importantly, the cerebrospinal fluid in patients with MS.[19,20]

Swank's diet significantly reduces the platelet adhesiveness and aggregation which is observed in atherosclerotic processes as well as in multiple sclerosis. Excessive platelet aggregation and micro-emboli are thought to result in the following abnormalities observed in MS – damage to the blood-brain barrier, alterations in the microcirculation of the brain and spinal cord and lack of oxygen to the brain.[21,22]

MS patients have been shown to have an abnormal blood-brain barrier, presumably as a result of excessive platelet adhesiveness and aggregation.[22,23] Damage to the blood-brain barrier may allow the influx to the cerebrospinal fluid of substances in the blood, such as bacteria, viruses, antibodies, toxic chemicals and other compounds, that are toxic to myelin. Lack of oxygen may also be a contributing factor in demyelination, by promoting both the release of cellular enzymes and cellular suffocation (death).[24]

The effect of diet on platelets is important in MS, but probably of greater importance is the effect that fatty aids have on the activity of the immune system. Compounds which suppress the immune system such as adrenal steroids, cyclophosphamide and various antimetabolites have yielded good short-term benefits in MS patients, but these drugs are of limited value due to their high toxicity and lack of demonstrable long-term effect.[1,3] Currently, new immunosuppressive drugs are being tested for use in MS. However, considering the lack of toxicity, Swank's dietary approach and supplementation with the essential fatty acids appear to be more appropriate and safer ways of reducing the immune response.

Supplementation with linoleic acid   Linoleic acid supplementation for the treatment of MS has been investigated in three double-blind trials.[25-7] Although the results of the studies were mixed (two showed an effect and one did not), combined analysis indicated that patients supplementing with linoleic acid had a smaller increase in disability and reduced severity and duration of relapses than did controls.[28,29] These studies used a sunflower seed oil emulsion at a sufficient dosage to provide a daily supplementation of 17.2 grams linoleic acid. Other vegetable oils which primarily contain linoleic acid include safflower and soy. Better results would probably have been attained in the double-blind studies if dietary saturated fatty acids had been restricted, larger amounts of linoleic acid had been used (at least 20 grams a day[26]) and the studies had been of longer duration (one study found that normalisation of erythrocyte fatty acid level requires at least two years of supplementation[30]).

The effectiveness of linoleic acid supplementation in MS is thought to be due to suppression of the immune system. As mentioned earlier, MS bears a strong resemblance to experimental allergic encephalomyelitis (EAE), an autoimmune disease induced in animals by immunisation with myelin.[31,32] Linoleic acid has been shown to inhibit greatly the severity of EAE in animals with less severe forms of the disease, paralleling the effect of linoleic acid supplementation in humans with MS, i.e. individuals with minimal disability respond better than those with severe disability. Polyunsaturated free fatty acids are known to influence cell-mediated immunity significantly.[33,34]

Evidence exists that the beneficial effects of essential fatty acid supplementation are mediated by prostaglandins and a factor from the spleen. Inhibitors of prostaglandin synthesis (such as aspirin and similar non-steroidal anti-inflammatory agents) and removal of the spleen have been shown to prevent the protective effect of linoleic acid in EAE.[35,36] The spleen is considered to be the major site for the production and release of immunologically active prostaglandins. Non-steroidal anti-inflammatory agents such as aspirin, indomethacin and ibuprofen should be avoided in patients with MS.

If the effect of essential fatty acid supplementation is related to correcting the lipid composition of oligodendrocytes, Schwann cells and other myelin-producing cells, several years of supplementation may be required before complete therapeutic benefits are observed. Mobility studies of red blood cells from subjects with MS indicate that treatment with unsaturated fatty acids must continue for at least two years before they regain normal reactivity.[30] Presumably, since myelin-producing cells have a much longer half life than erythrocytes, it could take several years before the total benefit of supplementation would be observed.

Other oils   Better results may be attained by using flaxseed oil as this oil contains both linoleic and alpha-linolenic acid (an omega-3 oil). Linolenic acid has a greater effect on platelets[37] and is required for normal CNS composition.[12,38]

It has been suggested that gamma-linolenic acid, as found in evening primrose oil, is more effective than linoleic acid alone, due to its more ready incorporation into brain lipids and its possibly greater effect on immune function.[39] However, due to its cost and the fact that relatively large amounts of the product would have to be consumed to exert a therapeutic effect, supplementation with evening primrose oil may not be indicated at this time. One study demonstrated that daily supplementation with only 340 mg of gamma-linolenic and 2.92 grams of linoleic acid (the ratio found in evening primrose oil) had no effect on the clinical course in MS patients.[26] In the same study, those receiving 23 grams of linoleic acid demonstrated reduced frequency and severity of acute attacks, even though the study was only 24 months in length.

There appears to be a strong rationale for supplementation with eicosapentaenoic acid (EPA) and docosahexanoic acid (DHA), the so-called fish oils, in the treatment of MS, although no direct clinical investigation has been done. EPA greatly inhibits platelet aggregation[40] and DHA is present in large concentration in lipids of the brain.[41] This is consistent with Swank's protocol, which included the liberal consumption of fish and supplementation with cod liver oil, a rich source of EPA and DHA.[10,18] Supplements may be used to increase EPA and DHA, particularly in areas where the availability of cold-water fish is limited.

433

Selenium and vitamin E   Selenium's role as the mineral portion of glutathione peroxidase is discussed above in regards to the increased lipid peroxidation observed in patients with MS. While selenium supplementation will not increase the activity of glutathione peroxidase in the majority of patients with MS, it is a relatively inexpensive supplement that may benefit some. Vitamin E supplementation is definitely indicated, due to the increase lipid peroxidation previously mentioned and the increased consumption of polyunsaturated fats, which increases vitamin E requirements.[41]

Other nutritional considerations

In general, supplementation of vitamins and minerals in patients with MS should be on an individual basis. Antioxidants and those nutrients which decrease platelet aggregation (see Chapter 18, Atherosclerosis) should be used at therapeutic levels. Wheat germ oil and octacosanol appear to be appropriate supplements for MS patients as well.

Malabsorption   A significant number of those with MS may have some degree of malabsorption.[42,43] In one study 42 per cent of MS patients were shown to have fat malabsorption, 42 per cent were shown to have high levels of undigested meat fibres in their faeces, 27 per cent had an abnormal D-xylose absorption and 12 per cent had malabsorption of vitamin B12.[42] Malabsorption appears to be an important factor to consider, since multiple subclinical deficiency may result.

Food allergy   The role of food allergies in the pathogenesis and treatment of MS has been popularised.[44] As mentioned earlier, the consumption of two common allergens, gluten and milk, has been implicated in the etiology of MS. Intestinal biopsy in a small group of MS patients indicated an increased frequency of significant intestinal damage similar to that which occurs in coeliac disease and food allergies.[43] Clinical evidence for a gluten-free diet is, however, minimal. A clinical trial of a gluten-free diet in 40 patients with MS indicated that the relapse rate was no better than average.[45] Another study demonstrated the absence of gluten antibodies in 35 out of 36 MS patients.[46] While there is no convincing evidence that gluten-free or allergy elimination diets are universally beneficial in the management of MS, it is certainly generally healthy to eliminate food allergens (as long as other dietary measures are also included, i.e. the Swank diet), and there is anecdotal evidence that specific individuals have been helped.

Other therapeutic considerations

Physical therapy   The patient should be encouraged to lead as normal and active a life as possible. Exercise is physically and psychologically beneficial; however, the patient should avoid overwork and fatigue. Passive movement and massage is indicated for weakened spastic limbs, both for comfort and circulation.

Hyperbaric oxygen   Early reports described promising results from the use of hyperbaric oxygen (HBO) in the treatment of MS.[47-9] However, these reports were largely anecdotal or from uncontrolled clinical trials. In 1970 one study reported a small, transient improvement in 16 out of 26 patients treated with HBO.[47] Another small study, in 1978, reported an improvement in 11 patients treated with HBO.[48] One year later a large study found minimal to dramatic improvement in 91 per cent of 250 patients treated with HBO.[49] Several other researchers published similarly encouraging results.

The first double-blind placebo-controlled trial of HBO indicated an apparent beneficial effect in the treatment of MS.[50] Objective improvement was noted in 12 out of 17 in the study group, compared to only one out of 20 in the placebo group. Although the improvements were mild and transient in most of the patients, it appeared that patients with milder forms of MS and a shorter duration of disease derived a more pronounced and longer-lasting benefit. This was an encouraging preliminary study, yet it was criticised for its small sample and short follow-up period.

Subsequently the Multiple Sclerosis Society commissioned further trials to be performed on a larger number of subjects, with longer periods of follow-up.[51,52] The results showed no significant improvement, apart from a subjective improvement in bowel and bladder functions in one of the studies. The results from these larger well designed studies cast much doubt on the efficacy of HBO treatment of MS.

Treatment

Treatment of MS with diet, lifestyle modification and supplementation should begin immediately, as the earlier in the disease process this therapy is initiated the better the results will be. Several non-specific measures are important, including avoidance of excessive fatigue, of emotional stress and of marked temperature changes.

The natural therapy of MS, while not proven highly effective, will help and poses no threat to the patient's health. Indeed, it is a healthy regime since the recommendations decrease the risk of atherosclerosis and other degenerative diseases. However, once MS has progressed to significant disability it is unlikely to be affected to any great degree by these measures.

Diet

Swank's dietary protocol is recommended:
- Saturated fat intake should be no more than 10 grams per day.
- Daily intake of polyunsaturated oils should be 40–50 grams (margarine, shortening and hydrogenated oils are not allowed).
- Normal amounts of protein are recommended.
- Fish should be eaten three or more times a week.

Fresh wholefoods should be emphasised and animal foods (with the exception of fish) should be reduced, if not completely eliminated.

Supplements

- Flaxseed oil, 1 tblsp a day.

- Cod liver oil, 1 tblsp a day.
- Eicosapentaenoic acid, 1 gram a day.
- Docosahexanoic acid, 750 mg a day.
- Selenium, 200 micrograms a day.
- Vitamin E, 600 iu per day.

- Greater than 10 per cent above 'normal' weight, or body fat percentage greater than 30 per cent for women and 25 per cent for men.

General considerations

Why do people get fat, and why can't people who are fat lose weight? These questions have baffled researchers for decades, yet no clearcut explanation exists, despite the fact that obesity is a major problem in our society. Estimates of the extent of the problem range from 10 per cent to 50 per cent or more of the adult population.[1-3]

Even more alarming is the fact that the number of obese children in the western countries in increasing dramatically[4]; in the US the number of markedly obese children nearly doubled between 1965 and 1980. The increase in childhood obesity will certainly result in an even greater frequency of adult obesity as these children grow up.

There are many myths and opinions concerning obesity. Most of these are simply not true. Many individuals (including physicians) erroneously still feel obesity is just a matter of slovenliness, poor eating habits and lack of proper education concerning health. In addition, in recent years the psychological aspects of obesity have been overstated at the expense of clarification of the biological basis of obesity.

The definition of obesity, body composition analysis, major classifications of obesity, as well as the treatment of obesity, are the topics of this chapter, in an effort to provide a comprehensive view of this complex issue.

Obesity defined

The simplest definition of obesity is an excessive amount of body fat. It must be distinguished from overweight, which refers to an excess of body weight relative to height. A muscular athlete may be overweight, yet have a very low body fat percentage. With this in mind it is obvious that using body weight alone as an index of obesity is not entirely accurate. None the less, obesity is classically identified as being a weight greater than

20 per cent more than the average desirable weight for men and women of a given height.

More precise estimations of body fat percentage enable the practitioner to determine obesity accurately. In terms of body fat percentage, obesity is defined as a body fat percentage greater than 30 per cent for women and 25 per cent for men.[1,2]

Determination of body composition

The significance of determining body fat composition and classifying obesity cannot be overstated. The most commonly used clinical methods are discussed below.

Anthropometric measurements

Anthropometric measurements involve determination of height and weight, determin-

Table 58.1 Guidelines for body weight

	Metric					
Height without shoes (m)	Men Weight without clothes (kg)			Women Weight without clothes (kg)		
	Acceptable average	Acceptable weight range	Obese	Acceptable average	Acceptable weight range	Obese
1.45				46.0	42–53	64
1.48				46.5	42–54	65
1.50				47.0	43–55	66
1.52				48.5	44–57	68
1.54				49.5	44–58	70
1.56				50.4	45–58	70
1.58	55.8	51–64	77	51.3	46–59	71
1.60	57.6	52–65	78	52.6	48–61	73
1.62	58.6	53–66	79	54.0	49–62	74
1.64	59.6	54–67	80	55.4	50–64	77
1.66	60.6	55–69	83	56.8	51–65	78
1.68	61.7	56–71	85	58.1	52–66	79
1.70	63.5	58–73	88	60.0	53–67	80
1.72	65.0	59–74	89	61.3	55–69	83
1.74	66.5	60–75	90	62.6	56–70	84
1.76	68.0	62–77	92	64.0	58–72	86
1.78	69.4	64–79	95	65.3	59–74	89
1.80	71.0	65–80	96			
1.82	72.6	66–82	98			
1.84	74.2	67–84	101			
1.86	75.8	69–86	103			
1.88	77.6	71–88	106			
1.90	79.3	73–90	108			
1.92	81.0	75–93	112			

Non-metric

Height without shoes (ft,in)	Men Weight without clothes (lb)			Women Weight without clothes (lb)		
	Acceptable average	Acceptable weight range	Obese	Acceptable average	Acceptable weight range	Obese
4 10				102	92–119	143
4 11				104	94–122	146
5 0				107	96–125	150
5 1				110	99–128	154
5 2	123	112–141	169	113	102–131	152
5 3	127	115–144	173	116	195–134	161
5 4	130	118–148	178	120	108–138	166
5 5	133	121–152	182	123	111–142	170
5 6	136	124–156	187	128	114–146	175
5 7	140	128–161	193	132	118–150	180
5 8	145	132–166	199	136	122–154	185
5 9	149	136–170	204	140	126–158	190
5 10	153	140–174	209	144	130–163	196
5 11	158	144–179	215	148	134–168	202
6 0	162	148–184	221	152	138–173	208
6 1	166	152–189	227			
6 2	171	156–194	233			
6 3	176	160–199	239			
6 4	181	164–204	245			

ation of various body circumferences or diameters (waist, chest or hip circumferences, distances between the iliac crests, greater trochanters or acromioclavicular joints) and measurements of skinfold thickness. In regard to the diagnosis of obesity, measurement of height and weight, body mass indices and skinfold thickness (alone and coupled with arm circumference data) are discussed below.

Height and weight   Height and weight indices are the most common measurements made in the determination of 'obesity'. Perhaps the indices receiving the widest use are the tables of 'desirable weight' provided by the life assurance companies (see Table 58.1).

However, the tables are often criticised for three major shortcomings:
- The stated weight ranges merely reflect the weights of those with lowest mortality of *insured* persons, which may not reflect the true population.
- Weight ranges for lowest mortality do not necessarily reflect optimal weight for height for health.
- The standard values make it difficult to assess degree of obesity, e.g. a person within the proper weight range may have excess body fat and lower than optimal lean body mass, or an individual with increased muscular development may be 'overweight', despite having an extremely low body fat percentage. Again it must be stated that weight alone is a poor reflector of body fat composition.

Skinfold thickness   By measuring the thickness of the subcutaneous fat (skinfold or fatfold thickness) the amount of total body fat can be estimated. Skinfold thickness is calculated with the aid of specialised skinfold calipers, and measurements are taken at several sites on the body to improve accuracy. The most common measurement sites are the triceps, biceps, just under the shoulder blade, and just above the hip bone.[1]

For most clinical purposes skinfold measurements provide the easiest and least expensive estimation of body fat percentage.

Classification and types of obesity

Obesity was initially classified as either exogenous, meaning that it is simply a result of excessive energy intake, or endogenous, meaning it is a result of an inherent metabolic defect that promotes obesity. It is not generally accepted that the term exogenous obesity is somewhat a misnomer as obesity can often be explained in terms of metabolic derangements in otherwise normal people.

Physiologically, obesity is often classified into three major categories based on the size and number of adipose cells. Fat cells may be increased in number (hyperblastic obesity), in size (hypertrophic obesity) or both (hyperblastic-hypertrophic obesity).

Hyperblastic obesity usually begins in childhood and tends to be associated with fewer metabolic aberrations than hypertrophic obesity, which usually develops later in life. This may reflect fat distribution, as hypertrophic obesity is generally associated with central adiposity or male-patterned (android) obesity. Hypertrophic obesity is associated more with the metabolic complications of obesity, i.e. diabetes, hyperin-sulinaemia, glucose intolerance, hypertension, hyperlipidaemia, etc.

Male-patterned (android) and female-patterned (gynoid) obesity refer to a classification of obesity based on fat distribution. In android obesity, fat is deposited primarily in the upper body, i.e. the abdomen and trunk. This type of obesity is typically seen in the obese male, hence the term android obesity. An increased waist to hip girth is diagnostic.[5,6]

In gynoid obesity the fat is distributed primarily in the lower body, i.e. the hip and thigh areas. This type of obesity pattern is most typically observed in females.[5,6]

In addition to the association of android obesity with diabetes (as discussed in Chapter 33, Diabetes mellitus), android obesity whether in the male or female has been shown to be predictive and strongly related to such major cardiovascular risk factors as hypertension and hyperglycaemia as well as female hormonal disturbances and gallstones.[7-10]

Therapy

Obesity is perhaps one of the most challenging health conditions to deal with. Few people want to be obese, yet only 5 per cent of markedly obese individuals are able to attain and maintain 'normal' body weight, while only 66 per cent of people just a few pounds or so overweight are able to do the same.

The successful programme for obesity is consistent with the basic tenets of naturo-pathic/holistic medicine – proper diet, adequate exercise and a positive mental attitude. All the components are interrelated, creating a system where no single component is more important than the other. Improvement in one facet may be enough to result in some positive changes, but working on all three components yields the greatest results.

There are literally hundreds of diets and diet programmes that claim to be the answer to the problem of obesity. Dieters are constantly bombarded with new reports of a wonder diet to follow. However, the basic equation for losing weight never changes. In order for an individual to lose weight, energy intake must be less than energy expenditure. This can be done by decreasing calorie intake (dieting) or by increasing the rate the calories are burned (exercising).

To lose 1 lb, a person must take in 3,500 fewer calories than he or she expends. To lose 1 lb each week there must therefore be a negative calorie balance of 500 calories a day. This can be achieved by decreasing the amount of calories ingested or by exercise. To reduce one's calorie intake by 500 calories is often extremely difficult, as is burning off an additional 500 calories per day by exercise (a person would need to jog for 45 minutes, play tennis for an hour, or take a brisk walk for one hour and 15 minutes). The most sensible approach to weight loss is to decrease calorie intake and increase energy expenditure.

Most individuals will begin to lose weight if they decrease their calorie intake below 1,500 calories per day and do aerobic exercise for 15 to 20 minutes three to four times per week. Starvation and crash diets usually result in rapid weight loss (largely muscle and water), but cause rebound weight gain. The most successful approach to weight loss is gradual weight reduction (0.5 to 1 pound per week) through adopting long-standing dietary and lifestyle modifications.

Psychological aspects of obesity

The psychological approach to obesity assumes that excessive eating is the primary cause of obesity. The main point of the psychological approach is that obese individuals eat in response to external cues (sight, smell and taste) and stimuli, even if they are satisfied.

For example, television watching has been linked very strongly to obesity; next to prior obesity, television watching is the strongest predictor of subsequent obesity.[3] Television watching has been demonstrated to be linked to the onset of obesity, and there is a dose effect (i.e. the more TV that is watched the greater the degree of obesity).[11] This fits very nicely with the psychological theory (increased sensitivity to external cues), as watching TV has been shown to result in increased food con-sumption. However, there are also several physiological effects of watching TV that promote obesity, such as reducing physical activity and actually lowering basal metabolic rate to a point similar to rates experienced during trance-like states. These factors clearly support the physiological view.

Psychological therapy is designed to offer different stimuli which will reduce food intake. Unfortunately, there has not been a great deal of success with this approach when used alone.[12] In addition, obese individuals often consume far less calories than their lean counterparts and still put weight on. This suggests a deeper physiological role in obesity than previously thought.

One thing that cannot be denied is the stigma that is attached to being obese. A group of children were once asked what they would rather be if given the choice of being fat or physically disabled. The results of the study were quite simple. Children would rather be physically disabled than fat. The obese individual experiences much psychological trauma. Fashion trends, insurance, college placements, employment opportunities all discriminate against the obese person. The obese person learns many self-defeating and self-degrading attitudes. They are led to believe that fat is 'bad' in our society, which often leads to a vicious cycle of low self-esteem, depression, over-eating for consolation, increased fatness, social rejection and further lowering of self-esteem. Counselling is necessary to change attitudes about being obese and aid in the improvement of self-esteem. If this is not dealt with, even the most perfect diet and exercise plan will fail. By improving the way overweight people feel about themselves, a change in eating behaviour may occur as a result.

A physiological view of obesity

While the psychological theory proposes that obese individuals are insensitive to internal cues of hunger and satiety, the biological theory states almost the opposite – obese individuals appear to be extremely sensitive to various internal clues. More and more research is supporting a biological basis for obesity and clarifying different types of obesity from this perspective.[13]

These biological/biochemical models of obesity are tied to the metabolism of the fat cells themselves; they explain why some people can eat very large quantities of food and not increase their weight substantially, and they also support the notion that obesity is not just a matter of overeating. It appears that each one of us has a programmed 'set point' weight. This was first displayed in animal studies and later in human studies. It has been suggested that individual fat cells control this set point. When the individual fat cell becomes smaller, it sends a message to the brain to eat. Since the obese individual often has fat cells which are larger in number and size, the result is an overpowering urge to eat.

This explains why most diets don't work. The obese individual can fight off the impulse for a time, but eventually the signal becomes too strong to ignore. The result is a rebound effect, with the individual often exceeding their previous weight. In addition, the result of the diet is that their set point is now set at an even higher level, making it even more difficult to lose weight the next time they go on a diet.[14]

The set point seems to be tied to how sensitive cells are to the hormone insulin. Obesity leads to insulin insensitivity and vice versa. The sensitivity of cells to insulin can be improved and the set point lowered by two simple measures – diet and exercise.

Dietary therapy

Hundreds of different diets are promoted for weight loss. In the author's opinion the best diet is a diet high in dietary fibre and high complex carbohydrate foods (60–70 per cent of the total calorie content of the diet), sufficient in protein (10–15 per cent) and low in fat (15–20 per cent). The recommended diet is outlined in Chapter 2, Basic principles of health.

Since fats have about 9 calories per gram while carbohydrates and proteins contain about 4 calories per gram, reduction of fat alone in the diet often results in significant weight loss. The typical western diet provides 50–60 per cent of its calorie intake from fats, 30 per cent from carbohydrates (mainly refined sugars) and 20 per cent from protein. Refined carbohydrates and saturated fats must be eliminated if the set point is to be reduced.

A diet low in fibre but high in refined carbohydrates and fats is believed to be the major factor responsible for the tremendous amount of obesity in the west. In contrast to the high rate of obesity in the west, obesity is extremely rare in those cultures that consume a diet high in fibre.[15]

Dietary fibre plays an important role in preventing and treating obesity by:
- Increasing the amount of necessary chewing, thus slowing the eating process.
- Increasing the excretion of fat in the faeces.
- Improving digestive hormone secretion and digestion.
- Improving glucose tolerance.
- Inducing satiety by giving a feeling of fullness and stimulating the release of intestinal hormones that reduce food intake.[16]

It is also important to eat set meals rather than snacks. Many studies have shown that obese individuals consume more after eating a snack than after consuming nothing. This is in contrast to normal-weight subjects, who significantly decrease their intake after a snack. If an individual must snack, it would be best to snack on good wholesome foods rather than processed foods. More natural snacks have less calories, are more nutritious and are more satisfying physiologically than their processed counterparts.

Protein-sparing modified fast   Low-calorie protein-sparing modified fasts typically utilise powdered formulas containing protein, carbohydrate, vitamins and minerals. Examples of commonly used formulas include Cambridge, Nu-day, Optifast, Medifast and Slim-fast.

In low-calorie protein-sparing modified fast programmes utilising these powders, the dieter is instructed to use the formula to replace meals. A strict approach is to limit calorie intake entirely to the formula. A number of clinical diets have documented the efficacy of the low-calorie protein-sparing modified fasts in producing significant weight loss.[17–20]

The diet is based on the idea that providing high-quality protein with a small amount of carbohydrate will have a sparing effect against the breakdown of muscle to meet energy needs. Instead weight loss will occur as a result of burning fat for energy. If an individual elects to use this approach it is recommended that they consult a physician prior to and during the programme. It is also recommended that an individual drink at least 2 litres of water a day while on the diet and include a supplemental dietary fibre to maintain bowel function.

Exercise

A diet high in fibre, complex carbohydrate and low in fat is the safest and most effective diet to achieve permanent weight loss, but for optimum results it must be combined with an appropriate exercise programme. The activity need not be strenuous: in fact, it is better to exercise at a moderate level for a longer period of time than it is to expend a lot of effort for a short period. Exercising at about 50 to 60 per cent of maximum intensity instead of at 70 to 80 per cent actually results in greater fat breakdown (see Chapter 2, Basic principles of health for information on how to determine exercise intensity). A walk at a good pace for 20 to 30 minutes a day is a good level to start at.[21]

Adjunctive therapy

Dietary fibre supplements Supplemented fibre formulas from grains, citrus, gluco-mannan (from konjac root), guar gum and other sources have been shown to reduce feelings of hunger and consequently reduce the intake of food. Several clinical trials have demonstrated that a daily supplement of 5 grams of supplemental fibre is of great value in the treatment of obesity.[22–25]

Pancreatin Pancreatin is a powdered preparation of dessicated and defatted raw pancreas that is often used to supplement digestive enzyme deficiencies. Pancreatin supplementation has been shown to result in decreased food intake and a significant loss of body weight in animals.[26]

Ma huang (Ephedra sinica), *Cola nut* (Cola nitida) *and green tea* (Camellia sinensis) A traditional approach to weight loss involves the use of isolated plant stimulants which promote fat breakdown. Although many stimulants are routinely abused in our current society, the use of plants as stimulants has a long history of use by the majority of cultures worldwide.

Three of these plants contain ingredients that are now widely used in prescription and over-the-counter medications; *Ephedra sinica* contains ephedrine and related alkaloids, and *Cola nitida* and *Camellia sinensis* contain caffeine, theophylline and other methylxanthines. If used in moderation these plants offer significant benefits in the obese individual. Although research has utilised the isolated constituents, it is appropriate to extrapolate the data to the crude herb or extract if similar content of active ingredients can be attained.

Ephedrine has been shown to reduce weight gain in experimental animal studies.[27,28] It appears to do this primarily by increasing the metabolic rate of adipose (fat) tissue. Its action, however, can be greatly enhanced when it is used in combination with caffeine and theophylline. These methylxanthines potentiate the action of ephedrine and other ephedra compounds. In one animal study, when ephedrine was used alone it resulted in losses of 14 per cent in body weight and 42 per cent in body fat; however, when used in combination with caffeine or theophylline there was a loss of 25 per cent in body weight and 75 per cent in body fat.[28] In contrast, when either caffeine or theophylline were used alone there was no significant loss in body weight. The reason for the decrease in body weight is an increased metabolic rate and fat cell breakdown promoted by ephedrine and enhanced by caffeine and theophylline. Human studies have also demonstrated that ephedrine/methylxanthine combinations are twice as effective as ephedrine alone in increasing the metabolic rate of the obese individual.[29]

Ephedrine's action is similar to that of adrenalin. It differs in that it can be given orally, has a much longer duration of action, a more pronounced effect on the central nervous system and is much less potent. Ephedra stimulates the circulatory system, increasing the force of contraction and output of the heart. It also increases blood pressure and the amount of blood flow to the brain.

It is recommended that green tea (*Camellia sinensis*) or extracts of *Cola spp.* be used for caffeine and theophylline content rather than coffee. Coffee contains many roasted hydrocarbons that are known to be potent carcinogens. Many feel that it is not the caffeine content of coffee that is detrimental; instead they contend that it is the roast hydrocarbons.[30]

Green tea is preferable to black tea as it is non-fermented while black tea is allowed to undergo fermentation. During fermentation, enzymes present in the tea convert many substances that possess outstanding therapeutic action to compounds with much less activity. With green tea, fermentation is not allowed to take place because the leaves are either steamed or subjected to low levels of dry heat after harvesting. The chemistry of tea is extremely complex. Green tea is extremely rich in flavonoid compounds which have very potent antioxidant and anti-allergy activity. Green tea also contains caffeine and related compounds. One cup of tea typically contains 50 mg of caffeine. Theophylline, a compound similar to caffeine, is also an important component of tea; it is used as a prescription drug in the treatment of asthma.

Use of these plants (ephedra, camellia and cola), like the isolated constituents contained in them, may produce insomnia, anxiety and hypertension. They should not be used alone, but only in conjunction with the diet and exercise as recommended here.

Supporting the liver

Liver function is disturbed in a large percentage of overweight individuals.[31] Nutritional factors which improve the liver's ability to break down and metabolise fat are very important components of a weight loss plan (see Chapter 8, Liver support, for detailed description). This includes the use of:

- Nutritional lipotropic agents, which by definition are compounds that hasten the removal or decrease the accumulation of fat in the liver.
- Herbal cholagogues and choleretics (cholagogues are herbs that stimulate the gallbladder to contract while choleretics are agents that stimulate bile flow into the gallbladder from the liver).

Dandelion root (*Taraxacum officinale*) is regarded as one of the finest liver remedies, both as food and as medicine. Dandelion has also been used historically as a weight loss aid in the treatment of obesity. This fact prompted researchers to investigate dandelion's effect on the body weight of experimental animals.[32] When these animals were administered the fluid extract of dandelion for one month, they lost as much as 30 per cent of their initial weights. However, much of the weight loss appeared to be a result of significant diuretic activity.

Treatment

This chapter has described currently accepted methods of defining and classifying obesity, as well as the natural therapy of obesity. Classification of obesity into android and gynoid fat distributions offers a significant non-invasive diagnostic aid in determining relative risk of serious disease. Specifically, android obesity is a risk factor for diabetes and cardiovascular disease.

The important thing to remember when beginning a weight loss programme is *be patient*. Better, more permanent results will be attained if the weight loss is achieved gradually in the context of developing healthy dietary and exercise habits. It takes time for the body to reset its programmed weight.

Diet

A 1,500 calories per day diet, high in fibre and complex-carbohydrate rich foods, adequate in protein and low in refined carbohydrate and fat. Avoid snacking.

Exercise

Daily exercise with the heart rate maintained in the 50–60 per cent intensity range for 15 to 20 minutes.

Supplements

- Pancreatin, 250–500 mg between meals.
- Fibre supplement, a minimum of 5 grams daily preferably in divided doses.
- Choline, 1 gram a day.
- L-methionine, 1 gram a day.

Botanical medicines

- Drink 1 cup of ephedra tea and green tea daily.
- Dandelion root (*Taraxacum officinale*):
    Dried root, 4 grams three times a day.
    Fluid extract (1:1), 4–8 ml three times a day.

Note: take basal body temperature to determine thyroid function (see Chapter 49, Hypothyroidism).

59

Osteoarthritis

- Mild early-morning stiffness, stiffness following periods of rest, pain that worsens on joint use, and loss of joint function.
- Local tenderness, soft tissue swelling, creaking and cracking of joints on movement, bony swelling, restricted mobility and other signs of degenerative loss of joint cartilage.

General considerations

Osteoarthritis or degenerative joint disease is the most common form of arthritis.[1-3] It is seen primarily, but not exclusively, in the elderly; surveys have indicated that 80 per cent of persons over the age of 50 have osteoarthritis. Under the age of 45, osteoarthritis is much more common in men; after age 45 it is ten times more common in women than men.[1-3]

The weight-bearing joints and joints of the hands are the joints principally affected by the degenerative changes associated with osteoarthritis. Specifically, there is much cartilage destruction, followed by hardening, and the formation of large bone spurs (calcified osteophytes) in the joint margins. Pain, deformity and limitation of motion in the joint results. Inflammation is usually minimal.[1,2]

Osteoarthritis is divided into two categories, primary and secondary osteoarthritis. In primary osteoarthritis, the degenerative wear-and-tear process occurs after the fifth and sixth decades, with no predisposing abnormality apparent. The cumulative effects of decades of use leads to the degenerative changes by stressing the integrity of the collagen matrix of the cartilage. Damage to the cartilage results in the release of enzymes that destroy collagen components. With aging, there is a decreased ability to restore and synthesise normal collagen structures.[1-3]

Secondary osteoarthritis is associated with some predisposing factor responsible for the degenerative changes.[1,2] Various predisposing factors in secondary osteoarthritis include congenital abnormalities in joint structure or function (e.g. excessive joint mobility and abnormally shaped joint surfaces), trauma (obesity, fractures along joint surfaces, surgery, etc.), crystal deposition, presence of abnormal cartilage, and previous inflammatory disease of joint (rheumatoid arthritis, gout, septic arthritis, etc.).

Causes of osteoarthritis

- Excessive mobility/joint instability.
- Age-related changes in collagen matrix repair mechanisms.
- Hormonal and sex factors.
- Altered biochemistry.
- Genetic predisposition.
- Inflammation.
- Fractures and mechanical damage.
- Inflammatory joint disease.
- Others.

Signs and symptoms

The onset of osteoarthritis can be very subtle, morning joint stiffness often being the first symptom. As the disease progresses, there is pain on motion of the involved joint, that is made worse by prolonged activity and relieved by rest. There are usually no signs of inflammation.[1,2]

The specific clinical picture varies with the joint involved. Disease of the hands leads to pain and limitation of use. Knee involvement produces pain, swelling and instability. Osteoarthritis of the hip causes local pain and a limp. Spinal osteoarthritis is very common and may result in compression of nerves and blood vessels, causing pain and vascular insufficiency.[1,2]

The classic presentation of osteoarthritis is easy to distinguish from other types of arthritis, especially rheumatoid arthritis, which is usually associated with much more inflammation of surrounding soft tissues.

Therapy

Data collected from the earliest signs of osteoarthritis to the most advanced stages suggest that cellular and tissue response to osteoarthritis (OA) is purposeful and is aimed at repair of the damaged joint structure; the process contributing to OA thus appears to be able to be arrested and sometimes reversed.[3,4] Therefore, the major therapeutic goal appears to be enhancing repair processes by various connective tissue cells.

Several studies have attempted to determine the 'natural course' of OA.[3,5] In one[15] the natural course of OA of the hip was studied over a ten-year period. All subjects had changes suggestive of advanced osteoarthritis, yet the researchers reported marked clinical improvement and radiologic recovery of the joint space in 14 of 31 hips. The authors purposely applied no therapy and regarded their results as reflecting the natural course of the disease.

These results as well as others raise some interesting questions. Does medical intervention in some way promote disease progression? Can various natural therapies enhance the body's own response towards health? The answer to both of these questions appears to be yes.

Aspirin and other non-steroidal anti-inflammatory drugs

The first drug generally employed in the treatment of osteoarthritis is aspirin. It is often quite effective in relieving both the pain and inflammation. It is also relatively inexpensive. However, since the therapeutic dose required is relatively high (2 to 4 grams per day), toxicity often occurs. Tinnitus (ringing in the ears) and gastric irritation are early manifestations of toxicity.[1,2]

Other non-steroidal anti-inflammatory drugs (NSAIDs) are often used as well, especially when aspirin is ineffective or intolerable – ibuprofen (Brufen, Motrin), fenoprofen (Fenopron), indomethacin (Indocid), naproxen (Naprosyn), tolmetin (Tolectin) and sulindac (Clinoril). These drugs are also associated with side effects including gastrointestinal upset, headaches and dizziness, and are therefore recommended for only short periods of time.[1,2]

One side effect of aspirin and other NSAIDs that is often not mentioned is their inhibition of cartilage repair (i.e. inhibition of collagen matrix synthesis) and acceleration of cartilage destruction in experimental studies.[6] Since osteoarthritis is caused by a degeneration of cartilage it appears that, while NSAIDs are fairly effective in suppressing the symptoms, they possibly worsen the condition by inhibiting cartilage formation and accelerating cartilage destruction. This has been upheld in studies which have shown that NSAIDs use is associated with acceleration of osteoarthritis and increased joint destruction.[7–10]

Simply stated, NSAIDs appear to suppress the symptoms but accelerate the progression of osteoarthritis.

Dietary considerations

Primary dietary therapy involves the achievement of normal body weight; excess weight means increased stress on weight-bearing joints affected with osteoarthritis.[11,12] A general healthy diet rich in complex carbohydrate and dietary fibre is recommended.

Childers, a horticulturist, popularised a diet in the treatment of osteoarthritis that eliminated foods from the genus *solanaceae* (nightshade family) after finding this simple dietary elimination cured his osteoarthritis.[13] Childers developed a theory that genetically susceptible individuals might develop arthritis, as well as a variety of other complaints, from long-term low level consumption of solanum alkaloids that are found in tomatoes, potatoes, eggplant, peppers and tobacco. Presumably these alkaloids inhibit normal collagen repair in the joints or promote the inflammatory degeneration of the joint. Although remaining to be proved, this diet may offer some benefit to certain individuals and is certainly worth a try.

Nutritional considerations

Niacinamide   Dr William Kaufman has reported very good clinical results in the treatment of hundreds of patients with rheumatoid and osteoarthritis using high dose niacinamide (i.e. 900 mg to 4 g in divided doses daily). Niacinamide at this high dose can result in significant side effects (glucose intolerance, liver damage) and should therefore be instituted under strict medical supervision.[14,15]

Methionine   The essential amino acid methionine, administered as S-adenosyl-methionine, was shown to be superior to ibuprofen (Motrin) in the treatment of osteoarthritis in a double-blind clinical trial.[16] The positive effect in this trial is consistent with several other clinical studies.[17] Methionine is a sulphur containing amino acid which is very important in cartilage structures, especially proteoglycans and glycosaminoglycans.[8]

Glycosaminoglycans   Injectable glycosaminoglycan polysulphate and activated acid-pepsin-digested calf tracheal cartilage as well as other glycosaminoglycan preparations have yielded positive results in controlled trials and experimental studies.[18–20] Results seem to indicate these compounds may address some of the underlying causes of the degenerative process characteristic of osteoarthritis.
  It must be pointed out that these studies have all utilised injectable formulas. It is highly unlikely similar results could be obtained with these formulations when administered orally, as intestinal absorption of glycosaminoglycans having a molecular weight greater than 4,000 is quite poor without the aid of special vehicles, such as liposomes, or possible enteric-coating.[21,22]
  Many commercial products are available that contain chondroitin sulphate (molecular weight 30,000). It must be pointed out the majority of these formulas are probably of no greater benefit than placebo as chondroitin sulphate is not absorbed to any significant degree.[21] Enteric coating or administering in the form of a liposome may increase bio-availability but this has yet to be fully determined.[21,22] In addition, it is possible that smaller fragments of the molecule may have some therapeutic effect, but again this has yet to be determined.

Superoxide dismutase   Like glycosaminoglycan preparations, intra-articular injection of superoxide dismutase (SOD) has demonstrated significant therapeutic effects in the treatment of OA.[23,24] Whether oral SOD preparations are absorbed orally has yet to be determined. Preliminary indications are that it is probably not.[25]

Vitamin E   A clinical trial using 600 iu of vitamin E in patients with osteoarthritis demonstrated significant benefit from the vitamin E.[26] The benefit was thought to be due to vitamin E's antioxidant and membrane stabilising actions. Later studies have shown that vitamin E has an ability to inhibit the enzymatic breakdown of cartilage as well as stimulate cartilage sysnthesis.[27]

Vitamin C   Deficient vitamin C intake is common in the elderly, resulting in altered collagen synthesis and compromised connective tissue repair.[28] Several studies have demonstrated that vitamin C has a positive effect on cartilage,[29,30] and one[29] confirmed the importance, indeed necessity, for an excess of ascorbic acid in human chondrocyte protein synthesis. In a study of experimental OA in guinea pigs[27] cartilage erosion was found to be much less and the overall changes in and around the OA joint milder in animals kept on high doses of vitamin C.

Vitamin C and E appear to possess synergistic effects.[27] Thus, both vitamins E and C appear to enhance the stability of sulfated proteoglycans in the complex structure comprising articular cartilage. Judicious use of these vitamins in the treatment of osteoarthritis, either alone or in combination with other therapeutic means, may thus be of great benefit to the patient population by retarding the erosion of cartilage.

Pantothenic acid   Acute deficiency of pantothenic acid in the rat causes a pronounced failure of cartilage growth and eventually produces similar lesions to osteoarthritis. This implicates low pantothenic acid levels in the development of human OA. Clinical improvements in OA symptomatology has been reported with the daily supplementation of 12.5 mg pantothenic acid,[31,32] although results often took 7–14 days before manifesting. (A larger double-blind study in patients with primarily rheumatoid arthritis displayed no significant benefit with 500 mg pantothenic acid administration.[33])

Vitamins A, B6 and E, zinc and copper   These nutrients are required for the synthesis of normal collagen and maintenance of cartilage structures.[11] A deficiency of any one of these would allow accelerated joint degeneration.

Physical therapy

Various physical therapies (exercise, heat, cold, diathermy, ultrasound, etc.) are often very beneficial in improving joint mobility and reducing pain in sufferers of OA. The importance of physical therapy appears to be quite significant, especially when administered regularly. Much of the benefit of physical therapy is thought to be a result of achieving a proper water content within the joint capsule.

Clinical and experimental studies seem to indicate short-wave diathermy may be of the greatest benefit.[34-6] Combining short-wave diathermy therapy with periodic ice massage, rest and appropriate exercises appears to be the most sensible approach. Proper exercises include isometric exercises and swimming; these types of exercises increase circulation to the joint and strengthen surrounding muscles without placing too much strain on the joint.

Botanical medicines

Yucca   A double-blind clinical trial indicated a saponin extract of yucca demonstrated a positive therapeutic effect.[37] Results were of gradual onset and no direct effects of the

451

yucca saponin were noted. It was suggested that effects were due to indirect effects on the gastrointestinal flora.

This is an interesting suggestion, since bacterial endotoxins have been shown to depress the biosynthesis of cartilage.[38] It is entirely possible yucca decreases bacterial endotoxin absorption and thus reduces this inhibition of cartilage synthesis. If this is the mechanism of action, other saponin containing herbs, as well as ways of reducing endotoxin load, may be appropriate.

Devil's claw (Harpagophytum procumbens)   Several studies utilising experimental models of inflammation in animals have reported devil's claw possesses an anti-inflammatory and analgesic effect comparable to the potent drug phenylbutazone.[39] However, other studies have indicated that devil's claw has little, if any, anti-inflammatory activity.[40,41]

The equivocal research results in experimental models may reflect a mechanism of action of devil's claw that is inconsistent with current anti-inflammatory drugs or a lack of quality control (standardisation) of the devil's claw preparations used. Since the main components of devil's claw are saponins, its therapeutic effect in OA may be similar to that observed for yucca.

Cherries, hawthorn berries and bilberries   Cherries, hawthorn berries, bilberries and other dark red-blue berries are rich sources of anthocyanidins and proanthocyanidins. These compounds are flavonoid molecules that give them their deep red-blue colour. These compounds are remarkable in their ability to enhance collagen matrix integrity and structure.[42–45] Liberal consumption of sources of collagen-stabilising flavonoids should be encouraged.

Treatment

Diet

All simple, processed and concentrated carbohydrates must be avoided, complex-carbohydrate, high-fibre foods should be stressed and fats should be kept to a minimum. Plants of the *solanaceae* family should be eliminated (tomatoes, potatoes, eggplant, peppers and tobacco).

Supplements

- Niacinamide, 500 mg four times a day (under strict supervision).
- Methionine, 250 mg four times a day.
- Vitamin E, 600 iu a day.
- Vitamin A, 10,000 iu a day.
- Vitamin C, 1–3 g a day.
- Vitamin B6, 50 mg a day.
- Pantothenic acid, 12.5 mg per day.

- Zinc, 45 mg a day.
- Copper, 1 mg a day.

Botanical medicines

- Yucca leaves 2–4 grams three times a day.
- *Harpagophytum procumbens*:
    Dried powdered root, 1–2 grams three times a day.
    Tincture (1:5), 4–5 ml three times a day.
    Dry solid extract (3:1), 400 mg three times a day.
- Liberal consumption of flavonoid rich berries or extracts.

Physical therapy and exercise

Daily exercises including isometric exercises and swimming. Short-wave diathermy and other physical therapy treatments may be helpful.

60

Osteoporosis

- Usually without symptoms until severe backache.
- Most common in postmenopausal white women.
- Decrease in height.
- Spontaneous fractures of the hip and vertebrae may occur.

General considerations

Osteoporosis literally means porous bones. Although the entire skeleton may be involved, bone loss is usually greatest in the spine, hips and ribs. Since these bones bear a great deal of weight, they are then susceptible to pain, deformity or fracture.

Normally there is a decline in bone mass after the age of 40. This bone loss is accelerated in patients with osteoporosis. Many factors can result in excessive bone loss and different variants of osteoporosis exist (see box). All of these other causes of accelerated bone loss should be ruled out before a diagnosis of osteoporosis is made. Post-menopausal osteoporosis is the most common form of osteoporosis.

Is osteoporosis preventable? Definitely yes! Recently there has been an incredible push for supplementing calcium in an effort to halt bone loss. While this appears to be sound medical advice, osteoporosis is much more than a lack of dietary calcium; it is a complex condition involving hormonal, lifestyle, nutritional and environmental factors.[1] A comprehensive plan that addresses these factors offers the greatest protection against developing osteoporosis. Such a plan is outlined in this chapter.

Osteoporosis versus osteomalacia

Osteoporosis involves both the mineral (inorganic) and the non-mineral (organic matrix composed primarily of protein) components of bone. This is the first clue that there is more to osteoporosis than a lack of dietary calcium. In fact, lack of dietary calcium in the adult results in a separate condition known as osteomalacia or softening of the bone. The two conditions, osteomalacia and osteoporosis, are different in that in osteomalacia there is only a deficiency of calcium in the bone. In contrast, in osteoporosis there is a lack of both calcium and other minerals, as well as a decrease in the non-mineral framework (organic matrix) of bone. Primarily composed of collagen and other proteins, little attention has been given to the important role that this organic matrix plays in maintaining bone structure.

Classification of osteoporosis

- Common forms unassociated with other diseases
    - Idiopathic osteoporosis (adult and juvenile)
    - Postmenopausal osteoporosis
    - Senile osteoporosis
- Endocrine
    - Cushing's syndrome
    - Thyrotoxicosis
    - Hyperparathyroidism
    - Hypergonadism
    - Hyperadrenocorticism
    - Diabetes mellitus
- Nutritional
    - Malnutrition, malabsorption
    - Calcium or vitamin D deficiency
    - Vitamin C deficiency
    - High acid ash diet (high protein diet)
    - High phosphate intake
    - Iron overload
- Heritable disorders
    - Osteogenesis imperfecta
    - Marfan's syndrome
    - Ehlers-Danlose syndrome
    - Homocystinuria
- Drug related
    - Alcoholism
    - Chronic heparin administration
    - Methotrexate
    - Corticosteroids
    - Cimetidine
- Miscellaneous
    - Rheumatoid arthritis
    - Immobilisation
    - Metabolic acidosis
    - Chronic obstructive pulmonary disease

Calcium metabolism and hormonal factors in osteoporosis

Normal bone metabolism is dependent on an intricate interplay of many nutritional and hormonal factors, with the liver and kidneys having a regulatory effect as well. In order to understand current theories on how osteoporosis develops it is necessary to take a brief look at normal calcium metabolism (absorption, storage and excretion).

Stomach acid

The absorption of calcium is dependent first on its being ionised in the intestines. In order for calcium carbonate, the most widely used form of calcium used for supplementation, and other insoluble calcium salts to be absorbed they must first be solubilised and ionised by stomach acid. And this is where the problem arises for many individuals.

In studies with postmenopausal women, it has been shown that about 40 per cent are severely deficient in stomach acid.[2] It has been shown that patients with insufficient stomach acid output can only absorb about 4 per cent of an oral dose of calcium as calcium carbonate, while a person with normal stomach acid can typically absorb about 22 per cent.[3] Patients with low stomach acid secretion need a form of calcium already in a soluble and ionised state, like calcium citrate, calcium lactate or calcium gluconate. About 45 per cent of the calcium is absorbed from calcium citrate in patients with reduced stomach acid, compared to 4 per cent absorption for calcium carbonate.[3]

This clearly demonstrates that ionised soluble calcium is much more beneficial than insoluble calcium salts like calcium carbonate in patients with reduced stomach acid secretion. It has also been demonstrated that calcium is more bioavailable from calcium citrate than the calcium carbonate in normal subjects.[4] In any event, calcium citrate and other soluble forms appear to be the best to supplement with for optimal absorption.

Vitamin D

Vitamin D stimulates the absorption of calcium. Since vitamin D can be produced in our bodies by the action of sunlight on 7-dehydrocholesterol in the skin, many experts consider it more of a hormone than a vitamin. The sunlight changes the 7-dehydrocholesterol into vitamin D_3 (cholecalciferol), which is then transported to the liver and converted by an enzyme into 25-hydroxycholecalciferol (25-OHD$_3$). The 25-hydroxycholecalciferol is then converted by an enzyme in the kidneys to 1,25-dihydroxycholecalciferol (1,25-(OH)$_2$D$_3$), which is ten times more potent than cholecalciferol and the most potent form of vitamin D (see Figure 60.1 for further explanation).

Disorders of the liver or kidneys results in impaired conversion of cholecalciferol to more potent vitamin D compounds. In many patients with osteoporosis there are high levels of 25-OHD$_3$ while the level of 1,25 (OH)$_2$D$_3$ is quite low. This signifies an impairment of renal conversion of 25-OHD$_3$ to 1,25-(OH)$_2$D$_3$ in osteoporosis.[5,6] Many theories have been proposed to account for this decreased conversion, including relationships to oestrogen and magnesium deficiency.

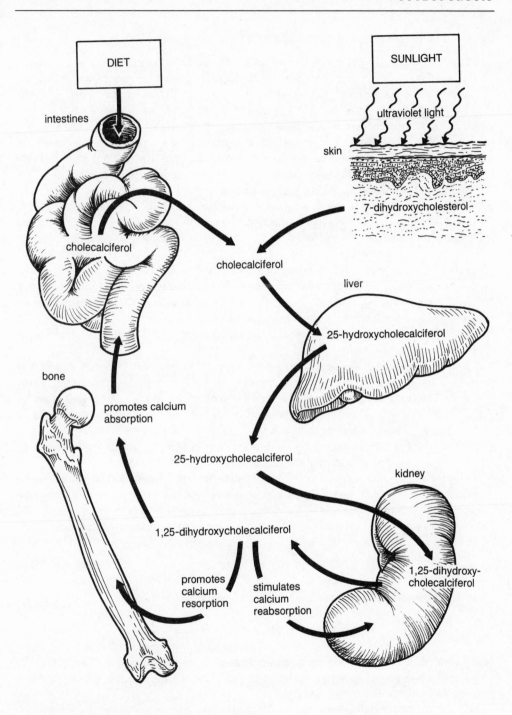

Figure 60.1 Vitamin D metabolism

Hormonal factors

The concentration of calcium in the blood is strictly maintained within very narrow limits. If levels start to decrease there is an increase in the secretion of parathyroid hormone by the parathyroid glands (there are four parathyroid glands nestled in the thyroid gland) and a decrease in the secretion of calcitonin by the thyroid and para-thyroids. If calcium levels in the blood start to increase there is a decrease in the secretion of parathyroid hormone and an increase in the secretion of calcitonin. An understanding of how these hormones increase (parathyroid hormone) and decrease (calcitonin) serum calcium levels is necessary in understanding osteoporosis.

Parathyroid hormone increases serum calcium levels primarily by increasing the activity of the cells that break down bone (osteoclasts), although it also decreases the excretion of calcium by the kidneys and increases the absorption of calcium in the intestines. In the kidneys, parathyroid hormone increases the conversion of 25-OHD_3 to $1,25\text{-(OH)}_2\text{D}_3$.

One of the theories relating bone loss to oestrogen deficiency is as follows. An oestrogen deficiency makes the cells that break down bone (osteoclasts) more sensitive to parathyroid hormone, resulting in increased bone breakdown, thereby raising serum calcium levels. This leads to a decreased parathyroid hormone level which results in diminished levels of active vitamin D and increased calcium excretion as well. Evidence seems to support this theory.[5,6,7]

Calcitonin acts on lowering serum calcium levels by increasing the activity of the cells that build bone (osteoblasts). Obviously this is a very desirable effect. Low calcitonin levels are found in postmenopausal osteoporosis and may be responsible for this type of bone loss. Calcitonin (isolated from salmon) has demonstrated remarkable effects in clinical studies and holds much promise in treating severe osteoporosis. Since calcitonin secretion can be increased by an elevation in serum calcium levels, this may be one of the ways calcium supplementation exerts its protective effect.

Although many physicians recommend oestrogen replacement for postmenopausal women, at present it is generally agreed that the risk outweighs the benefit in the majority of women who are at risk for osteoporosis. Instead, a greater emphasis should be placed on nutritional and lifestyle factors. In severe cases, improvement may result by the administration of oestrogen, $1,25\text{-(OH)}_2\text{D}_3$ or calcitonin (all of these are prescription medications).

Therapy

Diet

Many general dietary factors have been implicated in the development of osteoporosis – low calcium–high phosphorus intake, high protein diet, high acid-ash diet and trace mineral deficiencies, to name a few.[1]

Vegetarian and vegan diets are associated with a lower risk of osteoporosis.[8] Although bone mass in vegetarians does not differ significantly from omnivores in the third, fourth and fifth decades, there are significant differences in the later decades.[9]

This indicates that the decreased incidence of osteoporosis in vegetarians is not due to increased initial bone mass, but rather decreased bone loss.

Several factors are probably responsible for this decrease in bone loss observed in vegetarians. Most important is probably a lowered intake of protein and phosphorus.[1,7,10] A high-protein diet or a diet high in phosphates is associated with increasing the excretion of calcium in the urine. Raising daily protein from 47 to 142 grams doubles the excretion of calcium in the urine. A diet this high in protein is common in the west and may be a significant factor in the increased number of people suffering from osteoporosis.

Following sugar intake, there is an increase in the urinary excretion of calcium.[11] Considering that the average American consumes in one day 150 grams of sucrose, plus other refined simple sugars, and a glass of a carbonated beverage loaded with phosphates along with the high-protein, it is little wonder that there are so many suffering from osteoporosis. When lifestyle factors are also taken into consideration (discussed below), it is very apparent why osteoporosis has become a major medical problem.

Nutritional considerations

Calcium Supplementation of calcium has been shown to be effective in reducing age-related bone loss.[12,13] Many experts are recommending a daily calcium intake of 1.5 g. This typically means that supplementation in the range of 1 to 1.2 g is required. As mentioned above, the absorption and retention of calcium is dependent on a complex interplay of hormones and other factors. The initial approach is supplementation with the most bio-available form of calcium. At present, calcium citrate appears to be the best form of calcium to supplement with, both in regards to better absorption and decreased risk of developing kidney stone.[3,4,14]

Concern has arisen that increased calcium supplementation may result in increased calcium oxalate kidney stones. Calcium citrate appears to bypass this justifiable concern. While urinary calcium will rise in patients consuming calcium citrate, some of citrate'e effects inhibit the formation of kidney stones. Specifically citrate has the ability to reduce urinary saturation of calcium oxalate and calcium phosphate, and retard the nucleation and crystal growth of calcium salts.[14] The use of potassium of sodium citrate in the treatment of recurrent calcium oxalate stones has been shown to be quite effective in clinical studies, ceasing stone formation in nearly 90 per cent of the subjects.[15] In future magnesium citrate may prove to be the citrate of choice in the treatment of recurrent calcium oxalate kidney stones, due to magnesium's ability also to increase the solubility of calcium oxalate and inhibit the precipitation of both calcium phosphate and calcium oxalate.[16]

While the use of non-citrate calcium supplements may increase the risk of developing calcium oxalate kidney stones, the use of calcium citrate appears to reduce this risk of calcium overload greatly. Generally, over 95 per cent of the citrate ingested is used as an energy substrate, with the remainder being excreted in the urine. This citrate fulfils every requirement for an optimum calcium chelating agent:

- It is easily ionised.
- It is almost completely degraded.
- It has virtually no toxicity.
- It has been shown to result in increased absorption of calcium.

In addition citrate has some properties of its own that suggest further benefit. Included in these effects are its ability to chelate out heavy metals, prevent recurrent kidney stones, augment treatment of urinary tract infection and promote diuresis.

Magnesium   Magnesium supplementation is apparently as important as calcium supplementation. Individuals with osteoporosis have lower magnesium content, and other indicators of magnesium deficiency, than people without osteoporosis.[17] In human magnesium deficiency there is a decrease in serum concentration of the most active form of vitamin D (1,25-dihydroxycholecalciferol or 1,25-$(OH)_2D_3$) which has been observed in osteoporosis.[18] This could be either due to the enzyme responsible for the conversion of 25-OHD_3 to 1,25-$(OH)_2D_3$ being dependent on adequate magnesium levels or magnesium's ability to mediate parathyroid hormone and calcitonin secretion.

Intake of dairy foods fortified with vitamin D (as found in the US) results in decreased magnesium absorption.[19] This, combined with the higher number of osteoporotics that cannot tolerate milk (27–47 per cent), indicates that milk may not be an appropriate food to prevent osteoporosis.[20]

Vitamin B6, folic acid and vitamin B12   Low levels of these nutrients are quite common in the elderly population and may contribute to osteoporosis.[21,22] These vitamins are important in the conversion of the amino acid methionine to cysteine. If deficient in these vitamins, or if a defect exists in the enzymes responsible for this conversion, there will be an increase in homocysteine.[23] This compound has been implicated in a variety of conditions including arteriosclerosis (hardening of the arteries) and osteoporosis.

Increased homocysteine concentrations in the blood have been demonstrated in postmenopausal women and are thought to play a role in osteoporosis by interfering with collagen cross-linking leading to a defective bone matrix.[23] Since osteoporosis is known to be a loss of both the organic and inorganic phases of bone, this theory has much credence as it is one of the few that addresses both factors. Folic acid supplementation has been shown to reduce homocysteine levels, but vitamin B6 and B12 are necessary for this to occur.

Vitamin K   The major non-collagen protein in bone is osteocalcin. This protein is dependent on vitamin K in order to occur in its active form.[24] Vitamin K is necessary so that the osteocalcin can chelate the calcium and hold it in place within the bone. A deficiency of vitamin K could therefore lead to impaired mineralisation of the bone due to inadequate osteocalcin levels.

Vitamin K is found in green leafy vegetables and may be one of the protective factors of a vegetarian diet. Fat-soluble chlorophyll capsules are an excellent source of naturally occurring vitamin K. Vitamin K deficiency is quite high in individuals with chronic gastrointestinal disorders or poor fat absorption,[25] who are also at a greater risk of developing osteoporosis.

Boron The trace mineral boron has recently been shown to have a positive effect on calcium and active oestrogen levels in postmenopausal women. Supplementing the diet of postmenopausal women with 3 mg of boron per day reduced urinary calcium excretion by 44 per cent and increased dramatically the levels of 17-beta-oestradiol, the most biologically active oestrogen.[26]

It appears boron is require to activate certain hormones including oestrogen and vitamin D. It was mentioned previously that vitamin D is converted to its most active form (1,25-dihydroxyvitamin D_3) within the kidney. Boron is apparently required for this reaction to occur.

Fruits and vegetables are the main sources of boron, and diets inadequate in these foods may be deficient in boron.

Strontium Strontium occurs in relatively large concentrations in bones and teeth, where it contributes to bone strength. Awareness of the nutritional significance of strontium has been overshadowed by the fear of radioactive strontium, a component of nuclear fallout. Because strontium accumulates in bone tissue, radioactive strontium is extremely hazardous to humans. However, non-radioactive strontium occurs naturally in food, is extremely non-toxic and has a beneficial effect on bone health.

Strontium has been shown to improve signs and symptoms of osteoporosis significantly. In one study, 85 per cent of the subjects experienced a marked reduction in bone pain and 78 per cent displayed increased bone density on X-ray.[27]

Botanical medicines

Proanthocyanidins and anthocyanidins These types of flavonoids are responsible for the deep red-blue colour of many berries including hawthorn berries, blackberries, bilberries, cherries, raspberries, etc. Proanthocyanidins and anthocyanidins are remarkable in their ability to stabilise collagen structures.[26] Since collagen is the major protein structure in bone, stabilisation of its integrity and structure is very much indicated. Supplementation with concentrated extracts or eating plenty of those berries rich in these types of flavonoids may offer significant benefit in preventing osteoporosis.

Phytoestrogens Plant oestrogenic substances or phytoestrogens are components of many medicinal herbs with a historical use in conditions which are now treated by synthetic oestrogens. They may be suitable alternatives to oestrogens in the prevention of osteoporosis in menopausal women.

Menopausal women commonly receive oestrogens to help allay the hot flushes, nausea, bone loss and other symptoms of this decrease in the body's own natural hormone level. While generally effective, both synthetic and natural oestrogens may pose significant health risks, including increasing the risk of cancer, gallbladder disease and thromboembolic disease (strokes, heart attacks, etc.). Phytoestrogens have not been associated with these side effects.

Phytoestrogens are capable of exerting oestrogenic effects, although the activity compared to oestrogen is only 1:400. Because of this phytoestrogens tend to counteract extreme oestrogen levels. If oestrogen levels are low, since phytoestrogens have some oestrogenic activity they will cause an increase in oestrogen effect; if oestrogen levels are high, since phytoestrogens bind to oestrogen receptor binding sites, thereby competing with oestrogen, there will be a decrease in oestrogen effects.

Because of the balancing action of phytoestrogens on oestrogen levels, it is common to find the same plant recommended for conditions of oestrogen excess (like the premenstrual syndrome) as well as conditions of oestrogen deficiency (like menopause, menstrual abnormalities). Many of these herbs have been termed uterine tonics.

Herbs which possess both proven oestrogenic activity and a long historical use in treating various female complaints include dong quai (*Angelica sinensis*), liquorice (*Glycyrrhiza glabra*), unicorn root (*Aletris farinosa*), black cohosh (*Cimicifuga racemosa*), fennel (*Foeniculum vulgare*), and false unicorn root (*Helonias opulus*).[29-34]

Lifestyle

Coffee, alcohol and smoking induce a negative calcium balance and are associated with an increased risk of developing osteoporosis.[1,7,35,36] As smokers tend to drink more coffee and alcohol, and consume a diet high in refined carbohydrate, it is very difficult to control these other variables when trying to determine why smokers have a 15–30 per cent lower bone mineral content compared to non-smokers. Smoking in relation to osteoporosis probably constitutes one factor among the overall effects of someone's lifestyle rather than having a direct causal relationship.[35,36]

Physical exercise consisting of one hour of moderate activity three times a week has been shown to prevent bone loss[37,38] In fact, this type of exercise has actually been shown to increase the bone mass in postmenopausal women. Walking is probably the best exercise to start with. In contrast to exercise, immobilisation doubles the rate of urinary and faecal calcium excretion, resulting in a significant negative calcium balance.[39]

Treatment

A comprehensive programme to prevent osteoporosis begins with the adoption of a lifestyle designed not only to prevent osteoporosis but other significant diseases as well. Your healthcare practitioner may help in evaluating your risk of developing osteoporosis by taking a detailed medical history and performing appropriate tests. Outlined below is a suggested comprehensive prevention programme that takes into consideration all the factors discussed above, listed in order of relative importance.

Diet

A diet high in vegetables and fruits, but low in fat and animal products, should be adopted. Refined carbohydrate and alcohol intake should be held to a low level and carbonated beverages loaded with phosphates should be completely eliminated. Flavonoid-rich foods, like dark blue-black berries, citrus rinds and colourful fruits, should be liberally consumed.

Supplements

- Calcium (citrate), 1 g a day.
- Magnesium (citrate), 500 mg a day.
- Pyridoxine, 100 mg a day.
- Folic acid, 1 mg a day.
- Vitamin B12, 1 mg a day.
- Phylloquinone (K1), 1 mg a day.
- Boron, 3 mg a day.
- Strontium (lactate), 100 mg a day.

Botanical medicines

If symptoms of menopause or oestrogen deficiency are apparent, any of the following herbs, alone or in combination, can be used – dong quai (*Angelica sinensis*), liquorice (*Glycyrrhiza glabra*), unicorn root (*Aletris farinosa*), black cohosh (*Cimicifuga racemosa*), fennel (*Foeniculum vulgare*) and false unicorn root (*Helonias opulus*).

- Dried root (or as tea), 1 to 3 g a day.
- Freeze-dried root, 0.5 to 1 g a day.
- Tincture (1:5), 4 to 6 ml (1 to 1.5 tsp) a day.
- Fluid extract (1:1), 0.5 to 2.0 ml (¼ to ½ tsp) a day.
- Powdered solid extract (4:1), 250–500 mg a day.

Exercise

Physical exercise is vital in maintaining and restoring optimum bone density. Duration of the exercise is more important than the intensity. Walking is a very good exercise to prevent osteoporosis. A 45 minute to an hour's walk, three to five times a week, is the minimum exercise for this programme.

61

Periodontal disease

- Gingivitis – inflammation of the gums characterised by redness, contour changes, recession and bleeding.
- Periodontitis – localised pain, loose teeth, demonstration of dental pockets, redness, swelling and/or pus. X-ray may reveal jaw bone destruction.

General considerations

Periodontal disease describes an inflammatory condition of the gums (gingivitis) and/or the bone around the teeth (periodontitis). Periodontal disease usually progresses from gingivitis to periodontitis.[1,2] It may be a sign of a more systemic condition, such as diabetes mellitus, collagen diseases, leukaemia or other disorders of white cell function, anaemia, or vitamin deficiency.[1]

The rate of periodontal disease increases directly with age; it is approximately 15 per cent at age 10, 38 per cent at age 20, 46 per cent at age 35 and 54 per cent at age 50. As a group, men have more periodontal disease which is worse than that found in women. Periodontal disease is more common in those with a lower social and economic status and in rural people, who also have worse forms of the disease.[1]

Inflammatory periodontal disease is a condition that is probably best treated with combined expertise, i.e. a dentist or periodontist and a nutritionally-minded physician. Although oral hygiene is of great importance in treating and preventing periodontal disease, it is not sufficient in many cases. An individual's defences against the disease must be normalised if the progression of the disease is to be controlled.[1,3] To a large extent, the nutritional status of the individual determines their defence factors.

Causes

In periodontal disease understanding the normal protective factors in the periodontal area is vitally important. It has been concluded that 'Clearly bacteria are essential agents, but their presence is in itself insufficient; host factors must be involved if the disease is to develop and progress.'[3]

Bacterial factors　Bacterial plaque has long been considered the causative agent in most forms of periodontal disease.[1] However, an appreciation of host defence factors has developed.[1,3] Bacteria are known to produce and secrete numerous compounds that are detrimental to the status of the individual's defence mechanisms. These compounds include endotoxins and exotoxins, free radicals and connective tissue-destroying enzymes, white cell poisons, and bacterial antigens, waste products and toxic compounds.[1]

Immune system function　Neutrophils constitute a first line of defence against microbial overgrowth. Defects in neutrophil functions are catastrophic to the periodontium.[13] Neutrophil functions are depressed in older people, and in those with diabetes, Crohn's disease, Chediak-Higashi syndrome, Down's syndrome and juvenile periodontitis[1,3]; these individuals are at extremely high risk of developing rapidly progressing periodontal disease.

The complement system plays a critical role in immunological and non-specific resistance to infection. However, a side effect of complement activation is an increase in permeability of the gums, resulting in increased penetration of bacteria and bacterial byproducts.[1,3,4] Other effects of complement activation include solubilisation of immune complexes, cell membrane lysis, neutralisation of viruses and the killing of bacteria.[4] In periodontal disease, activation of complement is possibly the major factor in tissue destruction.

Mast cell release of histamine is also a major factor in periodontal disease.[1] This release can be initiated by IgE antibody-antigen complexes, complement components, mechanical trauma, bacterial toxins and free radicals. The finding of increased IgE concentrations in the gums of patients with periodontal disease suggests that allergic reactions may be a factor in the progression of the disease.[5]

Amalgam fillings　Faulty dental fillings and prostheses are common causes of gingival inflammation and periodontal destruction.[1] Overhanging margins provide an ideal location for the accumulation of plaque and the multiplication of bacteria. If the restoration is a silver amalgam filling there may be even more involvement, due to decreased activities of antioxidant enzymes. Mercury accumulation results in a depletion of the free radical-scavenging enzymes glutathione peroxidase, superoxide dismutase and catalase.[6] The connective tissue matrix is particularly sensitive to free radical damage.[7]

Miscellaneous local factors　Numerous local factors favour the progression of periodontal disease, including food impaction, unreplaced missing teeth, malocclusion, tongue thrusting, teeth grinding, toothbrush trauma and mouth breathing.

Tobacco　Tobacco smoking is associated with increased susceptibility to severe periodontal disease and tooth loss.[1,8,9] (Tobacco smoking is in fact associated with increased susceptibility to virtually every major chronic disease.) Many of the harmful effects of tobacco smoking are a result of free radical damage, particularly to the surface cells of the gums. Furthermore, smoking greatly reduces vitamin C levels, thereby aggravating its damaging effects.[10]

Structure and integrity of connective tissue   The collagen matrix of the periodontal membrane allows for the dissipation of the tremendous amount of pressure exerted during chewing.[11] The status of the collagen matrix of the periodontium determines the rate of diffusion and the permeability of inflammatory mediators, bacteria and their byproducts, and destructive enzymes from the oral cavity.[12,13] Due to the high rate of protein turnover in periodontal collagen, the collagen matrix in this area is extremely vulnerable to atrophy when the necessary nutrients for collagen synthesis are absent or deficient.[11]

Therapy

Nutritional considerations

Vitamin C   Vitamin C plays a major role in preventing periodontal disease.[1,14–18] The classical symptom of gingivitis seen in scurvy illustrates the vital function vitamin C plays in maintaining collagen integrity and immune system function. Deficiency is associated with defective formation and maintenance of collagen, retardation of bone matrix formation, impaired bone calcification and delayed wound healing.

Decreased vitamin C levels are also associated with increased permeability of the oral mucosa to toxins and bacterial byproducts, as well as impaired white cell functions.[19,20]

Vitamin A   A vitamin A deficiency predisposes to periodontal disease.[1] Vitamin A is necessary for collagen synthesis and wound healing, maintaining the integrity of the gums and enhancing numerous immune functions.[20] Beta-carotene may be a more advantageous supplement due to its affinity for gum tissue, potent antioxidant activity and increased safety.[21]

Zinc and copper   Zinc functions synergistically with vitamin A in many metabolic processes.[22] The severity of periodontal disease is directly associated with significantly decreased zinc levels while serum copper levels are increased.[23] Zinc's importance in treating periodontal disease cannot be overstated. In the United States, marginal zinc deficiency is widespread, particularly in the elderly.[23,24] This may be a factor in the increasing frequency of periodontal disease with age, although the geriatric population is at higher risk for development of a variety of nutrient deficiencies, some of which may also predispose to periodontal disease.[20]

Zinc functions in the gingiva and periodontium include stabilisation of membranes, antioxidant activity, collagen synthesis, inhibition of plaque growth, inhibition of mast cell release of histamine and numerous immune activities.[20,22,24–6] Zinc is also known to reduce wound healing time significantly.

Regular twice-daily use of a mouthwash that contains a 5 per cent zinc solution inhibits plaque growth.[25] However, the use of lower concentrations or less frequent mouth washing is not very effective.

Vitamin E and selenium   These two nutrients function synergistically as antioxidants and seem to potentiate each other's effect. Vitamin E alone has been demonstrated to be of considerable value in patients with severe periodontal disease.[1,28] This can largely be attributed to the decreased wound healing time associated with vitamin E supplementation.[29] The antioxidant effects of vitamin E are particularly needed if silver amalgams are present. As stated earlier, mercury depletes the tissues of the antioxidant enzymes superoxide dismutase, glutathione perioxidase and catalase. In animal studies this toxic effect of mercury is prevented by supplementation with vitamin E.[6] Selenium and vitamin E's antioxidant activities also deter periodontal disease, as the free radicals are extremely damaging to the gums.[7]

Flavonoids   As a group these compounds are very important components in the treatment of periodontal disease. Flavonoids are extremely effective in reducing inflammation and stabilising collagen structures. Flavonoids help maintain a healthy collagen structure by:
- Decreasing membrane permeability, thereby decreasing the load of inflammatory mediators and bacterial toxins.
- Preventing free radical damage through their potent antioxidant properties.
- Inhibiting enzymatic cleavage.
- Inhibiting mast cell release of histamine.
- Cross-linking with collagen fibres, making them stronger.[30–5]

The more biologically active flavonoids, i.e. quercetin, catechin, anthocyanidins and proanthocyanidins, can be supplemented or obtained through specific foods, but rutin has very little collagen-stabilising effect.

Folic acid   Double-blind studies have shown that folic acid, either topically or internally, produces significant reduction of gingival inflammation as determined by reduction in colour changes, bleeding tendency, gum exudates and plaque scores.[36–40] The folate mouthwash (0.1 per cent folic acid) is significantly more effective than oral supplementation of up to 5 mg per day, suggesting a local mechanism of action.[38,39] Folate has been demonstrated to bind toxins secreted by plaques.[38–40] The use of folate mouthwash is particularly indicated for pregnant women, oral contraceptive users, those using anti-folate drugs (e.g. phenytoin and methotrexate) and for other conditions associated with an exaggerated gingival inflammatory response.[38,39,41] The white blood cells of pregnant women and women taking oral contraceptives contain a molecule that binds folate, which, more than malabsorption or decreased intake, appears to be the major reason for their functional folate deficiency.[42] Folic acid deficiency is the most common nutritional deficiency in the world.[20]

Dietary considerations

Fibre   A diet high in dietary fibre may have a protective effect due to increased salivary secretion.[14] Avoidance of sugar and all refined carbohydrates is extremely important.

Sugar Sugar is known to increase plaque accumulation significantly while simultaneously decreasing white cell function.[1,43] This inhibition of white cell function is due, in part, to competition with vitamin C. Considering the fact that the average westerner consumes in excess of 150 grams of sucrose (plus other refined carbohydrates) a day, it is safe to say that most westerners have a chronically depressed immune system which puts them at increased risk for periodontal disease.[44]

Botanical medicines

Myrrh gum (Commiphora abyssinica) Myrrh has historically been used for periodontal disease.[45] It appears to be of some benefit when applied topically. Although the mechanism of action has not been elucidated, myrrh resins may function in binding toxins.

Flavonoid-containing plants Bilberries (*Vaccinium myrtillus*), hawthorn berries (*Crataegus oxycantha*) and grapes (*Vitis vinifera*) are all rich sources of flavonoids. Remarkable effects have been displayed by the flavonoid derivative 3-0-methyl-(+)-catechin in the treatment of hamsters with experimentally induced periodontitis; large doses significantly retarded plaque growth and jaw bone destruction.[4,5]

Treatment

The therapeutic goals in the treatment of periodontal disease are to:
- Decrease wound healing time (the time for wound healing is longer in patients who are more susceptible to periodontal disease[46]).
- Improve membrane and collagen integrity.
- Decrease inflammation and free radical damage.
- Enhance the function of the immune system.

Smoking must be stopped to allow rebuilding of the damaged tissues and, if possible, gold or plastic fillings should be used instead of silver amalgams. In addition, any structural defects of the mouth should be repaired and the teeth regularly cleaned by a dental hygienist, while significant periodontal disease requires the services of a dentist or periodentist.

Diet

Although no specific therapeutic diet has been developed for the treatment of periodontal disease, some recommendations are in order. As usual, a natural foods diet rich in nutrients and fibre is important. Simple sugars (white sugar, honey, fruit juice, dried fruit, etc.) and refined carbohydrates should be reduced as much as possible. Bioflavonoids-rich foods (dark blue-black fruits, onions, hawthorn berries, citrus rind, etc.) should be emphasised. Foods to which a person is known to be allergic should be avoided (as discussed in the Chapter 38, Food allergy, eating allergenic foods greatly decreases immune system function).

Nutritional supplements

- Vitamin C, 2–4 g per day in divided doses.
- Vitamin E, 200–400 iu a day.
- Beta-carotenes, 100,000 iu a day.
- Selenium, 200 micrograms per day.
- Zinc, 15 mg a day (picolinate form).
- Folic acid, 2 mg per day.
- Mixed bioflavonoids 500 mg three times a day.

Mouthwash

Wash mouth twice a day with 25 ml of a solution containing 5 per cent zinc and 0.1 per cent folic acid.

Premenstrual syndrome

- Recurrent signs and symptoms that develop during the 7–14 days prior to menstruation.
- Typical symptoms include decreased energy, tension, irritability, depression, headache, altered sex drive, breast pain, backache, abdominal bloating and oedema of the fingers and ankles.

General considerations

Premenstrual syndrome (PMS), also called premenstrual tension, is a recurrent condition of women, characterised by troublesome, yet often ill-defined, symptoms 7–14 days before menstruation. The syndrome affects about one-third of women between 30–40 years of age, about 10 per cent of whom may have a significantly debilitating form.[1]

Causes

Although there is a wide spectrum of symptoms, there are common hormonal patterns in PMS patients when compared to symptom-free control groups:

- Plasma oestrogens are elevated and plasma progesterone levels are reduced 5–10 days before the menses.[2]
- Prolactin levels are elevated in most, but not all, PMS patients.[3]
- Follicle stimulating hormone (FSH) levels are elevated 6–9 days prior to the onset of menses.[2]
- Aldosterone levels are marginally elevated 2–8 days prior to the onset of menses.[2]
- Hypothyroidism is common.

In an attempt to bring some order to the clinically and metabolically confusing picture of PMS, it has been subdivided into four distinct subgroups, each subgroup being linked to specific symptoms, hormonal patterns and metabolic abnormalities.[1] These are listed in Table 62.1 and are discussed separately below. The grading of symptoms was

Table 62.1 Premenstrual syndrome subgroups[1]

Subgroup	Symptoms	Mechanisms	Prevalence (%)
PMS-A (anxiety)	Anxiety Irritability Mood swings Nervous tension	High oestrogen Low progesterone	65–75
PMS-C (craving)	Increased appetite Headache Fatigue, dizziness or fainting Palpitations	Increased carbohydrate tolerance Low prostaglandin PGE1 in some	24–35
PMS-D (depression)	Depression Crying Forgetfulness Confusion Insomnia	Low serum oestrogen High progesterone Elevated adrenal Androgens if hirsute	23–37
PMS-H (hyperhydration)	Fluid retention Weight gain > 3 lb Swollen extremities Breast tenderness Abdominal bloating	Aldosterone	65–72

rated moderate in 85 per cent and severe in 15 per cent of the patients studied. Figure 62.1 shows a questionnaire useful for helping determine which subgroup best matches a woman's symptom pattern.

Premenstrual syndrome subgroups

PMS-A PMS-A is the most common symptom category and is found to be strongly associated with excessive oestrogen and deficient progesterone during the premenstrual phase.[1,2] Although symptom ratings correspond to the raised serum oestrogen levels, serum oestrogen-to-progesterone ratios give the best correlation. There is no significant correlation of symptoms with the decreased progesterone levels. The effect of the excess oestrogens is to alter the ratios and levels of important neurotransmitters. Women with PMS-A have increased levels of adrenaline, noradrenaline and serotonin and decreased levels of dopamine and phenylethylamine.[4,5]

The effects on mood and behaviour of these changes in the concentration of the neurotransmitters are well documented: adrenaline triggers anxiety; noradrenaline, hostility and irritability; and serotonin, at high levels, nervous tension, drowsiness, palpitations, water retention and inability to concentrate and perform.[5] Dopamine is believed to counteract the three other neurotransmitters by inducing a feeling of relaxation and increasing mental alertness.[1]

Oestrogens also affect mood by blocking the action of vitamin B6, inhibiting liver

Date: _____
Chart no.: _____

Name: _____ Age: _____ Ht : _____ Wt : _____
Marital status: ☐ Single ☐ Married ☐ Divorced ☐ Widowed   Present contraception: ☐ None ☐ Pill ☐ IUD ☐ Other
History of taking contraceptive pills: ☐ Yes ☐ No   If YES, months ago: _____   For how long _____ months
Your last period started _____(Date) Your last period lasted _____ days. Your last menstrual cycle was _____ days long.
Your last period was ☐ Light ☐ Moderate ☐ Heavy   Number of pregnancies _____ Children _____
Occupation: _____

GRADING OF SYMPTOMS

1 none.
2 mild-present but does not interfere with activities.
3 moderate-present and interferes with activities but not disabling.
4 severe disabling (unable to function)

Grade your symptoms for last menstrual cycle only

Symptoms	Week after period	Week before period
PMT-A Nervous tension, Mood swings, Irritability, Anxiety		
Total		
PMT-H Weight gain, Swelling of extremities, Breast tenderness, Abdominal bloating		
Total		
PMT-C Headache, Craving for sweets, Increased appetite, Heart pounding, Fatigue, Dizziness of fainting		
Total		
PMT-D Depression, Forgetfulness, Crying, Confusion, Insomnia		
Total		
TOTAL SCORE		

Other symptoms

Oily skin
Acne

During first two days of periods

Menstrual cramps
Menstrual backache

Figure 62.1 Menstrual symptom questionnaire

synthesis of serotonin and decreasing the body's ability to maintain normal blood glucose levels.[6,7]

Excessive levels of prolactin may also be implicated in PMS-A as oestrogens, both internally produced and ingested, are known to increase prolactin secretion by the pituitary gland. The symptoms of prolactin excess are similar to those of PMS-A and PMS-H, and a number of studies have shown such an excess.[3] However, other studies have failed to confirm these findings statistically,[8] possibly due to small sample size.

Another possible result of the increase in the oestrogen-to-progesterone ratio is impairment of endorphin activity. Endorphins are the body's own mood elevating and pain relieving substances. One study found a direct correlation between this ratio and endorphin activity in the brain.[9] This is significant considering the known ability of endorphins to normalise or improve mood and decrease pain sensitivity.

PMS-C   PMS-C is associated with increased appetite, craving for sweets, headache, fatigue, fainting spells and heart palpitations. Glucose tolerance tests (GTT) performed on PMS-C patients during the 5–10 days before their menses show a flattening of the early part of the curve (which usually implies excessive secretion of insulin in response to sugar consumption), whereas during other parts of the menstrual cycle their GTT is normal.[1,2,10] Currently there is no clear explanation for this phenomenon, although an increased cellular capacity to bind insulin has been postulated. This appears to be hormonally regulated, but other factors may also be involved. Salt (sodium chloride) enhances insulin response to sugar ingestion, and decreased pancreatic magnesium levels result in increased secretion of insulin in response to glucose.

A deficiency of the prostaglandin PGE1 in the pancreas and central nervous system may also be involved in PMS-C.[2,11] PGE1 inhibits glucose-induced insulin secretion in humans.[1]

PMS-D   This subgroup is the least prevalent and is relatively rare in its pure form. Its key symptom is depression, which is usually associated with low levels of neurotransmitters in the central nervous system. In PMS-D patients this is most likely due to increased breakdown of the neurotransmitters as a result of decreased levels of oestrogen (in contrast to PMS-A which shows just the opposite results).[1,2] The decreased ovarian oestrogen output has been attributed to a stress-induced increase in adrenal androgen secretion and/or progesterone.[1,2]

PMS-H   This subgroup is characterised by weight gain (greater than 3 pounds, 1.4 kg), abdominal bloating and discomfort, breast tenderness and congestion, and occasional swelling of the face, hands and ankles.[1] These symptoms are due to an increased fluid volume, secondary to an excess of the hormone aldosterone which causes increased fluid retention.[2] Aldosterone excess during the premenstrual phase of PMS-H patients may arise due to any of the following factors:

- Stress – secretion of the fluid retention hormone by the adrenal cortex is stimulated by the pituitary gland in response to stress, high serotonin levels and angiotensin II.
- Oestrogen excess – oestrogen increases excretion and production of angiotensin II.

- Dopamine deficiency – a relative dopamine deficiency has been demonstrated in PMS-H patients. Dopamine suppresses fluid retention hormone production by the adrenal glands and, in the kidneys, stimulates the elimination of salt and water.

Diagnosis

The recurrent signs and symptoms that develop during the 7–14 days prior to menses are listed in the accompanying box.

Signs and symptoms of premenstrual syndrome

- Behavioural
    Nervousness, anxiety and irritability.
    Mood swings and mild to severe personality change.
    Fatigue, lethargy and depression.
- Gastrointestinal
    Abdominal bloating.
    Diarrhoea and/or constipation.
    Change in appetite (usually craving of sugar).
- Female
    Tender and enlarged breasts.
    Uterine cramping.
    Altered libido.
- General
    Headache.
    Backache.
    Acne.
    Oedema of fingers and ankles.

Therapy

Nutritional considerations

Compared to symptom free women, PMS patients consume 62 per cent more refined carbohydrates, 275 per cent more refined sugar, 79 per cent more dairy products, 78 per cent more sodium, 53 per cent less iron, 77 per cent less manganese and 52 per cent less zinc.[1]

Multivitamin and mineral supplement In one small study, vitamin intake was significantly higher in the normal group due primarily to 12 out of the 14 normals taking nutritional supplements.[1] In contrast, only six out of 39 patients with PMS used nutritional supplements on a regular basis. When compared to normal women, the calculated intake of selected nutrients by the PMS patients was much lower. Although they consumed close to the recommended daily allowance, their intake levels were only

2.2 per cent as much for thiamin, 2.2 per cent for riboflavin, 16.7 per cent for niacin, 8.7 per cent for pantothenic acid and 2.7 per cent for pyridoxine.[1,2] PMS patients given a multivitamin and mineral supplement containing high doses of magnesium and pyridoxine in an uncontrolled study showed a 70 per cent reduction in both pre- and postmenstrual symptoms.[12]

Vitamin B complex   In the early 1940s an apparent relationship was observed between vitamin B complex deficiency and PMS, menstrual cramping, excessive menstrual bleeding and fibrocystic breast disease.[13] Patients with one or more of these complaints also had signs of B vitamin deficiency. B complex therapy resulted in an amelioration of the complaints.

Vitamin B6   The majority of clinical studies have demonstrated the efficacy of vitamin B6 supplementation in treating PMS.[14] For example, in one double-blind cross-over trial, 84 per cent of the subjects had a lower symptomatology score during the B6 treatment period. Although PMS has multiple causes, B6 supplementation alone appears to benefit most patients. In another study, premenstrual acne flare-up was reduced in 72 per cent of 106 affected young women taking 50 mg pyridoxine daily for one week prior and during the menstrual period.[2]

It is important to note, however, that not all double-blind studies of vitamin B6 have been positive.[15] These negative results may have been caused by many factors, such as the inability of some women to convert B6 to its active form due to a deficiency in another nutrient (e.g. vitamin B2) which was not supplemented. These results suggest that supplementing pyridoxine by itself may not result in adequate clinical results for all women suffering this disorder. Excessive supplementation (over 250 mg per day) should be avoided since it can cause neurological problems in some people.

Magnesium   Magnesium deficiency is strongly implicated as a causative factor in premenstrual syndrome. Red blood cell magnesium levels in PMS patients have been shown to be significantly lower than in normal subjects. The deficiency is characterised by excessive nervous sensitivity, with generalised aches and pains and a lower premenstrual pain threshold.[1,2] One clinical trial of magnesium in PMS showed a reduction of nervousness in 89 per cent, of breast tenderness in 96 per cent and of weight gain in 95 per cent.

Vitamin A   Vitamin A has been shown to be beneficial in reducing PMS symptoms when given in doses of 100,000 to 300,000 iu per day (a potentially toxic dose – *not recommended*) in the second half of the menstrual cycle.[2] Beta-carotenes may be better indicated since they are much less toxic and the body is able to regulate their conversion to vitamin A, thus maintaining more appropriate levels.[16]

Vitamin E   Although vitamin E research concerning PMS has focused primarily on breast tenderness, significant reduction of other PMS symptomatology has also been demonstrated in double blind studies.[1,17] Nervous tension, headache, fatigue, depression and insomnia were all significantly reduced.

Lactobacillus   *Lactobacillus acidophilus* has been shown to inhibit the faecal bacterial enzyme which converts oestrogens to more toxic forms and to decrease the reabsorption of excreted, detoxified oestrogens.[18]

Subgroup specific

PMS-A   When an apparent relationship was observed between B vitamin deficiency and PMS,[13] it was postulated that PMS was due to an excess in oestrogen levels caused by decreased detoxification and elimination in the liver. This supports the historic use of 'lipotropic factors' in PMS, since a B vitamin deficiency does result in depressed liver function.

A predisposing factor in brain dopamine depletion is a deficiency of intracellular magnesium.[1] Although PMS patients have been shown to have normal serum levels of magnesium, their intracellular levels are significantly depressed.[19] Diet surveys have shown that PMS-A patients consume five times more dairy products and three times more refined sugar than patients in other PMS subgroups.[1] This is significant, since dairy products and calcium interfere with magnesium absorption, while sugar increases the urinary excretion of magnesium.[1] The combined effects of these would lead to a chronic magnesium deficiency.

A pyridoxine deficiency also leads to decreased dopamine synthesis (the enzyme that synthesises dopamine is a pyridoxine-dependent enzyme), and high supplemental doses of vitamin B6 result in increased hypothalamic dopaminergic activity and the inhibition of prolactin secretion.[20] Zinc also inhibits prolactin release.[21] In addition, pyridoxine normalises low intracellular magnesium, lowers premenstrual oestradiol levels and increases progesterone levels.[2]

A high carbohydrate diet decreases hepatic clearance of oestradiol while a high protein diet increases hepatic clearance of oestradiol and may increase the half life of progesterone.[22]

The protein intake should, however, be derived largely from vegetable sources since vegetarian women are more able to clear oestrogen metabolites. These women excrete two to three times more oestrogen in their faeces and have 50 per cent lower mean plasma levels of unconjugated oestrogens than do omnivores.[23] This is due to the differing types of bacterial flora associated with these diets. Certain bacteria, common in the omnivore's colon, are capable of synthesising oestrogen as well as breaking the oestrogen-glucuronide linkages. This results in increased absorption and reabsorption of oestrogens from the intestines, and may be a significant cause of the increased oestrogen-to-progesterone ratio seen in PMS-A.

PMS-C   Important cofactors for prostaglandin PGE1 synthesis are pyridoxine, magnesium, zinc, vitamin C and niacin. PGE1 synthesis is inhibited by saturated animal fats, trans-fatty acids (such as those found in processed hydrogenated vegetable oils, e.g. shortening and margarine), alcohol and stress-induced rises in adrenal hormones.[1,2] Arachidonic acid (which comes only from animal fats in the diet) antagonises the anti-inflammatory PGE1 via increased formation of proinflammatory prostaglandins, such as PGF2-alpha and PGE2. Vitamin E is known to inhibit the formation of these arachidonic acid end products. Treatment of women with PMS using gamma-linolenic acid to promote PGE1 synthesis has shown good results in placebo-controlled studies.[11]

PMS-D   Lead may be important since it blocks the binding of oestrogen to receptor sites yet has no effect on progesterone. Magnesium may also be important; a deficiency results in increased lead absorption and retention, while decreasing resistance to stress. Hair mineral analysis has shown that, in general, PMS patients have higher heavy metal levels and lower magnesium levels than non-PMS controls.[2]

PMS-H   A deficiency in magnesium causes overgrowth of the adrenal cortex, elevated aldosterone levels and increased extracellular fluid volume. Aldosterone increases the urinary excretion of magnesium; hence a positive feedback mechanism results, which is aggravated since there is no renal mechanism for conserving magnesium.

In laboratory animals a vitamin B6 deficiency decreases the kidneys' ability to secrete sodium. Also, since pyridoxine requires magnesium for conversion to its active form, a magnesium deficiency can lead to decreased vitamin B6 activity.

Increased insulin secretion, in response to sugar consumption, results in sodium retention that is independent of aldosterone.

Botanical medicines

Although a wide variety of herbs have been used in folk medicine for the many disorders of menstruation, and many have been carefully evaluated for their oestrogenic effects, few have been specifically evaluated for their efficacy in relieving premenstrual symptoms. The herbs which are most likely to be useful are probably those which inhibit the formation of inflammatory prostaglandins, assist the body in balancing hormonal levels, improve liver function, relieve uterine cramping and/or have a long folk history of use.

*Unicorn root (*Aletris farinosa*)*   Unicorn root has been used in folk medicine for women who had 'poor ovarian function'. Research has confirmed that aletris does indeed have oestrogen-like activity, and diosgenin (a breakdown product of a glycoside extracted from aletris) is used in the manufacture of steroids.[24] It would probably be most useful in PMS-D.

Black haw (Viburnum prunifolium)   Black haw has demonstrated uterine antispasmodic properties, which are probably related to its content of scopoletin, a uterine sedative.[24] Black haw is related to *Viburnum opulus*, the guelder rose, which is appropriately also known as cramp bark, and both have a long folk history of use in this condition.[25]

Bromelain   Although not mentioned in the folk literature, this extract from the pineapple plant has been documented as relieving menstrual cramping.[26] Bromelain is believed to be a smooth muscle relaxant, since it decreases the spasms of the contracted cervix in these patients. This effect on the uterus is believed to be a result of decreasing the synthesis of prostaglandins of the 2-series, e.g. PGF2-alpha and PGE2, while increasing levels of PGE1-like compounds.[27] This balancing of prostaglandin synthesis is important in premenstrual tension, particularly PMS-C.

Milk thistle (Silybum marianum) Proper liver function is critical to maintaining normal hormone balance. The common milk thistle contains some of the most potent liver protecting and stimulating substances known.[28-30] The concentration of these components is highest in the fruit. Silybum's effects on the liver relate to its ability, in many instances, to inhibit the factors that are responsible for the damage, i.e. free radicals and leukotrienes, and to stimulate liver function by promoting protein metabolism.

Silybum components prevent free radical damage by acting as antioxidants.[28] These components are many times more potent in antioxidant activity than vitamin E. Perhaps the most interesting effect of silybum components on the liver is their ability to stimulate protein synthesis.[28] The result is an increase in the production of new liver cells to replace the damaged old ones. In human studies, silymarin has been shown to have significant positive effects in treating several liver diseases, including cirrhosis and chronic hepatitis.[29,39]

Treatment

Although using the general guidelines listed here will help most women, using the questionnaire in Figure 62.1 and, as necessary, laboratory tests, to determine the specific subgroup a woman belongs to will yield better results.

Diet

In general, limit consumption of refined carbohydrates (sugar, honey, white flour, etc.) and other concentrated carbohydrates such as maple syrup, dried fruit and fruit juice. Increase protein intake, particularly from vegetable sources such as legumes. Decrease milk and dairy products. Decrease intake of fats, especially natural and synthetically saturated fats, while increasing intake of vegetable oils (rich in linoleic and linolenic acids). Increase green leafy vegetables, except brassica family foods (cabbage, brussels sprouts and cauliflower). Use only hormone-free, organic red meat and fowl; fish is better. Decrease salt intake. Restrict alcohol and tobacco use. Restrict intake of methyl-xanthines (coffee, tea, chocolate and caffeine-containing foods and beverages).

Nutritional supplements

General recommendations
- B-complex, 25 mg complex once a day.
- Vitamin B6, 100 mg per day (double dose 10 days premenstrually if needed).
- Vitamin C, 500 mg per day.

- Vitamin E, 200 iu per day.
- Beta-carotene, 50,000 iu per day.
- Magnesium aspartate, 400–800 mg per day.
- Zinc picolinate, 15 mg per day.
- Linseed oil, 1–2 tblsp per day.
- *Lactobacillus acidophilus*, 1 tsp per day.

Subgroup-specific recommendations
- PMS-A
    Bioflavonoids, 500 mg two times a day.
- PMS-C
    Evening primrose oil, 500 mg two times a day.
    Hypoglycaemic diet.
- PMS-D
    Tyrosine, 300 mg per day.
    Check for lead toxicity.
- PMS-H
    Liquorice (*Glycyrrhiza glabra*) doses three times a day:
    - Dried root, or as tea, 1 to 2 grams.
    - Freeze-dried root, 500 to 1,000 mg.
    - Tincture (1:5), 4 to 6 ml (1 to 1.5 tsp).
    - Fluid extract (1:1), 0.5 to 2.0 ml (1/4 to 1/2 tsp).
    - Solid (dry, powdered) extract (4:1), 250 to 500 mg.

63

Prostate enlargement

- Symptoms of bladder obstruction (progressively increasing over time) – need to urinate more frequently, need to urinate at night, hesitancy and intermittency, with reduced force and calibre of urine stream.
- Enlarged, non-tender prostate.

General considerations

Nearly 60 per cent of men between the ages of 40 and 59 years have an enlarged prostate gland, a condition known as benign prostatic hyperplasia (BPH, also known in the past as benign prostatic hypertrophy).[1] The projected annual overall cost of hospital care and surgery for BPH is thus extremely high.[2]

Symptoms of BPH typically reflect obstruction of the bladder outlet (progressive urinary frequency, urgency and night-time awakening to empty the bladder, and hesitancy and intermittency with reduced force and calibre of urine). The condition, if left untreated, will eventually obstruct the bladder outlet, resulting in the retention of urine in the blood (uraemia).

Many physicians feel that surgery is the only solution to the problem. However, benign prostatic hyperplasia will often respond to nutritional and herbal support as described below. This is particularly important as the surgical procedure often results in complications. In addition, nutritional factors may offer significant protection against developing prostatic enlargement.

Hormonal factors

The normal aging process in men favours the development BPH due to a variety of factors, including age-related alterations in hormone levels.

BPH represents a male hormone (androgen) dependent disorder of metabolism. As men age there are many significant changes in hormone levels.[2] Testosterone and, in particular, free testosterone levels decrease with age after the fifth decade, while other hormones such as prolactin, oestradiol, sex hormone-binding ligand, luteinising hormone and follicle stimulating hormone levels are all increased. The ultimate effect of these changes is an increased concentration of dihydrotestosterone within the prostate. Dihydrotestosterone is a very potent androgen derived from testosterone, and is responsible for the overproduction of prostate cells which ultimately results in prostatic enlargement.

The increase of dihydrotestosterone within the prostatic cell is largely due to a decreased rate of removal.[2] Testosterone and dihydrotestosterone are normally metabolised by enzymes to compounds that have a reduced attraction for receptor molecules in the cells that bind these hormones. The metabolised testosterone and dihydrotestosterone are then able to be excreted. Since the hormones are not being metabolised and therefore excreted, levels of the hormones increase within the prostatic cells. Elevated oestrogen levels play a role in the development of BPH by inhibiting the enzymes that metabolise testosterone and dihydrotestosterone.

In addition to a decreased rate of excretion of the male hormones by the prostate in BPH, there is also an increase in the uptake of testosterone by the prostate. This appears to be the result of yet another hormone, prolactin, which increases the uptake of testosterone and increases the synthesis of dihydrotestosterone. The net result is that the more potent androgen, dihydrotestosterone, is greatly increased within the prostate in BPH.

Prolactin levels are increased by beer and stress. These factors may contribute greatly to BPH. Drugs that reduce prolactin levels reduce many of the symptoms of BPH. However, these drugs have severe side effects and are therefore not widely used. It appears that the trace mineral zinc and vitamin B6 can reduce prolactin levels as well, yet produce no side effects at prescribed doses.[3,4] As zinc and vitamin B6 are intricately involved in hormone metabolism, deficiency of one or both of these nutrients may be a contributing factor in the cause of BPH in many men.

In summary, it can be simply stated that in BPH there are several hormonal factors which cause an increase in the potent male hormone dihydrotestosterone within the prostate. This hormone is responsible for promoting excessive cellular reproduction in BPH. Several treatment measures will be discussed below which significantly reduce the dihydrotestosterone level in the prostate and hence reduce the signs and symptoms of BPH.

Therapy

Nutritional considerations

Zinc   Paramount to an effective BPH prevention and treatment plan is adequate zinc intake and absorption. Zinc has been shown to reduce the size of the prostate – as determined by rectal examination, X-ray and endoscopy – and to reduce symptomatology in the majority of patients.[5,6] The clinical efficacy of zinc is probably due to its critical involvement in many aspects of hormonal metabolism.

Zinc has been shown to inhibit the activity of 5-alpha-reductase, the enzyme that irreversibly converts testosterone to dihydrotestosterone.[7-10] Zinc also inhibits the binding of both male hormones to cellular receptor molecules, thereby allowing for increased excretion of these hormones.[11]

Zinc has also been shown to inhibit prolactin secretion and is believed to be the natural modulator for prolactin secretion by the pituitary.[3,12] The net result of all of zinc's actions is very apparent in BPH – a reduction in the dihydrotestosterone content of the prostate, causing a reduction in both the size of the prostate, and the symptoms of BPH.

The efficacy of oral zinc supplementation is dependent on absorption of the ingested zinc. Probably most important from a therapeutic standpoint is the choice of zinc chelate (or salt) used. It appears that zinc picolinate and perhaps zinc citrate are the best supplemental forms of zinc to use. Zinc absorption in humans is believed to proceed as follows: following ingestion of zinc, the pancreas secretes picolinic acid into the intestine; the picolinic acid then forms a complex with zinc that enhances the absorption of zinc from the intestine. In humans and animals, the quantity of zinc transported across the absorptive cells of the intestine is directly related to the availability of picolinic acid.[13] Picolinic acid is synthesised in our bodies from the amino acid tryptophan. Vitamin B6 is needed for this reaction to occur. Inborn errors in metabolism that affect the conversion of tryptophan to picolinic acid or a vitamin B6 deficiency will result in impaired zinc absorption.[14] In addition, vitamin B6 supplementation may also enhance zinc absorption.[14] Providing zinc as zinc picolinate bypasses the need for picolinic acid secretion by the pancreas.[13,14,15]

A decrease in the output of secretions by the pancreas would result in impaired zinc absorption. This is probably a major factor responsible for the decreased zinc levels in the elderly. Pancreatic insufficiency is a common condition with increasing age. This means that, even though an individual may be consuming high levels of zinc, a deficiency may result due to decreased absorption. Supplementation with zinc picolinate appears to be particularly indicated in individuals with even mild pancreatic insufficiency.[16]

Several other factors in BPH suggest the use of zinc picolinate. Intestinal uptake of zinc is impaired by oestrogens. Since oestrogen levels are increased in men with BPH, zinc uptake may be low despite adequate dietary intake. Providing zinc as zinc picolinate may compensate for oestrogen depression of zinc uptake. Alcohol also reduces zinc uptake and increases zinc excretion, leading to relative zinc deficiency. In addition, alcohol reduces active vitamin B6 levels which may further reduce zinc stores.

Essential fatty acids The administration of an essential fatty acid (EFA) complex containing linoleic, linolenic and arachidonic acids has resulted in significant improvement for many BPH patients.[17] All 19 subjects in an uncontrolled study showed diminution of residual urine, with 12 of the 19 having no residual urine by the end of several weeks of treatment. These effects appear to be due to the correction of an underlying essential fatty acid deficiency, since these patients' prostatic and seminal lipid levels and ratios are often abnormal.[18,19] Based on this evidence alone, supplementation with an essential fatty acid complex appears indicated.

Linseed oil, sunflower oil, evening primrose oil and soy oil are all appropriate vegetable oils to add to the diet to ensure the essential fatty acid requirement is being met. One teaspoon or 4 grams per day is usually a sufficient amount.

Amino acids   The combination of glycine, alanine and glutamic acid (in the form of two 6-grain capsules administered three times daily for two weeks and one capsule three times daily thereafter) has been shown in several studies to relieve many of the symptoms of BPH. In a controlled study of 45 men, night-time urination was relieved or reduced in 95 per cent, urgency reduced in 81 per cent, frequency reduced in 73 per cent and delayed micturition alleviated in 70 per cent.[20]

These results have also been reported in other controlled studies.[21] The mechanism of action is unknown, but may be due to glycine's role as an inhibitory neurotransmitter in the central nervous system. Amino acid therapy is probably only palliative and not curative.

Cholesterol   Cholesterol metabolites are damaging to cells and carcinogenic, and have been shown to accumulate in the hyperplastic or cancerous human prostate. These metabolites of cholesterol initiate degeneration of prostatic cells which can promote prostatic enlargement.

Drugs which lower cholesterol levels have been shown to have a favourable influence on BPH, preventing the accumulation of cholesterol in the prostatic cells and limiting subsequent formation of damaging cholesterol metabolites.[1] Every effort should be made to decrease serum cholesterol levels, principally because elevated cholesterol levels are implicated in so many diseases including the number one killer of westerners – heart disease (see Chapter 18, Atherosclerosis, for further discussion).

Environmental considerations

Drugs and pesticides   The diet should be as free as possible from pesticides and other contaminants, since many of these compounds (e.g. dioxin, polyhalogenated biphenyls, hexachlorobenzene and dibenzofurans) can increase the formation of dihydrotestos-terone in the prostate.[22] Diethylstilboestrol (DES) should also be avoided, since it produces changes in rat prostates similar to BPH.[1]

It is quite possible that the tremendous increase in the occurrence of BPH in the last few decades reflects an ever increasing effect that toxic chemicals have on our health. BPH is perhaps just one of many health problems that may be due to these toxic substances. A diet rich in natural wholefoods may offer some protection due to the presence of many protective substances. In particular, minerals (calcium, magnesium, zinc, selenium, germanium, etc.), vitamins, plant pigments (flavonoids, carotenes, chlorophyll, etc.), fibre (especially gel-forming and mucilaginous types) and sulphur-containing compounds all possess actions which help the body deal with toxic chemicals and heavy metals (see Chapter 3, Detoxification).

Botanical medicines

Saw palmetto (Serenoa repens)   This scrubby palm tree native to Florida bears a fruit that has a long folk history of use as an aphrodisiac and sexual rejuvenator. These berries have also been used for centuries in treating conditions of the prostate. Recently, the therapeutic effect of the liposterolic (fat and sterol) extract of saw palmetto berries has been shown to improve greatly the signs and symptoms of an enlarged prostate in clinical studies.[23-6] This effect appears to be due to its inhibition of dihydrotestosterone, the compound which causes the prostate cells to multiply excessively.

This inhibition of dihydrotestosterone occurs at its initial synthesis as well as at cellular binding sites, thereby greatly antagonising the effects of dihydrotestosterone on the prostate. This antagonism of dihydrotestosterone by saw palmetto extract has been demonstrated in experimental studies and further supports the therapeutic effect seen in clinical trials as well as the long folk use for this condition.[23-6]

Panax ginseng   Ginseng, one of the most widely used plants in oriental medicine, possesses a variety of pharmaceutical properties. In experimental animal studies, ginseng increases testosterone levels while decreasing prostate weight.[27] This suggests that ginseng should have favourable affects in BPH, since increased testosterone would improve intestinal zinc absorption, and decreased prostatic size would help alleviate the symptoms of BPH. However, no clinical trials have been reported to the authors' knowledge on ginseng in the treatment of BPH, despite a long historical folk use in BPH and other male conditions.

The consumer should be made aware of the fact that the quality of ginseng is extremely variable, although select ginseng products have been standardised for their 'ginsenoside' content.

Flower pollen   Flower pollen has been used to treat prostatitis and BPH in Europe since the early 1960s.[22] Although its mechanism of action has not been elucidated, it has been shown to be quite effective in several double-blind clinical studies.[28,29] Its effect is probably related to its high content of plant flavonoids.

Hydrotherapy

Hydrotherapy is the use of water in any of its forms (hot, cold, ice, steam, etc.) and methods of application (sitz bath, douche, spa and hot tub, whirlpool, sauna, shower, immersion bath, pack, poultice, foot bath, fomentation, wrap, colonic irrigations, etc.) in the maintenance of health or treatment of disease. It is one of the ancient methods of treatment, having been used to treat disease and injury by many different cultures, including the Egyptians, Assyrians, Persians, Greeks, Hebrews, Hindus and Chinese.

In the treatment of BPH, the most common hydrotherapy technique is the sitz bath which is a partial immersion bath of the pelvic region. It is more easily given in a specially constructed tub, but may also be performed in a regular bath tub. Often it is taken with the feet immersed in a separate tub of hot water before or during the bath. A sitz bath may be taken hot, neutral, cold, or contrast hot and cold (each discussed below). In the initial treatment of BPH, the hot sitz bath is the most useful and easiest to employ.

Hot sitz bath   The hot sitz bath is generally taken for 3 to 10 minutes at 105–15 °F (40.5–46 °C). A hot foot bath at 110–15 °F (43–46 °C) offers additional benefit. The hot sitz bath is followed by cool sponging of the pelvic area. Hot sitz baths are not indicated in cases of acute inflammation or infection of the prostate. The primary effect is relaxation and opening of the urinary passageway.

Neutral sitz bath   Neutral sitz baths are more appropriate for situations of acute inflammation of the prostate. They are given at 92–9 °F (33–35 °C) for 15 minutes to two hours. It is necessary to provide adequate coverings during this period to avoid chilling.

Cold sitz bath   The cold sitz bath is used mainly for its toning effects once a cure has been established. The cold sitz bath is given immediately following a warm-to-hot sitz bath of 1–3 minutes, and lasts (at a temperature of 55–75 °F, 12.5–24 °C) from 30 seconds to 8 minutes. It is important to make certain that the water level of the hot bath on the body is at least 1 inch (2.5 cm) above the level of the cold water. This ensures adequate warming of the area, thereby preventing chilling. Friction rubs to the hips during the cold sitz bath promote an increased reaction.

Contrast sitz bath   The contrast sitz bath (alternating hot and cold) increases pelvic circulation and tone of the smooth muscles of the region dramatically. It is probably the most beneficial of the sitz baths, but it is also the most difficult to employ.

Contrast sitz baths are given in groups of three; that is, three alterations of hot to cold. Two separate tubs are necessary; the hot is at 105–15 °F (40.5–46 °C), the cold at 55–85 °F (12.5–29.5 °C), with the temperatures being dependent on the condition and the strength of the patient. A standard treatment would be 3 minutes hot and 30 seconds cold. The water level in the hot tub is set 1 inch (2.5 cm) higher than in the cold. Adequate draping is necessary to prevent chilling. As with all hydrotherapy treatments, always finish with the cold.

Treatment

Several factors are of critical importance in a prevention plan for benign prostatic hyperplasia.

- Adequate zinc intake and absorption are required for normal prostatic function and hormonal metabolism.
- Adequate vitamin B6 intake.
- Elimination or reduction in the amount of beer and other alcohol consumed.
- Maintain serum cholesterol below 220 mg/dl.
- Consume an adequate intake, i.e. the equivalent of 1 teaspoon daily, of essential fatty acids (linseed, evening primrose, soy, walnut or sunflower oil).

- Limit dietary and environmental exposure to pesticides and other environmental contaminants.

In addition to these general factors, if an individual is already experiencing symptoms of prostatic enlargement, it may be appropriate to supplement the diet with the compounds listed below. Hydrotherapy, in the form of sitz baths, is often extremely beneficial. Herbal therapy may also be indicated, with saw palmetto, ginseng and flower pollen being appropriate therapeutic herbs to use both preventatively and thera-peutically.

Nutritional supplements

The following supplements are examples of those commonly used in the treatment of BPH of naturopathic physicians. There are several formulas available commercially that contain these critical nutrients.

- Zinc (picolinate), 60 mg per day (maximum of 6 months).
- Pyridoxine (vitamin B6), 100–250 mg per day.
- Linseed oil (essential fatty acid source), 1 teaspoon twice daily.
- Glycine, 200 mg per day.
- Glutamic acid, 200 mg per day.
- Alanine, 200 mg per day.
- Pumpkin seeds, ¼ to ½ cup per day for zinc and essential fatty acid content.

Botanical medicines

- Saw palmetto berries:

  The dosage for the liposterolic extract of saw palmetto berries (containing 85-95 per cent fatty acids and sterols) is 160 mg twice daily. To achieve a similar dose using the crude berries would require a dose of at least 10 grams twice daily. Dosages for fluid extracts and tinctures would result in extremely large quantities of alcohol and therefore cannot be recommended.

- *Panax ginseng*:

  Dried root, 2 to 4 grams three times daily.

  Extracts, equivalent to 25 to 50 mg ginsenosides daily.

- Flower pollen extracts.

- Sharply bordered reddened rash or plaques covered with overlapping silvery scales.
- Characteristically involves the scalp, the extensor surfaces of extremities (the backs of the wrists, elbows, knees and ankles) and sites of repeated trauma.
- Family history in 50 per cent of cases.
- Nail involvement results in characteristic 'oil drop' stippling.
- Possible arthritis.

General considerations

Psoriasis is an extremely common skin disorder, with a rate of occurrence between 2–4 per cent of the population. Psoriasis affects few blacks, and is rare in Indians and blacks in tropical zones. The condition is caused by a pile-up of skin cells that have replicated too rapidly. The rate at which skin cells divide in psoriasis is roughly 1,000 times greater than in normal skin; this is simply too fast for the cells to be shed, so they accumulate, resulting in the characteristic silvery scale.

The basic defect lies within the skin cells themselves. The rate at which cells divide is controlled by a delicate balance between two internal control compounds – cyclic AMP and cyclic GMP. Increases in cyclic GMP are associated with increased cell proliferation; conversely, increased levels of cyclic AMP are associated with enhanced cell maturation and decreased cell proliferation. Both decreased cAMP and increased cGMP have been measured in the skin of individuals with psoriasis.[1,2] The result is excessive cell proliferation. Rebalancing the cyclic AMP:GMP ratio is a prime therapeutic goal.

Therapy

A number of factors appear to be responsible for psoriasis, including incomplete protein digestion, bowel toxaemia, impaired liver function, alcohol consumption and excessive consumption of animal fats. Each one of these factors will be briefly discussed below, followed by additional therapeutic considerations.

Protein digestion

If protein digestion is incomplete or if there is inadequate intestinal absorption of amino acids, bacteria can break down the amino acids into many toxic compounds. A group of toxic amino acids known as polyamines (e.g. putrescine, spermidine and cadaverine) have been shown to be increased in individuals with psoriasis. These compounds inhibit the formation of cyclic AMP and therefore contribute greatly to the excessive rate of cell proliferation.[3-5] Lowered skin and urinary levels of polyamines are associated with clinical improvement in psoriasis.[3]

Vitamin A and compounds in goldenseal (*Hydrastis canadensis*) inhibit the formation of polyamines and are therefore indicated in the treatment of psoriasis.[6,7] However, the best way to prevent the excessive formation of polyamine is to make sure protein digestion is complete. This may involve the supplemention of hydrochloric acid and/or pancreatic enzymes with meals. (See Chapter 5, Digestion, for more complete information on ways to enhance protein digestion.)

Bowel toxaemia

Those guidelines discussed in Chapter 3, Detoxification, are appropriate in psoriasis. A number of gut-derived toxins are implicated in the development of psoriasis, including endotoxins (cell wall components of certain bacteria), streptococcal products, *Candida albicans*, yeast compounds and IgE and IgA immune complexes.[8] These compounds lead to increases in cyclic GMP levels within skin cells, thereby increasing the rate of proliferation dramatically.[9] *Candida albicans* overgrowth in the intestines (chronic candidiasis) may play a major role in many patients (see Chapter 21, Candidiasis).

A diet low in dietary fibre is associated with increased levels of gut-derived toxins.[8] Dietary fibre is of critical importance in maintaining a healthy colon; many fibre components are able to bind to bowel toxins and promote their excretion in the faeces. It is therefore essential that the diet of an individual with psoriasis be rich in fruits and vegetables.

An aqueous extract of Honduran sarsaparilla has been found to be effective in psoriasis, particularly the more chronic, large plaque-forming variety.[10] This is apparently due to an ability to bind bacterial endotoxins.

The liver and psoriasis

Correcting abnormal liver function is of great benefit in the treatment of psoriasis.[11] The connection between the liver and psoriasis relates to one of the liver's basic tasks – filtering the blood. As mentioned above, psoriasis has been linked to several microbial byproducts. If the liver is overwhelmed by an increased number of these toxins, or if there is a decrease in the liver's ability to filter these toxins, the level of these compounds circulating in the blood will be increased and the psoriasis will get much worse.

Alcohol consumption is known to worsen psoriasis considerably.[12] Alcohol's negative effects are a result of increasing the absorption of toxins from the gut, along with impairing liver function. Alcohol intake must be eliminated in individuals with psoriasis.

Silymarin, the flavonoid component of milk thistle (*Silybum marianum*), has been reported to be of value in the treatment of psoriasis.[11] Presumably this is a result of its ability to improve liver function, inhibit inflammation and reduce excessive cellular proliferation.[13,14]

Nutritional considerations

The aqueous extract of bitter melon or balsam pear (*Momardica charantia*) is an inhibitor of guanylate cyclase (resulting in lower levels of cyclic GMP) and has been shown to inhibit rapid proliferation.[15] The amino acid cysteine also reduces cyclic GMP levels, and antioxidants suppress free radical-induced elevations in cyclic GMP.[16]

Zinc seems particularly indicated due to its anti-inflammatory effects and the fact that there is an increased serum copper:zinc ratio (both high copper and low zinc) in psoriatic patients.[17,18]

Insulin insensitivity is speculated in psoriasis, due to the increased serum levels of both insulin and glucose.[19] Chromium supplementation may be indicated to increase insulin receptor sensitivity.

Glutathione peroxidase (GP) levels are low in psoriatic patients, possibly due to such factors as alcohol abuse, malnutrition and the excessive skin loss of the hyperproliferative disease. The depressed levels of GP normalise with oral selenium and vitamin E therapy.[20]

Psoriatic patients improved on a fasting and vegetarian regime at a Swedish hospital where the effect of such diets on chronic inflammatory disease was being studied.[21] The improvement was probably due to decreased levels of gut-derived toxins and polyamines. Patients have also benefited from a gluten-free diet.[22]

Dietary oils   Dietary oils are extremely important in the management of psoriasis. Of particular benefit are the fish oils, specifically eicosapentaenoic acid (EPA). Several double-blind clinical studies have demonstrated that supplementing the diet with 10–12 grams of EPA results in significant improvement.[23-5] This would be equivalent to the amount of EPA in about 150 grams of mackerel or herring.

The improvement with EPA supplementation is largely due to inhibition of the production of inflammatory compounds. In the skin of individuals with psoriasis the production of inflammatory leukotrienes from arachidonic acid (oil found only in animal tissues) is many times greater than normal. It is therefore necessary to limit the intake of animal products, particularly animal fats and dairy products.

Psychological aspects

A high number (39 per cent) report a specific stressful event occurring within one month prior to their initial episode. Such patients have a better prognosis.[26] A few case histories have been reported which document the successful treatment of psoriasis with hypnosis and biofeedback.[27]

Physical therapeutics

Sunlight (ultraviolet light) is extremely beneficial for individuals with psoriasis. The standard medical treatment of psoriasis typically involves the use of the drug psoralen and ultraviolet A (PUVA therapy). However, ultraviolet B (UVB) exposure alone leads to inhibition of cell proliferation and has been shown to be as effective as PUVA therapy without the side effects.[28-31]

The induction of localised elevation of temperature (42–5 °C, 108–13 °F) to the affected area by ultrasound and heating pads has been shown to be an effective therapy in psoriasis.[32,33]

Treatment

Despite the complexity of this disease, the therapeutic approach is fairly straight-forward.

Diet

Limit sugar, meat, animal fats and alcohol. Increase fibre and cold-water fishes and, if necessary, bring weight to normal levels.

Supplements

- Folic acid, 0.5 mg a day.
- Vitamin A, 50,000 iu a day.
- Vitamin E, 400 iu a day.
- Selenium, 200 micrograms a day.
- Zinc (picolinate), 25 mg a day.
- Flaxseed oil, 1–2 tablespoons a day.
- Eicosapentaenoic acid – 1 tblsp cod liver oil a day or 10–12 grams EPA or 150 grams of mackerel, herring or salmon per day.

Botanical medicines

Doses three times a day.
- Bitter melon, balsam pear (*Momardica charantia*), 2–4 oz (50–100 g) fresh juice.
- *Sarsaparilla spp.*:
    Dried root or by decoction, 1–4 g.
    Liquid extract (1:1), 8–16 ml (2–4 tsp).
    Solid extract (4:1), 250–500 mg.
- Silymarin (from *Silybum marianum*), 70–210 mg.

Physical medicine

- Aerobic exercise, 30 minutes three times a week.
- Warm sunlight, 1 hour per day.

Psychological

If stress is a significant factor it is necessary to utilise stress reduction techniques.

Topical treatment

A number of natural proprietary formulas as well as over-the-counter drugs exist which can be used to provide symptomatic relief. Especially effective are those containing allantoin (from comfrey), glycyrrhetinic acid (from liquorice) and camomile extracts.

65

Rheumatoid arthritis

- Fatigue, low grade fever, weakness, joint stiffness and vague joint pain may proceed the appearance of painful, swollen joints by several weeks.
- Severe joint pain with much inflammation that begins in small joints, but progressively affects all joints in the body.

General considerations

Rheumatoid arthritis (RA) is a chronic inflammatory condition that affects the entire body, including the synovial membranes in the joints. The joints typically involved are the hands and feet, wrists, ankles and knees. Somewhere between 1 and 3 per cent of the population is affected, female patients outnumber males almost 3:1 and the usual age of onset is 20–40 years, although rheumatoid arthritis may begin at any age.[1,2] Standard medical treatment of RA involves the use of physical therapy along with drugs, the physical therapy including exercise, heat, cold, massage and the use of special equipment such as diathermy, lasers and paraffin baths.[1,2]

The first drug generally employed is aspirin. It is often quite effective in relieving both the pain and inflammation. It is also relatively inexpensive. However, since the therapeutic dose required is relatively high, toxicity often occurs; tinnitus (ringing in the ears) and gastric irritation are early manifestations of toxicity.[1,2]

Other non-steroidal anti-inflammatory drugs (NSAIDs) are often used as well, especially when aspirin is ineffective or is intolerable, the following being representative: ibuprofen (Motrin), fenoprofen (Fenopron), indomethacin (Indocid), naproxen (Naprosyn), tolmetin (Tolectin) and sulindac (Clinoril). While more expensive, none of the drugs have demonstrated superior efficacy than aspirin; in addition these drugs are also associated with side effects including gastrointestinal upset, headaches and dizziness.[1,2]

If conservative therapy does not offer benefit, more aggressive and potentially more toxic treatments are available. Gold salt injections aid about 60 per cent of patients, but severe side effects occurs in nearly one-third of patients. Other powerful drugs are used

492

including d-penicillamine and hydroxychloroquine, but benefit often does not substantiate toxicity. Corticosteroids are also used during acute worsenings of the disease. Long-term use of corticosteroids in RA is not advised due to side effects. Joint surgery and replacement are reserved for the most severe cases.[1,2]

Diagnosis

The onset of RA is usually gradual, but occasionally it is quite abrupt. Fatigue, low grade fever, weakness, joint stiffness and vague joint pain may proceed the appearance of painful, swollen joints by several weeks. Several joints are usually involved in the onset, typically in a symmetrical fashion, i.e. both hands, wrists or ankles. In about one-third of persons with RA, initial involvement is confined to one or a few joints.[1,2]

Involved joints will characteristically be quite warm, tender and swollen. The skin over the joint will take on a ruddy purplish hue. As the disease progresses joint deformities result in the hands and feet. Terms used to describe these deformities include swan neck, *boutonnière* and cockup toes.[1,2]

There are a variety of abnormal laboratory findings in RA including elevated erythrocyte sedimentation rate characteristic of inflammatory conditions, anaemia, serum protein abnormalities and antibodies to altered immunoglobulins. Examination of the joint fluid usually reflects the degree of inflammation. X-ray findings usually show soft tissue swelling, erosion of cartilage and joint space narrowing.[1,2]

Causes of rheumatoid arthritis

There is abundant evidence that RA is an autoimmune reaction, where antibodies develop against components of joint tissues. Yet what triggers this autoimmune reaction remains largely unknown. Speculation and investigation has centred around genetic susceptibility, lifestyle factors, nutritional factors, food allergies and micro-organisms.[1]

An interesting association between rheumatoid arthritis and abnormal bowel function exists that may provide a unified theory as to the cause of RA. What is currently known is that individuals with RA have increased intestinal permeability to dietary and bacterial antigens as well as alterations in bacterial flora.[3,4,5] This altered permeability and bacterial flora could result in the absorption of antigens that are very similar to antigens in joint tissues. Antibodies formed to bind these antigens would cross-react with the antigens in the joint tissues. Increasing evidence appears to support this concept.

Therapy

Diet

Diet has been strongly implicated in many forms of arthritis for many years, both in regards to cause and cure. Various practitioners have recommended all sorts of specific diets for arthritis. In general, since RA is not found in societies that eat a more 'primitive' diet and is found at a relative high rate in societies consuming the so-called western diet, a generally healthy diet rich in wholefoods, vegetables and fibre and low in sugar, meat, refined carbohydrate and saturated fat appears to be indicated in the prevention and possibly the treatment of RA. In addition, there appears to be strong scientific support for the roles that food allergies and dietary fats play in the inflammatory process.[6–14]

Food allergy

Elimination of allergic foods has been shown to offer significant benefit to some individuals with rheumatoid arthritis.[7,8,9] An elimination or hypoallergenic diet followed by systematic reintroduction is often an effective method of isolating offending foods (see Chapter 38, Food allergy, for more information). Virtually any food can result in aggravating RA, but the most common offending foods are wheat, corn, milk and other dairy products, beef and nightshade family foods (tomato, potato, eggplants, peppers and tobacco).

Dietary fats

Fatty acids are important mediators of inflammation through their ability to form prostaglandins, thromboxanes and leukotrienes. Manipulation of dietary oil intake can significantly increase or decrease inflammation, depending on the type of oil being increased.

Arachidonic acid is a fatty acid that is derived almost entirely from animal sources (meat, dairy products, etc.). It contributes greatly to the inflammatory process through its conversion to inflammatory prostaglandins and leukotrienes. Vegetarian diets are often beneficial in the treatment of inflammatory conditions, presumably as a result of decreasing the availability of arachidonic acid for conversion to inflammatory prostaglandins.[6,10,11,12]

Another important way of decreasing the inflammatory response is the consumption of coldwater fish such as mackerel, herring, sardines and salmon. These fish are rich sources of eicosapentaenoic acid (EPA) which competes with arachidonic acid for prostaglandin and leukotriene production. The net effect of consumption of these fish is a significantly reduced inflammatory/allergic response. In a double-blind study of patients with RA, it was shown that a diet rich in polyunsaturated fats and low in saturated fat supplemented daily with 1.8 grams of eicosapentaenoic acid (EPA) brought about significant improvement. Supplementation may not be necessary if a serving of one these coldwater fish is consumed at least once daily.[6,13,14,15] In another study, individuals with arthritis who supplemented their diets with cod liver oil showed major clinical improvement.[16] Cod liver oil may be a less expensive way of administering EPA.

Fasting

Patients with RA have benefited from fasting, although this should only be done under direct medical supervision. Fasting presumably decreases the absorption of allergenic food components, although it may also have an effect on the immune system.[17,18]

Nutritional considerations

EPA In a double-blind study of patients with RA, it was shown that a diet rich in polyunsaturated fats and low in saturated fat supplemented daily with 1.8 grams of eicosapentaenoic acid (EPA) brought about significant improvement.[13] Prostaglandins and leukotrienes formed from EPA are significantly less inflammatory than those prostaglandins and leukotrienes formed from arachidonic acid. Supplementing the diet with EPA appears warranted in the treatment of RA and other inflammatory conditions.[6,13,14,15]

Selenium Serum selenium levels are low in patients with RA.[19-21] This may be a significant factor, as selenium plays a valuable role as an antioxidant and serves as the mineral cofactor in the free radical scavenging enzyme glutathione peroxidase. This enzyme is also important in reducing the production of inflammatory prostaglandins and leukotrienes.

Free radicals, oxidants, prostaglandins and leukotrienes cause much of the damage to tissues seen in RA. A deficiency of selenium would result in even more significant damage. Clinical studies have not yet demonstrated clearly that selenium supplementation alone improves the signs and symptoms of RA; however, one clinical study indicated that selenium combined with vitamin E had a positive effect. Supplementation appears to be appropriate due to increased demand for selenium in RA and selenium's synergistic effect with other antioxidant mechanisms.

Vitamin E Vitamin E is an important antioxidant, working synergistically with glutathione peroxidase and other antioxidant enzymes (superoxide dismutase, catalase). Vitamin E also has a slight anti-inflammatory action due to its effect on prostaglandin and leukotriene synthesis. Vitamin E combined with selenium supplementation has been shown to improve RA[21,22]

Zinc Zinc is also an antioxidant and functions in the antioxidant enzyme superoxide dismutase (copper-zinc SOD). Zinc levels are typically reduced in patients with RA and several studies have been done using zinc sulphate in the treatment of RA, with some of the studies demonstrating a slight therapeutic effect. For these reasons, zinc supplementation appears to be indicated for individuals suffering from RA.[23,24,25]

Manganese Manganese also functions in the antioxidant enzyme superoxide dismutase (manganese SOD), which is deficient in patients with RA. Manganese supplementation has been shown to increase SOD activity indicating increased antioxidant activity. No trials have yet been done with manganese and RA, but supplementation appears to be indicated.[26,27]

Vitamin C Vitamin C functions as an important antioxidant. Supplementation with vitamin C increases SOD activity, decreases histamine levels and provides anti-inflammatory action.[28,29]

Betaine HCl   Many individuals with RA are deficient in stomach acid and other digestive factors. Supplementation with betaine HCl with meals will aid in protein digestion and possibly reduce food sensitivities through improved digestion.[30,31]

Proteolytic enzymes   Pancreatic enzyme preparations and the protein digesting enzyme of the pineapple, bromelain, have been demonstrated to be an effective anti-inflammatory agent in both clinical studies and experimental models.[32,33,34] Their major effects are to reduce swelling and help the body eliminate the immune complexes which can be deposited within the joints. For best results as anti-inflammatory agents, pancreatic enzymes and bromelain should be taken between meals.

Flavonoids   Several bioflavonoids have demonstrated effects in experimental studies that indicate that they may be beneficial to individuals with RA. Specifically, some flavonoids inhibit the release of histamine and the production of the potent inflammatory compounds, the leukotrienes.[35,36] For best results, flavonoids should be taken with pancreatic enzymes or bromelain between meals. A combination of the pancreatic enzymes chymotrypsin and trypsin, flavonoids and vitamin C has displayed a broader spectrum of action than the non-steroidal drugs like aspirin, indomethacin, phenylbutazone, etc.[37]

DLPA (D,L-phenylalanine   DLPA is a mixture of the natural form of phenylalanine (the L form) with its mirror image (the D form). The D form has been shown to be an effective pain reliever against the chronic pain of osteoarthritis, rheumatoid arthritis, low back pain and migraine headaches.[38] Its mode of action appears to inhibit the breakdown of endorphins, thereby increasing the effect of these components of the body's own pain relieving system. (Endorphins are morphine-like compounds that act as mild mood elevators and potent pain relievers.)

Niacinamide   Very good clinical results have been reported in the treatment of hundreds of patients with rheumatoid and osteoarthritis using high dose niacinamide (i.e. 900 to 4,000 mg in divided doses daily).[39,40] Niacinamide at this high dose can result in significant side effects (e.g. glucose intolerance and liver damage) and should therefore be instituted under strict medical supervision.

Tryptophan   Tryptophan is an amino acid that is often deficient in individuals with RA. It is the precursor to the neurotransmitter serotonin. One of serotonin's functions is to dampen the perception of pain. Tryptophan also increases endorphin activity. Tryptophan supplementation has been shown to reduce the level of pain in patients suffering from acute as well as chronic pain.[41,42] Best results are obtained if patients also consume a diet consisting of 80 per cent carbohydrate, 10 per cent protein and 10 per cent fat.

Copper   Copper aspirinate (salicylate) is a form of aspirin that yields better results in reducing pain and inflammation than standard aspirin preparations. These copper containing substances may be indicated in patients with RA requiring aspirin.[43,44]

The wearing of copper bracelets has been a long-time folk remedy which appears to have some scientific support, as found in a double-blind study performed in Australia. Presumably copper is absorbed through the skin and chelated to another compound which is able to exert anti-inflammatory action.[45]

Copper is a component, along with zinc, in one type of superoxide dismutase (copper-zinc SOD). Deficiency may result in significant susceptibility to free radical damage as a result of decreased SOD levels. However, an excess intake of copper may be detrimental due to copper's ability to combine with peroxides and damage joint tissues.[44,46]

Superoxide dismutase This antioxidant enzyme protects cells and tissues from free radical damage. The injectable form of this enzyme has been shown to be effective in the treatment of RA and osteoarthritis; however, it is not clear if any orally administered SOD can escape digestion in the intestinal tract and exert a therapeutic effect.[47,48] In one study, oral SOD was not shown to affect tissue SOD levels.

Botanical medicines

Many herbs possess significant anti-inflammatory action and are appropriate in the treatment of RA. The suggestions below represent some of the more effective of these herbs. Several are discussed in relation to their ability to enhance the function or secretion of the body's own cortisone as well as prevent or reverse some of the negative effects of orally administered cortisone.

Feverfew (Tanacetum parthenium) As feverfew has a long folk history in the treatment of fever, arthritis and migraine, it would be only natural to assume that feverfew acts in a similar fashion to aspirin. Researchers have actually shown extracts of feverfew to have greater activity in inhibiting inflammation and fever than aspirin in experimental studies.[49,50,51] They have specifically shown feverfew extracts to inhibit the synthesis of many pro-inflammatory compounds at their initial stage of synthesis. In addition, feverfew also decreases the secretion of inflammatory particles from platelets and white blood cells.

The net effect of feverfew's action is a significantly decreased inflammatory response. These experimental studies provide insight to the exact healing effect of feverfew in the treatment of arthritis.

Devil's claw (Harpagophytum procumbens) Devil's claw has been advocated in the treatment of a variety of diseases, including rheumatoid arthritis. Several pharmacological studies in animals and clinical trials in human beings have reported that devil's claw possesses an anti-inflammatory and analgesic effect comparable to the potent drug phenylbutazone.[52,53] However, other studies have indicated that devil's claw has little anti-inflammatory activity.[54,55] In addition to relieving joint pain in the positive clinical trials, serum cholesterol and uric acid were reduced.

Bilberries, cherries and hawthorn berries These berries are rich sources of flavonoid molecules, particularly proanthocyanidins, the flavonoids that give them their deep red/ blue colour. These flavonoids exhibit membrane and collagen stabilising, antioxidant, anti-inflammatory actions as well as many other actions that are very beneficial in the treatment of RA.[56,57,58] These berries or extracts of them should be consumed liberally.

Chinese thoroughwax (Bupleuri falcatum) Bupleuri root is an important component in various prescriptions in Chinese traditional medicine, particularly in remedies for inflammatory conditions. Recently these formulas have not only been used alone to relieve inflammation, but also in combination with corticosteroid drugs like prednisolone and prednisone.[59] Bupleuri has been shown to enhance the activity of glucocorticoids.

The active ingredients of bupleuri are steroid-like compounds known as saikosaponins. These compounds have diverse pharmacological activity including significant anti-inflammatory action.[59,60] The anti-inflammatory activity of the saikosaponins is related to an increase in the release of glucocorticoid hormones by the adrenal gland and a potentiation of their effects.

The release of glucocorticoids by the adrenal gland is stimulated by the pituitary hormone adrenocorticotropic hormone (ACTH). Bupleuri increases the release of glucocorticoids by increasing the pituitary release of ACTH.[61] This is very important, as ACTH increases the functional ability of the adrenal cortex. In contrast, when corticosteroid drugs are given, the adrenal glands get smaller and lose much activity. Saikosaponins have been shown to prevent adrenal gland atrophy caused by corticosteroid drugs. If an individual is on corticosteroid drugs, taking this formula along with their medication would be of great benefit.[59]

Bupleuri saikosaponins have other therapeutic activities including lowering cholesterol levels, preventing liver damage, improving liver functions in chronic hepatitis and mild sedative/pain relieving action.

Liquorice (Glycyrrhiza glabra) Liquorice appears to enhance the action of bupleuri and the two are almost always used together in traditional Chinese herbal formulas. Liquorice is used effectively in the treatment of Addison's disease, a condition of severe adrenal insufficiency. Liquorice also has significant anti-inflammatory and anti-allergy activity. Liquorice components are able to bind to glucocorticoid receptors on cells and exert glucocorticoid-like effects.[62,63,64]

Perhaps liquorice's major effect is its ability to inhibit the breakdown of adrenal hormones by the liver.[62,63] When used in combination with bupleuri, the net effect is increased corticosteroids in the circulation as a result of bupleuri promoting secretion of these hormones by the adrenal glands combined with liquorice's ability to inhibit the breakdown of these hormones by the liver.

Although liquorice enhances many actions of cortisol, there are several actions of cortisol that are inhibited by liquorice. Liquorice inhibits cortisol's ability to promote thymus atrophy, increase cholesterol levels, inhibit ACTH secretion and its effect on several different enzymes.[64]

Liquorice has been used historically in the treatment of inflammation, allergy, asthma and other conditions that put added stress on the adrenals.[62,63] Long-term use of liquorice is, however, contraindicated since it can cause an elevation of blood pressure.

Curcumin (Curcuma longa) Curcumin, the yellow pigment of *Curcuma longa* (turmeric), has significant anti-inflammatory action.[65,66,67] In animal studies it was discovered that curcumin was not as effective in animals that had their adrenal glands removed. Curcumin is thought to 'prime' or sensitise cellular receptor sites to the adrenal hormones, thereby potentiating adrenal hormone action. Curcumin has been shown to be as effective as cortisone or phenylbutazone in certain models of inflammation. Curcumin also exhibits many beneficial effects on liver functions.

Korean ginseng (Panax ginseng) Korean ginseng is referred to as an 'adaptogen.' Specifically, an adaptogen is an agent that:
- Protects against both mental and physical fatigue.
- Provides non-specific resistance against stress.
- Normalises an abnormal state caused by some excess or deficient physiological factor.[69]

Much of ginseng's 'adaptogenic' activity relates to its influence on the adrenal gland.

Ginseng components have been shown to increase the release of ACTH, thus causing an increase in the release of adrenal hormones as well.[68,69] It appears, based on extensive research, that gingseng acts through nervous system control mechanisms to adjust metabolic and functional systems that maintain homoeostasis during the challenge of stresses.[68,69] This is very similar to how a thermostat maintains temperature.

Like bupleuri, ginseng potentiates adrenal gland function and counteracts any shrinkage of the adrenal gland by the corticosteroid drugs which are often used in the treatment of rheumatoid arthritis.[68,69] Many of the historical uses of ginseng, particularly that as a tonic, relate to its ability to enhance adrenal gland function and improve reactions against a variety of stresses.

Siberian ginseng (Eleutherococcus senticosus) Like Korean ginseng, Siberian ginseng is also an adaptogen.[70,71] Generally regarded as an even more effective adaptogen by the Russians, Siberian ginseng has also been shown to protect against the effects of physical and mental stress.[70,71]

Siberian ginseng has been shown to improve the ability of humans to withstand extremely stressful conditions (heat, noise, motion, work load increase, exercise, decompression), to increase mental alertness and work output and to improve both the quality of work under stress and athletic performance.[70,71] Many of these effects are thought to be a result of improved adrenal function.

Chinese skullcap (Scutellaria baicalensis) Chinese skullcap has confirmed anti-arthritic and anti-inflammatory actions, similar in effect to the prescription drugs phenylbutazone and indomethacin.[72] However, while these drugs are associated with toxicity and adverse effects, Chinese skullcap does not appear to have any adverse effects at therapeutic levels.

Its therapeutic action appears to be related to its high content of flavonoid molecules.[73] These flavonoids inhibit the formation of compounds that are over 1,000 times more potent in their allergic and inflammatory effect than histamine. These flavonoids function similarly to the flavonoid drug sodium chromoglycate (Intal) which is used as an anti-asthmatic. In addition these flavonoids are extremely potent anti-oxidants and free-radical scavenging compounds.

Treatment

RA represents a disease known to have many contributing factors. Natural treatment involves reducing as many of these factors as possible. Foremost is the use of dietary measures known to reduce greatly the signs and symptoms of RA. Standard physical therapy measures are also quite important (i.e. exercise, heat, cold, massage, and the use of special physical therapy equipment such as diathermy, lasers and paraffin baths).

The following guidelines for diet, supplementation and herbal therapy are offered in summary.

Diet

The first step is using therapeutic fasting or an elimination diet (low in allergic foods), followed by careful reintroduction of foods and noting any symptom-producing foods. Virtually any food can result in aggravating RA, but the most common offending foods are wheat, corn, milk and other dairy products, beef and nightshade family foods (tomato, potato, eggplants, peppers and tobacco).

After isolating and eliminating all allergens, a generally healthy diet rich in whole-foods, vegetables and fibre and low in sugar, meat, refined carbohydrate and saturated fat is indicated. Special foods for the sufferer of RA include coldwater fish (mackerel, herring, sardines and salmon), cod liver oil and flavonoid rich berries or their extracts (cherries, hawthorn berries, bilberries, blackberries, etc.).

Supplements

The following are appropriate supplements to consume in the aggressive treatment of rheumatoid arthritis:
- EPA, 1.8 grams per day.
- Selenium, 200 micrograms per day.
- Vitamin E, 400 iu per day.
- Zinc, 45 mg per day.
- Manganese, 15 mg per day.
- Vitamin C, 1 to 3 grams per day in divided doses.
- Betaine HCl, 5 to 10 grains with meals.
- Pancreatin (10 × USP), 350 mg between meals, three times a day.
- Bromelain, 250 mg (2,000 mcu) between meals three times a day.
- Quercetin, 250 mg between meals three times a day.

- DLPA, 400 mg three times a day.
- Tryptophan, 400 mg three times a day.
- Copper, 1 mg per day.
- Niacinamide, 500 mg four times a day (under doctor's supervision).

Botanical medicines

Any of the herbs discussed above would be appropriate to use individually or in combination with other herbs in the treatment of RA. Your naturopathic physician can be invaluable in selecting the herb or formula best suited. Usually, the more severe the inflammation and joint destruction, the more aggressive the herbal therapy.

In individuals with a history of corticosteroid use (e.g. prednisone) or those desiring to reduce the dosage, it is necessary to utilise herbs which prevent and/or reverse the shrinking effect on the adrenal glands of these drugs (see Chapter 10, Stress). The following herbs possess a positive effect on the adrenal glands:

- *Bupleuri falcatum* (Chinese thoroughwax).
- *Glycyrrhiza glabra* (liquorice).
- *Curcuma longa* (turmeric).
- *Panax ginseng* (Korean ginseng).
- *Eleutherococcus senticosus* (Siberian ginseng).

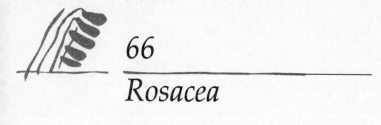

66

Rosacea

- Chronic acne-like eruption on the face of middle-aged and older adults associated with facial flushing.
- The primary involvement occurs over the flushed areas of the cheeks and nose.
- More common in women (3:1), but more severe in men.

General considerations

Rosacea is a relatively common skin disorder in adults between the ages of 30 and 50, with women being affected about three times as often as men.

Many factors have been suspected of causing acne rosacea – alcoholism, menopausal flushing, local infection, B-vitamin deficiencies and gastrointestinal disorders. Most cases are associated with moderate to severe seborrhoea (excess flow of sebum).

Therapy

Hypochlorhydria

Gastric analysis of rosacea patients has led to the postulate that it is the result of hypochlorhydria or reduced gastric acid output.[1] Psychological factors, i.e. worry, depression, stress, etc., often reduce gastric acidity.[2] Hydrochloric acid supplementation results in marked improvement in those rosacea patients who have insufficient hydrochloric acid secretion.[1,2] Rosacea patients have also been shown to have decreased secretion of the pancreatic enzyme lipase and to benefit from pancreatic supplementation.[3]

Food allergy

The high incidence of migraine headaches in individuals with rosacea points to food intolerance.

B-vitamins

The administration of large doses of B-vitamins has been shown to be quite effective in the treatment of rosacea,[4] with riboflavin appearing to be the key factor.[5] The mite *Demodex folliculorum* has been considered a causative factor; it is interesting to note that researchers were able to infect the skin of riboflavin deficient rats with demodex, but not the skin of normal rats.[5]

Treatment

Although the cause(s) has not yet been determined, sufficient information is available to treat most patients adequately. The control of hypochlorhydria and food intolerance forms the basis of therapy. This is supported with B-complex supplementation and the avoidance of vasodilating foods.

Diet

Avoid coffee, alcohol, hot beverages, spicy foods and any other food or drink that causes a flush.

Supplements

- B-complex vitamins, 100 mg a day (avoid niacin).
- Hydrochloric acid, as directed in Chapter 5, Digestion.
- Pancreatin (8 × USP), 1–2 tablets per meal.
- Ox-bile salts, 1 tablet per meal.

67

Seborrhoeic dermatitis

- Superficial reddened bumps and scaly eruptions occurring on the scalp, cheeks and skinfolds of the axilla (armpit), groin and neck.
- Usually non-itchy.
- Seasonal; worse in winter.

General considerations

Seborrhoeic dermatitis is a common condition that may be associated with excessive oiliness (seborrhoea) and dandruff. The scale of seborrhoea may be yellowish and either dry or greasy. The scaly bumps may coalesce to form large plaques or patches. Seborrhoeic dermatitis usually occurs either in infancy (usually between two and twelve weeks of age) or in the middle-aged or elderly and has a prognosis of lifelong recurrence.

Therapy

Food allergy

Seborrhoeic dermatitis usually begins as 'cradle cap' and, although not primarily an allergic disease, has been associated with food allergy (67 per cent develop some form of allergy by 10 years of age).[1]

Biotin

The underlying factor for seborrhoeic dermatitis in infants appears to be a biotin deficiency.[2] A syndrome clinically similar to seborrhoeic dermatitis has been produced by feeding rats a diet high in raw egg white (high in avidin, a protein that binds biotin, making it unavailable for absorption). Since a large portion of the human biotin supply is provided by intestinal bacteria, it has been postulated that the absence of normal intestinal flora may be responsible for biotin deficiency in infants.[2] A number of articles have demonstrated successful treatment of seborrhoeic dermatitis with biotin in both the nursing mother and the infant.[2,3]

In adults, treatment with biotin alone is usually of no value. It has been postulated that long chain fatty acid synthesis is impaired in seborrhoeic lesions. B-vitamins (biotin, pyridoxine, pantothenic acid, niacin and thiamin and the lipotropics) are vital for fatty acid metabolism.

Vitamin B6 (pyridoxine)

Both the administration of deoxypyridoxine, which induces pyridoxine deficiency in humans, and the placing of rats on a pyridoxine-deficient diet cause skin lesions indistinguishable from seborrhoeic dermatitis.[4] Despite these results, oral and topical applications of pyridoxine have shown little success. However, in the sicca form of the disorder (involvement of the scalp (dandruff), brow, nasolabial folds, and bearded area with varying degrees of greasy adherent scales on an erythematous base), all patients cleared completely within 10 days with local application of a water-soluble ointment containing 50 mg/g of pyridoxine. These results are clouded, however, by the results of another study which indicate that the improvement from topical application may be due more to reduction in sebaceous secretion rate from the ointment itself, the added pyridoxine having no effect.[5]

Folic acid and vitamin B12

Oral treatment with folic acid has been only moderately successful; patients with the sicca form were unresponsive.[6] Injections of vitamin B12, both synthetic and liver-extracted, have been shown to be very effective in many cases.[7]

Miscellaneous factors

Other B-vitamins have also been shown to be involved in seborrhoeic dermatitis; experimentally induced ariboflavinosis produces the sicca form of the disorder.[8]

Treatment

Although the optimal approach to treating all patients with seborrhoeic dermatitis is not clear at this time, effective therapy is available for most patients. In infants, alleviation of the biotin deficiency and control of the food allergies are the keys. For adults, correcting the impaired long chain fatty acid synthesis by supplementing with large doses of vitamin B-complex is the primary therapy. To maximise therapeutic results, we recommend a broad spectrum approach. (Note that the following dosages are for adults; children's doses should be modified according to weight.)

Diet

Detect and treat food allergens. In nursing infants, the food allergies of the mother should be considered.

Supplements

- Biotin, 3 mg two times a day.
- B-complex, 50 mg two times a day.
- Zinc (picolinate), 25 mg a day.
- Flaxseed oil, 1 tblsp a day.

Topical treatment

- Pyridoxine ointment, 50 mg/g in a water soluble base.

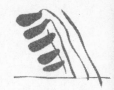

68

Sinus infection

- History of acute viral respiratory infection, dental infection or nasal allergy.
- Nasal congestion and discharge.
- Fever, chills and frontal headache.
- Pain, tenderness, redness and swelling over the involved sinus.
- Chronic infection may produce no symptoms other than mild postnasal discharge, a musty odour or a nonproductive cough.

General considerations

The most common predisposing factor in acute bacterial sinusitis is viral upper respiratory tract infection (e.g. the common cold). Allergies and other factors which interfere with normal protective mechanisms may precede the viral infection and therefore are also likely predisposing factors. Any factor which induces swelling and fluid retention of the mucous membranes of the sinuses may cause blockage of drainage; bacterial overgrowth then occurs, with streptococci, pneumococci, staphylococci and *Haemophilus influenzae* being most commonly cultured.

In chronic sinus infections (sinusitis) an allergic background is commonly present, and in 25 per cent of chronic maxillary sinusitis there is an underlying dental infection. Although antihistamines cause transient relief, their chronic use is not indicated since there is usually a reflex reaction following continual administration.

Treatment

In acute sinusitis the therapeutic goals are to establish drainage and clear up the acute infection. Various measures can be used – local application of heat, local use of volatile oils and botanicals with antibacterial properties, and immune system support (see Chapter 6, Immune support).

Since chronic sinusitis is associated with allergy, long-term control is dependent on isolation and elimination of the food or airborne allergens and correction of the underlying problem which allowed the allergy to develop (see Chapter 38, Food allergy, and Chapter 17, Asthma and hayfever). During the acute phase, elimination of the common food allergens (milk, wheat, eggs, citrus, corn and peanut butter) is indicated until a more definitive diagnosis can be made.

Local applications of heat have been shown to be very effective in alleviating both short- and long-term symptoms of allergic rhinitis.[1]

General measures in an acute infection

- Rest (bed rest better).
- Drink large amount of fluids (preferably diluted vegetable juices, soups and herb teas).
- Limit simple sugar consumption (including fruit sugars) to less than 50 grams a day.
- Elimination of the common food allergens (milk, wheat, eggs, citrus, corn and peanut butter).

Supplements

- Vitamin C, 500 mg every two hours.
- Bioflavonoids, 1 g per day.
- Vitamin A, 25,000 iu per day.
- Beta-carotene, 200,000 iu per day.
- Zinc lozenges, one lozenge containing 23 mg elemental zinc every two waking hours for one week. (Note: prolonged supplementation at this dose is not recommended as it may lead to immunosuppression.)
- Thymus extract, 500 mg twice daily.

Botanicals for acute infection

Hydrastis canadensis (goldenseal) is the most effective botanical for acute bacterial sinus infections. The therapeutic effect can be enhanced by combining it with 250–500 mg of bromelain, the proteolytic enzyme from pineapple. Take goldenseal in one of the forms below every two waking hours.

- Dried root (or as tea), 1 to 2 g.
- Freeze-dried root, 0.5 to 1 g.
- Tincture (1:5), 4 to 6 ml (1 to 1.5 tsp).
- Fluid extract (1:1), 0.5 to 2.0 ml (¼ to ½ tsp).
- Powdered solid extract (4:1), 250–500 mg.

Local treatment

- Intranasal douche with hydrastis tea.
- Swab passages with oil of bitter orange.

- Menthol or eucalyptus packs over sinuses.

Care should be taken to avoid irritation.

Physical therapy

- Local applications of hot packs.
- Diathermy for 30 minutes.

Discontinue if pain increases without drainage.

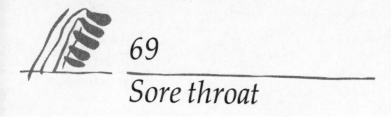

69

Sore throat

- Abrupt onset of sore throat, fever, malaise, nausea and headache.
- Throat red and swollen, with or without exudation.
- Tender lymph nodes along the neck.
- Group A streptococci on throat culture (strep throat).
- Throat culture negative for group A streptococci (usually viral pharyngitis).

General considerations

In adults, over 90 per cent of sore throats are viral in origin. None the less a throat culture is indicated since signs and symptoms of 'strep throat' are indistinguishable from a viral throat infection (viral pharyngitis), although it must be remembered that 10–25 per cent of the general population are carriers for group A streptococci.[1]

Strep throat and viral pharyngitis are usually self-limiting diseases, i.e. the individual does not require specific therapy. Controlled trials in individuals with strep throat showed clinical recovery in similar cases with and without use of antibiotics.[2] The 'streptophobia' associated with the risk of rheumatic fever and after-strep-throat glomerulonephritis (inflammation of the kidneys) is probably unwarranted today, although proper care is still important.[3]

Antibiotic administration does not reduce the incidence of after-strep-throat glomerulonephritis,[4] and the dramatic decrease in the incidence of rheumatic fever began before the advent of effective antibiotics.[5] Improved social and economic conditions, hygiene and nutritional factors were, as in most infectious diseases, more important than the liberal use of penicillin. The present attack rates after a streptococcal infection are 0.4 to 2.8 per cent for rheumatic fever and 0.2 to 20 per cent for glomerulonephritis. Obviously, such a wide range of reported sequelae makes accurate evaluation of the risk difficult.

The use of antibiotics should probably be reserved for those individuals with strep throat who are unresponsive to conservative therapy (i.e. no response after a week of therapy) and those with a prior history of rheumatic fever or glomerulonephritis. Even then, penicillin fails to eliminate the streptococci in over 20 per cent of patients.[6]

Therapy

The guidelines for enhancing the immune system, as presented in Chapter 6, Immune support, are particularly well indicated for both strep throat and viral pharyngitis, particularly the botanicals *Hydrastis canadensis* and *Echinacea angustifolia*.

Vitamin C

During the 1930s there was considerable interest in the relationship of malnutrition and the development of the sequelae of strep throat (i.e. rheumatoid arthritis and glomerulonephritis). Both experimental animal work and population surveys demonstrate a correlation between vitamin C deficiency and the development of sequelae. Rheumatic fever is virtually nonexistent in the tropics where vitamin C intake is higher, and 18 per cent of children in high risk groups have subnormal serum vitamin C levels.

Vitamin C supplementation of streptococcal-infected vitamin C-deficient guinea pigs totally prevents the development of rheumatic fever.[7,8] Uncontrolled clinical studies demonstrated very positive results when children were given orange juice supplementation. Unfortunately, this promising line of research appears to have been dropped, probably due to the advent of, supposedly effective, antibiotics.

Garlic

The antibacterial properties of *Allium sativum* have been recognised for centuries and are well documented in the literature.[9] In particular, the allicin fraction is an effective antimicrobial agent for streptococci.[10]

Goldenseal

Goldenseal (*Hydrastis canadensis*) is particularly indicated in strep throat due to its confirmed antibiotic activity against streptococcal bacteria.[11]

Treatment

The treatment of strep throat and viral pharyngitis involves the use of nutritional and botanical measures to support the body's immune system. (See Chapter 6, Immune support, for a complete approach to infection.)

General measures

- Rest (bed rest better).
- Drink large amounts of fluids (preferably diluted vegetable juices, soups and herb teas).
- Limit simple sugar consumption (including fruit sugars) to less than 50 grams a day.

Supplements

- Vitamin C, 500 mg every two hours.
- Bioflavonoids, 1 g per day.
- Vitamin A, 25,000 iu per day.
- Beta-carotene, 200,000 iu per day.
- Zinc lozenges, one lozenge containing 23 mg elemental zinc every two waking hours for one week. (Note: prolonged supplementation at this dose is not recommended as it may lead to immunosuppression.)
- Thymus extract, 500 mg twice daily.

Botanicals

Echinacea angustifolia and *Hydrastis canadensis* (goldenseal) can be taken at the following dosages (all doses three times a day).
- Dried root (or as tea), 1 to 2 g.
- Freeze-dried root, 0.5 to 1 g.
- Tincture (1:5), 4 to 6 ml (1 to 1.5 tsp).
- Fluid extract (1:1), 0.5 to 2.0 ml (¼ to ½ tsp).
- Powdered solid extract (4:1), 250–500 mg.

70

Tendinitis and bursitis

Tendinitis:

- Acute or chronic pain localised to a tendon.
- Insidiously developing local dull or draggy sensation after exercise.
- Limited range of motion.

Bursitis:

- Severe pain in the affected joint, particularly on movement.
- Limited range of motion.

General considerations

Tendinitis is an inflammatory condition of a tendon, usually resulting from a strain. Although acute tendinitis usually heals within a few days to two weeks, it may become chronic, in which case calcium salts will typically deposit along the tendon fibres. The tendons most commonly affected are the Achilles (back of ankle), the biceps (front of shoulder), the pollicis brevis and longus (thumb), the upper patella (knee), the posterior tibial (inside of foot) and the rotator cuff (shoulder).

Bursitis is inflammation of the bursa, the sac-like membrane which contains fluid which lubricates the joints. Bursitis may be secondary to trauma, strain, infection or arthritic conditions. The most common locations are shoulder, elbow, hip, seat and lower knee. Occasionally the bursa can develop calcified deposits and become a chronic problem.

Cause

The most common cause is sudden excessive tension on a tendon or bursa, although repeated trauma, such as from intense sports, can result in similar injury. Some tendinitis may have an anatomical basis, in that the grooves in which the tendons move may develop bone spurs or other mechanical abnormalities. Proper stretching and warming-up before exercise are important preventive measures.

Therapy

After an injury or sprain, immediate injury first-aid is very important. The acronym RICE summarises the approach:

- Rest the injured part as soon as it is hurt, to avoid further injury.
- Ice the area of pain to decrease swelling and bleeding.
- Compress the area with an elastic bandage, also to limit swelling and bleeding.
- Elevate the part above the level of the heart to increase drainage of fluids out of the injured area.

Proper application of these procedures is important for optimal results.

When icing, first cover the injury with a towel, then place an ice pack on it. It is important not to wrap the injured part so tightly that circulation is impaired. The ice and compress should be applied for 30 minutes, followed by 15 minutes without to allow recirculation. Of course, for any serious injury a physician should be consulted immediately; indications for a physician include severe pain, injuries to the joints, loss of function and pain which persist for more than two weeks.[1]

Nutritional considerations

Vitamin C   Ascorbic acid plays a major role in the prevention and repair of injuries. Deficiency of vitamin C is associated with defective formation and maintenance of collagen, ground substance and intercellular cement substance, all important for the formation of tendon and bursal tissues.[2]

Vitamin A   Vitamin A is necessary for collagen synthesis and wound healing.[3] Beta-carotene may be more advantageous, due to its potent antioxidant and anti-inflammatory activity and increased safety.[4]

Zinc   Zinc functions along with vitamin A in many metabolic processes. An increased copper-to-zinc ratio is found in individuals with chronic inflammatory conditions[5] Zinc functions relevant to tissue repair include stabilisation of membranes, antioxidant activity, collagen synthesis and inhibition of mast cell release of mediators in inflammation. Zinc supplementation is also known to reduce wound healing time significantly.[3,5]

Vitamin E and selenium   These two nutrients function synergistically in antioxidant mechanisms (thus quenching free radicals) and seem to potentiate each other's effect. Decreasing free radicals is important in the body's control of inflammatory processes. Decreased wound healing time is also found with vitamin E supplementation.[6]

Flavonoids   Flavonoids are extremely effective in reducing inflammation and stabilising collagen structures. Flavonoids help maintain a healthy collagen structure by:

- Decreasing membrane permeability, thereby decreasing the influx of inflammatory mediators.

- Preventing free radical damage with their potent antioxidant properties.
- Inhibiting enzymatic cleavage of collagen tissue.
- Inhibiting mast cell release of inflammatory chemicals.
- Cross-linking with collagen fibres to make them stronger.[7,8,9]

The more biologically active flavonoids, i.e. quercetin, citrus bioflavonoids, catechin, anthocyanidins and proanthocyanidins, should be used as rutin has very little collagen-stabilising effect.

Quercetin is particularly effective since it limits the release of histamine and other mediators of inflammation, has antioxidant activity, inhibits important inflammatory pathways, and limits the tissue destruction associated with injury.[7–10]

Double-blind placebo-controlled studies have shown that supplemental citrus bioflavonoids cut in half the time needed to recover from sports injuries.[11,12]

Vitamin B12 An uncontrolled study found that intramuscular injections of vitamin B12 (daily for the first week and then less frequently according to response) gave rapid relief of bursitis pain for most patients. Subsequent X-rays of those patients with calcific bursitis showed considerable reabsorption of the calcium deposits.[13]

Botanical medicines

*Turmeric (*Curcuma longa*)* Turmeric (also known as Indian saffron) has been used in the Indian and Chinese systems of medicine for the treatment of many forms of inflammation. Its efficacy is probably due to its well-documented anti-inflammatory properties and vitamin C content.[14] The volatile oil fraction has been demonstrated to possess anti-inflammatory activity in a variety of experimental models, where its effects were shown to be comparable to hydrocortisone and phenylbutazone.[15,16] These anti-inflammatory effects are believed due to anti-histamine activity in early inflammation.

Even more potent in acute inflammation is the yellow pigment of turmeric, curcumin.[17–19] Curcumin, or the alcoholic extract of the curcuma root, is used in several indigenous systems of medicine in the treatment of sprain and inflammation. This use seems to be substantiated by recent investigations where curcumin has been found as effective as cortisone or phenylbutazone in models of acute inflammation, but only half as effective in chronic models. While phenylbutazone is associated with significant toxicity (ulcer formation and decreased white cell levels), curcumin displays no significant toxicity.

The more potent sodium curcuminate is produced in a poultice made from turmeric mixed with slaked lime, an ancient household remedy for sprains, muscular pain and inflamed joints.[19]

Bromelain The proteolytic enzyme of *Ananas comosus* (pineapple) has well-documented efficacy in virtually all inflammatory conditions, regardless of cause. The effect of orally administered bromelain on the reduction of oedema, bruising, healing time and pain following various injuries and surgical procedures has been demonstrated in several clinical studies.[20–23]

Physical therapy

Transcutaneous electrical nerve stimulation   The use of transcutaneous electrical nerve stimulation (TENS) to control pain has been well documented. Patients with tendinitis have been found to respond well to TENS.[11]

Ultrasound   Ultrasound is a form of high frequency sound vibrations used to heat an area and increase its blood supply and lymphatic drainage. Although its usefulness during the acute stage (the first 24 to 48 hours) of an injury has not been definitively determined, it has well documented efficacy in the recovery and remobilisation phases. It is also particularly useful in the treatment of calcific bursitis and tendinitis and in the stretching and removal of the adhesions and contractures that can develop in tissues after injury.[24]

Treatment

Treatment of the muscle, joint, tendon or bursal damage caused by acute and chronic injuries involves two phases: inflammation inhibition and protection of the injured tissues, followed by remobilisation after the acute phase has resolved. For any serious injury, a physician should be consulted immediately. Indications for a physician include severe pain, injuries to the joints, loss of function and pain which persist for more than two weeks.

RICE

- Rest the injured part.
- Ice the area of pain.
- Compress the area with an elastic bandage.
- Elevate the part above the level of the heart.

The ice and compress should be applied for 30 minutes, followed by 15 minutes without to allow recirculation. After the acute inflammatory stage, gradually increasing range of motion exercises should be used to maintain and improve mobility and prevent adhesions and contractures.

Nutritional supplements

- Vitamin C, 3–5 g a day.
- Beta-carotene, 50,000 iu a day.
- Bioflavonoids, 500 mg three times a day.
- Vitamin E, 200 iu a day.
- Zinc (picolinate form), 15 mg a day.

Botanical medicines

- Curcumin (from turmeric), 250 to 500 mg between meals.
- Bromelain (2,000 mcu), 250 mg three times a day between meals.

Physical treatment

- TENS, if needed for pain control.
- Ultrasound, three times per week during the recovery phase and if adhesions or contractures develop.

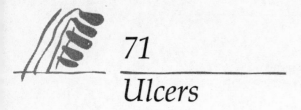

71

Ulcers

- Upper abdominal pain 45–60 minutes after meals or during the night. Pain is relieved by food, antacids or vomiting.
- Diagnosis confirmed by X-ray or fibre-optic examination.

General considerations

The terms ulcer, peptic ulcer and gastric ulcer are loosely used to refer to a group of ulcerative disorders of the upper gastrointestinal tract. The major forms of ulcer are chronic duodenal and gastric ulcer. Although duodenal and gastric ulcerations occur at different locations (see Fig. 71.1), they appear to be the result of similar mechanisms. Specifically, the development of a duodenal or gastric ulcer is generally thought to be the result of the digestive enzyme pepsin and stomach acids damaging the lining of the duodenum or stomach. Normally there are enough protective factors to prevent the ulcer formation; however, when there is a decrease in the integrity of these protective factors ulceration occurs.

Although symptoms of a peptic ulcer may be absent or quite vague, most often peptic ulcers are associated with abdominal discomfort noted 45–60 minutes after meals or during the night. In the typical case, the pain is described as gnawing, burning, cramplike or aching, or as 'heartburn'. Eating or using antacids usually results in great relief.

Current medical treatment of peptic ulcer focuses on reducing gastric acidity with antacids and/or histamine-2 receptor blockers like cimetidine and ranitidine which decrease stomach acid secretion. Though effective, these treatments are relatively expensive, carry some risk of toxicity, disrupt normal digestive processes, and alter the structure and function of the cells that line the digestive tract. The latter factor is responsible for an increase in the recurrence rate for peptic ulcers if the medications are discontinued. Cimetidine (trade name Tagamet) is currently the second most commonly prescribed drug. While cimetidine is effective in healing peptic ulcers, there is a higher relapse rate if maintenance treatment (usually 400 mg at bedtime) is discontinued than with any other anti-ulcer medication.[1]

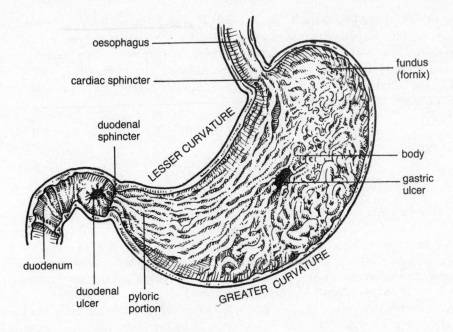

Figure 71.1   Sites of duodenal and gastric ulcers

Rather than focusing on eliminating stomach acid, an alternative approach appears to involve increasing the integrity of the lining of the stomach and duodenum. The principles of this approach are outlined in this chapter.

Description of ulcers

Duodenal ulcer   Duodenal ulcer is an extremely common condition. It is four times more common in men than in women and four to five times more common than clinically evident gastric ulcer. As a group, patients with duodenal ulcers have twice as many cells in their stomachs that secrete hydrochloric acid (parietal cells) than individuals without peptic ulcers. Many also secrete more acid than normal, although one-third to one-half of patients with duodenal ulcers have normal gastric acid secretory rates. The ulcers are usually less than 1 cm in diameter, with more than 95 per cent occurring in the first 5 cm of the duodenum.[2]

The clinical picture of duodenal ulcer is characterised by abdominal distress, typically occurring 45–60 minutes after a meal. The pain is relieved by food or antacids. The symptoms are chronic and periodic.

Gastric ulcer   The clinical picture in gastric ulcer is very similar to that in duodenal ulcer, although a greater number of gastric ulcer patients will be without symptoms and/or will have a less characteristic history. As acid secretion is normal or reduced in most patients, decreased tissue resistance plays a particularly important role in the development of this form of peptic ulcer. The use of alcohol, aspirin and other non-steroidal anti-inflammatory drugs (Motrin, Indocid, etc.), tobacco or coffee (both caffeinated and decaffeinated) is often the causative factor.[2] As mentioned earlier, gastric ulcers are not as common as duodenal ulcers.

Therapy

Nutritional factors

Food allergy   Strange as it may seem, clinical and experimental evidence points to food allergy as a prime causative factor in peptic ulcer.[3-6] The lesions of peptic ulcers and those caused by classic allergic reactions (e.g. the Arthus reaction) show the same microanatomical changes.[3] The association between allergy and peptic ulcer has been investigated in several studies; in one study, 98 per cent of patients with radiographic evidence of peptic ulcer had coexisting lower and upper respiratory tract allergic disease,[3] while in another, 25 of 43 allergic children had X-ray-diagnosed peptic ulcers.[6]

Clinically, an elimination diet has been used with great success in treating and preventing recurrent ulcers.[4,5] Food allergy is also consistent with the high recurrence rate of peptic ulcers. If food allergy is the cause, the ulcer will continue to recur until the food has been eliminated from the diet. It is ironic that many people with peptic ulcers soothe themselves by consuming inordinate amounts of milk, a highly allergic food.

Fibre   A diet rich in fibre is associated with a reduced rate of duodenal ulcers as compared with a low-fibre diet. The therapeutic use of a high-fibre diet in patients with recently healed duodenal ulcers reduces the recurrence rate by half.[7] This is probably a result of fibre's ability to promote mucin secretion and delay gastric emptying, counteracting the rapid movement of food into the duodenum normally seen in ulcer patients. If digestion of protein is not initiated in the stomach, the risk of developing an allergy to food proteins is very high.

Aspirin   Aspirin is a gastric irritant that damages the lining of the stomach and predisposes individuals to ulcer development when taken regularly. The combination of aspirin and smoking may be particularly harmful to the ulcer patient.[8]

Antacids   Many popular antacids should not be used by individuals with peptic ulcers. The calcium carbonate antacids (Tums, Alka-2, etc.) actually produce a rebound effect on gastric acid secretion and may cause kidney stones, while the sodium bicarbonate antacids (Rolaids, Alka-Seltzer, Bromo-Seltzer, etc.) have a tendency to induce systemic alkalosis and interfere with heart and kidney function.

The type of antacids typically used in the treatment of peptic ulcers are aluminium-magnesium compounds (Maalox, Mylanta, Digel, etc.) which may cause calcium and phophorus depletion as well as possibly causing aluminium toxicity or the accumulation of aluminium in the brain. Although antacids are currently the mainstay of peptic ulcer therapy, their use does pose certain risks.[2]

Miscellaneous nutritional factors   Vitamins A and E have been shown to inhibit the development of stress ulcers in rats and are important factors in maintaining the integrity of the lining of the digestive tract.[9,10] Zinc increases mucin production, and has been shown to have a protective effect on peptic ulcers in animals[11] and a positive effect in humans.[12]

Smoking

Another factor strongly linked to peptic ulcers is smoking. Increased frequency, decreased response to peptic ulcer therapy and an increased mortality due to peptic ulcer are all related to smoking. Three postulated mechanisms for this association are decreased pancreatic bicarbonate secretion (an important neutraliser of gastric acid), increased reflux of bile salts into the stomach and acceleration of gastric emptying into the duodenum.[2,11]

Bile salts are extremely irritating to the stomach and the initial portions of the duodenum; bile salts reflux induced by smoking therefore appears to be the most likely factor responsible for the increased peptic ulcer rate in smokers. However, the psychological aspects of smoking are also important, since the chronic anxiety and psychological stress associated with smoking appear to worsen ulcer activity.

Stress and emotional factors

Ulcer patients as a group have been characterised as tending to repress emotions. The idea that a specific personality trait (in this case the excessive wish for dependency) is responsible for the development of peptic ulcers was first popularised in the 1930s. A study in 1957 offered support for this approach by attempting to predict which individuals would develop gastric ulcers over a given period of time. Based on a battery of psychological tests, 10 out of 120 military recruits thought to have an 'oral dependent' psychic conflict (characterised by an excessive wish to be fed, loved and cared for, leading to feelings of shame, anger and guilt) were identified. Using radiographic analysis, 7 of the 10 recruits were shown either to have or to have developed an ulcer during the 12-week study.[13]

Stress is universally believed to be an important factor in the development of peptic ulcers. However, this belief is based on uncontrolled observations. In the medical literature the role of stress in the development of peptic ulcer is controversial, and every substantial attempt to examine this assumption has been fraught with methodological errors.[13]

This problem is further complicated by the observation that men and women with peptic ulcers appear to have distinctly different psychological profiles. In addition, several studies have shown that the number of stressful events is not significantly different in peptic ulcer patients as compared to carefully selected ulcer-free controls. This data suggests that it is not simply the amount of stress, but rather an individual's response to stress that is the significant factor. It is probable that psychological factors are important in some individuals with peptic ulcer disease, but not in others.

Botanical medicines

Many herbs and herbal formulas have been used over the years in the therapy of peptic ulcers. Due to the limited amount of space, only the special liquorice preparation of deglycyrrhizinated liquorice and Robert's formula will be discussed in this chapter. Herbal remedies for peptic ulcers share a similar effect in stimulating the body's own natural defences against ulceration. Specifically, natural compounds within the herbs are thought to stimulate the production and secretion of mucus compounds that coat the digestive tract and prevent tissue damage.

Liquorice (Glycyrrhiza glabra)   A constituent of liquorice, glycyrrhizinic acid, was the first compound proven to promote the healing of gastric and duodenal ulcers.[14] Its mode of action is different to the current medications used for the treatment of peptic ulcers. Rather than inhibiting the release of acid, liquorice stimulates the normal defence mechanisms that prevent ulcer formation. This includes increasing the number of mucus secreting cells, thereby increasing the amount of protective mucosubstances secreted, improving the quality of mucus produced, increasing the life-span of the surface intestinal cells and enhancing the microcirculation of the gastrointestinal tract lining.

Carbenoxolone, a derivative of glycyrrhizinic acid, has been marketed throughout the world for the treatment of both gastric and duodenal ulcers. It has been shown to normalise the disturbance in the structure and function of the intestinal cells caused by cimetidine and have a better effect in preventing ulcer recurrences.[15,16] Carbenoxolone has been associated with side effects, though, including oedema, hypertension and low potassium levels. However, due to the known side effects of carbenoxolone and glycyrrhizinic acid, a procedure was developed to remove glycyrrhizinic acid from liquorice to form deglycyrrhizinated liquorice (DGL). The result is a very successful anti-ulcer agent without any known side effects. This is quite interesting and provides further support for the idea that a herbal medicine is more than just an active ingredient enclosed in a natural base.

Numerous studies over the years have found DGL to be an effective anti-ulcer compound. Most of the clinical trials of DGL utilised a product called Caved-S, shown to be very effective in healing peptic ulcers. This form of DGL is supplied in a chewable tablet. It appears that DGL must mix with saliva in order to be effective, as another product, called Ulcedal, containing DGL in capsule form was generally ineffective. Ulcedal was subsequently removed from the market. DGL may promote the release of salivary compounds like urogastrone or epithelial cell growth factors which stimulate the growth and regeneration of stomach and intestinal cells.

DGL in gastric ulcer   Gastric ulcers are often a result of the use of alcohol, aspirin or other non-steroidal anti-inflammatory drugs, caffeine and other factors that decrease the integrity of the gastric lining. As DGL has been shown to reduce the gastric bleeding caused by aspirin, DGL is strongly indicated for the prevention of gastric ulcers in patients requiring long-term treatment with ulcerogenic drugs, such as aspirin, non-steroidal anti-inflammatory agents and corticosteroids.[17]

In one study of DGL in gastric ulcer there was a significantly greater reduction in ulcer size in the DGL group (78 per cent) than in the placebo group (34 per cent), and complete healing occurred in 44 per cent of those receiving DGL but in only 6 per cent of the placebo group.[18] In another study, DGL promoted healing as effectively as carbenoxolone.[19] DGL was also superior to antacids, with nearly twice as many patients showing complete healing after six weeks. This difference, however, was not statistically significant.

DGL has been shown to be as effective as cimetidine (Tagamet) for both short term treatment and maintenance therapy of gastric ulcer,[20] while in another study DGL was as effective as ranitidine (Zantac) in the treatment of gastric ulcer.[21]

DGL in duodenal ulcer   In one study, 40 patients with chronic duodenal ulcers of 4 to 12 years duration and more than six relapses during the previous year were treated with DGL.[22] All the patients had been referred for surgery because of relentless pain, sometimes with frequent vomiting, despite treatment with bed rest, antacids and anticholinergic drugs. Half of the patients received 3 grams of DGL daily for 8 weeks; the other half received 4.5 grams per day for 16 weeks. All 40 patients showed substantial improvement, usually within five to seven days, and none required surgery during the one year follow-up. Although both dosages were effective, the higher dose was significantly more effective than the lower dose.

In another study the therapeutic effect of DGL was compared to that of antacids, geranylferensylacetate or cimetidine in 874 patients with endoscopically confirmed chronic duodenal ulceration.[23] There was no significant difference in healing rate in the four groups. However, there were fewer relapses in the DGL group than in those receiving cimetidine, geranylferensylacetate or antacids. These results, coupled with DGL's protective effects, suggest that DGL may be a more advantageous treatment of duodenal ulcers.

Cabbage   Raw cabbage juice has been well documented as having remarkable success in treating peptic ulcers.[24,25] One litre per day of the fresh juice, taken in divided doses, resulted in total ulcer healing in an average of only 10 days. Further research has shown that the high glutamine content of the juice is probably responsible for the efficacy of cabbage in treating these ulcers.[26] Although the mechanism is not known, it may be due to the role of glutamine in the biosynthesis of the hexosamine moiety in certain mucoproteins. This could stimulate mucin synthesis which would benefit peptic ulcer patients greatly.

Modified Robert's formula   Although no research has been done to document its efficacy, an old naturopathic remedy, Robert's formula, has a long history of use in peptic ulcer. Legend has it that a sailor named Robert had a severe peptic ulcer and every time he visited a new port he would add a new plant remedy to his self-made formula. Eventually Robert healed his ulcer.

Robert's formula has undergone several revisions, and is described in some detail in Chapter 30, Crohn's disease and ulcerative colitis.

Treatment

Patients with any symptoms of a peptic ulcer need competent medical care. Peptic ulcer complications – haemorrhage, perforation and obstruction – represent medical emergencies that require immediate hospitalisation. Patients with peptic ulcer must be carefully evaluated to determine which of the above factors is most relevant to their health problem. The following general approach can be instituted in the majority of cases.

The first step is to identify and eliminate or reduce all factors implicated in the development of peptic ulcers – food allergy, cigarette smoking, stress and drugs, especially aspirin and other non-steroidal analgesics. Once the causative factors have been controlled and/or eliminated, attention should be directed at healing the ulcers and promoting tissue resistance. This includes eating a diet high in fibre and low in allergic foods, avoiding those factors known to promote ulcer formation such as smoking, alcohol, coffee and aspirin, and incorporating an effective stress reduction plan. Once this has been done it may be appropriate to supplement the diet with those nutrients which heal and prevent ulcer recurrences (vitamins A and E, and zinc). It also may be wise to use a deglycyrrhizinated liquorice preparation, cabbage juice or the modified Robert's formula to soothe the damaged digestive tract lining.

- Deglycyrrhizinated liquorice, two to four 380 mg tablets between, or 20 minutes before, meals. Dosage should be continued for 8 to 16 weeks, depending on the clinical response.
- Cabbage juice, 1 litre per day.
- Modified Robert's formula – the dosage for the formula below would be ¼ to ½ teaspoon or 1 to 2 capsules between meals (three times per day). Equal amounts of:
  American cranesbill (*Geranium maculatum*)
  Cabbage (*Brassica oleracea*)
  Marsh mallow (*Althaea officinalis*)
  Slippery elm (*Ulmus fulva*)
  Okra (*Hibiscus esculentus*)
  Echinacea angustifolia
  Goldenseal (*Hydrastis canadensis*)

72

Vaginitis[1]

- Increased volume of vaginal secretions.
- Abnormal colour, consistency or odor of vaginal secretions.
- Vulval and/or vaginal itching, burning or irritation.
- Painful urination and/or painful intercourse may be present.

General considerations

Vaginitis is one of the most common reasons for women to seek healthcare, accounting for approximately 7 per cent of all visits to gynaecologists[2]; a study reported that 72 per cent of young sexually active females had one or more forms of vaginitis.[3] Another study of 821 women found vaginal infections to be six times more common than urinary tract infections.[4] In fact, women with painful urination are more likely to have vaginitis than a urinary tract infection. Most women can distinguish between the internal painful urination of a urinary tract infection and the external pain felt when urine passes over inflamed labial tissues.[4]

In addition to causing physical discomfort and embarrassment, vaginitis may be a symptom of a more serious underlying problem such as chronic inflammation of the cervix or a sexually transmitted disease. If infectious in nature, the agent may cause an ascending infection of the genital tract, leading to endometritis, salpingitis and pelvic inflammatory disease. These may in turn lead to tubal scarring, infertility or ectopic pregnancies. Chronic vaginal infections without symptoms have been implicated in recurrent urinary tract infections by their action as a reservoir for the infectious agent.[5,6] In addition, evidence is accumulating which links some forms of vaginitis to cervical cellular abnormalities and increased risk of cervical dysplasia.

Some women are hesitant to mention symptoms of vaginitis to their doctors out of embarrassment, associating them with poor personal hygiene or venereal disease. Because of the relative frequency of occurrence, and the potential for serious consequences if untreated, all women should seek a physician's help if they have itching, vaginal discharge, painful urination or other symptoms of vaginitis.

Diagnosis

There are three general types of vaginitis – hormonal, irritant and infectious. Each is further divided into several specific subgroups based on cause. These are listed in the accompanying box.

Types of vaginitis

- Hormonal vaginitis
     Atrophic vaginitis
     Increased vaginal discharge
- Irritant vaginitis
     Chemical vaginitis
     Allergic vaginitis
     Traumatic vaginitis
     Foreign body vaginitis
- Infectious vaginitis
     Trichomonas vaginalis
     Candida albicans
     Non-specific vaginitis
     Gonorrhoea
     Herpes simplex
     Chlamydia trachomatis

Atrophic vaginitis This is primarily a problem of postmenopausal women and those whose ovaries have been surgically removed. The vaginal epithelium becomes thin due to the lack of oestrogenic stimulation, which may result in formation of adhesions, painful intercourse and increased susceptibility to infection. The most commonly reported symptoms are itching or burning and a thin watery discharge that may occasionally be blood-tinged. (NB: any vaginal bleeding in a post-menopausal woman requires a complete check-up to rule out the presence of cancer.)

Increased vaginal discharge When increased quantities of normal secretions exist in the absence of other symptomatology, the diagnosis of physiological vaginitis is often applied. This is inappropriate, since no inflammation actually exists. The increased discharge frequently reflects increased hormonal stimulation, such as occurs during pregnancy or at some stages of the menstrual cycle. It is primarily a diagnosis of exclusion after ruling out other causes. In most cases no further treatment is required. Over-zealous douching or washing will briefly alleviate symptoms, but may ultimately aggravate the situation by causing an irritant vaginitis.

Chemical vaginitis This type is due to the use of medications or hygiene products which directly irritate the delicate membranes of the vagina. A variant of this subgroup is allergic vaginitis, where the damage is elicited by an immunologic reaction to a product rather than direct toxic reaction.

Traumatic vaginitis   Injury caused by physical agents or sexual activity can cause vaginitis.

Foreign body vaginitis   A foul-smelling discharge may indicate the presence of a foreign body in the vagina – most commonly a forgotten tampon. Contraceptive devices, pessaries and a wide variety of other items may also be found upon examination.

Infectious vaginitis   Infectious vaginitis may be sexually transmitted or may arise from a disturbance to the ecology of the healthy vagina. Vaginal infections frequently involve common organisms found in the cervix and vagina of many healthy, asymptomatic women.[7] Factors influencing the vaginal environment include the pH, glycogen content, glucose level, the presence of other organisms (particularly lactobacilli), the natural flushing action of vaginal secretions, the presence of blood and the presence of antibodies and other compounds in the vaginal secretions. Many of these factors are, in turn, affected by the woman's internal milieu and general health.

Immune dysfunction will predispose a woman to increased infections, including vaginal infections. Depressed immunity may occur as a result of nutritional deficiencies, medications (e.g. steroids), pregnancy or serious illness. Other factors may predispose to infectious agents – diabetes mellitus, the wearing of synthetic underwear or tights (which tend to retain moisture) and a suspected but still unproven link between birth control pills and candida infections.[8]

Risk factors for sexually transmitted infections include increased numbers of sexual partners, unusual sexual practices and the type of birth control (barrier methods, e.g. condoms, reduce risk of infection).

Approximately 90 per cent of vulvovaginitis will be associated with one of three organisms – *Trichomonas vaginalis*, *Gardnerella vaginalis* or *Candida albicans*[9] The relative frequency of each form varies with the population studied, as well as with sexual activity levels. Less frequent causes of vaginitis include *Neisseria gonorrhoea*, *Herpes simplex* and chamydia. Each is described more fully below.

Trichomonas vaginalis   Trichomonas is a flagellated protozoan found in the lower urogenital tract of both men and women. Humans appear to be its only host, and sexual transmission appears to be its primary mode of dissemination. Trichomonas does not invade tissues and rarely causes serious complications. The most frequent symptom is an abnormal discharge associated with itching and burning. The discharge is frequently malodorous, greenish yellow and frothy.

Trichomonads grow optimally at an acid pH of 5.5 to 5.8[10–12] Thus, conditions which elevate the pH (make it alkaline), such as increased progesterone, will favour overgrowth of trichomonas. Conversely, a vaginal pH of 4.5 in a woman with vaginitis is suggestive of an agent other than trichomonas.

Candida albicans   Both the relative frequency and the toal incidence of candidal vaginitis have increased two and a half times since the late 1960s, paralleling a declining incidence of gonorrhoea and trichomonas.[8] Several factors have contributed to this increased incidence, chief among them being the increased use of antibiotics. The alterations antibiotics cause in both intestinal and vaginal ecology favour the growth of candida. One study found a 100 per cent correlation between genital and gastrointestinal candida cultures, leading to the suggestion that significant intestinal colonisation with candida may be the single most important predisposing factor in vulvovaginal candidiasis.[8,12] Steroids, oral contraceptives and the continuing increase in diabetes mellitus all contribute to the problem.

Candida is 10–20 times more frequent during pregnancy, due to the elevated vaginal pH, increased vaginal epithelial glycogen, elevated blood glucose and intermittent glycosuria. Yeast infections are three times more prevalent in women wearing tights than those wearing cotton underwear, because the synthetic fabric prevents drying of the area.[13] The predisposing factors for candidal vaginitis are summarised in the box.

Predisposing factors for candidal vaginitis

- Allergies
- Antibiotics
- Diabetes mellitus
- Elevated vaginal pH
- Gastrointestinal candidiasis
- Oral contraceptives
- Nylon tights
- Pregnancy
- Steroids

Most cases of recurrent candidal vaginitis are due either to autoinoculation from the gastrointestinal tract or failure to recognise and treat the presence of one or more predisposing factors. In extremely persistent cases, sexual partners may be a source of reinfection. Allergies have been reported to cause recurrent candidiasis, which resolves when the allergies are treated.[14]

The primary symptom of candidal vaginitis is vulval itching, which can be quite severe. This is associated with the presence of a thick, curdy or 'cottage cheese' discharge, which may reveal pinpoint bleeding when removed. The presence of such a discharge is strong evidence of a yeast infection, but its absence does not rule out candida.[3]

Non-specific vaginitis   This is defined as vaginitis not due to trichomonas, gonorrhoea or candida. Whereas itching is the predominant symptom of candidal vaginitis, the presence of a discharge and odour are the key to non-specific vaginitis (NSV). The odour is variously described as fishy, foul or rotten. The discharge is non-irritating, grey and homogeneous, and may occasionally be frothy, or even thick and pasty. The pH will be elevated to 5.0–5.5 in most cases, and there appears to be a correlation between elevated pH and the presence of odour.[15]

The organism most frequently cited as responsible for NSV is *Gardnerella vaginalis* (formerly called *Haemophilus vaginalis*). Although it is recovered from 95 per cent of women with NSV, gardnerella may also be recovered from 40 per cent of asymptomatic women.[2] When purified cultures of gardnerella were placed in the vaginas of 13 volunteers, 10 showed neither symptoms of vaginitis nor positive cultures. Two women showed positive cultures for two to three months but developed no symptoms, and the thirteenth volunteer developed signs of vaginitis.[16] Evidence continues to mount indicating that gardnerella is a secondary bacteria which prospers in the conditions of NSV, but that the responsible organism may be the anaerobic microorganisms found in the condition, or the combination of gardnerella and the vaginal anaerobes.[16–18]

Gonorrhoea   *Neisseria gonorrhoea* is an uncommon cause of vaginitis, responsible for less than 4 per cent of cases.[4] Gonococcal vaginitis is more common in young girls because the vaginal epithelium is thinner before puberty. During reproductive years, purulent cervicitis is the primary symptom. Spread of the infection frequently causes other symptoms such as urethritis, bartholinitis or salpingitis, which finally prompt the seeking of medical treatment. Gonorrhoea, either alone or in combination with other organisms, is cultured in 40 to 60 per cent of cases of pelvic inflammatory disease (PID), a major cause of infertility. Because of the potential for serious sequelae, and the fact that up to 80 per cent of gonorrhoeal infections in women are asymptomatic, all examinations for vaginitis should include a routine gonorrhoea culture.[4]

Herpes simplex   *Herpes simplex* infection is the most common cause of genital ulcers in the United States. Other causes to be ruled out include syphilis, chancroid, lympho-granuloma venereum and granuloma inguinale. (For a more thorough discussion see Chapter 45, *Herpes simplex*.)

Chlamydia trachomatis   *Chlamydia trachomatis* is an intracellular parasite which rarely causes vaginitis but is frequently found in association with other common infectious agents. With the availability of better culture techniques and antibody tests, chlamydia is now recognised as a major health problem in most western countries. Chlamydia infects 5 to 10 per cent of women and is usually asymptomatic until the development of complications such as cervicitis, salpingitis or urethritis. Certain populations have infection rates as high as 25 per cent.[19] Chlamydia is the organism most frequently recovered in cultures of women with pelvic inflammatory disease,[20] and tubal scarring appears to be more frequent after chlamydial infection than gonorrhoea. Thus, chlamydia may be far more important in causing infertility and ectopic pregnancy than has been previously recognised.

Chlamydial infection during pregnancy increases risk of prematurity and neonatal death. If a healthy baby is born to an infected woman, there is a 50 per cent chance it will develop chlamydial conjunctivitis and a 10 per cent chance of pneumonia.[19] Because of the considerable risks of untreated chlamydia, all women with vaginitis, particularly those who are also pregnant, should be tested.

Therapy

Dietary considerations

The internal environment of the vagina is a reflection of the condition of the entire body. Vaginal secretions are continuously released which affect, and are affected by, the microbial flora; these secretions contain water, nutrients, electrolytes and proteins; the quantity and character of these components is altered by hormonal and dietary factors. A generally healthy diet is recommended in all cases to assure availability of all nutrients in sufficient quantity to optimise the body's ability to respond to changing conditions. A well-balanced diet, low in fats, sugars and refined foods, is particularly important in cases due to infectious organisms, particularly candida.

A diet high in lysine-containing foods and low in arginine-containing foods will reduce the number and severity of herpetic outbreaks. However, many of the foods high in lysine are animal products which are also high in fats. A low-arginine diet combined with lysine supplements will ensure adequate levels of lysine without excessive intake of fats.

Nutritional considerations

Vitamin A and beta-carotene   Both of these nutrients are necessary for normal growth and integrity of epithelial tissues, such as the vaginal mucosa. Vitamin A is essential for adequate immune response and resistance to infection. Secretory IgA, a major factor in resistance to infection of the mucous membranes, is lower in vitamin A-deficient subjects.[21] Beta-carotene is a source of non-toxic vitamin A precursors. In addition, it has been shown to enhance immunologically active T cell numbers and to alter their ratios favourably.[22] (NB: excessive vitamin A can be toxic and teratogenic. This is of particular concern in women of reproductive age. If large doses of vitamin A are used, particular care should be paid to contraception.)

B Vitamins   B vitamins are needed for carbohydrate metabolism, protein catabolism (breakdown) and synthesis, cell replication and immune function. Vitamins B2 and B6 have been shown to have oestrogen-like effects and act synergistically with oestradiol. Vitamin B1 and pantothenic acid enhance the action of oestradiol, although they have no oestrogenic activity themselves.[23] This suggests that B vitamins may be of use in oestrogen deficiency conditions such as atrophic vaginitis, especially if combined with phytoestrogens.

Vitamin C and bioflavonoids   These nutrients are essential in any process related to immune function. Deficiency of vitamin C reduces the bacteria-destroying activity of white cells. Both vitamin C and bioflavonoids improve connective tissue integrity, thus reducing spread of infection. Both nutrients are also useful in reducing the frequency and severity of *Herpes simplex* outbreaks.[24–8]

Vitamin E   Lack of vitamin E depresses the immune response. Several experiments have shown increased resistance to chlamydial infection when subjects were supplemented with vitamin E. Vitamin E also regulates vitamin A metabolism in humans.[29] Vitamin E has beneficial effects upon many of the symptoms of menopause without the risks of oestrogen therapy; symptoms reported to be improved in various studies included hot flushes, vaginal atrophy, chills, headaches, vaginal infection rates and diabetic vulvolvaginitis. Vitamin E is thought to exert its effects in many of these hormonally related problems because it reduces the breakdown of progesterone.[30-7] Topical applications combined with oral doses appear to offer the best results.

Excessive vitamin E intake (above 1,200 iu per day) may, however, be immunosuppressive and may transiently elevate blood pressure. Thus, extra caution should be exercised in those with diabetes, hypoglycaemia, hypertension or heart disease.

Zinc Low levels of zinc are associated with depressed immunity and thymus gland function, both of which are corrected when zinc is replenished. Zinc is also essential for proper utilisation of vitamin A. Many otherwise well-nourished adults receive less than 50 per cent of the recommended daily amount of zinc from their diets and have one or more measurable signs of deficiency.[38-40]

Treatment with topical and oral zinc has been shown to reduce the duration and severity of herpes outbreaks. This effect may be due either to the effect of the zinc on production of prostaglandins, or to the direct antiviral activity of the zinc ion. High levels of zinc are also toxic to chlamydia and trichomonas and have been used successfully in cases which did not respond to antibiotic therapy.[45-5]

Lysine Oral supplementation with lysine has been shown to decrease the frequency and severity of herpes outbreaks but not necessarily to shorten healing time. The postulated mechanism of action is that the lysine becomes incorporated into the virus in place of arginine, resulting in an inactive virus. Lysine should be taken preventatively at low doses and at higher doses at the first sign of symptoms, which correspond to the time of greatest viral replication. Effectiveness is dose-related, and best results are obtained if combined with the low-arginine diet.[46,47]

Lithium Lithium ointments can be used for the topical treatment of *Herpes simplex* lesions. Lithium interferes with replication of the herpes virus, without affecting host cells. Lithium succinate (8 per cent solution) may be combined with zinc in a topical ointment, or it may be used alone.[48,49]

Botanical medicines

Liquorice (Glycyrrhiza glabra) Liquorice has anti-viral activity and has been used successfully in the treatment of herpes. The number and severity of recurrences may be reduced by repeated applications of the gel to active lesions.[50,51] The isoflavonoid compounds in liquorice are also reported to be effective against candida.[50]

Chlorophyll Chlorophyll is bacteriostatic and is soothing to inflamed mucous membranes. Water soluble chlorophyll may be added to douching solutions for symptomatic relief.[52,53,54]

Garlic (Allium sativum)   Garlic is antibacterial, antiviral and antifungal, and has even been shown to be effective against some antibiotic-resistant organisms. Garlic may be added to douching solutions or may be wrapped in gauze and placed as a tampon/suppository for most forms of infectious vaginitis.[55-9]

Goldenseal (Hydrastis canadensis) *and Oregon grape* (Berberis vulgaris)   Goldenseal and Oregon grape contain the alkaloid berberine, which has significant effects against many bacteria. Berberine enhances immune function when taken internally as a tea and offers symptomatic local relief when used in douching solutions, as it is soothing to inflamed mucous membranes.[60-3]

Oestrogenic plants   Atrophic vaginitis may be treated by the use of phytoestrogens. These compounds have a molecular structure similar to that of oestrogen and have an effect similar to, but weaker than, that of oestrogen. Phytoestrogenic plants include fennel, anise, ginseng, dong quai, alfalfa, red clover and liquorice. These plants may be used as teas, in salads or in capsules.[64-8]. The simultaneous advantage and disadvantage of phytoestrogens is that they lack the potency of synthetic oestrogens. Thus their benefits will be slower to be noticed, but they are also less likely to produce undesirable side effects.

Tea tree oil (Maleluca alternafolia)   An alcoholic extract of tea tree oil diluted to 1 per cent in water exerts a strong antibacterial and antifungal action. It has been shown to be effective in the treatment of trichomoniasis, candidiasis and cervicitis. Treatment consists of daily douching combined with saturated tampons used weekly. No adverse reactions were reported, and patients comment favourably on its soothing effect.[69]

Other agents

Lactobacillus acidophilus   These desirable bacteria are an integral component of the normal vaginal flora. Lactobacilli help to maintain a healthy vaginal ecology by preventing the overgrowth of less desirable species. They do this by the production of lactic acid, natural antibiotic substances and peroxides. In addition they compete with other bacteria for the utilisation of glucose. Whenever there is a disturbance of the vaginal flora, reestablishment of these organisms is important. This may be accomplished by the insertion of live lactobacillus-culture yogurt (careful reading of labels is important since most commercially available yogurts do not use lactobacilli), but a more efficient and less messy method is to insert one capsule of lactobacillus into the vagina twice daily for one to two weeks. Whenever antibiotics (particularly broad spectrum) are taken for any reason, regular use of lactobacillus will reduce the risk of complications, such as candida overgrowth.[2,70]

Iodine   Iodine used topically as a douche is effective against a wide range of organisms, including trichomonas, candida, chlamydia and non-specific vaginitis. Povidone-iodine (Betadine) has all the advantages of iodine without the disadvantages of stinging and staining; a study published in 1969 found povidone-iodine to be effective in treating 100 per cent of cases of candidal vaginitis, 80 per cent of trichomonas and 93 per cent of combination infections. A douching solution diluted to one part iodine in 100 parts water used twice daily for 14 days is effective against most organisms.[71-8] However, excessive use must be avoided since some iodine will be absorbed into the system and can cause suppression of thyroid function.

Boric acid   Capsules of boric acid inserted into the vagina have been used to treat candidiasis with success rates equal to or better than those of nystatin. This treatment offers an inexpensive, easily accessible therapy for vaginal yeast infections.[79,80]

Gentian violet   Swabbing the vagina with gentian violet has been called 'as close to a specific treatment for candida as exists'.[8]

Treatment

Since approximately 90 per cent of all vaginitis is due to candida, trichomonas or gardnerella infections, the following recommendations are primarily directed towards treatment of these organisms. Due to their infectious nature, immune support (through proper diet, nutritional supplementation and botanical medicines) is an important aspect of the therapy.

For general maintenance of health and immune competence, a high quality multivitamin and multimineral supplement will provide low-cost compensation for most dietary inadequacies. In addition, the following nutrients may be useful in one or more types of vaginitis.

Diet

For all causes of vaginitis a nutrient-dense diet is recommended. All refined foods and simple carbohydrates should be eliminated and fats kept to a minimum. If food allergies are suspected, they should be determined and eliminated.

Nutritional supplements

- Vitamin A 25,000 iu a day or beta-carotene, 200,000 iu a day.
- Vitamin C, 0.5–1 g every 4 hours.
- B-complex vitamins, a good balanced B-complex averaging 10 times the recommended daily allowance.
- Zinc (picolinate is best), 15 mg a day.
- Vitamin E, 200 iu a day of d-alpha-tocopherol.
- *Lactobacillus spp.*, ½ teaspoon twice daily.

Botanical medicines

Echinacea angustifolia and *Hydrastis canadensis* (goldenseal) can be taken at the following doses (doses three times a day):
- Dried root (or as tea), 1 to 2 g.
- Freeze-dried root, 0.5 to 1 g.
- Tincture (1:5), 4 to 6 ml (1 to 1.5 tsp).
- Fluid extract (1:1), 0.5 to 2.0 ml (¼ to ½ tsp).
- Powdered solid extract (4:1), 250–500 mg.

Topical treatment

Douches and saturated tampons are effective methods of achieving high concentrations of therapeutic agents in the vagina. The following agents are useful in treatment of the common forms of vaginitis. In general, only one of these agents should be used at once. The variety provides alternatives for use in resistant cases.
- Betadine – various gels, pessaries and fluids are available. A 1:100 dilution in a retention douche kills most organisms within 30 seconds.
- Boric acid caps, 600 mg placed in capsules and inserted into the vagina. NB: repeated use may cause irritation, and use for more than seven days may result in problems from systemic absorption.
- Garlic – chopped garlic may be added to any douching solution or a clove can be peeled, wrapped in gauze and then inserted as a vaginal suppository. If irritation results, remove immediately.
- Hydrastis tea, made of 2 tsp per cup of hot water, for douching.
- *Lactobacillus spp.*, ½ tsp in a cup of warm water.
- Liquorice – use the tea (2 tsp per cup) in douches or apply the gel locally.
- Lithium sulphate, 8 per cent solution applied topically.
- Tea tree oil, use a 1 per cent dilution as a douche, combined with insertion of a saturated tampon for 24 hours once a week. NB: repeated use may result in sensitivity in some women.
- White vinegar – this traditional naturopathic formula for treatment of vaginitis consists of 1–2 tablespoons of white vinegar and 2 tablespoons of green clay added to a pint of water and used as a douche.
- Zinc sulphate, one tablespoon of a 2 per cent solution in 1 pint of water may be used as a douche.

General recommendations
- In all cases of vaginitis, lactobacillus capsules or lactobacillus-culture yogurt should be used daily to reinoculate the vagina with these desirable organisms.
- Treatment failures may be due to incorrect diagnosis, reinfection, failure to treat predisposing factors or resistance to the treatment used.
- Sexual activity should be avoided during treatment to avoid reinfection and to reduce trauma to inflamed tissues. If this is not possible, at least ensure that condoms are used.

- In recurrent cases the sexual partner(s) should be treated.
- Cotton underwear, particularly for candidal vaginitis, should be worn.
- Early symptomatic relief of pruritis and burning is often possible with the use of warm sitz baths, either plain or with herbs or Epsom salts.
- In severe cases it is often helpful to cleanse the vagina thoroughly with a calendula succus-saturated cotton swab to remove the microbe-saturated discharge.

Specific recommendations

Candida   Due to the high correlation of vaginal candida with intestinal overgrowth of the same organism, it is suggested that the internal condition be treated simultaneously to prevent recurrences. Treatment of candida should continue for at least one full menstrual cycle. Some authors suggest therapy for another three to four months during the week preceding the menses.
- Betadyne, two times a day.
- Boric acid caps, inserted daily for 14 days.
- Liquorice, daily.

Trichomonas
- Betadyne, two times a day.
- Zinc sulphate, daily.
- Tea tree oil, daily.

Chlamydia
- Betadyne, daily.
- Zinc sulphate, daily.

Herpes
- Avoid arginine-rich foods.
- Lysine, 2 g a day maintenance dose, double during outbreak, increase if arginine-rich foods are consumed.
- Zinc sulphate, daily.
- Lithium sulphate, add to the zinc sulphate douching solution.

Non-specific vaginitis
- Betadyne, daily.
- Hydrastis, daily.

Atrophic vaginitis
- B-complex vitamins, 100 mg a day.
- Vitamin E, 400 iu a day.
- Topical vitamin E cream.
- Phytoestrogenic herbs.

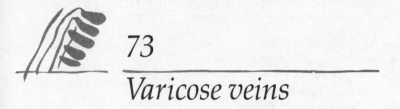

73

Varicose veins

- Dilated, tortuous, superficial veins in the legs.
- May be without symptoms or may be associated with fatigue, aching discomfort, feeling of heaviness or pain.
- Swelling, pigmentation and ulceration of the skin of the leg may develop.
- Women are affected four times as frequently as men.

General considerations

Veins are fairly frail structures. Defects in the wall of a vein lead to dilation of the vein and damage to the valves.[1] When the valves become damaged, the increased static pressure results in the bulging veins known as varicose veins.

Varicose veins affect nearly 50 per cent of middle-aged adults. The veins just under the skin of the legs are the veins most commonly affected, due to the tremendous strain that standing has on these veins. When an individual stands for long periods, the pressure exerted against the vein can increase by up to ten times. Hence, individuals with occupations that require long periods of standing are at greatest risk of developing varicose veins.

Women are affected about four times as frequently as men; obese individuals have a much greater risk; and the risk increases with age due to loss of tissue tone, loss of muscle mass and weakening of the walls of the veins. Pregnancy may also lead to the development of varicose veins, as pregnancy increases venous pressure in the legs.[2]

In general, varicose veins pose little harm if the involved vein is near the surface. These types of varicose veins are, however, cosmetically unappealing. Although significant symptoms are not common, the legs may feel heavy, tight and tired. A more serious form of varicose vein involves obstruction and valve defects of the deeper veins of the leg. This type of varicose vein can lead to problems such as thrombophlebitis, pulmonary embolism, myocardial infarction and stroke.

Cause of varicose veins

Several theories exist to explain the cause of varicose veins: genetic weakness of the veins or venous valves; excessive venous pressure due to a low-fibre induced increase in straining during defaecation; long periods of standing and/or heavy lifting; damage to the veins or venous valves secondary to thrombophlebitis; and weakness of the vascular walls due to either abnormalities in the protein structures that support the vein including the intercellular cement (ground substance), or excessive release of cellular enzymes which break down the ground substance, resulting in increased capillary permeability and loss of integrity of the venous structure.

Therapy

Dietary considerations

In contrast to the west, varicose veins are rarely seen in parts of the world where high-fibre unrefined diets are consumed.[3,4] A low-fibre diet, high in refined foods, contributes to the development of varicose veins. Individuals consuming a low-fibre diet tend to strain more during bowel movements, since their smaller and harder stools are more difficult to pass. This straining increases the pressure in the abdomen, which obstructs the flow of blood up the legs. The increased pressure may, over a period of time, significantly weaken the vein wall, leading to the formation of varicose veins or haemorrhoids, or may weaken the wall of the large intestine and produce diverticuli in the large intestine.[5]

A high-fibre diet is the most important component in the treatment and prevention of varicose veins (and haemorrhoids). A diet rich in vegetables, fruits, legumes and grains promotes peristalsis, and many fibre components attract water and form a gelatinous mass which keeps the faeces soft, bulky and easy to pass. The net effect of a high-fibre diet is significantly less straining during defaecation.

Bulking agents

Natural bulking compounds can also be used. These substances, particularly psyllium seed, oat bran and guar gum, possess mild laxative action due to their ability to attract water and form a gelatinous mass. This, as mentioned above, keeps the faeces soft and promotes peristalsis, significantly reducing straining during defaecation. These types of fibres are generally less irritating than wheat bran and other cellulose fibre products.

Physical measures

Exercise and the avoidance of standing for long periods of time will reduce the risk of development of varicose veins. Exercise, especially walking, riding a bike or jogging, is particularly beneficial, as the contraction of the leg muscles pushes pooled blood back into circulation.

Elastic compression stockings are occasionally beneficial. Surgical stripping of the vein can be performed in severe cases.

Botanical medicines

Centella asiatica When given orally, a purified extract of centella, containing the triterpenic acids, asiatic acid, madecassic acid and asiatoside, has demonstrated impressive clinical results in the treatment of venous insufficiency of the lower limbs and varicose veins.[6-10] Its effect in venous insufficiency and varicose veins appears to be related to its ability to enhance connective tissue structure, reduce sclerosis and improve the blood flow through the affected limbs.[6-10]

Several experimental studies have discovered that centella exerts a normalising action on the metabolism of connective tissue. Specifically, it possesses an ability to enhance connective tissue integrity by stimulating glycosaminoglycan synthesis.[7] Glycosaminoglycans are the major components of the amorphous intercellular matrix (ground substance) which surrounds the vein and helps give it structure.

*Horse chestnut (*Aesculus hippocastanum*)* Aescin is a compound isolated from the seeds of the *Aesculus hippocastanum,* which has a long folk history of use in the treatment of varicose veins and haemorrhoids.[11] It has anti-oedema and anti-inflammatory properties and decreases capillary permeability by reducing the number and size of the small pores of the capillary walls.[12,13] The reduction in capillary permeability and oedema appears to be due to inhibition of the lysosomal enzymes (mentioned above) which break down the ground substance.

Investigators have also demonstrated that aescin has venotonic activity.[14] A venotonic is a substance which improves venous tone by increasing the contractile potential of the elastic fibres in the vein wall. As mentioned earlier, relaxation of the venous wall contributes greatly to the development of varicose veins. Aescin's venotonic activity has been confirmed in clinical trials that demonstrate a positive effect in the treatment of varicose veins and thrombophlebitis.[12,15]

In the treatment of varicose veins, aescin can be given orally or an aescin/cholesterol complex can be applied topically. The topical formula is also of benefit in the treatment of bruises, due to aescin's ability to decrease capillary fragility and swelling.

*Butcher's broom (*Ruscus aculeatus*)* Butcher's broom is a subshrub of the lily family, and the rhizome from butcher's broom has a long history of use in treating venous disorders such as haemorrhoids and varicose veins.[16]

The active ingredients in butcher's broom are ruscogenins. These compounds have demonstrated a wide range of pharmacological actions, including anti-inflammatory and vasoconstrictor effects.[17,18] Butcher's broom extracts are used extensively, both internally and externally, in the treatment of varicose veins and haemorrhoids.

Flavonoid-rich extracts Since increasing the integrity of the wall of the vein may also reduce the risk of developing varicose veins, it appears that flavonoid-rich berries, such as hawthorn berries, cherries, bilberries and blackberries, are beneficial in the prevention and treatment of varicose veins. These bioflavonoids give the berries their blue-red colour.

The berries are very rich sources of proanthocyanidins and anthocyanidins.[19–21] Proanthocyanidins and anthocyanidins also improve the integrity of ground substance and the vascular system. Extracts of several of these berries are medications used widely for various circulatory conditions.[19–21] The efficacy of these extracts is related to their ability to:

- Reduce capillary fragility.
- Increase the integrity of the venous wall.
- Inhibit the breakdown of the compounds composing the ground substance.
- Increase the muscular tone of the vein.[19–21]

Consumption of these berries or of their extracts is indicated for individuals with varicose veins, as well as for those who wish to prevent them.

Bromelain and other fibrinolytic compounds   Individuals with varicose veins have a decreased ability to break down fibrin.[22] This is extremely important, as fibrin is deposited in the tissue near the varicose veins; the skin then becomes hard and 'lumpy' due to the presence of the fibrin and fat. In addition, decreased fibrinolytic activity increases the risk of thrombus formation, which may result in thrombophlebitis, myocardial infarction, pulmonary embolism or stroke.

Herbs that increase the fibrinolytic activity of the blood are therefore indicated. Capsicum (cayenne),[23] garlic,[24] onion[25] and ginger[26] all increase fibrin breakdown. Liberal consumption of these spices in foods is recommended for individuals with varicose veins and other disorders of the cardiovascular system.

The proteolytic enzyme from pineapple, bromelain, also appears indicated in the treatment of varicose veins. Vein walls are an important source of plasminogen activator, which promotes the breakdown of fibrin. Veins that have become varicosed have decreased levels of plasminogen activator. Bromelain acts in a similar manner to plasminogen activator to cause fibrin breakdown.[27] Bromelain may help prevent the development of the hard and lumpy skin (lipodermatosclerosis) found around varicosed veins.

Treatment

Varicose veins are extremely common in our society, largely due to dietary and lifestyle factors. The supplements and botanicals are recommended in order to strengthen the walls of the vein and increase fibrinolytic activity. To treat and reduce risk of varicose veins, it is important to:

- Consume a diet high in fibre.
- Exercise regularly.
- Avoid standing in one place for long periods of time (use elastic support stockings if standing is necessary).
- Avoid obesity.

- Employ measures which increase the integrity of the connective tissue and vein wall.
- Enhance fibrinolytic activity.

Diet

Indicated is a high-complex carbohydrate diet rich in dietary fibre. The diet should contain liberal amounts of proanthocyanidin- and anthocyanidin-rich foods, such as blackberries, cherries, bilberries, etc. Garlic, onions, ginger and cayenne should also be consumed liberally.

Supplements

- Vitamin A, 10,000 iu a day.
- Vitamin B-complex, 10–100 mg a day.
- Vitamin C, 0.5–3 g a day.
- Vitamin E, 200–600 iu a day.
- Bioflavonoids, 0.1–1 g a day.
- Zinc, 15–30 mg a day.

Botanical medicines

- *Aesculus hippocastanum,* horse chestnut:
    Bark of root, 500 mg three times a day.
    Aescin, 10 mg three times a day.
    An aescin/cholesterol complex may be applied topically in a 1 per cent concentration.
- *Centella asiatica,* gotu kola:
    Dried leaves, 2–4 grams daily.
    Tincture (1:5), 10–20 ml (1–2 tbsp) daily.
    Fluid extract (1:1), 2–4 ml (½–1 tsp) daily.
    The preferred form is a standardised extract containing asiaticoside (40 per cent), asiatic acid (29–30 per cent) and madecassoside (1–2 per cent), 60–120 mg daily.
- *Ruscus aculeatus* (butcher's broom) extract (9–11 per cent ruscogenin content), 100 mg three times daily.
- *Vaccinium myrtillus,* bilberry:
    Fresh berries, 2–4 oz three times a day.
    Extract containing 25 per cent anthocyanoside, 80–160 mg three times a day.
- Bromelain (minimum 1,500 mcu), 500–750 mg three times a day between meals.

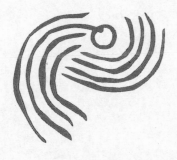

Appendices

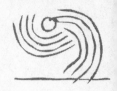

Glossary

abscess   A localised collection of pus and liquefied tissue in a cavity.

acetylcholine   One of the chemicals which transmits impulses between nerves and between nerves and muscle cells.

achlorhydria   Absence of hydrochloric acid in the stomach.

acute   Having a rapid onset, severe symptoms and a short course; not chronic.

adrenaline   Hormone secreted by the adrenal gland which produces the 'fight or flight' response. Also called epinephrine.

aldosterone   A hormone secreted by the adrenal gland which causes the retention of sodium and water.

alkaloids   A group of nitrogen-containing substances found in plants.

allopathy   A term that describes the conventional method of medicine which combats disease by using substances and techniques specifically against the disease.

amino acids   A group of nitrogen-containing chemical compounds which form the basic structural units of proteins.

amoebiasis   An intestinal infection characterised by severe diarrhoea caused by the parasite *Entamoeba histolytica*.

anaemia   A condition in which the oxygen-carrying pigment haemoglobin in the blood is below normal limits.

analgesic   A substance which reduces the sensation of pain.

androgen   Hormone which stimulates male characteristics.

anorexia   The medical term for loss of appetite.

anthocyanidin   A particular class of flavonoids which gives plants, fruits and flowers colours ranging from red to blue.

antibody   Protein manufactured by the body which binds to antigens to neutralise, inhibit or destroy them.

antidote   A substance which neutralises or counteracts the effects of a poison.

antigen   Any substance or microorganism that, when introduced into the body, causes the formation of antibodies against it.

antihypertensive   Blood-pressure lowering effect.

antioxidant   A compound which prevents free radical or oxidative damage.

anxiety   An unpleasant emotional state ranging from mild unease to intense fear.

artery   A blood vessel which carries oxygen-rich blood away from the heart.

atherosclerosis   A process in which fatty substances (cholesterol and triglycerides) are deposited in the walls of medium to large arteries, eventually leading to blockage of the artery.

atopy   A predisposition to various allergic conditions including eczema and asthma.

autoimmune   A process in which antibodies develop against the body's own tissues.

balm   A soothing or healing medicine applied to the skin.

basal metabolic rate   The rate of metabolism when the body is at rest.

basophil   A type of white blood cell which is involved in allergic reactions.

benign   A mild disorder that is usually not fatal.

beta-carotene   Pro-vitamin A. A plant carotene which can be converted to two vitamin A molecules.

beta cells   The cells in the pancreas which manufacture insulin.

bilirubin   The breakdown product of the haemoglobin molecule of red blood cells.

biofeedback   A technique for developing conscious control of various involuntary functions like heart rate, intestinal mobility and body temperature.

biopsy   A diagnostic test in which tissue or cells are removed from the body for examination under a microscope.

bleeding time   The time required for the cessation of bleeding from a small skin puncture as a result of platelet disintegration and blood vessel constriction. Ranges from 1 to 4 minutes.

blood-brain barrier   A barrier which prevents the passage of materials from the blood to the brain.

blood pressure   The force exerted by blood as it is pumped by the heart and presses against and attempts to stretch blood vessels.

bromelain   The protein digesting enzyme found in pineapple.

bursa   A sac or pouch which contains a special fluid which lubricates joints.

bursitis   Inflammation of a bursa.

Calorie   A unit of heat. A nutritional Calorie is the amount of heat necessary to raise 1 kg of water 1 °C.

Candida albicans   A yeast common to the intestinal tract.

candidiasis   A complex medical syndrome produced by a chronic overgrowth of the yeast *Candida albicans*.

carbohydrate   Sugars and starches.

carcinogen   Any agent or substance capable of causing cancer.

carcinogenesis   The development of cancer caused by the actions of certain chemicals, viruses and unknown factors on primarily normal cells.

cardiac output   The volume of blood pumped from the heart in 1 minute.

cardiopulmonary   Pertaining to the heart and lungs.

cardiotonic   A compound which tones and strengthens the heart.

carotene   Fat-soluble plant pigments, some of which can be converted into vitamin A by the body.

cartilage   A type of connective tissue which acts as a shock absorber at joint interfaces.

cathartic   A substance which stimulates the movement of the bowels, more powerful than a laxative.

cholagogue   A compound which stimulates the contraction of the gallbladder.

cholecystitis   Inflammation of the gallbladder.

cholelithiasis   Gallstones.

choleretic   A compound which promotes the flow of bile.

cholestasis   The stagnation of bile within the liver.

cholinergic   Pertaining to the parasympathetic portion of the autonomic nervous system and the release of acetylcholine as a transmitter substance.

chronic   Long-term or frequently recurring.

cirrhosis   A severe disease of the liver characterised by the replacement of liver cells with scar tissue.

coenzyme   A necessary non-protein component of an enzyme, usually a vitamin or mineral.

cold sore   A small skin blister anywhere around the mouth caused by the *Herpes simplex* virus.

colic   Severe, spasmodic pain that occurs in waves of increasing intensity, reaches a peak, then abates for a short time before returning.

colitis   Inflammation of the colon which is usually associated with diarrhoea with blood and mucus.

collagen   The protein which is the main component of connective tissue.

compress   A pad of linen applied under pressure to an area of skin and held in place.

congestive heart failure   Chronic disease that results when the heart is not capable of supplying the oxygen demands of the body.

connective tissue   The type of tissue which performs the function of providing support, structure and cellular cement to the body.

contagious   A disease which can be transferred from one person to another by direct contact.

coronary artery disease   A condition when the heart receives an inadequate blood and oxygen supply due to atherosclerosis.

corticosteroid drugs   A group of drugs similar to the natural corticosteroid hormones which are used predominantly in the treatment of inflammation and to suppress the immune system.

corticosteroid hormones   A group of hormones produced by the adrenal glands that control the body's use of nutrients and the excretion of salts and water in the urine.

cyst   An abnormal lump or swelling, filled with fluid or semisolid material, in any body organ or tissue.

cystitis   Inflammation of the inner lining of the bladder. It is usually caused by a bacterial infection.

dehydration   Excessive loss of water from the body.

dementia   Senility. Loss of mental function.

demineralisation   Loss of minerals from the bone.

dermatitis   Inflammation of the skin, sometimes due to allergy.

dialysis   A technique using sophisticated machinery to remove waste products from the blood and excess fluid from the body in the treatment of kidney failure.

diastolic   The second number in a blood pressure reading. It is the measure of the pressure in the arteries during the relaxation phase of the heart beat.

disaccharide   A sugar composed of two monosaccharide units.

diuretic   A compound which causes increased urination.

diverticuli   Saclike outpouchings of the wall of the colon.

double-blind study   A way of controlling against experimental bias by ensuring that neither the researcher nor the subject know when an active agent or placebo is being used.

douche   Introduction of water and/or a cleansing agent into the vagina with the aid of a bag with a tubing and nozzle attached.

dysfunction   Abnormal function.

dysplasia   Any abnormality of growth.

eicosapentaenoic acid (EPA)   A fatty acid found primarily in cold-water fish.

electrocardiogram (ECG)   Machine which measures and records the activity of the heart.

electroencephalogram (EEG)   A machine which measures and records brain waves.

elimination diet   A diet which eliminates allergic foods.

emulsify   The dispersement of large globules into smaller uniformly distributed particles. Usually refers to fat globules.

encephalitis   Inflammation of the brain, usually due to viral infection.

endometrium   The membrane lining the uterus.

enteric-coated   A special way of coating a tablet or capsule to ensure that it does not dissolve in the stomach and so can reach the intestinal tract.

enzyme   An organic catalyst which speeds chemical reactions.

epidemiology   The study of disease as it affects a particular population.

epithelium   The cells that cover the entire surface of the body and that line most of the internal organs.

Epstein-Barr virus   The virus which causes infectious mononucleosis and is associated with Burkitt's lymphoma and nasopharyngeal cancer.

essential fatty acid (EFA)   Fatty acids which the body cannot manufacture – linoleic and linolenic acids.

excretion   The elimination of waste products from a cell, tissue or the entire body.

extracellular   The space outside the cell, composed of fluid.

exudate   Escaping fluid or semifluid material that oozes from a space that may contain serum, pus and cellular debris.

faruncle   Another name for a boil that involves a hair follicle.

fibrin   A white insoluble protein formed by the clotting of blood which serves as the starting point for wound repair and scar formation.

fibrinolysis   The dissolution of fibrin or a blood clot by the action of enzymes which convert insoluble fibrin into soluble particles.

flavonoid   Plant pigments which exert a wide variety of physiological effects in the human body.

free radicals   Highly reactive molecules that can bind to and destroy cellular compounds.

giardiasis   An infection of the small intestine caused by the protozoan (single-celled) *Giardia lamblia*.

gingivitis   Inflammation of the gums.

glaucoma   A condition in which the pressure of the fluid in the eye is so high it causes damage.

glucose   A monosaccharide which is found in the blood and is one of the body's primary energy sources.

gluten   One of the proteins in wheat and certain other grains that gives dough its tough, elastic character.

goblet cell   A goblet-shaped cell which secretes mucus.

ground substance   The thick, gel-like material in which the cells, fibres and blood capillaries of cartilage, bone and connective tissue are embedded.

haemorrhoids   Distended veins in the lining of the anus.

helper T cell   White blood cells which help in the immune response.

hepatic   Pertaining to the liver.

hepatomegaly   Enlargement of the liver.

holistic medicine   A form of therapy aimed at treating the whole person, not just the part or parts in which symptoms occur.

hormone   A secretion of an endocrine gland that controls and regulates functions in other parts of the body.

hyperglycaemia   High blood sugar level.

hyperlipidaemic   Elevation of cholesterol and triglycerides in the blood.

hypersecretion   Excessive secretion.

hypertension   High blood pressure.

hypochlorhydria   Insufficient gastric acid output.

hypoglycaemia   Low blood sugar.

hypotension   Low blood pressure.

hypoxia   An inadequate supply of oxygen.

iatrogenic   Meaning literally 'physician produced', the term can be applied to any medical condition, disease or other adverse occurrence that results from medical treatment.

idiopathic   Of unknown cause.

immunoglobulins   Antibodies

incidence   The number of new cases of a disease that occurs during a given period (usually years) in a defined population.

incontinence   The inability to control urination or defaecation.

infarction   Death of a localised area of tissue due to lack of oxygen supply.

insulin   A hormone secreted by the pancreas which lowers blood sugar levels.

interferon   A potent immune enhancing substance that is produced by the body's cells.

jaundice   A condition caused by elevation of bilirubin in the body and characterised by yellowing of the skin.

keratin   An insoluble protein found in hair, skin and nails.

lactase   An enzyme which breaks down lactose into the monosaccharides glucose and galactose.

lactose   One of the sugars present in milk. It is a disaccharide.

lesion   Any localised, abnormal change in tissue formation.

lethargy   A feeling of tiredness, drowsiness or lack of energy.

leucocyte   White blood cell.

leucoplakia   A precancerous lesion usually seen in the mouth that is characterised by a white coloured patch.

leukotrienes   Inflammatory compounds produced when oxygen interacts with polyunsaturated fatty acids.

lipid   Fat, phospholipid, steroid or prostaglandin.

lipotropic   Promoting the flow of lipids to and from the liver.

lymph   Fluid contained in lymphatic vessels which flows through the lymphatic system to be returned to the blood.

lymphocyte   A type of white blood cell found primarily in lymph nodes.

malabsorption   Impaired absorption of nutrients, most often due to diarrhoea.

malaise   A vague feeling of being sick or of physical discomfort.

malignant   A term used to describe a condition that tends to worsen and eventually causes death.

manipulation   As a therapy, the skilful use of the hands to move a part of the body or a specific joint or muscle.

mast cell   A cell found in many tissues of the body which contributes greatly to allergic and inflammatory processes by secreting histamine and other inflammatory chemicals.

menorrhagia   Excessive loss of blood during periods.

metabolism   A collective term for all the chemical processes that take place in the body.

metabolite   A product of a chemical reaction.

metalloenzyme   An enzyme which contains a metal at its active site.

microbe   A popular term for microorganism.

microflora   The microbial inhabitants of a particular region, e.g. colon.

mites   Small, eight-legged animals, less than one twentieth of an inch (1.2 mm) long, similar to tiny spiders.

molecule   The smallest complete unit of a substance that can exist independently and still retain the characteristic properties of the substance.

monoclonal antibodies   Genetically engineered antibodies specific for one particular antigen.

monosaccharide   A simple one-unit sugar like fructose and glucose.

mortality rate   The number of deaths per 100,000 of the population per year.

mucosa   Another term for mucous membrane.

mucous membrane   The soft, pink, tissue which lines most of the cavities and tubes in the body, including the respiratory tract, gastrointestinal tract, genitourinary tract and eyelids. The mucous membranes secrete mucus.

mucus   The slick, slimy fluid secreted by the mucous membranes which acts as a lubricant and mechanical protector of the mucous membranes.

mycotoxins   Toxins from yeast and fungi.

myelin sheath   A white fatty substance which surrounds nerve cells and aids in nerve-impulse transmission.

neoplasia   A medical term for a tumour formation, characterised by a progressive, abnormal replication of cells.

neurofibrillary tangles   Clusters of degenerated nerves.

neurotransmitters   Substances which modify or transmit nerve impulses.

night blindness   The inability to see well in dim light or at night.

nocturia   The disturbance of a person's sleep at night by the need to pass urine.

oedema   Accumulation of fluid in tissues, causing swelling.

oestrogen   Hormone which affects female characteristics.

oligoantigenic diet   Elimination diet.

pancreatin   A product obtained from the pancreas of pigs which contains a potent concentration of digestive enzymes.

papain   The protein digesting enzyme of papaya.

pathogen   Any agent, particularly a microorganism, that causes disease.

pathogenesis   The process by which a disease originates and develops, particularly the cellular and physiologic processes.

peristalsis   Successive muscular contractions of the intestines which move food through the gastrointestinal tract.

physiology   The study of the functioning of the body, including the physical and chemical processes of its cells, tissues, organs and systems.

physostigmine   A drug which blocks the breakdown of acetylcholine.

phytoestrogen   Plant compound which exerts oestrogen-like effects.

picolinic acid   An amino acid secreted by the pancreas that facilitates zinc absorption and transport. Forms picolinates.

piles   A common name for haemorrhoids.

placebo   An inert or inactive substance used to test the efficacy of another substance.

polysaccharide   A molecule composed of many sugar molecules linked together.

prostaglandin   Hormone-like compounds manufactured from essential fatty acids.

psychosomatic   Pertaining to the relationship between the mind and body. Commonly used to refer to those physiological disorders thought to be caused entirely or partly by psychological factors.

putrefaction   The process of breaking down protein compounds by rotting.

RDA   Recommended dietary allowance.

saccharide   A sugar molecule.

satiety   A feeling of fullness or gratification.

saturated fat   A fat whose carbon atoms are bonded to the maximum number of hydrogen atoms; found in animal products like meat, milk, milk products and eggs.

sclerosis   The process of hardening or scarring.

senile dementia   Mental deterioration associated with aging.

slow reacting substance of anaphylaxis (SRSA)   A potent allergic mediator produced and released by mast cells.

submucosa   The tissue just below the mucous membrane.

suppressor T cell   Lymphocytes controlled by the thymus gland which suppress the immune response.

syndrome   A group of signs and symptoms that occur together in a pattern characteristic of a particular disease or abnormal condition.

systolic   The first number in a blood pressure reading. The pressure in the arteries during the contraction phase of the heart beat.

T cell   A lymphocyte which is under the control of the thymus gland.

tonic   A substance which exerts a gentle strengthening effect on the body.

trans-fatty acid   The type of fat found in margarine.

uraemia   The retention of urine by the body and the presence of high levels of urine components in the blood.

urinalysis   The analysis of urine.

vasoconstriction   The constriction of blood vessels.

vitamin   An essential compound necessary to act as a catalyst in normal processes of the body.

western diet   A diet characteristic of western societies, i.e. high in fat, refined carbohydrate and processed foods, and low in dietary fibre.

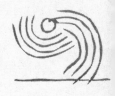

References

1 What is natural medicine?

1. Orr, J., Wilson, K., Bodiford, C. *et al.*, 'Nutritional status of patients with untreated cervical cancer, II. Vitamin assessment', *Am.J.Ob.Gyn.*, 1985, 151, pp. 632–5.
2. Dawson, E., Nosovitch, J. and Hannigan, E., 'Serum vitamin and selenium changes in cervical dysplasia', *Fed.Proc.*, 1984, 46, p. 612.
3. Krupp, M.A. and Chatton, M.J., *Current Medical Diagnosis and Treatment*, Lange Medical Publishing, Los Altos, CA, 1984, p. 199.
4. Pizzorno, J.E. and Murray, M.A., *A Textbook of Natural Medicine*, John Bastyr College Publications, Seattle, WA, 1988, p. VI: HyprTn-1-7.
5. Rafsky, H.A. and Weingarten, M., 'A study of the gastric secretory response in the aged', *Gastroent.*, 1946, May, pp. 348–52.
6. Davies, D. and James, T.G., 'An investigation into the gastric secretion of a hundred persons over the age of sixty', *Br.Med.J.*, 1930, i, pp. 1–14.
7. Hunt, J. and Johnson, C., 'Relation between gastric secretion of acid and urinary excretion of calcium after oral supplements of calcium', *Dig.Dis.Sci.*, 1983, 28, pp. 417–21.
8. Lust, B., *Universal Naturopathic Director and Buyer's Guide*, American Naturopathic Association, 1918.
9. Cody, G., 'History of naturopathic medicine', in Pizzorno, J.E. and Murray, M.A., *A Textbook of Natural Medicine*, John Bastyr College Publications, Seattle, WA, 1985, p. I:HistNM-1-24.
10. Clarke, E., Hatcher, J., McKeown-Essyen, G. and Liekrish, G., 'Cervical dysplasia: association with sexual behaviour, smoking, and oral contraceptive use', *Am.J.Ob.Gyn.*, 1985, 151, pp. 612–16.
11. Van Niekerk, W., 'Cervical cytological abnormalities caused by folic acid deficiency', *Acta Cytol.*, 1966, 10, pp. 67–73.
12. Romney, S., Duttagupta, C., Basu, J., *et al.*, 'Plasma vitamin C and uterine dysplasia', *Am.J.Ob.Gyn.*, 1985, 151, pp. 978–80.
13. Ramaswamy, P. and Natarajan, R., 'Vitamin B6 status in patients with cancer of the uterine cervix', *Nutr.Cancer*, 1984, 6, pp. 176–80.
14. Pizzorno, J.E. and Murray, M.A., *op.cit.*, p. A:VagPac-1-2.
15. Meneely, G. and Battarbee, 'High sodium–low potassium environment and hypertension', *Am.J.Card.*, 1976, 38, pp. 768–81.
16. Fries, E., 'Salt, volume and the prevention of hypertension', *Circ.*, 1976, 53, pp. 589–95.
17. Khaw, K.T. and Barrett-Connor, 'Dietary potassium and blood pressure in a population', *Am.J.Clin.Nutr.*, 1984, 39, pp. 963–8.
18. McCarron, D., Morris, C. and Cole, C., 'Dietary calcium in human hypertension', *Science*, 1982, 217, pp. 267–9.
19. Belizan, J., Villar, J., Pineda, O. *et al.*, 'Reduction of blood pressure with calcium supplementation in young adults', *J.A.M.A.*, 1983, 249, pp. 1,161–15.
20. Resnick, L.M., Gupta, R.K. and Laragh, J.H., 'Intracellular free magnesium in erythrocytes of essential hypertension: relationship to blood pressure and serum divalent cations', *Proc. Natl. Acad. Sci.*, 1984, 81, pp. 6,511–15.
21. Dyckner, T. and Wester, O., 'Effect of magnesium on blood pressure', *Br.Med.J.*, 1983, 286, pp. 1,847–9.
22. Vergroesen, A., Fleischman, A., Comberg,H., *et al.*, 'The influence of increased dietary linoleate on essential hypertension in man', *Acta Biol.Med.Germ.Band.*,1978, 37, pp. 879–83.
23. Rao, R., Rao, U. and Srikantia, S., 'Effect of polyunsaturated vegetable oils on blood pressure in essential hypertension', *Clin.Exp.Hypertension*, 1981, 3, pp. 27–38.
24. Yoshioka, M., Matsushita, T. and Chuman, Y., 'Inverse association of serum ascorbic acid level and blood pressure on rate of hypertension in male adults aged 30–39 years', *Int.J.Vit.Nutr.Res.*, 1984, 54, pp. 343–7.
25. Hodges, R. and Rebello, T., 'Carbohydrates and blood pressure', *Ann.Int.Med.*, 1983, 98, pp. 838–41.
26. Lang, T., Degoulet, P., Aime, F., *et al*, 'Relationship between coffee drinking and blood pressure: analysis of 6,321 subjects in the Paris region', *Am.J.Card.*, 1983, 52, pp. 1,238–42.
27. Gruchow, H.W., Sobocinski, M.S. and Barboriak, J.J., 'Alcohol, nutrient intake and hypertension in US adults', *J.A.M.A.*, 1985, 253, pp. 1,567–70.
28. Kershbaum, A., Pappajohn, D., Bellet, S., *et al*, 'Effect of smoking and nicotine on adrenocortical secretion', *J.A.M.A.*, 1968, 203, pp. 113–16.
29. Havlik, R., Hubert, H., Fabsitz, R. and Feinleib, M., 'Weight and hypertension', *Ann.Int.Med.*, 1983, 98, pp. 855–9.
30. Ford, M., 'Biofeedback treatment for headaches, Raynaud's disease, essential hypertension and irritable bowel syndrome: a review of the long term follow-up literature', *Biof.Self-Reg.*, 1982, 7, pp. 521–35.
31. Henry, H.J., McCarron, D.A., Morris, C.D. and Parrott-Garcia, M., 'Increasing calcium intake lowers blood pressure: the literature reviewed', *J.Am.Diet.Assoc.*, 1985, 85, pp. 182–5.

32   Glauser, S., Bello, C. and Glauser, E., 'Blood-cadmium levels in normotensive and untreated hypertensive humans', *Lancet*, 1976, i, pp. 717–18.

33   Foushee, D., Ruffin, J. and Banerjee, U., 'Garlic as a natural agent for the treatment of hypertension: a preliminary report', *Cytobios*, 1982, 34, pp. 145–52.

34   Petkov, V., 'Plants with hypotensive, antiatheromatous and coronary dilating action', *A.J.Chinese Med.*, 1979, 7, pp. 197–236.

35   *ibid.*

36   Pizzorno, J. and Murray, M. *op.cit.*, p. VI:HyprTn-5.

37   Fahim, M., Fahim, Z., Der, R. and Harman, J., 'Zinc treatment for the reduction of hyperplasia of the prostate', *Fed.Proc.*, 1976, 35, p. 361.

38   Boyd, E.M. and Berry, N.E., 'Prostatic hypertrophy as part of a generalised metabolic disease. Evidence of the presence of lipopenia', *J.Urol.*, 1939, 41, pp. 406–11.

39   Burkitt, D. and Trowell, H., *Western Diseases: Their Emergence and Prevention*, Harvard University Press, Cambridge, MA, 1981.

40   Steinberg, M., 'Chromium deficiency and the glucose tolerance factor', *J.John Bastyr Coll.Nat.Med.*, 1976, 1, pp. 32–6.

41   Offenbacher, E. and Stunyer, F., 'Beneficial effects of chromium-rich yeast on glucose tolerance and blood lipids in elderly patients', *Diabetes*, 1980, 26, pp. 919–25.

42   Coggeshall, J.C., Heggers, J.P., Robson, M.C. and Baker, H., 'Biotin status and plasma glucose in diabetics', *Ann.NY.Acad.Sci.*, 1986, 447, pp. 389–92.

43   Pizzorno, J. and Murray, M., *op.cit.*, p. VI:DiabMe-1-17.

2 Basic principles of health

1   Ross, C.E. and Hayes, D., 'Exercise and psychologic well-being in the community', *Am.J.Epidemiology*, 1988, 127, pp. 762–71.

3 Detoxification and heavy metal elimination

1   Passwater, R.A. and Cranton, E.M., *Trace Elements, Hair Analysis and Nutrition*, Keats, New Canaan, CT, 1983.

2   Rutter, M. and Russell-Jones, R.(eds), *Lead versus Health: Sources and Effects of Low Level Lead Exposure*, John Wiley, New York, NY, 1983.

3   Yost, K.J., 'Cadmium, the environment and human health: an overview', *Experentia*, 1984, 40, pp. 157–64.

4   Gerstner, B.G. and Huff, J.E., 'Clinical toxicology of mercury', *J.Toxicol.Environ.Health*, 1977, 2, pp. 471–526.

5   Nation, J.R., Hare, M.F., Baker, D.M., *et al.*, 'Dietary administration of nickel: effects on behaviour and metallothionein levels', *Physiol.Behavior*, 1985, 34, pp. 349–53.

6   Editorial, 'Toxicologic consequences of oral aluminum', *Nutrition Reviews*, 1987, 45, pp. 72–4.

7   Marlowe, M., Coissairt, A., Welch,K. and Errera, J., 'Hair mineral content as a predictor of learning disabilities', *J.Learn Disabil.*, 1977, 17, pp. 418–21.

8   Pihl, R. and Parkes, M., 'Hair element content in learning disabled children', *Science*, 1977, 198, pp. 204–6.

9   David, O., Clark, J. and Voeller, K., 'Lead and hyperactivity', *Lancet*, 1972, ii, pp. 900–3.

10   David, O., Hoffman, S. and Sverd, J. 'Lead and hyperactivity. Behavioral response to chelation: a pilot study', *Am.J.Psychiatry*, 1976, 133, pp. 1,155–88.

11   Benignus, V., Otto, D., Muller, K. and Seipple, K., 'Effects of age and body lead burden on CNS function in young children. EEG spectra', *EEG and Clin.Neurophys.*, 1981, 52, pp. 240–8.

12   Rimland, B. and Larson, G., 'Hair mineral analysis and behaviour: an analysis of 51 studies', *J.Learn.Disabil.*, 1983, 16, pp. 279–85.

13   Flora, S.J.S., Jain, V.K., Behari, J.R. and Tandon, S.K., 'Protective role of trace metals in lead intoxication', *Toxicology Letters*, 1982, 13, pp. 51–6.

14   Hsu, H.S., Krook, L., Pond, W.G. and Duncan, J.R., 'Interaction of dietary calcium with toxic levels of lead and zinc in pigs', *J.Nutrit.*, 1975, 105, pp. 112–68.

15   Petering, H.G., 'Some observations on the interaction of zinc, copper and iron metabolism in lead and cadmium toxicity', *Environ.Health Perspect.*, 1978, 25, pp. 141–5.

16   Papaioannou, R., Sohler, A. and Pfeiffer, C.C., 'Reduction of blood lead levels in battery workers by zinc and vitamin C', *J.Orthomol.Psychiatry*, 1978, 7, pp. 94–106.

17   Flora, S.J.S., Singh, S. and Tandon, S.K., 'Role of selenium in protection against lead intoxication', *Acta Pharmacol.et Toxicol.*, 1983, 53, pp. 28–32.

18   Tandon, S.K., Flora, S.J.S. Behari, J.R. and Ashquin, M., 'Vitamin B complex in treatment of cadmium intoxication', *Annals Clin.Lab.Sci.*, 1984, 14, pp. 487–92.

19   Bratton, G.R., Zmudzki, J., Bell, M.C. and Warnock, L.G., 'Thiamin (vitamin B1) effects on lead intoxication and deposition of lead in tissue. Therapeutic potential', *Toxicol.Appl.Pharmacol.*, 1981, 59, pp. 164–72.

20   Flora, S.J.S., Singh, S. and Tandon, S.K., 'Prevention of lead intoxication by vitamin B complex', *Z.Ges.Hyg.*, 1984, 30, pp. 409–11.

21   Ballatori, N. and Clarkson, T.W., 'Dependence of biliary excretion of inorganic mercury on the biliary transport of glutathione', *Biochem.Pharmacol.*, 1984, 33, pp. 1,093–8.

22   Murakami, M. and Webb, M.A., 'A morphological and biochemical study of the effects of L-cysteine on the renal uptake and nephrotoxicity of cadmium', *Br.J.Exp.Pathol.*, 1981, 62, pp. 115–30.

23   Cha, C.W., 'A study on the effect of garlic to the heavy metal poisoning of rat', *J.Korean Med.Sci.*, 1987, 2, pp. 213–23.

24   Hunter, B., 'Some food additives as neuroexcitors and neurotoxins', *Clinical Ecology*, 1984, 2, pp. 83–9.

25   Cullen, M.R.(ed.), *Workers with Multiple Chemical Sensitivities*, Hanley & Belfus, Philadelphia, PA, 1987.

26   Stayner, L.T., Elliott, L., Blade, L., *et al.*, 'A retrospective cohort mortality study of workers exposed to formaldehyde in the garment industry', *Am.J.Ind.Med.*, 1988, 13, pp. 667–81.

27   Kilburn, K.H., Warshaw, R., Boylen, C.T.,*et al.*, 'Pulmonary and neurobehavioural effects of formaldehyde exposure', *Archiv.Environ.Health*, 1985, 40, pp. 254–60.

28   Sterling, T.D. and Arundel, A.V., 'Health effects of phenoxy herbicides', *Scand.J.Work Environ.Health*, 1986, 12, pp. 161–73.

29   Dickey, L.(ed.), *Clinical Ecology*, C.C. Thomas, Springfield, IL, 1976.

30   Lindstrom, K., Riihimaki, H. and Hannininen, K., 'Occupational solvent exposure and neuropsychiatric disorders', *Scan.J.Work Environ.Health*, 1984, 10, pp. 321–3.

31   Donovan, P., 'Bowel toxemia', in Pizzorno, J.E. and Murray, M.T., *A Textbook of Natural Medicine*, John Bastyr College Publications, Seattle, WA, 1985.

32   Murray, M.T., 'Alternative complement pathway', in Pizzorno, J.E. and Murray, M.T., *A Textbook of Natural Medicine*, John Bastyr College Publications, Seattle, WA, 1985.

33   Kroker, G.F., 'Chronic candidiasis and allergy', in Brostoff, J. and Challacombe, S.J. (eds), *Food Allergy and Intolerance*, W.B. Saunders, Philadelphia, PA, 1987, pp. 850–72.

34   Liehr, H. and Grun, M., 'Endotoxins in liver disease', in *Progress in Liver Disease*, Grune & Stratton, New York, NY,1979, pp. 313–26.

35   Kasting, N. and Martin, J., 'Altered release of growth hormone and thyrotropin induced by endotoxin in the rat', *Am.J.Physiol.*, 1982, 243, pp. 332–7.

36   Ballard, J. and Shiner, M., 'Evidence of cytotoxicity in ulcerative colitis from immunofluorescent staining of the rectal mucosa', *Lancet*, 1974, i, pp. 1,014–17.

37   Belew, P.W., Rosenberg, E.W., Skinner, R.B., *et al.*, 'Endotoxemia in psoriasis', *Arch.Dermatol.*, 1982, 118, pp. 142–3.

38   Foulis, A.K., Murray, W.R., Galloway, D., *et al.*, 'Endotoxemia and complement activation in acute pancreatitis', *Gut*, 1982, 23, pp. 656–61.

39   Stephansson, K., Dieperink, M.E., Richman, D.P., *et al.*, 'Sharing of antigenic determinants between the nicotinic acetylcholine receptor and proteins in Escherichia coli, Proteus vulgaris, and Klebsiella pneumoniae', *N.Eng.J.Med.*, 1985, 312, pp. 221–5.

40   LeRoith, D., Shiloach, J., Roth, J. and Lesniak, M., 'Insulin or a closely related molecule is native to Escherichia coli', *J.Biochem.*, 1981, 256, pp. 6,533–6.

41   Weiss, M. and Ingbar, S.H., 'Demonstration of a saturable binding site for thyrotropin in Yersinia enterocolitica', *Science*, 1983, 219, pp. 1,331–5.

42   For information write IAPNH, c/o Mark A. Huberman, 204 Stambaugh Bldg, Youngstown, OH 44503, USA.

43   Salloum, T.K., 'Therapeutic fasting', in Pizzorno, J.E. and Murray, M.T., *A Textbook of Natural Medicine*, John Bastyr College Publications, Seattle, WA, 1988.

44   Bloom, W.L., 'Fasting as an introduction to the treatment of obesity', *Metabolism*, 1959, 8, pp. 214–20.

45   Duncan, G.G., Jenson, W.K., Cristofori, F.C. and Schless, G.L., 'Intermittent fasts in the correction and control of intractable obesity', *Am.J.Med.Sci.*, 1963, 245, pp. 515–20.

46   Duncan, G.G., Duncan, T.G., Schless, G.L. and Cristofori, F.C., 'Contraindications and therapeutic results of fasting in obese patients', *Ann.NY.Acad.Sci.*, 1965, 131, pp. 632–6.

47   Sorbris, R., Aly, K.O., Nilsson-Ehle, P., *et al.*, 'Vegetarian fasting of obese patients: a clinical and biochemical evaluation', *Scand.J.Gastroenterol.*, 1982, 17, pp. 417–24.

48   Gresham, G.A., 'Is atheroma a reversible lesion', *Atherosclerosis*, 1976, 23, pp. 379–91.

49   Suzuki, J., Yamauchi, Y., Horikawa, M. and Yamagata, S., 'Fasting therapy for psychosomatic disease with special reference to its indications and therapeutic mechanism', *Tohoku J.Exp.Med.*, 1976, 118 (Suppl.), pp. 245–59.

50   Imamura, M. and Tung, T., 'A trial of fasting cure for PCB poisoned patients in Taiwan', *Am.J.Ind.Med.*, 1984, 5, pp. 147–53.

51   Lithell, H., Bruce, A., Gustafsson, I.B., *et al.*, 'A fasting and vegetarian diet treatment trial on chronic inflammatory disorders', *Acta Derm.Venereol.*, 1983, 63, pp. 397–403.

52   Skoldstam, L., Larsson, L. and Lindstrom, F.D., 'Rheumatoid arthritis', *Scand.J.Rheumatol.*, 1979, 8, pp. 249–55.

53   Skoldstam, L., Lindstrom, F.D. and Lindblom, B., 'Impaired con A suppressor cell activity in patients with rheumatoid arthritis shows normalisation during fasting', *Scand.J.Rheumatol.*, 1983, 12, 4, pp. 369–73.

54   Sundquist, T., Lindstrom, F., Magnusson, K. and Skoldstam, L., 'Influence of fasting on intestinal permeability and disease activity in patients with rheumatoid arthritis shows normalisation during fasting', *Scand.J.Rheumatol.*, 1982, 11, pp. 33–8.

55   Kroker, G.F., Stroud, R.M., Marshall, R., *et al.*, 'Fasting and rheumatoid arthritis: a multicentre study', *Clin.Ecology*, 1984, 2, 3, pp. 137–44.

56   Boehme, D.L., 'Preplanned fasting in the treatment of mental disease: survey of the current Soviet literature', *Schizophr.Bull.*, 1977, 3, 2, pp. 288–96.

57   Shakman, R.A., 'Nutritional influences on the toxicity of environmental pollutants: a review', *Arch.Env.Health.*, 1974, 28, pp. 105–33.

4 Dietary fibre: its importance in the maintenance of health and prevention of disease

1   Linder, P.G., '"Junk foods" and medical education', *Obes.Bar.Med.*, 1982, 11, p. 109.

2   Burkitt, D. And Trowell, H., *Western Diseases: Their Emergence and Prevention*, Harvard University Press, Cambridge, MA, 1981.

3   Vahouny, G. and Kritchevsky, D., *Dietary Fiber in Health and Disease*, Plenum Press, New York, NY, 1982.

4   Worthington-Roberts, B., *Contemporary Developments in Nutrition*, C.V.Mosby, St Louis, MO, 1981.

5   Goodhart, R. and Young, V.R., *Modern Nutrition in Health and Disease*, Lea & Febiger, Philadelphia, PA, 1988.

6   Price, W., *Nutrition and Physical Degeneration*, Price-Pottinger Foundation, La Mesa, CA, 1970.

7   Selvendran, R.R., 'The plant cell wall as a source of dietary fiber: chemistry and structure', *Am.J.Clin.Nutr.*, 1984, 39, pp. 320–37.

8   Watt, J. and Marcus, R., 'Harmful effects of carrageenan fed to animals', *Canc.Det.Prev.*, 1981, 4, pp. 129–34.

9   Aldercreutz, H., 'Does fibre-rich food containing animal lignin precursors protect against both colon and breast cancer? An extension of the "fiber hypothesis"', *Gastroenterol.*, 1984, 86, pp. 761–6.

10   National Research Council, *Diet, Nutrition and Cancer*, National Academy Press, Washington DC, 1982.

11   Trowell, H., 'Definition of dietary fiber and hypothesis that it is a protective factor in certain diseases', *Am.J.Clin.Nutr.*, 1976, 29, pp. 417–27.

12   Sommer, H. and Kasper, H., 'Effect of long-term administration of dietary fiber on the exocrine pancreas in the rat', *Hepato-gastroenterol.*, 1984, 31, pp. 176–9.

13   Prasa, K.N., 'Butyric acid: a small fatty acid with diverse biological functions', *Life Sci.*, 1980, 27, pp. 1,351–8.
14   Novogrodsky, A., Dvir, A., Ravid, A., *et al.*, 'Effect of polar organic compounds on leukemic cells', *Cancer*, 1983, 51, pp. 9–14.

5 Digestion

1   The authors wish to acknowledge Dr Stephen Barrie, whose chapter 'Heidelberg pH capsule gastric analysis', in Pizzorno, J.E. and Murray, M.A., *A Textbook of Natural Medicine*, John Bastyr College Publications, Seattle, WA, 1988, formed the basis for parts of this chapter.
2   Guyton, A.C., *Textbook of Medical Physiology*, W.B. Saunders, Philadelphia, PA, 1985.
3   Bray, G.W., 'The hypochlorhydria of asthma in childhood', *Br.Med.J.*, 1930, i, pp. 181–97.
4   Hosking, D.J., Moody, F., Stewart, I.M. and Atkinson, M., 'Vagal impairment of gastric secretion in diabetic autonomic neuropathy', *Br.Med.J.*, 1975, i, pp. 588–90.
5   Rabinowitch, I.M., 'Achlorhydria and its clinical significance in diabetes mellitus', *Am.J.Dig.Dis.*, 1949, 18, pp. 322–33.
6   Carper, W.M., Butler, T.J., Kilby, J.O. and Gibson, M.J., 'Gallstones, gastric secretion and flatulent dyspepsia', *Lancet*, i, pp. 413–15.
7   Rawls, W.B. and Ancona, V.C., 'Chronic urticaria associated with hypochlorhydria or achlorhydria', *Rev.Gastroent.*, 1950, Oct., pp. 267–71.
8   Gianella, R.A., Broitman, S.A. and Zamcheck, N., 'Influence of gastric acidity on bacterial and parasitic enteric infections', *Ann.Int.Med.*, 1973, 78, pp. 271–6.
9   De Witte, T.J., Geerdink, P.J. and Lamers, C.B., 'Hypochlorhydria and hypergastrinaemia in rheumatoid arthritis', *Ann.Rheum.Dis.*, 1979, 38, pp. 14–17.
10   Ryle, J.A. and Barber, H.W., 'Gastric analysis in acne rosacea', *Lancet*, 1920, ii, pp. 1,195–6.
11   Ayres, S., 'Gastric secretion in psoriasis, eczema and dermatitis herpetiformis', *Arch.Derm.*, 1929, Jul., pp. 854–9.
12   Dotevall, G. and Walan, A., 'Gastric secretion of acid and intrinsic factor in patients with hyper and hypothyroidism', *Acta.Med.Scand.*, 1969, 186, pp. 529–33.
13   Howitz, J. and Schwartz, M., 'Vitiligo, achlorhydria, and pernicious anemia', *Lancet*, 1971, i, pp. 1,331–4.
14   Rafsky, H.A. and Weingarten, M., 'A study of the gastric secretory response in the aged', *Gastroent.*, 1946, May, pp. 348–52.
15   Davies, D. and James, T.G., 'An investigation into the gastric secretion of a hundred normal persons over the age of sixty', *Brit.Med.J.*, 1930, i, pp. 1–14.
16   Baker, H., Frank, O. and Jaslow, S.P., 'Oral versus intramuscular vitamin supplementation for hypovitaminosis in the elderly', *J.Am.Geriat.Soc.*, 1980, 48, pp. 42–5.
17   Steinberg, W.J., Mina, F.A. and Pick, P.G., 'Heidelberg capsule. In vitro evaluation of a new instrument for measuring intragastric pH', *J.Pharm.Sci.*, 1965, 54, pp. 772–8.
18   Stavney, L.S., Hamilton, T. and Sircus, W., 'Evaluation of the pH-sensitive telemetry capsule in the estimation of gastric secretory capacity', *Am.J.Dig.Dis.*, 1966, ii, p. 10.
19   Dabney, R., Yarbrough, I. and McAlhany, J.C., 'Evaluation of the Heidelberg capsule method of tubeless gastric analysis', *Am.J.Surgery*, 1969, 117, p. 185.
20   Mojaverian, P., *et al.*, 'Estimation of gastric residence time of the Heidelberg capsule in humans', *Gastroenterology*, 1985, 89, pp. 392–7.
21   Wright, J., 'A proposal for standardized challenge testing of gastric acid secretory capacity using the Heidelberg capsule radiotelemetry system', *J. John Bastyr Col.Nat.Med.*, 1979, 1, 2, pp. 3–11.
22   Rubinstein, E., Mark, Z., Haspel, J., *et al.*, 'Antibacterial activity of the pancreatic fluid', *Gastroenterol.*, 1985, 88, pp. 927–32.
23   Gilman, A.G., Goodman, A.S. and Gilman, A., *The Pharmacological Basis of Therapeutics*, Macmillan, New York, NY, 1980.
24   Taussig, S., Yokoyama, M., Chinen, A., *et al.*, 'Bromelain, a proteolytic enzyme and its clinical application. A review', *Hiroshima J.Med.Sci.*, 1975, 24, pp. 185–93.
25   Taussig, S., 'The mechanism of the physiological action of bromelain', *Med.Hypothesis*, 1980, 6, pp. 99–104.
26   Messer, M., Anderson, C.M. and Hubbard, L., 'Studies on the mechanism of destruction of the toxic action of wheat gluten in coeliac disease by crude papain', *Gut*, 1964, 5, pp. 295–303.
27   Krainick, H.G. and Mohn, G., 'Weitere Untersuchungen uber den schadlichen Weizenmehleffekt bei del Coliakie. 2. Die Wirkung der enzymatischen Abbauprodukte des Gliadin', *Helv.Paediatr.Acta.*, 1959, 14, pp. 124–40.
28   Messer, M. and Baume, P.E., 'Oral papain in gluten intolerance', *Lancet*, 1976, ii, p. 1,022.
29   Innerfield, I., *Enzymes in Clinical Medicine*, McGraw Hill, New York, NY, 1960.
30   Ransberger, K., 'Enzyme treatment of immune complex diseases', *Arthritis Rheuma.*, 1986, 8, pp. 16–19.
31   Stauder, G., Ransberger, K., Streichhan, P., *et al.*, 'The use of hydrolytic enzymes as adjuvant therapy in AIDS/ARC/LAS patients', *Biomed.Pharmacother.*, 1988, 42, pp. 31–4.
32   Nyrenn, O., Adami, H.O., Bates, S., *et al.*, 'Absence of therapeutic benefit from antacids or cimetidine in non-ulcer dyspepsia', *New Eng.J.Med.*, 1986, 314, pp. 339–43.
33   Glatzell, H., 'Treatment of dyspeptic disorders with spice extracts', *Hippokrates*, 40, pp. 916–19.
34   Deininger, R., 'Amarum-bitter herbs: common bitter principle remedies and their action', *Krankenpflege*, 1975, 29, pp. 99–100.

6 Immune support

1   Pizzorno, J.E. and Murray, M.T., *A Textbook of Natural Medicine*, John Bastyr College Publications, Seattle, WA, 1985.
2   Beisel, W., Edelman, R., Nauss, K. and Suskind, R., 'Single-nutrient effects of immunologic functions', *J.A.M.A.*, 1981, 245, pp. 53–8.
3   Dieter, M., 'Further studies on the relationship between vitamin C and thymic hormonal factor', *Proc.Soc.Exp.Biol.Med.*, 1971, 136, pp. 316–22.
4   Seifter, E., Rettura, G., Seiter, J., *et al.*, 'Thymotrophic action of vitamin A', *Fed.Proc.*, 1973, 32, p. 947.
5   Dardenne, M., Pleau, J., Nabarra, B., *et al*, 'Contribution of zinc and other metals to the biological activity of the serum thymic factor', *Proc.Natl Acad.Sci.*, 1982, 79, pp. 5,370–3.

6   Pandolfi, F., Quinti, I., Montella, F., *et al.*, 'T-dependent immunity in aged humans. II. Clinical and immunological evaluation after three months of administering a thymic extract', *Thymus*, 1983, 5, pp. 235–40.

7   Valesini, G., Barnaba, V., Levrero, M. *et al.*, 'Clinical improvement and partial correction of the T-cell defects of acquired immunodeficiency syndrome (AIDS) and lymphadenopathy syndrome (LAS) by a calf thymus lysate', *Eur.J.Clin.Oncol.*, 1986, 22, pp. 531–2.

8   Cazzola, P., Mazzanti, P. and Bossi, G., 'In vivo modulating effect of a calf thymus acid lysate on human T lymphocyte subsets and CD4+/ CD8+ ratio in the course of different diseases', *Curr.Ther.Res.*, 1987, 42, pp. 1,011–17.

9   Fiocchi, A., Borella, E., Riva, E., *et al.*, 'A double-blind clinical trial for the evaluation of the therapeutic effectiveness of a calf thymus derivative (Thymomodulin) in children with recurrent respiratory infections', *Thymus*, 1986, 8, pp. 831–9.

10 Wagner, H. and Proksch, A., 'Immunostimulatory drugs of fungi and higher plants', *Economic Medicinal Plant Research*, 1985, 1, pp. 113–53.

11 Wagner, V.H., Proksch, A., Riess-Maurer, I., *et al.*, 'Immunostimulating polysaccharides (heteroglycans) of higher plants', *Arzneim-Forsch*, 1985, 35, pp. 1,069–75.

12 Abe, N., Ebina, T. and Ishida, N., 'Interferon induction by glycyrrhizin and glycyrrhetinic acid in mice', *Microbial Immunol.*, 1982, 26, pp. 535–9.

13 Kumagai, A., Nanaboshi, M., Asanuma, Y., *et al.*, 'Effects of glycyrrhizin on thymolytic and immunosuppressive action of cortisone', *Endocrinol.Japan*, 1967, 14, pp. 39–42.

14 Bloksma, N., Van Dijk, H., Korst, P., *et al.*, 'Cellular and humoral adjuvant activity of a mistletoe extract', *Immunobiol.*, 1979, 156, pp. 309–19.

15 Bloksma, N., Schmiermann, P., de Reuver, M., *et al.*, 'Stimulation of humoral and cellular immunity by viscum preparations', *Planta Medica*, 1982, 46, pp. 221–7.

16 Kumazawa, Y., Itagaki, A., Fukumoto, M., *et al.*, 'Activation of peritoneal macrophages by berberine-type alkaloids in terms of induction of cytostatic activity', *Int.J.Immunopharmac.*, 1984, 6, pp. 587–92.

17 Minter, M.M., 'Agranulocytic angina: treatment of a case with fetal calf spleen', *Texas State J.Med.*, 1933, 2, pp. 338–43.

18 Sabir, M. and Bhide, N., 'Study of some pharmacologic actions of berberine', *Ind.J.Phys.Pharm.*, 1971, 15, pp. 111–32.

19 Vomel, V., 'Influence of a non-specific immune stimulant on phagocytosis of erythrocytes and ink by the reticuloendothelial system of isolated perfused rat livers of different ages', *Arzneim-Forsch.*, 1985, 35, pp. 1,069–75.

20 Stimpel, M., Proksch, A., Wagner, H., *et al.*, 'Macrophage activation and induction of macrophage cytotoxicity by purified polysaccharide fractions from the plant Echinacea purpurea', *Infection Immunity*, 1984, 46, pp. 845–9.

21 Mose, J., 'Effect of echinacin on phagocytosis and natural killer cells', *Med.Welt.*, 1983, 34, pp. 1,463–7.

22 Yunde, H., Guoliang, M., Shuhua, W., *et al.*, 'Effects of Radix astragalus seuhedysari on the interferon system', *Chin.Med.J.*, 1981, 94, pp. 35–40.

23 Moldofsky, H., Lue, F.A., Eisen, J., *et al.*, 'The relationship of interleukin-1 and immune functions to sleep in humans', *Psychosomatic Medicine*, 1986, 48, pp. 309–15.

24 Leevy, C., Cardi, L., Frank, O., *et al.*, 'Incidence and significance of hypovitaminemia in a randomly selected municipal hospital population', *Am.J.Clin.Nutr.*, 1965, 17, pp. 259–71.

25 Saxena, Q., Saxena, R. and Adler, W., 'Effect of feeding a diet with half of the recommended levels of all vitamins on the natural and inducible levels of cytotoxic activity in mouse spleen cells', *Immunol.*, 1984, 52, pp. 41–8.

26 Chandra, R. and Newberne, R., *Nutrition, Immunity, and Infection*, Plenum Press, New York, NY, 1977.

27 Sanchez, A., Reeser, J., Lau, H., *et al.*, 'Role of sugars in human neutrophilic phagocytosis', *Am.J.Clin.Nutr.*, 1973, 26, pp. 1,180–4.

28 Ringsdorf, W., Cheraskin, E. and Ramsay, R., 'Sucrose, neutrophil phagocytosis and resistance to disease', *Dent.Surv.*, 1976, 52, pp. 46–8.

29 Bernstein, J., Alpert, S., Nauss, K. and Suskind, R., 'Depression of lymphocyte transformation following oral glucose ingestion', *Am.J.Clin.Nutr.*, 1977, 30, p. 613.

30 Mann, G., 'Hypothesis: the role of vitamin C in diabetic angiopathy', *Pers.Biol.Med.*, 1974, 17, pp. 210–17.

31 Mann, G. and Newton, P., 'The membrane transport of ascorbic acid', *Ann.N.Y.Acad.Sci.*, 1975, 258, pp. 243–51.

32 Palmblad, J., Hallberg, D. and Rossner, S., 'Obesity, plasma lipids and polymorphonuclear (PMN) granulocyte functions', *Scand.J.Haematol.*, 1977, 19, pp. 293–303.

33 Simone, D., Ferrari, M., Meli, D., *et al.*, 'Reversibility by L-carnitine of immunosuppression induced by an emulsion of soya bean oil, glycerol and egg lecithin', *Arzneim-Forsch.*, 1982, 32, pp. 1,488–9.

34 Simone, C., Ferrari, M., Lozzi, A., *et al.*, 'Vitamins and immunity: II Influence of L-carnitine on the immune system', *Acta Vit.Enz.*, 1982, 4, pp. 135–40.

35 Demetriou, A., Franco, I., Bark, S., *et al.*, 'Effects of vitamin A and beta carotene on intra-abdominal sepsis', *Arch.Surg.*, 1984, 119, pp. 161–5.

36 Tachibana, K., Sone, S., Tsubura, E. and Kishino, Y., 'Stimulation effect of vitamin A on tumoricidal activity of rat alveolar macrophages', *Br.J.Cancer*, 1984, 49, pp. 343–8.

37 Reinhardt, A., Auperin, D. and Sands, J., 'Mechanism of viricidal activity of retinoids: protein removal from bacteriophage 6 envelope', *Antimicrob.Agents Chemother.*, 1980, 17, pp. 1,034–7.

38 Retura, G., Stratford, F., Levenson, S. and Seifter, E., 'Prophylactic and therapeutic actions of supplemental B-carotene in mice inoculated with C3HBA adenocarcinoma cells: lack of therapeutic action of supplemental ascorbic acid', *J.N.C.I.*, 1982, 69, pp. 73–7.

39 Rhodes, J., 'Human interferon action: reciprocal regulation by retinoic acid and B-carotene', *J.N.C.I.*, 1983, 70, pp. 833–7.

40 Rhodes, J., Stokes, P. and Abrams, P., 'Human tumor-induced inhibition of interferon action in vitro: reversal of inhibition by B-carotene (pro-vitamin A)', *Cancer Immunol.Immunother.*, 1984, 16, pp.189–92.

41 Burton, G. and Ingold, K., 'B-carotene: an unusual type lipid antioxidant', *Science*, 1984, 224, pp. 569–73.

42 Alexander, M., Newmark, H. and Miller, R., 'Oral beta-carotene can increase the number of OKT4+ cells in human blood', *Immunology Letters*, 1985, 9, pp. 221–4.

43 Baird, I., Hughes, R., Wilson, H., *et al.*, 'The effects of ascorbic acid and flavonoids on the occurrence of symptoms normally associated with the common cold', *Am.J.Clin.Nutr.*, 1979, 32, pp. 1,686–90.

44 Anderson, T., Reid, D. and Beaton, G., 'Vitamin C and the common cold: a double blind trial', *Can.Med.Assoc.J.*, 1972, 107, pp. 503–8.

45 Cheraskin, E., Ringsdorf, W.M. and Sisley, E.L., *The Vitamin C Connection*, Bantam Books, New York, NY, 1983.

46 Anderson, T.W., 'Large scale trials of vitamin C', *Ann.N.Y.Acad.Sci.*, 1975, 258, pp. 494–505.

47 Scott, J., 'On the biochemical similarities of ascorbic acid and interferon', *J.Theor.Biol.*, 1982, 98, pp. 235–8.

48 Schwerdt, P. and Schwerdt, C., 'Effect of ascorbic acid on rhinovirus replication in WI-38 cells', *Proc.Soc.Exp.Biol.Med.*, 1975, 148, pp. 1,237–43.

49 Prasad, A., 'Clinical, biochemical and nutritional spectrum of zinc deficiency in human subjects: an update', *Ntr.Rev.*, 1983, 41, pp. 197–208.

50 Gershwin, M., Beach, R. and Hurley, L., 'Trace metals, aging, and immunity', *J.Am.Ger.Soc.*, 1983, 31, pp. 374–8.

51 Bogden, J.D., Oleske, J.M., Munves, E.M., *et al.*, 'Zinc and immunocompetence in the elderly: baseline data on zinc nutriture and immunity in unsupplemented subjects', *Am.J.Clin.Nutr.*, 1987, 46, pp. 101–9.

52 Katz, E. and Margalith. E., 'Inhibition of vaccinia virus maturation by zinc chloride', *Antimicrob.Agents Chemother.*, 1981, 19, pp. 213–17.

53 Eby, G.A., Davis, D.R., and Halcomb, W.W., 'Reduction in duration of common colds by zinc gluconate lozenges in a double-blind study', *Antimicrob.Agents Chemother.*, 1984, 25, pp. 20–4.

54 Al-Nakib, Higgins, P.G., Barrow, I., *et al.*, 'Prophylaxis and treatment of rhinovirus colds with zinc gluconate lozenges', *J.Antimicrob.Chemother.*, 1987, 20, pp. 893–901.

55 Dowd, P. and Heatley, R., 'The influence of undernutrition on immunity', *Clin.Sci.*, 1984, 66, pp. 241–8.

56 Stockman, J., 'Infections and iron: too much of a good thing', *Am.J.Dis.Child.*, 1981, 135, pp. 18–20.

57 Wacker, A. and Hilbig, W., 'Virus inhibition by echinacea purpurea', *Planta Medica*, 1978, 33, pp. 89–102.

58 Leung, A., *Encyclopedia of Common Natural Ingredients Used in Food, Drugs, and Cosmetics*, John Wiley & Sons, New York, NY, 1980.

59 Hahn, F. and Ciak, J., 'Berberine', *Antibiotics*, 1976, 3, pp. 577–84.

60 Mahajan, V.M., Sharma, A. and Rattan, A., 'Antimycotic activity of berberine sulphate: an alkaloid from an Indian medicinal herb', *Sabouraudia*, 1982, 20, pp. 79–81.

61 Pompeii, R., Pani, A., Flore, O. *et al.*, 'Antiviral activity of glycyrrhizic acid', *Experentia*, 1980, 36, pp. 304–5.

62 Mitscher, L., Park, Y. and Clark, D., 'Antimicrobial agents from higher plants. Antimicrobial isoflavonoids from glycyrrhiza glabre L. var. typica', *J.Nat.Products*, 1980, 43, pp. 259–69.

7 Life extension

1   Pearson, D. and Shaw, S., *Life Extension. A Practical Scientific Approach*, Warner Books, New York, NY, 1982.

2   Wolford, R.L., *Maximum Life Span*, Avon Books, New York, NY, 1983.

3   Hendler, S.S., *The Complete Guide to Anti-Aging Nutrients*, Simon & Schuster, New York, NY, 1985.

4   Schneider, E.L. and Reed, J.D., 'Life extension', *New Eng.J.Med.*, 1985, 312, pp. 1,159–68.

5   Harper, A.E., 'Nutrition, aging, and longevity', *Am.J.Clin.Nutr.*, 1982, 36, pp. 737–49.

6   Mazess, R.B. and Forman, S.H., 'Longevity and age exaggeration in Vilcabamba, Ecuador', *J.Gerontol.*, 1979, 34, pp. 94–8.

7   Medvedev, Z.A., 'Myths about the Caucasian mountain centers of longevity', *Geriatric Med.Today*, 1986, 5, pp. 96–112.

8   Masoro, E.J., 'Biology of aging. Current state of knowledge', *Arch.Intern.Med.*, 1987, 147, pp. 166–9.

9   Taubman, L.B., 'Theories of aging', *Resident and Staff Physician*, 1986, 32, pp. 31–7.

10 Hayflick, L., 'The cell biology of human aging', *N.Eng.J.Med.*, 1976, 295, pp. 302–8.

11 Cutler, R.G., 'Peroxide-producing potential of tissues: inverse correlation with longevity of mammalian species', *Proc.Natl Acad.Sci.*, 1985, 82, pp. 4,798–802.

12 Harman, D., 'Free radical theory of aging: the free radical diseases', *Age*, 1984, 7, pp. 111–31.

13 Cross, C.E., Halliwell, B., Borish, E.T., *et al.*, 'Oxygen radicals and human disease', *Annals Intern.Med.*, 1987, 107, pp. 526–45.

14 Yu, B.P. Masoro, E.J. and McMahan, C.A., 'Nutritional influences on aging of fischer 344 rats: I. Physical, metabolic, and longevity characteristics', *J.Gerontol.*, 1985, 40, pp. 657–70.

15 Cutler, R.G., 'Carotenoids and retinol: their possible importance in determining longevity of primate species', *Proc.Natl Acad.Sci.*, 1984, 81, pp. 7,627–31.

16 Pizzorno, J.E. and Murray, M.T., 'Vitamin A, beta-carotene and other carotenoids', in *A Textbook of Natural Medicine*, John Bastyr College Publications, Seattle, WA, 1986.

17 Burton, G. and Ingold, K., 'Beta-carotene: an unusual type of antioxidant', *Science*, 1984, 224, pp. 569–73.

18 Alexander, M., Newmark, H. and Miller, R.G., 'Oral beta-carotene can increase the number of OKT4+ cells in human blood', *Immunol.Letters*, 1985, 9, pp. 221–4.

19 Cody, V., Middleton, E. and Harborne, J.B., *Plant Flavonoids in Biology and Medicine – Biochemical, Pharmacological, and Structure-activity Relationships*, Alan R. Liss, New York, NY, 1986.

20 Kuhnau, J., 'The flavonoids: a class of semi-essential food components: their role in human nutrition', *Wld Rev.Nutr.Diet*, 1976, 24, pp. 117–91.

21 Havsteen, B., 'Flavonoids, a class of natural products of high pharmacological potency', *Biochem.Pharmacol.*, 1983, 32, pp. 1,141–8.

22 Middleton, E., 'The flavonoids', *Trends in Pharmaceut.Sci.*, 1984, 5, pp. 335–8.

23 Vogel, G., Trost, W., Braatz, R., *et al.*, 'Studies on pharmacodynamics, site and mechanism of action of silymarin, the antihepatotoxic principle from Silybum marianum (L.), *Gaert.Arzneim-Forsch.*, 1975, 25, pp. 179–85.

24 Hikino, H., Kiso, Y., Wagner, H. and Fiebig, J., 'Antihepatotoxic actions of flavonolignans from silybum marianum', *Planta Medica*, 1984, 50, pp. 248–50.

25 Brunello, N., Racagni, G., Clostre, F., *et al.*, 'Effects of an extract of ginkgo biloba on noradrenergic systems of rat cerebral cortex', *Pharmacol.Res.Commun.*, 1985, 17, pp. 1,063–72.

26 Chatterjee, S.S. and Gabard, B., 'Studies on the mechanism of action of an extract of Ginkgo biloba, a drug for the treatment of ischemic vascular diseases', *Naunyn-Schmiedeberg's Arch.Pharmacol.*, 1982, 320, p. R52.

27 Vorberg, G., 'Ginkgo biloba extract (GBE): a long-term study of chronic cerebral insufficiency in geriatric patients', *Clinical Trials Journal*, 1985, 22, pp. 149–57.

8 Liver support

1   Regenstein, L., *America the Poisoned*, Acropolis, Washington DC, 1982.

2   Petersdorf, R., *Harrison's Principles of Internal Medicine*, McGraw-Hill, New York, NY, 1983.

3   Robbins, S., Cotran, R. and Kumar, V., *Pathologic Basis of Disease*, W.B. Saunders, Philadelphia, PA, 1984.

4   Dreisbach, R. H., *Handbook of Poisoning*, 11th edition, Lange Medical Publications, Los Altos, CA, 1983, pp. 80–3.

5   Pizzorno, J.E. and Murray, M.T., *A Textbook of Natural Medicine*, Chapter IV: Hepatoprotection, John Bastyr College Publications, Seattle, WA, 1988.

6   Nutrition Review, *Present Knowledge in Nutrition*, Nutrition Foundation, Washington DC, 1984.

7   Baraona, E. and Lieber, C., 'Effects of ethanol on lipid metabolism', *J.Lipid Res.*, 1979, 20, pp. 289–315.

8   Martin, D., Mayes, P. and Rodwell, V., *Harper's Review of Biochemistry*, Lange, Los Altos, CA, 1983.

9   Montgomery, R., Dryer, R., Conway, T. and Spector, A., *Biochemistry, a Case-Oriented Approach*, C.V. Mosby, St Louis, MO, 1980.

10 Padova, C., Tritapepe, R., Padova, F., *et al.*, 'S-adenosyl-L-methionine antagonizes oral contraceptive-induced bile cholesterol supersaturation in healthy women: preliminary report of a controlled randomized trial', *Am.J.Gastroenterol.*, 1984, 79, pp. 941–4.

11 Frezza, M., Pozzato, G., Chiesa, L., *et al.*, 'Reversal of intrahepatic cholestasis of pregnancy in women after high dose S-adenosyl-L-methionine (SAMe) administration', *Hepatology*, 1984, 4, pp. 274–8.

12 Bombardieri, G., Milani, A., Bernardi, L. and Rossi, L., 'Effects of S-adenosyl-methionine (SAMe) in the treatment of Gilbert's syndrome', *Curr.Ther.Res.*, 1985, 37, pp. 580–5.

13 Mazzanti, R., Arcangeli, A., Salvadori, G., *et al.*, 'On the antisteatosic effects of S-adenosyl-L-methionine in various chronic liver diseases. A multicenter study', *Curr.Ther.Res.*, 1979, 25, pp. 25–32.

14 Wisniewska-Knypl, J., Sokal, J., Klimczak, J., *et al.*, 'Protective effect of methionine against vinyl chloride-mediated depression of non-protein sulfhydryls and cytochrome P-450', *Toxicology Letters*, 1981, 8, pp. 147–52.

15 Stanko, R.T., Mendelow, H., Shinozuka, H. and Adibi, S.A., 'Prevention of alcohol-induced fatty liver by natural metabolites and riboflavin', *J.Lab.Clin.Med.*, 1978, 91, pp. 228–35.

16 Hartroft, W.S., Porta, E.A. and Suzuki, M., 'Effects of choline chloride on hepatic lipids after acute ethanol intoxication', *Q.J.Stuc.Alcohol.*, 1964, 25, pp. 427–37.

17 Sachan, D.S., Rhew, T.H. and Ruark, R.A., 'Ameliorating effects of carnitine and its precursors on alcohol-induced fatty liver', *Am.J.Clin.Nutr.*, 1984, 39, pp. 738–44.

18 Hosein, E.A. and Bexton, B., 'Protective action of carnitine on liver lipid metabolism after ethanol administration to rats', *Biochem.Pharm.*, 1975, 24, pp. 1,859–63.

19 Sachan, D.A. and Rhew, T.H., 'Lipotropic effect of carnitine on alcohol-induced hepatic stenosis', *Nutr.Rep.Int.*, 1983, 27, pp. 1,221–6.

20 Gilbert, A. and Carnot, P., 'Note preliminaire sur l'opotherapie hepatique', *Compt.Rend.Soc.Biol.*, 1896, 48, pp. 934–7.

21 Nagai, K., 'A study of the excretory mechanism of the liver – effect of liver hydrolysate on BSP excretion', *Jap.J.Gastroenterol.*, 1970, 67, pp. 633–8.

22 Ohbayashi, A., Akioka, T. and Tasaki, H., 'A study of effects of liver hydrolysate on hepatic circulation', *J.Therapy*, 1972, 54, pp. 1,582–5.

23 Hirayama, S., Kishikawa, H., Kume, T. and Tada, H., 'Therapeutic effect of liver hydrolysate on experimental liver cirrhosis', *Nisshin Igaku*, 1978, 45, pp. 528–33.

24 Sanbe, K., Murata, T., Fujisawa, K., *et al.*, 'Treatment of liver disease – with particular reference to liver hydrolysates', *Jap.J.Clin.Exp.Med.*, 1973, 50, pp. 2,665–76.

25 Fujisawa, K., Suzuki, H., Yamamoto, S., *et al.*, 'Therapeutic effects of liver hydrolysate preparation on chronic hepatitis – a double blind, controlled study', *Asian Med.J.*, 1984, 26, pp. 497–526.

26 Leung, A.Y., *Encyclopedia of Common Natural Ingredients Used in Food, Drugs and Cosmetics*, John Wiley & Sons, New York, NY, 1980.

27 Duke, J.A., *Handbook of Medicinal Herbs*, CRC Press, Boca Raton, FL, 1985.

28 Mowrey, D.B., *The Scientific Validation of Herbal Medicine*, Cormorant Books, Lehi, UT, 1986.

29 Faber, K., 'The dandelion – *Taraxacum officinale Weber*', *Pharmazie*, 1958, 13, pp. 423–35.

30 Hikino, H., Kiso, Y., Wagner, H. and Fiebig, M., 'Antihepatotoxic actions of flavonolignans from Silybum marianum fruits', *Planta Medica*, 1984, 50, pp. 248–50.

31 Vogel, G., Trost, W., Braatz, R., *et al.*, 'Studies on pharmacodynamics, site and mechanism of action of silymarin, the antihepatotoxic principle from Silybum marianum (L.) Gaert'., *Arzneim-Forsch.*, 1975, 25, pp. 179–85.

32 Wagner, H., 'Antihepatotoxic flavonoids', in Cody, V., Middleton, E. and Harbourne, J.B. (eds), *Plant Flavonoids in Biology and Medicine: Biochemical, Pharmacological, and Structure-Activity relationships*, Alan R. Liss, New York, NY, 1986, pp. 545–58.

33 Wagner, H., 'Plant constituents with antihepatotoxic activity', in Beal, J.L. and Reinhard, E. (eds), *Natural Products as Medicinal Agents*, Hippokrates-Verlag, Stuttgart, 1981.

34 Sarre, H., 'Experience in the treatment of chronic hepatopathies with silymarin', *Arzneim-Forsch.*, 1971, 21, pp. 1,209–12.

35 Canini, F., Bartolucci, A., Cristallini, E., *et al.*, 'Use of silymarin in the treatment of alcoholic hepatic stenosis', *Clin.Ther.*, 1985, 114, pp. 307–14.

36 Salmi, H.A. and Sarna, S., 'Effect of silymarin on chemical, functional, and morphological alteration of the liver. A double-blind controlled study', *Scand.J.Gastroenterol.*, 1982, 17, pp. 417–21.

37 Scheiber, V. and Wohlzogen, F.X., 'Analysis of a certain type of 2 X 3 tables, exemplified by biopsy findings in a controlled clinical trial', *Int.J.Clin.Pharmacol.*, 1978, 16, pp. 533–5.

38 Boari, C., Montanari, M., Galleti, G.P., *et al.*, 'Occupational toxic liver diseases. Therapeutic effects of silymarin', *Min.Med.*, 1985, 72, pp. 2,679–88.

39 Maros, T., Racz, G., Katonaj, B. and Kovacs, V., 'The effects of Cynara scolymus extracts on the regeneration of the rat liver', *Arzneim-Forsch.*, 1966, 16, pp. 127–9; 1968, 18, pp. 884–6.

40 Montini, M., Levoni, P., Angoro, A. and Pagani, G., 'Controlled trial of cynarin in the treatment of the hyperlipemic syndrome', *Arzneim-Forsch.*, 1975, 25, pp. 1,311–14.

41 Pristautz, H., 'Cynarin in the modern treatment of hyperlipemias', *Wiener Medizinische Wocheschrift*, 1975, 1,223, pp. 705–9.

42 Kiso, Y., Suzuki, Y., Watanabe, N., *et al.*, 'Antihepatotoxic principles of Curcuma longa rhizomes', *Planta Medica*, 1983, 49, pp. 185–7.

9 Pain control

1 The authors wish to acknowledge Dr Rick Kitaeff, MA, ND, DAc, from whose chapter on the non-pharmacological control of pain in *A Textbook of Natural Medicine*, part of this chapter was derived.

REFERENCES

2   Loeser, J.D., 'Perspectives on pain', in Turner, P. (ed.), *Clinical Pharmacology and Therapeutics*, University Park Press, Baltimore, MD, 1980, p. 313.

3   Melzack, R. and Wall, P.D., 'Pain mechanisms: a new theory', *Science*, 1965, 150, pp. 971–9.

4   Kitzinger, S., 'Pain in childbirth', *J.Medical Ethics*, 1978, 4, pp. 119–21.

5   Willis, A., 'Dihomo-gamma-linolenic acid as the endogenous protective agent for myocardial infarction', *Lancet*, 1984, ii, p. 697.

6   Lee, T., Hoover, R., Williams, J., *et al.*, 'Effects of dietary enrichment with eicosapentaenoic and docosahexanoic acids on in vitro neutrophil and monocyte leukotriene generation and neutrophil generation', *N.E.J.M.*, 1985, 312, pp. 1,217–24.

7   Strasser, T., Rischer, S. and Weber, P., 'Leukotriene B5 is formed in human neutrophils after dietary supplementation with eicosapentaenoic acid', *Proc.Natl Acad.Sci.*, 1985, 82, pp. 1, 540–3.

8   Boublik, J.H., 'Coffee contains potent opiate receptor binding activity', *Nature*, 1983, 301, pp. 246–8.

9   Budd, K., 'Use of D-phenylalanine, an enkephalinase inhibitor, in the treatment of intractable pain', *Adv.Pain Res.Therapy*, 1983, 5, pp. 305–8.

10 Wash, N.E., *et al.*, 'Analgesic effectiveness of D-phenylalanine in chronic pain patients', *Phys.Med.Rehabil.*, 1986, 67, pp. 436–9.

11 Werbach, M.R., *Nutritional Influences on Illness: A Sourcebook of Clinical Research*, Third Line Press, Tarzana, CA, 1987, pp. 336–9.

12 Liberman, H.R., *et al.*, 'Mood, performance and pain sensitivity: changes induced by food constituents', *J.Psychiat.Res.*, 1983, 17, pp. 135–45.

13 Seltzer, S., *et al.*, 'The effects of dietary tryptophan on chronic maxillofacial pain and experimental pain tolerance', *J.Psychiat.Res.*, 1983, 17, pp. 181–6.

14 Seltzer, S., *et al.*, 'Alteration of human pain thresholds by nutritional manipulation and L-tryptophan supplementation', *Pain*, 1982, 13, pp. 385–93.

15 King, R.B., 'Pain and tryptophan', *J.Neurosurg.*, 1980, 53, pp. 44–52.

16 Shpeen, S.E., *et al*, 'The effect of tryptophan on postoperative endodontic pain', *Oral Surg.Oral Med.Oral Pathol.*, 1984, 58, pp. 446–9.

17 Bicknell, F. and Prescott, F., *The Vitamins in Medicine*, Lee Foundation for Nutrition Research, Milwaukee, WI, 1953, p. 251.

18 Leung, A.Y., *Encyclopedia of Common Natural Ingredients Used in Food*, John Wiley & Sons, New York, NY, 1980.

19 Editorial, 'Hot peppers and substance P', *Lancet*, 1983, i, p. 1,198.

20 Buck, S.H. and Burks, T.F., 'The neuropharmacology of capsaicin: review of some recent observations', *Pharm.Rev.*, 1986, 38, pp. 179–226.

21 Goth, A., *Medical Pharmacology*, C.V. Mosby, St Louis, MO, 1984, p. 367.

22 Pervin, L., 'The need to predict and control under conditions of threat', *J.Person.*, 1963, 31, pp. 570–85.

23 Staub, E., Tursky, B. and Schwartz, G., 'Self-control and predictability: their effects on reactions to aversive stimulation', *J.Person. and Soc.Psych.*, 1971, 18, pp. 157–62.

24 Johnson, J., 'Effects of accurate expectations about sensations on the sensory and distress components of pain', *J.Person. and Soc.Psych.*, 1973, 25, pp. 381–9.

25 Stevens, R.J. and Heide, F., 'Analgesic characteristics of childbirth techniques', paper at Congress on Psychosomatic Medicine and Gynaecology, Rome, November, 1977.

26 Stevens, R.J. and Heide, F., 'Analgesic characteristics of childbirth techniques', *J.Psychos.Res.*, 1977, 21, pp. 429–38.

27 Kanfer, F. and Goldfoot, D., 'Self-control and tolerance of noxious stimulation', *Psych.Reports*, 1966, 18, pp. 79–85.

28 Evans, M. and Paul, G., 'Effects of hypnotically suggested analgesia on physiological and subjective responses to cold stress', *J.Consul.Clin.Psych.*, 1970, 35, pp. 362–71.

29 Anand, B.K., Chhina, E.S. and Singh, B., 'Some aspects of electroencephalographic studies in yogis', *EEG Clin.Neurophysio.*, 1961, 13, pp. 452–6.

30 Pelletier, K. and Peper, E., 'The Chutzpah factor in altered states of consciousness', *J.Humanis.Psych.*, 1977, 17, pp. 63–73.

31 Benson, H., *The Relaxation Response*, Avon, New York, NY, 1976.

32 Zilman, F.G., 'Biofeedback in chronic pain', in Bonica, J. J., Lindblom, U. and Iggo, A.(eds), *Advances in Pain Research and Therapy*, Vol.5, Raven Press, New York, NY, 1983, p. 795.

33 Beecher, H.K., 'Relationship of significance of wound to pain experienced', *J.A.M.A.*, 1956, 161, pp. 1,609–13.

34 Cassels, E.J., 'The nature of suffering and the goals of medicine', *N.E.J.M.*, 1982, 306, pp. 639–45.

35 Evans, F.J., 'Unraveling placebo effects', *Advances*, 1984, 1, pp. 11–19.

36 Beecher, H.K., *Measurement of Subjective Responses: Quantitative Effect of Drugs*, Oxford University Press, New York, NY, 1959.

37 Engstrom, D., 'Cognitive behavioral therapy methods in chronic pain treatment', in Bonica, J.J., Lindblom, U. and Iggo, A. (eds), *Advances in Pain Research and Therapy*, vol.5, Raven Press, New York, NY, 1983, p. 829.

38 Augustinsson, Lars-Erik, Bohlin, P., Bundsea, P., *et al.*, 'Pain during delivery by transcutaneous electrical nerve stimulation', *Pain*, 1977, 4, pp. 59–65.

39 Shealy, C.N. and Maurer, D., 'Transcutaneous nerve stimulation for control of pain', *Surg.Neurol.*, 1974, 2, pp. 45–57.

40 Oliveri, A.C., Clelland, J.A., Jackson, J. and Knowles, C., 'Effects of auricular transcutaneous electrical nerve stimulation on experimental pain threshold', *Phys.Ther.*, 1986, 66, p. 1,216.

41 Grim, L.C. and Morey, S.H., 'Transcutaneous electrical nerve stimulation for relief of parturition pain: a clinical report', *Phys.Ther.*, 1985, 65, pp. 337–40.

42 Saveriano, G., Lioretti, P., Maiolo, F. and Battista, E., 'Our experience in the use of a new objective pain measuring system in rheumarthropatic subjects treated with transcutaneous electroanalgesia and ultrasound', *Minerva Med.*, 1986, 77, pp. 745–52.

43 Estrin, V.A. and Mkrtchian, V.R., 'Central electroanalgesia in arresting the acute pain-ischemic syndrome at the prehospital stage', *Kardilogiia*, 1981, 21, pp. 81–5.

44 Lewith, G.T. and Machin, D., 'On the evaluation of the clinical effects of acupuncture', *Pain*, 1983, 16, pp. 111–27.

45 Mayer, D.J., Price, D.D. and Rafii, A., 'Antagonism of acupuncture analgesia in man by the narcotic antagonist naloxone', *Brain Res.*, 1977, 121, pp. 368–72.

46 Chapman, C.R., Colpitts, Y.M., Benedetti, C., *et al*, 'Evoked potential assessment of acupuncture analgesia: attempted reversal with naloxone', *Pain*, 1980, 9, pp. 183–97.

10 Stress

1   Seyle, H., *Stress in Health and Disease*, Butterworths, London, 1976.
2   Guyton, A.C., *Textbook of Medical Physiology*, W.B. Saunders, Philadelphia, PA, 1985, pp. 944–58.
3   Tortora, G.J. and Anagnostakos, N.P., *Principles of Anatomy and Physiology*, 4th ed., Harper & Row, New York, NY, 1984, pp. 427–9.
4   Holmes, T.H. and Rahe, R.H., 'The social readjustment scale', *J.Psychosomatic Res.*, 1967, 11, pp. 213–18, reproduced in Table 10.1 with permission.
5   Benson, H., *The Relaxation Response*, William Morrow, New York, NY, 1975.
6   Brown, B.B., *Stress and the Art of Biofeedback*, Harper & Row, New York, NY, 1977.
7   Nutrition Foundation, *Present Knowledge in Nutrition*, 5th ed., Washington DC, 1984.
8   Pizzorno, J.E. and Murray, M.T., *A Textbook of Natural Medicine*, John Bastyr College Publications, Seattle, WA, 1988.
9   Shibata, S., Tanaka, O., Shoji, J. and Saito, H., 'Chemistry and pharmacology of Panax', *Economic and Medicinal Plant Research*, 1985, 1, pp. 217–84.
10 Leung, A.Y., *Encyclopedia of Common Natural Ingredients Used in Food, Drugs and Cosmetics*, John Wiley & Sons, New York, NY, 1980, pp. 186–9.
11 Duke, J.A., *Handbook of Medicinal Herbs*, CRC Press, Boca Raton, FL, 1985, pp. 337–8.
12 Brekhman, I.I. and Dardymov, I.V., 'New substances of plant origin which increase nonspecific resistance', *Ann.Rev.Pharmacol.*, 1969, 9, pp. 419–30.
13 Brekhman, I.I. and Dardymov, I.V., 'Pharmacological investigation of glycosides from ginseng and Eleutherococcus', *Lloydia*, 1969, 32, pp. 46–51.
14 Hallstrom, C., Fulder, S. and Carruthers, M., 'Effect of ginseng on the performance of nurses on night duty', *Comp.Med.East and West*, 1982, 6, pp. 277–82.
15 D'Angelo, L., Grimaldi, R., Caravaggi, M., *et al.*, 'A double-blind, placebo controlled clinical study on the effect of a standardized ginseng extract on psychomotor performance in healthy volunteers', *J.Ethnopharmacol.*, 1986, 16, pp. 15–22.
16 Bombardelli, E., Cirstoni, A. and Lietti, A., 'The effect of acute and chronic (Panax) ginseng saponins treatment on adrenal function; biochemical and pharmacological', *Proceedings 3rd International Ginseng Symposium*, 1980, pp. 9–16.
17 Fulder, S.J., 'Ginseng and the hypothalamic-pituitary control of stress', *Am.J.Chin.Med.*, 1981, 9, pp. 112–18.

11 Acne

1   Pizzorno, J.E. and Murray, M.T., *A Textbook of Natural Medicine*, John Bastyr College Publications, Seattle, WA, 1985, pp. IV:HepPro-3, V:Silybm-1-4, VI:Acne1-4.
2   Schiavone, F., Rietschel, R., Squotas, D. and Harris, R., 'Elevated free testosterone levels in women with acne', *Arch.Dermatol.*, 1983, 119, pp. 799–802.
3   Darley, C., Moore, J., Besser, G., *et al.*, 'Androgen status in women with late onset or persistent acne vulgaris', *Clin.Exp.Dermatol.*, 1984, 9, pp. 28–35.
4   Pochi, P., 'Acne: endocrinological aspects', *Cutis*, 1982, 30, pp. 212–22.
5   Sansone, G. and Reisner, R., 'Differential rates of conversion of testosterone to dihydrotestosterone in acne and normal human skin – a possible pathogenic factor in acne', *J.Invest.Dermatol.*, 1971, 56, pp. 366–72.
6   Kappas, A., Anderson, K., Conney, A., *et al*, 'Nutrition-endocrine interactions: induction of reciprocal changes in the delta-5-alpha-reduction of testosterone and the cytochrome P-450-dependent oxidation of estradiol by dietary macronutrients in man', *Proc.Natl Acad.Sci.*, 1983, 80, pp. 7,646–9.
7   Juhlin, L. and Michaelsson, G., 'Fibrin microclot formation in patients with acne', *Acta Derm.Venerol.*, 1983, 63, pp. 538–40.
8   Etzel, K., Swerdel, M., Swerdel, J. and Cousins, R., 'Endotoxin-induced changes in copper and zinc metabolism in the syrian hamster', *J.Nutr.*, 1982, 112, pp. 2,363–73.
9   Semon, H. and Herrmann, F., 'Some observations on the sugar metabolism in acne vulgaris, and its treatment by insulin', *Br.J.Derm.*, 1940, 52, pp. 123–8.
10 Grover, R. and Arikan, N., 'The effect of intralesional insulin and glucagon in acne vulgaris', *J.Invest.Derm.*, 1963, 40, pp. 259–61.
11 Abdel, K.M., El Mofty, A., Ismail, A. and Bassili, F., 'Glucose tolerance in blood and skin of patients with acne vulgaris', *Ind.J.Derm.*, 1977, 22, pp. 139–49.
12 Cohen, J. and Cohen, A., 'Pustular acne staphyloderma and its treatment with tolbutamide', *Can.Med.Assoc.J.*, 1959, 80, pp. 629–32.
13 Offenbach, E. and Pistunyer, F., 'Beneficial effect of chromium-rich yeast on glucose tolerance and blood lipids in elderly patients', *Diabetes*, 1980, 29, pp. 919–25.
14 McCarthy, M., 'High chromium yeast for acne?' *Med.Hypoth.*, 1984, 14, pp. 307–10.
15 Kugman, A., Mills, O., Leyden, J., *et al*, 'Oral vitamin A in acne vulgaris', *Int.J.Dermatol.*, 1981, 20, pp. 278–85.
16 Thomas, R., Cooke, J. and Winkelmann, R., 'High-dose vitamin A therapy in Darier's disease', *Arch.Dermatol.*, 1982, 118, pp. 891–4.
17 Randle, H., Diaz-Perez, J. and Winkelmann, R., 'Toxic doses of vitamin A for pityriasis rubra pilaris', *Arch.Dermatol.*, 1980, 116, pp. 888–92.
18 Mulay, A. and Urbach, F., 'Local therapy of oral leukoplakia with vitamin A', *Arch.Dermatol.*, 1958, 78, pp. 637–8.
19 Peck, S., Glick, A., Sobotka, H. and Chargin, L., 'Vitamin A studies in cases of keratosis folliculitis (Darier's disease)', *Arch.Dermatol.Syph.*, 1943, 48, pp. 17–31.
20 Michaelson, G., Juhlin, L. and Ljunghall, K., 'A double blind study of the effect of zinc and oxytetracycline in acne vulgaris', *Br.J.Dermatol.*, 1977, 97, pp. 561–5.
21 Weimar, V., Puhl, S., Smith, W. and Broeke, J., 'Zinc sulphate in acne vulgaris', *Arch.Dermatol.*, 1978, 114, pp. 1,776–8.
22 Barrie, S.A., Wright, J.V., Pizzorno, J.E., Kutter, B. and Barron, P.C., 'Comparative absorption of zinc picolinate, zinc citrate and zinc gluconate in humans', *Agents and Actions*, 1987, 21, pp. 223–8.

23 Boosalis, M., Evans, G. and McClain, C., 'Impaired handling of orally administered zinc in pancreatic insufficiency', *Am.J.Clin.Nutr.*, 1983, 37, pp. 268–71.

24 Leake, A., Chisholm, G. and Habib, F., 'The effect of zinc on the 5-alpha-reduction of testosterone by the hyperplastic human prostate gland', *J.Steroid.Biochem.*, 1984, 20, pp. 651–5.

25 Michaelsson, G., Vahlquist, A. and Juhlin, L., 'Serum zinc and retinol-binding protein in acne', *Br.J.Dermatol.*, 1977, 96, pp. 283–6.

26 Michaelsson, G. and Edqvist, L., 'Erythrocyte glutathione peroxidase activity in acne vulgaris and the effect of selenium and vitamin E treatment', *Acta Derm.Venerol.*, 1984, 64, pp. 9–14.

27 Snider, B. and Dieteman, D., 'Pyridoxine therapy for premenstrual acne flare', *Arch.Dermatol.*, 1974, 110, pp. 103–11.

28 Symes, E., Bender, D., Bowen, J. and Coulson, W., 'Increased target tissue uptake of, and sensitivity to, testosterone in the vitamin B6 deficient rat', *J.Steroid Biochem.*, 1984, 20, pp. 1,089–93.

29 Ayres, S. and Mihan, R., 'Acne vulgaris: therapy directed at pathophysiological defects', *Cutis*, 1981, 28, pp. 41–2.

30 Tyler, V., Brady, L. and Robbers, J., *Pharmacognosy*, 8th ed., Lea & Febiger, Philadelphia, PA, 1981, pp. 480–1.

31 Mose, J., 'Effect of echinacin on phagocytosis and natural killer cells', *Med.Welt.*, 1983, 34, pp. 1,463–7.

32 Wagner, V., Proksch, A., Riess-Maurer, I, *et al.*, 'Immunostimulating polysaccharides (heteroglycanes) of higher plants – preliminary communications', *Arzneim-Forsch.*, 1984, 34, pp. 659–60.

33 Duke, J.A., *Handbook of Medicinal Herbs*, CRC Press, Boca Raton, FL, 1985.

34 Leung, A.Y., *Encyclopedia of Common Natural Ingredients Used in Food, Drugs, and Cosmetics*, John Wiley & Sons, New York, NY, 1980, pp. 52–3, 189–90.

35 Hahn, F.E., and Ciak, J., 'Berberine', *Antibiotics*, 1976, 3, pp. 577–88.

36 Amin, A.H., Subbaiah, T.V. and Abbasi, K.M., 'Berberine sulfate: antimicrobial activity, bioassay, and mode of action', *Can.J.Microbiol.*, 1969, 15, pp. 1,067–76.

37 Choudry, V.P., Sabir, M. and Bhide, V.N., 'Berberine in giardiasis', *Ind.Pediatr.*, 1972, 9, pp. 143–6.

38 Subbaiah, T.V and Amin, A.H., 'Effect of berberine sulfate on Entamoeba histolytica', *Nature*, 1967, 215, pp. 527–8.

39 Ghosh, A.K., 'Effect of berberine chloride on Leishmania donovani', *Ind.J.Med.Res.*, 1983, 78, pp. 407–16.

40 Majahan, V.M., Sharma, A. and Rattan, A., 'Antimycotic activity of berberine sulphate: an alkaloid from an Indian medicinal herb', *Sabouraudia*, 1982, 20, pp. 79–81.

41 Sabir, M. and Bhide, N., 'Study of some pharmacologic actions of berberine', *Ind.J.Physiol.Pharm.*, 1971, 15, pp. 111–32.

42 Chan, M.Y., 'The effect of berberine on bilirubin excretion in the rat', *Comp.Med.East West*, 1977, 5, pp. 161–8.

43 Watanabe, A., Obata, T. and Nagashima, H., 'Berberine therapy of hypertyraminemia in patients with liver cirrhosis', *Acta Med.Okayama*, 1982, 36, pp. 277–81.

44 Sanbe, K., Murata, T., Fujisawa, K., *et al.*, 'Treatment of liver disease – with particular reference to liver hydrosylates', *J.Clin.Exp.Med.*, 1973, 50, pp. 2,665–76.

45 Faber, K., 'The dandelion – Taraxacum officinale Weber', *Pharmazie*, 1958, 13, pp. 423–35.

12 Acquired immunodeficiency syndrome

1 The authors wish to acknowledge Drs Patrick Donovan NM and Herb Joiner-Bey ND, from whose excellent chapter on the acquired immuno deficiency syndrome in *A Textbook of Natural Medicine* this chapter was derived (Pizzorno, J.E. and Murray, M.A., *A Textbook of Natural Medicine*, John Bastyr College Publications, Seattle, WA, 1988).

2 Gold, J.W., 'Clinical spectrum of infections in patients with HTLV-III associated diseases', *Cancer Res.(suppl.)*, 1985, 45, pp. 4,652s–4s.

3 Fauci, A.S. and Lane, H.C., 'The acquired immunodeficiency syndrome (AIDS): an update', *Int.Arch.Allergy Appl.Immunol.*, 1985, 77, pp. 81–8.

4 Curran, J.W., Morgan, W.M., Starcher, E.T., *et al.*, 'Epidemiological trends of AIDS in the United States', *Cancer Res.(suppl.)*, 1985, 45, pp. 4,602s–4s.

5 'Pneumocystis pneumonia-Los Angeles', *M.M.W.R.*, 1981, 30, pp. 250–2.

6 Lui, K.J., Darrow, W.W. and Rutherford, G.W., 'A model-based estimate of the mean incubation period for AIDS in homosexual men', 1988, 240, pp. 133–5.

7 Curran, J., 'The epidemiology and prevention of the acquired immunodeficiency syndrome', *Ann.Int.Med.*, 1985, 103, pp. 657–62.

8 Groopman, J.E., 'Clinical spectrum of HTLV-III in humans', *Cancer Res. (suppl.)*, 1985, 45, pp. 4,649s–54s.

9 Ranki, A., Valle, S., Antonen, J., *et al.*, 'Immunosuppression in homosexual men seronegative for HTLV-III', *Cancer Res.(suppl.)*, 1985, 45, pp. 4,616s–8s.

10 Crook, W.G., *The Yeast Connection*, Professional Books, Jackson, TN, 1984.

11 Hauser, W.E. and Remington, J.S., 'Effect of antibiotics on the immune response', *Am.J.Med.*, 1982, 72, pp. 711–16.

12 Sanchez, A., Reeser, J., Lau, H., *et al.*, 'Role of sugars in human neutrophilic phagocytosis', *Am.J.Clin.Nutr.*, 1973, 26, pp. 1,180–4.

13 Ringsdorf, W., Cheraskin, E. and Ramsay, R., 'Sucrose, neutrophil phagocytosis and resistance to disease', *Dent.Surv.*, 1976, 52, pp. 46–8.

14 Johnston, D.V. and Marshall, L.A., 'Dietary fat, prostaglandins and the immune response', *Prog.Food, Nutr.Sci.*, 1984, 8, pp. 3–25.

15 Palmblad, J., Hallberg, D. and Rossner, S., 'Obesity, plasma lipids and polymorphonuclear (PMN) granulocyte functions', *Scand.J.Haematol.*, 1977, 19, pp. 293–303.

16 Brayton, R., Stokes, P., Schwartz, M. and Louaia, D., 'Effect of alcohol and various diseases on leukocyte mobilization, phagocytosis and intracellular bacterial killing', *N.E.J.M.*, 1970, 282, pp. 123–8.

17 Saxena, A.K., Singh, K.P., Srivastava, S.N., *et al.*, 'Immunomodulating effects of caffeine (1,3,7-trimethylxanthine) in rodents', *Indian J.Exp.Biol.*, 1984, 22, pp. 293–301.

18 Kotler, D.P., Gaetz, H.P., Lange, M. and Holt, P.R., 'Enteropathy associated with the acquired immunodeficiency syndrome', *Ann.Int.Med.*, 1984, 101, pp. 421–8.

19 Dworkin, B., Wormser, G.P., Rosenthal, W.S., *et al.*, 'Gastrointestinal manifestations of the acquired immune deficiency syndrome: a review of 22 cases', *Am.J.Gastroenterology*, 1985, 80, pp. 774–84.

20   Archer, D.L. and Glinsman, W.H., 'Intestinal infection and malnutrition initiate acquired immune deficiency syndrome (AIDS)', *Nutrition Res.*, 1985, 5, pp. 9–19.
21   Warshaw, A.L., Walker, W.A. and Isselbacher, K.J., 'Protein uptake by the intestine: evidence of intact macromolecules', *Gastroenterology*, 1974, 66, pp. 987–92.
22   Walker, W.A. and Isselbacher, K.J., 'Uptake and transport of macromolecules by the intestine: possible role in clinical disorder', *Gastroenterology*, 1974, 67, pp. 531–50.
23   Mavligitt, G.M., Talpax, M., Hsia, F.T., *et al.*, 'Chronic immune stimulation by sperm alloantigens', *J.A.M.A.*, 1984, 251, pp. 237–41.
24   Russel, M.W., Brown, T.A., Clafin, J.L., *et al.*, 'Immunoglobulin A-mediated hepatobiliary transport constitutes a natural pathway for disposing of bacterial antigens', *Infect.Immunity*, 1983, 42, pp. 1,041–8.
25   Triger, D.R., Alp, M.H. and Wright, R., 'Bacterial and dietary antibodies in liver disease', *Lancet*, 1972, i, pp. 60–3.
26   Glasgow, B.J., Anders, K., Layfield, L.J., *et al.*, 'Clinical and pathological findings of the liver in the acquired immune deficiency syndrome (AIDS)', *Am.J.Clin.Pathol.*, 1985, 83, pp. 582–8.
27   Selye, H., *The Physiology and Pathology of Exposure to Stress*, Acta Inc.Medical Publications, Montreal, 1950.
28   Dilley, J.W., Ochitill, H.N., Perl, M., *et al.*, 'Findings in psychiatric consultations with patients with acquired immune deficiency syndrome', *Am.J.Psychiatry*, 1985, 142, pp. 82–6.
29   Tecoma, E.S. and Huey, L.Y., 'Psychic distress and the immune response', *Life Sciences*, 1985, 36, pp. 1,799–812.
30   Dillon, K.M., Minchoff, B. and Baker, K.H., 'Positive emotional states and enhancement of the immune system', *Int.J.Psychiatry Med.*, 1985–6, 15, pp. 13–17.
31   Miller, L.G., Goldstein, G., Murphy, M. and Ginns, L., 'Reversible alterations in immunoregulatory T-cells in smoking', *Chest*, 1982, 82, pp. 526–9.
32   Beisel, W., Edelman, R., Nauss, K. and Suskind, R., 'Single-nutrient effects of immunologic functions', *J.A.M.A.*, 1981, 245, pp. 53–8.
33   Chondra, R.K., Heresi, G. and Au, B., 'Serum thymic factor activity in deficiencies of calories, zinc, vitamin A and pyridoxine', *Clin.Exp.Immunol.*, 1980, 42, pp. 332–5.
34   Moldofsky, H., Lue, F.A., Eisen, J., *et al.*, 'The relationship of interleukin-1 and immune functions to sleep in humans', *Psychosomatic Medicine*, 1986, 48, pp. 309–19.
35   Viti, A., Muscettola, M., Paulesu, L., *et al.*, 'Effect of exercise on plasma interferon levels', *J.Appl.Phys.*, 1985, 59, pp. 426–8.
36   Alexander, M., Newmark, H. and Miller, R.G., 'Oral beta-carotene can increase the number of OKT4+ cells in human blood', *Immunol.Letters*, 1985, 9, pp. 221–4.
37   Heywood, R., Palmer, A.K., Gregson, R.L., *et al.*, 'The toxicity of beta-carotene', *Toxicology*, 1985, 36, pp. 91–100.
38   Scott, J., 'On the biochemical similarities of ascorbic acid and interferon', *J.Theor.Biol.*, 1982, 98, pp. 235–8.
39   Hoffer, A., 'Ascorbic acid and kidney stones', *Can.Med.Assoc.J.*, 1985, 132, p. 320.
40   Kaul, T.N., Middleton, E. and Ogra, P., 'Antiviral effect of flavonoids on human viruses', *J.Med.Virol.*, 1985, 15, pp. 71–9.
41   Blum, A., Dolle, W., Kortum, K., *et al.*, 'Treatment of acute viral hepatitis with (+)-cyanidanol-3', *Lancet*, 1977, ii, pp. 1,153–5.
42   Schomerus, H., Wieman, K., Dolle, W., *et al.*, '(+)-cyanidanol-3 in the treatment of acute viral hepatitis: a randomized controlled trial', *Hepatology*, 1984, 4, pp. 331–5.
43   Abonyi, M., Kisfolody, S. and Szalay, F., 'Therapeutic effect of (+)-cyanidanol-3 (catechin) in chronic alcoholic liver disease', *Acta Physiol.Hung.*, 1984, 64, pp. 455–60.
44   Stimpel, M., Proksch, A., Wagner, H. and Lohmann-Matthes, M.L., 'Macrophage activation and induction of macrophage cytotoxicity by purified polysaccharide fractions from the plant Echinacea purpurea', *Infect.Immun.*, 1984, 46, pp. 845–9.
45   Wagner, V., Proksch, A., Riess-Maurer, I., *et al.*, 'Immunostimulating polysaccharides (heteroglycans) of higher plants/preliminary communications', *Arzneim-Forsch.*, 1984, 34, pp. 659–60.
46   Wacker, A. and Hilbig, W., 'Virus-inhibition by Echinacea purpurea', *Planta Medica*, 1978, 33, pp. 89–102.
47   Kumazawa, Y., Itagaki, A., Fukumoto, M., *et al.*, 'Activation of peritoneal macrophages by berberine-type alkaloids in terms of induction of cytostatic activity', *Int.J.Immunopharm.*, 1984, 6, pp. 587–92.
48   Desai, A.B., Shah, K.M. and Shah, D.M., 'Berberine in treatment of diarrhea', *Indian Ped.*, 1971, 8, pp. 462–5.
49   Reinhardt, A., Auperin, D. and Sands, J., 'Mechanism of viricidal activity of retinoids: protein removal from bacteriophage 6 envelope', *Antimicrob.Agents Chemother.*, 1984, 17, pp. 1,034–7.
50   Fletcher, R., Albers, A., Chen, A. and Albertson, J., 'Ascorbic acid inhibition of Campylobacter jejuni growth', *App.Env.Micro.*, 1983, 45, pp. 792–5.
51   Schwerdt, P. and Schwerdt, C., 'Effect of ascorbic acid on rhinovirus replication in WI-38 cells', *Proc.Soc.Exp.Biol.Med.*, 1975, 148, pp. 1,237–43.
52   Yunde, H., Guoliang, M., Shuhua, W., *et al*, 'Effect of Radix astragalis seuhedysari on the interferon system', *Chin.Med.J.*, 1981, 94, pp. 35–40.
53   Alstat, E.K., 'Lomatium dissectum', *Comp.Med.*, 1987, May/June, pp. 32–4.
54   Abe, N., Ebina, T. and Ishida, N., 'Interferon induction by glycyrrhizin and glycyrrhetinic acid in mice', *Microbiol.Immunol.*, 1982, 26, pp. 535–9.
55   Pompeii, R., Pani, A., Flore, O., *et al.*, 'Antiviral activity of glycyrrhizic acid', *Experientia*, 1980, 36, p. 304.
56   Pompeii, R., Flore, O., Marccialis, M.A., *et al.*, 'Glycyrrhizic acid inhibits virus growth and inactivates virus particles', *Nature*, 1979, 281, pp. 689–90.

13 Alcoholism

1   Rubenstein, E. and Federman, D., *Scientific American Textbook of Medicine*, Scientific American, New York, NY, 1985, pp. 13:III:1–14.
2   Cruz-Coke, R., 'Genetics and alcoholism', *Neurobeh.Toxicol.Teratol.*, 1983, 5, pp. 179–80.
3   Krupp, M.A. and Chatton, M.J., *Current Medical Diagnosis and Treatment*, Lange Medical Publishers, Los Altos, CA, 1984, pp. 662–5.
4   Dreisbach, A.H., *Handbook of Poisoning*, 7th ed., Lange Medical Publishers, Los Altos, CA, 1983, pp. 185–9.
5   Montgomery, R., *Biochemistry: A Case-Oriented Approach*, C.V. Mosby, St Louis, MO, 1980.

REFERENCES

6   Tipton, K.F., Heneman, G.T.M. and McCrodden, J.M., 'Metabolic and nutritional aspects of alcohol', *Biochem.Soc.Trans.*, 1983, 11, pp. 59–61.

7   Lieber, C.S. and Decarli, L.M., 'Quantitive relationship between amount of dietary fat and severity of alcoholic fatty liver', *Am.J.Clin.Nutr.*, 1970, 23, pp. 474–8.

8   Williams, R.J., *Physician Handbook of Nutritional Science*, C.C. Thomas, Springfield, IL, 1978, p. 79.

9   Das, I., Burch, R.E. and Hahn, H.K.J., 'Effects of zinc deficiency on ethanol metabolism and alcohol and aldehyde dehydrogenase activities', *J.Lab.Clin.Med.*, 1984, 104, pp. 610–17.

10 Silverman, B. and Rivlin, R., 'Ethanol provoked disturbances in the binding of zinc to rat jejunal mucosal proteins', *J.Nutr.*, 1982, 112, p. 744.

11 Wu, C.T., Lee, J.N., Shen, W.W. and Lee, S.L., 'Serum zinc, copper, and ceruloplasmin levels in male alcoholics', *Biol.Psy.*, 1982, 19, pp. 1,333–8.

12 Scholmerich, J., Lohle, E., Kottgen, E. and Gerok, W., 'Zinc and vitamin A deficiency in liver cirrhosis', *Hepato-Gastroenterol.*, 1983, 30, pp. 119–25.

13 Yunice, A.A. and Lindeman, R.D., 'Effect of ascorbic acid and zinc sulphate on ethanol toxicity and metabolism', *Proc.Soc.Exp.Biol.Med.*, 1977, 154, pp. 146–50.

14 Messiha, F.S., 'Vitamin A, gender and ethanol interactions', *Neurobehav.Toxicol.Teratol.*, 1983, 5, pp. 233–6.

15 Morin, L.P. and Forger, N.G., 'Endocrine control of ethanol intake by rats or hamsters: relative contributions of the ovaries, adrenals and steroids', *Pharmac.Biochem.Behav.*, 1982, 17, pp. 529–37.

16 Suematsu, T., Matsumura, T., Sato, N., *et al.*, 'Lipid peroxidation in alcoholic liver disease in humans', *Alcoholism Clin.Exp.Res.*, 1981, 5, pp. 427–30.

17 DiLuzio, N.R., 'A mechanism of the acute ethanol-induced fatty liver and the modification of liver injury by antioxidants', *Lab.Invest.*, 1966, 15, pp. 50–61.

18 Stanko, R.T., Mendelow, H., Shinozuka, H. and Adibi, S.A., 'Prevention of alcohol-induced fatty liver by natural metabolites and riboflavin', *J.Lab.Clin.Med.*, 1978, 91, pp. 228–35.

19 Hartroft, W.S., Porta, E.A. and Suzuki, M., 'Effects of choline chloride on hepatic lipids after acute ethanol intoxication', *Q.J.Stud.Alcohol*, 1964, 25, pp. 427–37.

20 Sachan, D.S., Rhew, T.H. and Ruark, R.A., 'Ameliorating effects of carnitine and its precursors on alcohol-induced fatty liver', *Am.J.Clin.Nutr.*, 1984, 39, pp. 738–44.

21 Hosein, E.A. and Bexton, B., 'Protective action of carnitine on liver lipid metabolism after ethanol administration to rats', *Biochem.Pharm.*, 1975, 24, pp. 1,859–63.

22 Sachan, D.A. and Rhew, T.H., 'Lipotropic effect of carnitine on alcohol-induced hepatic stenosis', *Nutr.Rep.Int.*, 1983, 27, pp. 1,221–6.

23 Majumdar, S.K., Shaw, G.K. and Thomson, A.D., 'Changes in plasma amino acid patterns in chronic alcoholic patients during ethanol withdrawal syndrome: their clinical applications', *Med.Hypoth.*, 1983, 12, pp. 239–51.

24 Branchey, L., Branchey, M., Shaw, S. and Lieber, C.S., 'Relationship between changes in plasma amino acids and depression in alcoholic patients', *Am.J.Psych.*, 1984, 141, pp. 1,212–15.

25 Rosen, H.M., Yoshimura, N., Hodgman, J.M. and Fischer, J.E., 'Plasma amino acid patterns in hepatic encephalopathy of differing etiology', *Gastro.*, 1977, 72, pp. 483–7.

26 Fischer, J.E., Rosen, H.M., Ebeid, A.M., *et al.*, 'The effect of normalization of plasma amino acids on hepatic encephalopathy', *Surgery*, 1976, 80, pp. 77–91.

27 Baines, M., 'Detection and incidence of B and C vitamin deficiency in alcohol-related illness', *Ann.Clin.Biochem.*, 1978, 15, pp. 307–12.

28 Yunice, A.A., Hsu, J.M., Fahmy, A. and Henry, S., 'Ethanol-ascorbate interrelationship in acute and chronic alcoholism in the guinea pig', *Proc.Soc.Exp.Biol.Med.*, 1984, 177, pp. 262–71.

29 Ireland, M.A., Vandongen, R., Davidson, L., *et al.*, 'Acute effects of moderate alcohol consumption on blood pressure and plasma catecholamines', *Clin.Sci.*, 1984, 66, pp. 643–8.

30 Lumeng, L., 'The role of acetaldehyde in mediating the deleterious effect of ethanol on pyridoxal 5'-phosphate metabolism', *J.Clin.Invest.*, 1978, 62, pp. 286–93.

31 Burch, G.E. and Giles, T.D., 'The importance of magnesium deficiency in cardiovascular disease', *Am.Heart J.*, 1977, 94, pp. 649–57.

32 Dutta, S.K., Miller, P.A., Greenberg, L.B. and Levander, O.A., 'Selenium and acute alcoholism', *Am.J.Clin.Nutr.*, 1983, 38, pp. 713–18.

33 Anggard, E., Alling, C., Becker, W. and Jones, A.W., 'Chronic ethanol exposure enhances essential fatty acid deficiency in rats', *Adv.Prost.Thromb.Leuko.Res.*, 1983, 12, pp. 217–22.

34 Rogers, L.L. and Pelton, R.B., 'Glutamine in the treatment of alcoholism', *J.Biol.Chem.*, 1955, 214, pp. 503–6.

35 Rogers, L.L. and Pelton, R.B., 'Glutamine in the treatment of alcoholism', *Q.J.Studies in Alcoholism*, 1957, 18, pp. 581–7.

36 Ravel, J.M., Felsing, B., Lansford, E., *et al.*, 'Reversal of alcohol toxicity by glutamine', *J.Biol.Chem.*, 1955, 214, pp. 497–502.

37 Rogers, L.L., Pelton, R.B. and Williams, R.J., 'Voluntary alcohol consumption by rats following administration of glutamine', *J.Biol.Chem.*, 1955, 214, pp. 503–7.

38 Wagner, H., 'Antihepatotoxic flavonoids', in Cody, V., Middleton, E. and Harbourne, J.B.(eds), *Plant Flavonoids in Biology and Medicine: Biochemical, Pharmacological, and Structure-Activity Relationships*, Alan R. Liss, New York, NY, 1986, pp. 545–58.

39 Wagner, H., 'Plant constituents with antihepatotoxic activity', in Beal, J.L. and Reinhard, E.(eds), *Natural Products as Medicinal Agents*, Hippokrates-Verlag, Stuttgart, 1981.

40 Canini, F., Bartolucci, Cristallini, E., *et al.*, 'Use of silymarin in the treatment of alcoholic hepatic steatosis', *Clin.Ter.*, 1985, 114, pp. 307–14.

41 Salmi, H.A. and Sarna, S., 'Effect of silymarin on chemical, functional, and morphological alteration of the liver. A double-blind controlled study', *Scand.J.Gastroenterol.*, 1982, 17, pp. 417–21.

42 Boari, C., Montanari, M., Galleti, G.P., *et al.*, 'Occupational toxic liver diseases. Therapeutic effects of silymarin', *Min.Med.*, 1985, 72, pp. 2,679–88.

43 Branchey, L., Shaw, S. and Lieber, C.S., 'Ethanol impairs tryptophan transport into the brain and depresses serotonin', *Life Sci.*, 1981, 29, pp. 2,751–5.

44 Bode, J.C., Bode, C., Heidelbach, R., *et al.*, 'Jejunal microflora in patients with chronic alcohol abuse', *Hepato-gastro.*, 1984, 31, pp. 30–4.

45 Worthington, B.S., Meserole, L. and Syrotuck, J.A., 'Effect of daily ethanol ingestion on intestinal permeability to macromolecules', *Dig.Dis.*, 1978, 23, pp. 23–32.

46 Sinyor, D., Brown, T., Rostant, L. and Seraganian, P., 'The role of a physical fitness program in the treatment of alcoholism', *J.Stud.Alcohol.*, 1982, 43, pp. 380–6.

14 Alzheimer's disease

1 Garcia, C.A., Reding, M.J. and Blass, J.P., 'Over diagnosis of dementia', *J.Am.Ger.Soc.*, 1981, 29, pp. 407–10.
2 Wells, C., *Dementia*, F.A. Davis, Philadelphia, PA, 1977.
3 Terry, R.D. and Katzman, R., 'Senile dementia of the Alzheimer type', *Ann.Neurol.*, 1983, 14, pp. 497–506.
4 Editorial, 'Problems with prescription drugs among elderly', *Am.Fam.Phys.*, 1986, 28, p. 236.
5 Heyman, A., Wilkenson, W.E., Hurwitz, B.J., *et al.*, 'Alzheimer's disease: genetic aspects and associated clinical disorders', *Ann.Neurol.*, 1983, 14, pp. 507–15.
6 Fabris, N., Amadio, L., Licastro, F., *et al.*, 'Thymic hormone deficiency in normal ageing and Down's syndrome: is there a primary failure of the thymus?' *Lancet*, 1984, i, pp. 983–6.
7 Nordstrom, J.W., 'Trace mineral nutrition in the elderly', *Am.J.Clin.Nutr.*, 1982, 36, pp. 788–95.
8 Boosalis, M.G., Evans, G.W. and McClain, C.J., 'Impaired handling of orally administered zinc in pancreatic insufficiency', *Am.J.Clin.Nutr.*, 1983, 37, pp. 268–71.
9 Burnet, F.M. 'A possible role of zinc in the pathology of dementia', *Lancet*, 1981, i, pp. 186–8.
10 Lott, I.T., 'Down's syndrome, aging, and Alzheimer's disease: a clinical review', *Ann.N.Y.Acad.Sci.*, 1982, 396, pp. 15–27.
11 Weinreb, H.J., 'Fingerprint patterns in Alzheimer's disease', *Arch.Neurol.*, 1985, 42, pp. 50–4.
12 King, R.G., 'Do raised brain aluminum levels in Alzheimer's Dementia contribute to cholinergic neuronal deficits?', *Med.Hypoth.*, 1984, 14, pp. 301–6.
13 Hershey, C.O., Hershey, L.A., Varnes, A., *et al.*, 'Cerebrospinal fluid trace element content in dementia: clinical, radiologic, and pathologic correlations', *Neurol.*, 1983, 33, pp. 1,350–3.
14 Candy, J.M., Klinowski, J., Perry, R.H., *et al.*, 'Aluminosilicates and senile plaque formation in Alzheimer's disease', *Lancet*, 1986, i, pp. 354–7.
15 Cole, M.G. and Prchal, J.F., 'Low serum vitamin B12 in Alzheimer-type dementia', *Age Aging*, 1984, 13, pp. 101–5.
16 Abalan, F. and Delile, J.M., 'B12 deficiency in presenile dementia', *Biol.Psychiatry*, 1985, 20, pp. 1,247–51.
17 Craig, G.M., Elliot, C. and Hughes, K.R., 'Masked vitamin B12 and folate deficiency in the elderly', *Br.J.Nutr.*, 1985, 54, pp. 613–19.
18 Vorberg, G., 'Ginkgobiloba extract (GBE): a long-term study of chronic cerebral insufficiency in geriatric patients', *Clinical Trials Journal*, 1985, 22, pp. 149–57.
19 Hindmarch, I. and Subhan, Z., 'The psychopharmacological effects of ginkgobiloba extract in normal healthy volunteers', *Int.J.Clin.Pharmacol.Res.*, 1984, 4, pp. 89–93.
20 Gebner, B., Voelp, A. and Klasser, M., 'Study of the long-term action of a ginkgobiloba extract on vigilance and mental performance as determined by means of quantitative pharmaco-EEG and psychometric measurements', *Arzneim-Forsch.*, 1985, 35, pp. 1,459–65.
21 Rosenberg, G. and Davis, K.L., 'The use of cholinergic precursors in neuropsychiatric diseases', *Am.J.Clin.Nutr.*, 1982, 36, pp. 709–20.
22 Levy, R., Little, A., Chuaqui, P. and Reith, M., 'Early results from double blind, placebo controlled trial of high dose phosphatydylcholine in Alzheimer's disease', *Lancet*, 1982, i, pp. 474–6.
23 Sitaram, N., Weingartner, B., Gaine, E.D. and Cillin, J.C., 'Choline: selective enhancement of serial learning and encoding of low imagery words in man', *Life Sci.*, 1978, 22, pp. 1,555–60.

15 Anaemia

1 Krause, M.V. and Mahan, K.L., *Food, Nutrition and Diet Therapy*, 7th ed., W.B. Saunders, Philadelphia, PA, 1984, pp. 128–31, 157–64, 585–99.
2 Petersdorf, R., *et al.*(eds), *Harrison's Principles of Internal Medicine*, McGraw-Hill, New York, NY, 1983, pp. 1,848–60.
3 Morley, J.E., 'Nutritional status of the elderly', *Am.J.Med.*, 1986, 81, pp. 679–95.
4 Jacobs, A.M. and Owen, G.M., 'The effect of age on iron absorption', *J.Gerontol.*, 1969, 24, pp. 95–6.
5 Bezwoda, W., Charlton, R., Bothwell, T., *et al.*, 'The importance of gastric hydrochloric acid in the absorption of nonheme iron', *J.Lab.Clin.Med.*, 1978, 92, pp. 108–16.
6 Carmel, R., Weiner, J.M. and Johnson, C.S., 'Iron deficiency occurs frequently in patients with pernicious anemia', *J.A.M.A*, 1987, 257, pp. 1,081–3.
7 Davis, R.E. and Nichol, D.J., 'Folic acid', *Int.J.Biochem.*, 1988, 20, pp. 133–9.
8 Gordeuk, V.R., Brittenham, G.M., Hughes, M., *et al.*, 'High dose carbonyl iron deficiency anemia: a randomized double-blind trial', *Am.J.Clin.Nutr.*, 1987, 46, pp. 1,029–34.
9 Danisi, M., Guerresi, E., Landucci, G., *et al.*, 'Serum iron concentration following administration of two different iron preparations', *J.Int.Med.Res.*, 1987, 15, pp. 374–8.
10 Fochi, F., Ciampini, M. and Ceccarelli, G., 'Efficacy of iron therapy: a comparative evaluation of four iron preparations administered to anaemic pregnant women', *J.Int.Med.Res.*, 1985, 13, pp. 1–11.
11 Minot, G.R. and Murphy, W.P., 'Treatment of pernicious anemia by special diet', *J.A.M.A.*, 1926, 87, pp. 470–6.
12 Deininger, R., 'Amarum-bitter herbs: common bitter principle remedies and their action', *Krankenpfledge*, 1975, 29, pp. 99–100.
13 Duke, J.A., *Handbook of Medicinal Herbs*, CRC Press, Boca Raton, FL, 1985.

16 Angina pectoris

1 Bamji, M. 'Nutritional and health implications of lysine carnitine relationship', *Wld Rev. Nutr. Diet.*, 1984, 44, pp. 185–211.
2 Silverman, N.A., Schmitt, G., Vishwanath, M., *et al.*, 'Effect of carnitine on myocardial function and metabolism following global ischemia', *Annals Thoracic Surg.*, 1985, 40, pp. 20–5.

3   Cherchi, A., Lai, C., Angelino, F., *et al.*, 'Effects of L-carnitine on exercise tolerance in chronic stable angina: a multicenter, double-blind, randomized, placebo controlled crossover study', *Int. J. Clin. Pharm. Ther. Toxicol.*, 1985, 23, pp. 569–72.

4   Orlando, G. and Rusconi, C., 'Oral L-carnitine in the treatment of chronic cardiac ischaemia in elderly patients', *Clin. Trials J.*, 1986, 23, pp. 338–44.

5   Kamikawa, T., Suzuki, Y., Kobayashi, A., et al., 'Effects of L-carnitine on exercise tolerance in patients with stable angina pectoris', *Jap. Heart. J.*, 1984, 25, pp. 587–97.

6   Kosolcharoen, P., Nappi, J., Peruzzi, P., *et al.*, 'Improved exercise tolerance after administration of carnitine', *Curr. Ther. Res.*, 1981, 30, pp. 753–64.

7   Pola, P., Savi, L., Serricchio, M., *et al.*, 'Use of physiological substance, acetyl-carnitine, in the treatment of angiospastic syndromes', *Drugs Exptl. Clin. Res.*, 1984, X, pp. 213–17.

8   Dal Negro, R., Plmari, G., Zoccatelli, O. and Turco, P., 'Changes in physical performance of untrained volunteers: effects of L-carnitine', *Clin. Trials J.*, 1986, 23, pp. 242–8.

9   Opie, L.H., 'Role of carnitine in fatty acid metabolism of normal and ischemic myocardium', *Am. Heart. J.*, 1979, 97, pp. 373–8.

10 Rebuzzi, A.G., Schiavoni, G., Amico, C.M., *et al.*, 'Beneficial effects of L-carnitine in the reduction of the necrotic area in acute myocardial infarction', *Drugs Exptl Clin. Res.*, 1984, 10, pp. 219–23.

11 Arsenio, L., Bodria, P., Magnati, G., *et al.*, 'Effectiveness of long-term treatment with pantethine in patients with dyslipidemias', *Clin. Ther.*, 1986, 8, pp. 537–45.

12 Avogaro, P., Bittolo, B.G. and Fusello, M., 'Effect of pantethine on lipids, lipoproteins and apolipoproteins in man', *Curr. Ther. Res.*, 1983, 33, pp. 488–93.

13 Miccoli, R., Marchetti, P., Sampietro, T., *et al.*, 'Effects of pantethine on lipids and apolipoproteins in hypercholesterolemic diabetic and non-diabetic patients', *Curr. Ther. Res.*, 1984, 36, pp. 545–90.

14 Maggi, G., Donati, C. and Criscuoli, G., 'Pantethine: a physiological lipo-modulating agent in the treatment of hyperlipidemias', *Curr. Ther. Res.*, 1982, 32, pp. 380–6.

15 Galeone, F., Scalabrino, A., Giuntoli, F., *et al.*, 'The lipid lowering effect of pantethine in hyperlipidemic patients: a clinical investigation', *Curr. Ther. Res.*, 1983, 34, pp. 383–90.

16 Gaddi, A., Descovich, G., Noseda, G., *et al.*, 'Controlled evaluation of pantethine, a natural hypolipidemic compound, in patients with different forms of hyperlipoproteinemia', *Atheroscl.*, 1984, 50, pp. 73–83.

17 Hayashi, H., Kobayashi, A., Terad, H., *et al.*, 'Effects of pantethine on action potential of canine papillary muscle during hypoxic perfusion', *Jap. Heart. J.*, 1985, 26, pp. 289–96.

18 Folkers, K., Yamamura, Y., Ito, Y., (eds), *Biomedical and Clinical Aspects of Coenzyme Q10*, volumes 1–4, Elsevier Science Publishers, Amsterdam: vol. 1, 1977; vol. 2, 1980; vol. 3, 1982; vol. 4, 1984.

19 Folkers, K., Vadhanavikit, S. and Mortensen, S., 'Biochemical rationale and myocardial tissue data on the effective therapy of cardiomyopathy with coenzyme Q10', *Proc. Natl Acad. Sci.*, 1985, 82, pp. 901–4.

20 Mortensen, S.A., Vadhanavikit, S. and Folkers, K., 'Deficiency of coenzyme Q10 in myocardial failure', *Drugs Exptl Clin. Res.*, 1984, 10, pp. 487–502.

21 Kitamura, N., Yamaguchi, A., Otaki, M., Sawatani, O., *et al.*, 'Myocardial tissue level of coenzyme Q10 in patients with cardiac failure', in Folkers, K., Yamamura, Y., Ito, Y. (eds) *Biomedical and Clinical Aspects of Coenzyme Q10*, vol. 4, Elsevier Science Publishers, Amsterdam, 1984, pp. 243–52.

22 Littarru, G.P., Ho, L. and Folkers, K., 'Deficiency of coenzyme Q10 in human heart disease. Part II', *Int. J. Vit. Nutr. Res.*, 1972, 42, p. 413.

24 Kamikawa, T., Kobayashi, A., Yamashita, T., *et al.*, 'Effects of coenzyme Q10 on exercise tolerance in chronic stable angina pectoris', *Am. J. Cardiol.*, 1985, 56, p. 247.

25 Yamasawa, I., Nohara, Y., Konno, S., *et al.*, 'Experimental studies on effects of coenzyme Q10 on ischemic myocardium', in Yamamura, Y., Folkers, K., Ito, Y. (eds), *Biomedical and Clinical Aspects of Coenzyme Q10*, vol. 2, Elsevier/North-Holland Biomedical Press, Amsterdam, 1980, pp. 333–47.

26 Turlapaty, P.D.M.V. and Altura, B.M., 'Magnesium deficiency produces spasms of coronary arteries: relationship to etiology of sudden death ischemic heart disease', *Sci.*, 1980, 208, pp. 199–200.

27 Seelig, M.S. and Heggtveit, H.A., 'Magnesium interrelationship in ischemic heart disease: a review', *Am. J. Clin. Nutr.*, 1974, 27, pp. 59–79.

28 Iseri, L.T., 'Magnesium and cardiac arrhythmias', *Magnesium*, 1986, 5, pp. 111–26.

29 Altura, B.M. and Altura, B.T., 'New perspectives on the role of magnesium in the pathophysiology of the cardiovascular system', *Magnesium*, 1985, 4, pp. 226–44.

30 Petkov, V., 'Plants with hypotensive, antiatheromatous and coronarodilating action', *Am. J. Chin. Med.*, 1979, 7, pp. 197–236.

31 Ammon, H.P.T. and Handel, M., 'Crataegus, toxicology and pharmacology', *Planta Medica*, 1981, 43, pp. 101–20, 318–22.

32 Wegrowski, J., Robert, A.M. and Moczar, M., 'The effect of procyanidolic oligomers on the composition of normal and hypercholesterolemic rabbit aortas', *Biochem. Pharm.*, 1984, 33, pp. 3,491–7.

33 Mavers, V.W.H. and Hensel, H., 'Changes in local myocardial blood flow following oral administration of a crataegus extract to non-anesthetized dogs', *Arzniem-Forsch.*, 1974, 24, pp. 783–5.

34 Roddewig, V.C. and Hensel, H., 'Reaction of local myocardial blood flow in non-anesthetized dogs and anesthetized cats to oral and parenteral application of a crataegus fraction (oligomere procyanidins)', *Arzneim-Forsch.*, 1977, 27, pp. 1,407–10.

35 Rewerski, V.W., Piechocki, T., Tyalski, M. and Lewak, S., 'Some pharmacological properties of oligomeric procyanidin isolated from hawthorn (Crataegus oxyacantha)', *Arzneim-Forsch.*, 1967, 17, pp. 490–1.

36 Hammerl, H., Kranzl, C., Pichler, O. and Studlar, M., 'Klinixch-experimentelle toffwechseluntersuchungen mit einem crataegus-extrakt', *Arzniem-Forsch.*, 1971, 21, pp. 261–3.

37 Vogel, V.G., 'Predictability of the activity of drug combinations – yes or no?', *Arzniem-Forsch.*, 1975, 25, pp. 1,356–65.

38 O'Conolly, V.M., Jansen, W., Bernhoft, G. and Bartsch, G., 'Treatment of cardiac performance (NYHA stages I to II) in advanced age with standardized crataegus extract', *Fortschr. Med.*, 1986, 104, pp. 805–8.

39 Petkov, E., Nikolov, N. and Uzunov, P., 'Inhibitory effect of some flavonoids and flavonoid mixtures on cyclic AMP phosphodiesterase activity of rat heart', *Planta Medica*, 1981, 43, pp. 183–6.

17 Asthma and hayfever

1   Pizzorno, J.E. and Murray, M.T., *A Textbook of Natural Medicine*, John Bastyr College Publications, Seattle, WA, 1985, p. VI: Asthma-1-7.
2   Kay, A.B., 'Mediators of hypersensitivity and inflammatory cells in the pathogenesis of bronchial asthma', *Euro. J. Resp. Dis. Suppl.*, 1983, 129, pp. 1–45.
3   Bock, S.A., 'Food-related asthma and basic nutrition', *J. Asthma*, 1983, 20, pp. 377–81.
4   Oehling, A., 'Importance of food allergy in childhood asthma', *Allergol. Immunopathol. Suppl.*, 1981, IX, pp. 71–3.
5   Ogle, K.A. and Bullocks, J.D., 'Children with allergic rhinitis and/or bronchial asthma treated with elimination diet: a five-year follow-up', *Ann. Allergy*, 1980, 44, pp. 273–8.
6   Pelikan, Z., 'Nasal response to food ingestion challenge', *Arch. Otolaryngol. Head Neck Surg.*, 1988, 114, pp. 525–30.
7   Bray, G.W., 'The hypochlorhydria of asthma in childhood', *Quart. J. Med.*, 1931, 24, pp. 181–97.
8   Personal communication with Jonathan Wright MD.
9   Freedman, B.J., 'A diet free from additives in the management of allergic disease', *Clin. Allergy*, 1977, 7, pp. 417–21.
10   Stevenson, D.D. and Simon, R.A., 'Sensitivity to ingested metabisulfites in asthmatic subjects', *J. Allergy Clin. Immunol.*, 1981, 68, pp. 26–32.
11   Lindahl, O., Lindwall, L., Spangberg, A., *et al.*, 'Vegan diet regimen with reduced medication in the treatment of bronchial asthma', *J. Asthma*, 1985, 22, pp. 45–55.
12   Dahlen, S.E., Hansson, G., Hedqvist, P., *et al.*, 'Allergen challenge of lung tissue from asthmatics elicits bronchial contraction that correlates with the release of leukotrienes C_4, D_4 and E_4 *Proc. Natl. Acad. Sci.*, 1983, 80, pp. 1,712–16.
13   Bisgaard, H., 'Leukotrienes and prostaglandins in asthma, *Allergy*, 1984, 39, pp. 413–20.
14   Yen, S.S. and Morris, H.G., 'An imbalance of arachidonic acid metabolism in asthma', *Biochem. Biophys, Res. Com.*, 1981, 103, pp. 774–9.
15   Unge, G., Grubbstrom, J., Olsson, P., *et al.*, 'Effect of dietary tryptophan restrictions on clinical symptoms in patients with endogenous asthma', *Allergy*, 1983, 38, pp. 211–12.
16   Collip, P.J., Goldzier III, S., Weiss, N., *et al.*, 'Pyridoxine treatment of childhood asthma', *Ann. Allergy*, 1975, 35, pp. 93–7.
17   Reynolds, R.D. and Natta, C.L., 'Depressed plasma pyridoxal phosphate concentrations in adult asthmatics', *Am. J. Clin. Nutr.*, 1985, 41, pp. 684–8.
18   Simon, S.W., 'Vitamin B_{12} therapy in allergy and chronic dermatoses', *J. Allergy*, 1951, 2, pp. 183–5.
19   Garrison, R. and Somer, E., *The Nutrition Desk Reference*, Ch. 5, 'Vitamin research: selected topics', Keats Publications, New Canaan, CN, 1985, pp. 93–4.
20   Olusi, S.O., Ojutiku, O.O., Jessop, W.J.E., and Iboko, M.I., 'Plasma and white blood cell ascorbic acid concentrations in patients with bronchial asthma', *Clinica Chimica Acta*, 1979, 92, pp. 161–6.
21   Anderson, R., Hay, I., Van Wyk, H.A. and Theron, A., 'Ascorbic acid in bronchial asthma', *S.A. Med. J.*, 1983, 63, pp. 649–52.
22   Mohsenin, V., Dubois, A.B. and Douglas, J.S., 'Effect of ascorbic acid on response to methylcholine challenge in asthmatic subjects', *Am. Rev. Respir. Dis.*, 1983, 127, pp. 143–7.
23   Buck, M.G. and Zadunaisky, J.A., 'Stimulation of ion transport by ascorbic acid through inhibition of 3':5'-cyclic-AMP phosphodiesterase in the corneal epithelium and other tissues', *Biochemica Biophysica Acta*, 1975, 389, pp. 251–60.
24   Anah, C.O., Jarike, L.N. and Baig, H.A., 'High dose ascorbic acid in Nigerian asthmatics', *Trop. Geogr. Med.*, 1980, 32, pp. 132–7.
25   Spannhake, E.W. and Menkes, H.A., 'Vitamin C – new tricks for an old dog', *Am. Rev. Resp. Dis.*, 1983, 127, pp. 139–41.
26   Grosch, W. and Laskawy, G., 'Co-oxidation of carotenes requires one soybean lipoxygenase isoenzyme', *Biochem. Biophys. Acta*, 1979, 575, pp. 439–45.
27   Panganamala, R.V. and Cornwell, D.G., 'The effects of vitamin E on arachidonic acid metabolism', *Ann. N.Y. Acad. Sci.*, 1982, 393, pp. 376–91.
28   McCarty, M., 'Can dietary selenium reduce leukotriene production?', *Med. Hypoth.*, 1984, 13, pp. 45–50.
29   Trendelenburg, P., 'Physiologische und pharmakologische untersuchungen an der isolierten bronchial muskulatur', *Arch. Exp. Pharmacol. Ther.*, 1912, 69, p. 79.
30   Haury, V.G., 'Blood serum magnesium in bronchial asthma and its treatment by the administration of magnesium sulfate', *J. Lab. Clin. Med.*, 1940, 26, pp. 340–4.
31   Brunner, E.H., Delabroise, A.M. and Haddad, Z.H., 'Effect of parenteral magnesium on pulmonary function, plasma cAMP, and histamine in bronchial asthma', *J. Asthma*, 1985, 22, pp. 3–11.
32   Duke, J.A., *Handbook of Medicinal Herbs*, CRC Press, Boca Raton, FL, 1985.
33   Duke, J.A. and Ayensu, E.S., *Medicinal Plants of China*, Reference Publications, Algonac, MI, 1985.
34   Gilman, A.G., Goodman, A.S. and Gilman, A., *The Pharmacologic Basis of Therapeutics*, Macmillan Publishing, New York, NY, 1980.
35   Kasahara, Y., Hikino, H., Tsuru, F., *et al.*, 'Anti-inflammatory actions of ephedrines in acute inflammations', *Planta Medica*, 1985, 54, pp. 325–31.
36   Kubo, M., Matsuda, H., Tanaka, M., *et al.*, 'Studies on Scutellariae radix. VII. Anti-arthritic and anti-inflammatory actions of methanolic extract and flavonoid components from Scutellaria radix', *Chem. Pharm. Bull.*, 1984, 32, pp. 2,724–9.
37   Kimura, Y., Okuda, H. and Arichi, S., 'Studies on Scutellariae radix; VIII. Effects of various flavonoids on arachidonate metabolism in leukocytes', *Planta Medica*, 1985, 54, pp. 132–6.
38   Hikino, H., 'Recent research on Oriental medicinal plants', *Economic Medicinal Plant Research*, 1985, 1, pp. 53–86.
39   Sung, C., Baker, A.P., Holden, D.A., *et al.*, 'Effect of extracts of Angelica polymorpha on reaginic antibody production', *J. Natural Products*, 1982, 45, pp. 398–406.
40   Cyong, J., 'A pharmacological study of the anti-inflammatory activity of Chinese herbs. A review', *Int. J. Acupunct. Electro-Ther. Research*, 1982, 7, pp. 173–202.
41   Tanaka, S., Ikeshiro, Y., Tabata, M. and Konoshima, M., 'Anti-nociceptive substances from the roots of Angelica acutiloba', *Arzneim-Forsch.*, 1977, 27, pp. 2,039–45.
42   Leung, A.Y., *Encyclopedia of Common Natural Ingredients Used in Food, Drugs, and Cosmetics*, John Wiley & Sons, New York, NY, 1980.
43   Tamura, Y., Nishikawa, T. and Yamada, K., 'Effects of glycyrrhetinic acid and its derivatives on delta-4-5-alpha- and 5-beta-reductase in rat liver', *Arzneim-Forsch.*, 1979, 29, pp. 647–9.
44   Suzuki, H., Ohta, Y., Takino, T., *et al.*, 'Effects of glycyrrhizin on biochemical tests in patients with chronic hepatitis – double-blind trial', *Asian Med. J.*, 1984, 26, pp. 423–38.

45   Vanderhoek, J., Makheja, A. and Bailey, J., 'Inhibition of fatty acid lipoxygenases by onion and garlic oils. Evidence for the mechanism by which these oils inhibit platelet aggregation', *Bioch. Pharmacol.*, 1980, 29, pp. 3,169–73.

46   Dorsch, W. and Weber, J., 'Prevention of allergen-induced bronchial constriction in sensitized guinea pigs by crude alcohol onion extract', *Agents Actions*, 1984, 14, pp. 626–30.

47   Dorsch, W., Adam, O., Weber, J. and Ziegeltrum, T., 'Antiasthmatic effects of onion extracts – detection of benzyl- and other isothiocyanates in mustard oils as antiasthmatic compounds of plant origin', *Euro. J. Pharmacol.*, 1985, 107, pp. 17–24.

48   Halmagyi, D.F.J., Kovacs, A. and Neumann, P., 'Adrenalcortical pathway of lobeline protection in some forms of experimental lung edema in the rat', *Dis. Chest*, 1958, 33, pp. 285–96.

49   Mitchell, W., *Naturopathic Applications of the Botanical Remedies*, W. Mitchell, Seattle, WA, 1983.

50   Lundberg, J.M. and Saria, A., 'Capsaicin-induced desensitization of airway mucosa to cigarette smoke, mechanical and chemical irritants', *Nature*, 1983, 302, pp. 251–3.

51   Tan, Y. and Collins-Williams, C., 'Aspirin-induced asthma in children', *Ann. Allergy*, 1982, 48, pp. 1–5.

52   Vanderhoek, J.Y., Ekborg, S.L. and Bailey, J.M., 'Nonsteroidal anti-inflammatory drugs stimulate 15-lipoxygenase/leukotriene pathway in human polymorphonuclear leukocytes', *J. Allergy Clin. Immunol.*, 1984, 74, pp. 412–7.

18 Atherosclerosis

1   Petersdorf, R., *Harrison's Principles of Internal Medicine*, 10th ed., McGraw-Hill, New York, NY, 1983.

2   Robbins, S.A. and Cotran, R., *Pathologic Basis of Disease*, W.B. Saunders, New York, NY, 1974.

3   Elliot, W.J., 'Ear lobe crease and coronary artery disease', *Am. J. Med.*, 1983, 75, pp. 1,024–32.

4   McCully, K.S. and Wilson, R.B., 'Homocysteine theory of arteriosclerosis', *Atherosclerosis*, 1975, 22, pp. 215–27.

5   Levene, C.I. and Murray, J.C., 'The aetiological role of maternal B6 deficiency in the development of atherosclerosis', *Lancet*, 1977, i, pp. 628–9.

6   Lam, S.C.-T., Harfenist, E.J., Packham, M.A., *et al.*, 'Investigation of possible mechanisms of pyridoxal 5'-phosphate inhibition of platelet reactions', *Thrombosis Res.*, 1980, 20, pp. 633–45.

7   Bendit, E., 'The origin of atherosclerosis', *Sci. Am.*, 1977, 236, pp. 74–85.

8   Curtiss, L.K. and Plow, E.F., 'Interaction of plasma lipoproteins with human platelets', *Blood*, 1984, 64, pp. 365–74.

9   Ross, R. and Vogel, A., 'The platelet derived growth factor', *Cell*, 1978, 14, pp. 203–10.

10   Gerrard, J.M., White, J.G., and Krivit, W., 'Labile aggregation stimulating substance, free fatty acids and platelet aggregation', *J. Lab. Clin. Med.*, 1976, 87, pp. 73–82.

11   Gillman, A.G., Goodman, L.S. and Gillman, A., *The Pharmacological Basis of Medicine*, Macmillan, New York, NY, 1980.

12   Sanders, T.A.B. and Roshanai, F., 'The influence of different types of omega-3 polyunsaturated fatty acids on blood lipids and platelet function in healthy volunteers', *Clin. Sci.*, 1983, 64, pp. 91–9.

13   Connor, W.E., Harris, W.S., Rothrock, D.W., *et al.*, 'Reduction of plasma lipids, lipoproteins, and apoproteins by dietary fish oils in patients with hypertriglyceridemia', *N. Eng. J. Med.*, 1985, 312, pp. 1,210–16.

14   Von Schacky, C., 'Prophylaxis of atherosclerosis with marine omega-3 fatty acids. A comprehensive strategy', *Ann. Int. Med.*, 1987, 107, pp. 890–9.

15   Simons, L.A., Hickie, J.B. and Balasubramaniam, S., 'On the effects of dietary n-3 fatty acids (Maxepa) on plasma lipids and lipoproteins in patients with hyperlipidemia', *Atherosclerosis*, 1985, 54, pp. 75–88.

16   Kato, H., Tillotson, M.Z. and Nichamai, G.G., 'Epidemiological studies of CHD and stroke in Japanese men living in Japan, Hawaii and California: serum lipids and diet', *Am. J. Epid.*, 1973, 97, pp. 372–85.

17   Fromhout, D., Bosschieter, E.B., and Coulander, C.D.L., 'The inverse relationship between fish consumption and 20-year mortality from coronary heart disease', *N. Eng. J. Med.*, 1985, 312, pp. 1,205–9.

18   Snowdon, D.A., Phillips, R.L. and Fraser, G.E., 'Meat consumption and fatal heart disease', *Prev. Med.*, 1984, 13, pp. 490–500.

19   Fisher, M., Levine, P.H., Weiner, B., *et al.*, 'The effect of vegetarian diets on plasma lipid and platelet levels', *Arch. Int. Med.*, 1986, 146, pp. 1,193–7.

20   Robertson, J., Brydon, W.G., Tadesse, K., *et al.*, 'The effect of raw carrot on serum lipids and colon function', *Am. J. Clin. Nutr.*, 1979, 32, pp. 1,889–92.

21   Rosenthal, M.B., Barnard, R.J., Rose, D.P., *et al.*, 'Effects of a high-complex-carbohydrate, low-fat, low-cholesterol diet on levels of serum lipids and estradiol', *Am. J. Med.*, 1985, 78, pp. 23–7.

22   Vahouny, G. and Kritchevsky, D., *Dietary Fiber in Health and Disease*, Plenum Press, New York, NY, 1982.

23   Kirby, R.W., Anderson, J.W., Sieling, R.D., *et al.*, 'Oat-bran intake selectively lowers serum LDL concentration of hypercholesterolemic men', *Am. J. Clin. Nutr.*, 1981, 34, pp. 824–9.

24   Anderson, J.W., and Chen, W.L., 'Plant fiber: carbohydrate and lipid metabolism', *Am. J. Clin. Nutr.*, 1979, 32, pp. 346–63.

25   Redgrave, T.G., 'Dietary proteins and atherosclerosis', *Atherosclerosis*, 1984, 52, pp. 349–51.

26   Yudin, J., 'Dietary factors in atherosclerosis: sucrose', *Lipids*, 1978, 13, pp. 370–2.

27   Alexander, J.C., 'Chemical and biological properties related to toxicity of heated fats', *J. Tox. Env. Health.*, 1981, 7, pp. 125–38.

28   Editorial, 'Atherogenicity of trans-fatty acids in rabbits', *Nutr. Rev.*, 1984, 42, pp. 197–8.

29   Hill, E.G., Johnson, S. and Holman, R., 'Intensification of essential fatty acid deficiency in the rat by dietary trans-fatty acids', *J. Nutr.*, 1979, 109, pp. 1,759–67.

30   Renaud, S. and Nordoy, A., '"Small is beautiful": alpha-linolenic acid and eicosapentaenoic acid in man', *Lancet*, 1983, i, p. 1,169.

31   Saynor, R., 'Effects of omega-3 fatty acids on serum lipids', *Lancet*, 1984, ii, p. 696.

32   Willis, A.L., 'Dihomo-gamma-linolenic acid as the endogenous protective agent for myocardial infarction', *Lancet*, 1984, ii, pp. 697.

33   Heine, R.J., Schouten, J.A., van Gent, C.M., *et al.*, 'The effect of dietary linoleic acid and pectin on lipoprotein and apolipoprotein A1 concentrations in rhesus monkeys', *Ann. Nutr. Metab.*, 1984, 28, pp. 201–6.

34   Horrobin, D.F. and Manku, M.S., 'How do polyunsaturated fatty acids lower plasma cholesterol levels?', *Lipids*, 1983, 18, pp. 558–62.

35   Wood, D.A., Butler, S., Riemersma, R.A., *et al.*, 'Adipose tissue and platelet fatty acids and coronary heart disease in Scottish men', *Lancet*, 1984, ii, pp. 117–21.

36   Editorial, 'Evidence of prostaglandin 13 formation in vivo from dietary eicosapentaenoic acid', *Nutr. Rev.*, 1984, 42, pp. 317–21.

37   Ginter, E. *et al.*, 'Effect of ascorbic acid in the regulation of cholesterol metabolism and the pathogenesis of atherosclerosis', *Int. J. Vit. Nutr. Res.*, 1977, 47, pp. 1–18.

38   Turley, S., West, C. and Horton, B., 'Role of ascorbic acid in the regulation of cholesterol metabolism and the pathogenesis of atherosclerosis', *Atherosclerosis*, 1976, 24, pp. 1–18.

39   Krumdieck, C. and Butterworth, C.E., 'Ascorbate-cholesterol-lecithin interactions: factors of potential importance in the pathogenesis of atherosclerosis', *Am. J. Clin. Nutr.*, 1974, 27, pp. 866–76.

40   Cordova, C., Musca, A., Viola, F., *et al.*, 'Influence of ascorbic acid on platelet aggregation in vitro and in vivo', *Atherosclerosis*, 1982, 41, pp. 15–19.

41   Okuma, N., Takayama, H. and Uchino, H., 'Generation of prostacyclin-like substance and lipid peroxidation in vitamin E deficient rats', *Prostaglandins*, 1980, 19, pp. 527–36.

42   Nakamura, M., 'Effect of vitamin E deficiency on the level of SOD, glutathione peroxidase, catalase and lipid peroxide', *Int. J. Vit. Nutr. Res.*, 1976, 46, pp. 187–91.

43   Steiner, M. and Anastasi, J., 'Vitamin E – an inhibitor of platelet release reaction', *J. Clin. Invest.*, 1976, 57, pp. 732–7.

44   Watanabe, J., Umeda, F., Wakasugi, H. and Ibayashi, H., 'Effect of vitamin E on platelet aggregation in diabetes mellitus', *Thromb. Haemostas.* (Stuttgart), 1984, 51, pp. 313–16.

45   Galli, C. and Socini, A., 'Biological actions and possible uses of vitamin E', *Acta Vitaminol. Enzymol.*, 1982, 4, pp. 245–52.

46   Mower, R. and Steiner, M., 'Biochemical interaction of arachidonic acid and vitamin E in human platelets', *Prostaglandins Med.*, 1983, 10, pp. 389–403.

47   Hermann, W.J., Ward, K. and Faucett, J., 'The effect of tocopherol on high-density lipoprotein cholesterol', *Am. J. Clin. Path.*, 1979, 72, pp. 848–52.

48   Vermaak, W.J.H., Barnard, H.C., Potgeiter, G.M. and Theron, H.T., 'Vitamin B6 and coronary artery disease', *Atherosclerosis*, 1987, 63, pp. 235–8.

49   Altura, B.M. and Altura, B.T., 'New perspectives on the role of magnesium in the pathophysiology of the cardiovascular system', *Magnesium*, 1985, 4, pp. 226–44.

50   Turlapaty, P.D.M.V. and Altura, B.M., 'Magnesium deficiency produces spasms of coronary arteries: relationship to etiology of sudden death ischemic heart disease', *Sci.*, 1980, 208, pp. 199–200.

51   Seelig, M.S., 'Magnesium deficiency with phosphate and vitamin D excess: role in pediatric cardiovascular disease', *Card. Med.*, 1978, 3, pp. 637–50.

52   Iseri, L.T., 'Magnesium and cardiac arrhythmias', *Magnesium*, 1986, 5, pp. 111–26.

53   Davis, W.H., Leary, W.P., Reyes, A.J. and Olhaberry, J.V., 'Monotherapy with magnesium increases abnormally low high density lipoprotein cholesterol: a clinical assay', *Curr. Ther. Res.*, 1984, 36, pp. 341–5.

54   Hughes, A. and Tonks, R.S., 'Platelets, magnesium, and myocardial infarction', *Lancet*, 1965, i, pp. 1,044–6.

55   Jeppesen, B.B., Blach, A. and Harvald, B., 'Serum magnesium in Greenland eskimos', *Acta Med. Scand.*, 1984, 215, pp. 477–9.

56   Bierenbaum, M.L., Fleischman, A.I. and Raichelson, R.I., 'Long term human studies on the lipid effects of oral calcium', *Lipids*, 1972, 7, pp. 202–6.

57   Allen, K.G.D. and Klevay, L.M., 'Hyperlipoproteinemia in rats due to copper deficiency', *Nutr. Rep. Int.*, 1980, 22, pp. 295–9.

58   Freland-Graves, J.H., Friedman, B.J., Han, W.H., *et al.*, 'Effect of zinc supplementation on plasma high-density lipoprotein cholesterol and zinc', *Am. J. Clin. Nutr.*, 1982, 35, pp. 988–92.

59   Philip, B., Nampoothiri, V.K. and Kurup, P.A., 'Zinc and metabolism of lipids in normal and atheromatous rats', *Ind. J. Exp. Biol.*, 1978, 16, pp. 46–50.

60   Klevay, L.M., 'Dietary copper: a powerful determinant of cholesterolemia', *Med. Hypothesis*, 1987, 24, pp. 111–19.

61   Editorial, 'Activation of lysyl oxidase by copper', *Nutr. Rev.*, 1979, 37, pp. 330–1.

62   Mertz, W., 'Trace minerals and atherosclerosis', *Fed. Proc.*, 1982, 41, pp. 2,807–12.

63   Riales, R. and Albrink, M.J., 'Effect of chromium chloride supplementation on glucose tolerance and serum lipids including high-density lipoprotein of adult men', *Am. J. Clin. Nutr.*, 1981, 34, pp. 2,670–8.

64   Offenbacher, E.G. and Pi-Sunyer, F.X., 'Beneficial effect of chromium-rich yeast on glucose tolerance and blood lipids in elderly subjects', *Diabetes*, 1980, 29, pp. 919–25.

65   Salonen, J.T., 'Association between cardiovascular death and myocardial infarction and serum selenium in a matched-pair longitudinal study', *Lancet*, 1982, 2, pp. 175–9.

66   Schone, N.W., Morris, V.C. and Levander, O.A., 'Effects of selenium deficiency on aggregation and thromboxane formation in rat platelet', *Fed. Proc.*, 1984, 43, p. 477.

67   Kosolcharoen, P., Nappi, J., Peruzzi, P., *et al.*, 'Improved exercise tolerance after administration of carnitine', *Curr. Ther. Res.*, 1981, 30, pp. 753–64.

68   Pola, P., Savi, L., Serricchio, M., *et al.*, 'Use of physiological substance, acetyl-carnitine, in the treatment of angiospastic syndromes', *Drugs Exptl Clin. Res.*, 1984, X, pp. 213–17.

69   Pola, P., Savi, M., Grilli, R., *et al.*, 'Carnitine in the therapy of dyslipidemic patients', *Curr. Ther. Res.*, 1980, 27, pp. 208–15.

70   Rossi, C.S. and Siliprandi, N., 'Effect of carnitine on serum HDL-cholesterol: report of two cases', *Johns Hopkins Med. J.*, 1982, 150, pp. 51–4.

71   Pola, P., Tondi, P., Dal Lago, A., *et al.*, 'Statistical evaluation of long-term L-carnitine therapy in hyperlipoproteinaemias', *Drugs Exptl Clin. Res.*, 1983, IX, pp. 925–34.

72   Tripp, M.E., Katcher, M.L., Peters, H.A., *et al.*, 'Systemic carnitine deficiency presenting as familial endocardial fibroelastosis', *Med. Intel.*, 1981, 305, pp. 385–90.

73   Heinicke, R.M., van der Wal, L. and Yokoyama, M., 'Effect of bromelain (Ananase) on human platelet aggregation', *Experientia*, 1972, 28, pp. 844–5.

74   Taussig, S.J. and Nieper, H.A., 'Bromelain: its use in prevention and treatment of cardiovascular disease – present status', *J. Int. Ac. Prev. Med.*, 1979, VI, pp. 139–50.

75   Baghurst, K.I., Raj, M.J. and Truswell, A.S., 'Onions and platelet aggregation', *Lancet*, 1977, i, p. 101.

76   Louria, D.B., MacAnally, J.F., Lasser, N., *et al.*, 'Onion extract in treatment of hypertension and hyperlipidemia: a preliminary communication', *Curr. Ther. Res.*, 1985, 37, pp. 127–31.

77   Norwell, D.Y. and Tarr, R.S., 'Garlic, vampires, and CHD', *Osteopath. Ann.*, 1984, 12, pp. 276–80.

78   Bordia, A.K., Josh, H.K. and Sanadhya, Y.K., 'Effect of garlic oil on fibrinolytic activity in patient with CHD', *Atherosclerosis*, 1977, 28, pp. 155–9.

79   Gujaral, S., Bhumra, H. and Swaroop, M., 'Effect of ginger (zinger officinale roscoe) oleoresin on serum and hepatic cholesterol levels in cholesterol fed rats', *Nutr. Rep. Int.*, 1978, 17, pp. 183–9.

80   Srivastava, K.C., 'Effects of aqueous extracts of onion, garlic and ginger on platelet aggregation and metabolism of arachidonic acid in the blood vascular system: in vitro study', *Prostaglandins Med.*, 1984, 13, pp.227–35.

81   Malinow, M.R., 'Alfalfa', *Atherosclerosis*, 1973, 30, pp. 27–43.

82   Brook, J.G., Linn, S. and Aviram, J., 'Dietary soya lecithin decreases plasma triglyceride levels and inhibits collagen- and ADP-induced platelet aggregation', *Biochem. Med. Metabol. Biol.*, 1986, 35, pp. 31–9.

83   Stevens, R.L., Colombo, M., Gonzales, J., *et al.*, 'The glycosaminoglycans of the human artery and their changes in atherosclerosis', *J. Clin. Invest.*, 1976, 58, pp. 470–81.

84   Tammi, M., Seppala, P.O., Lehtonen, A. and Mottonen, M., 'Connective tissue components in normal and atherosclerotic human coronary arteries', *Atherosclerosis*, 1978, 29, pp. 191–4.

85   Day, C.E., Powell, J.R. and Levy, R.S., 'Sulfated polysaccharide inhibition of aortic uptake of low density lipoproteins', *Artery*, 1975, 1, pp. 126–37.

86   Pernigotti, L.M., Orso, L., Romagnoli, R. and Fabris, F., 'Effect of mesoglycan on clotting, fibrinolysis and platelet aggregation in normal subjects and hyperaggregating arteriosclerosis', in Widhalm, K. and Sinzinger, H. (eds), *Current Aspects of Atherosclerosis, Lipids, Lipoproteins, Platelets, Prostaglandins, and Experimental Findings*, Verlag Wilhelm, Madrich, 1983, pp. 164–75.

87   Postiglione, A., De Simone, B., Rubba, P., *et al.*, 'Effect of oral mesoglycan-sulphate on plasma lipoprotein concentration and on lipoprotein concentration in primary hyperlipidemia', *Pharmacol. Res. Commun.*, 1984, 16, pp. 1–8.

88   Saba, P., Galeone, F., Guintoli, F., *et al.*, 'Hypolipidemic effect of mesoglycan in hyperlipidemic patients', *Current Therapeutic Research*, 1986, 40, pp. 761–8.

89   Zanolo, G., Giachetti, C., Mascellani, G., *et al.*, 'Pharmacokinetic aspect of tritium-labeled glycosaminoglycans (mesoglycan) their absorption in rat and monkey and tissue distribution in rat', *Boll. Chim. Farm.*, 1984, 123, pp. 223–35.

90   Sangrigoli, V., Carra, G., Lazzara, N., *et al.*, 'Our experience in therapy with mesoglycan in the treatment of peripheral chronic arterial insufficiency', *Proceedings of the IX National Congress of the Italian Society of Vascular Pathology*, Copanello, Italy, 6–9 June, 1987.

91   Mansi, D., Sinisi, L., De Michelle, G., *et al.*, 'Open trial of mesoglycan in the treatment of cerebrovascular ischemic disease', *Acta Neurologica*, 1988, 10, pp. 108–12.

92   Catalini, R., Sturbini, S., Rimatori, C. and Russo, P., 'Echographic monitoring of atheromatous injuries after chronic administration of mesoglycan', *Proceedings of the IX National Congress of the Italian Society of Vascular Pathology*, Copanello, Italy, 6–9 June, 1987.

93   Arsenio, L., Bodria, P., Magnati, G., *et al.*, 'Effectiveness of long-term treatment with pantethine in patients with dyslipidemias', *Clin. Ther.*, 1986, 8, pp. 537–45.

94   Avogaro, P., Bittolo, B.G. and Fusello, M., 'Effect of pantethine on lipids, lipoproteins and apolipoproteins in man', *Curr. Ther. Res.*, 1983, 33, pp. 488–93.

95   Miccoli, R., Marchetti, P., Sampietro, T., *et al.*, 'Effects of pantethine on lipids and apolipoproteins in hypercholesterolemic diabetic and non-diabetic patients', *Curr. Ther. Res.*, 1984, 36, pp. 545–9.

96   Maggi, G., Donati, C. and Criscuoli, G., 'Pantethine: a physiological lipo-modulating agent in the treatment of hyperlipidemias', *Curr. Ther. Res.*, 1982, 32, pp. 380–6.

97   Galeone, F., Scalabrino, A., Giuntoli, F., *et al.*, 'The lipid lowering effect of pantethine in hyperlipidemic patients: a clinical investigation', *Curr. Ther. Res.*, 1983, 34, pp. 383–90.

98   Gaddi, A., Descovich, G., Noseda, G., *et al.*, 'Controlled evaluation of pantethine, a natural hypolipidemic compound, in patients with different forms of hyperlipoproteinemia', *Atheroscl.*, 1984, 50, pp. 73–83.

99   Hayashi, H., Kobayashi, A., Terad, H., *et al.*, 'Effects of pantethine on action potential of canine papillary muscle during hypoxic perfusion', *Jap. Heart. J.*, 1985, 26, pp. 289–96.

100   Higuchi, M., Hashimoto, I., Yamakawa, K., *et al.*, 'Effect of exercise training on plasma high-density lipoprotein cholesterol levels at a constant weight', *Clin. Physiol.*, 1984, 4, pp. 125–33.

101   Danner, S.A., Wieling, W., Havekes, L., *et al.*, 'Effect of physical exercise on blood lipids and adipose tissue composition of young healthy men', *Atherosclerosis*, 1984, 53, pp. 83–90.

102   Sedgwick, A.W., Taplin, R.E., Davidson, A.H. and Thomas, D.W., 'Relationships between physical fitness and risk factors for coronary heart disease in men and women', *Aust. N.Z. J. Med.*, 1984, 14, pp. 208–14.

103   Hartung, G.H., Foreyt, J.P., Mitchell, R.E., *et al.*, 'Relation of diet to high-density-lipoprotein cholesterol in middle-aged marathon runners, joggers, and inactive men', *N. Eng. J. Med.*, 1980, 302, pp. 357–61.

104   Morris, J.N., Schave, S.P.W., Adam, C., *et al.*, 'Vigorous exercise in leisure-time and the incidence of coronary heart-disease', *Lancet*, 1973, i, pp. 333–9.

105   Arnesen, E., Forde, O.H. and Thelle, D.S., 'Coffee and serum cholesterol', *Br. Med. J.*, 1984, 288, p. 1,960.

106   Anonymous, 'Coffee drinking and acute myocardial infarction', *Lancet*, 1972, ii, pp. 1,278–9.

19 Boils

1   Krupp, M.A. and Chatton, M.J., *Current Medical Diagnosis and Treatment*, Lange Medical Publishing, Los Altos, CA, 1984, pp. 70–1.

2   Sanchez, A., Reeser, J., Lau, H., *et al.*, 'Role of sugars in human neutrophilic phagocytosis', *Am. J. Clin. Nutr.*, 1973, 26, pp. 1,180–4.

3   Ringsdorf, W., Cheraskin, E. and Ramsay, R., 'Sucrose, neutrophil phagocytosis and resistance to disease', *Dent. Surv.*, 1976, 52, pp. 46–8.

4   Wright, J.V., *Healing with Nutrition*, Rodale, Emmaus, PA, 1984.

5   Hahn, F.E. and Ciak, J., 'Berberine', *Antibiotics*, 1976, 3, pp. 577–88.

6   Johnson, C.C., Johnson, G. and Poe, C.F., 'Toxicity of alkaloids to certain bacteria', *Acta Pharmacol. Toxicol.*, 1952, 8, pp. 71–8.

7   Kumazawa, Y., Itagaki, A., Fukumoto, M., *et al.*, 'Activation of peritoneal macrophages by berberine alkaloids in terms of induction of cytostatic activity', *Int. J. Immunopharmacol.*, 1984, 6, pp. 587–92.

8   Sabir, M., Akhter, M.H. and Bhide, N.K., 'Further studies on pharmacology of berberine', *Ind. J. Physiol. Pharmacol.*, 1978, 22, pp. 9–23.

9   Leung, A.Y., *Encyclopedia of Common Natural Ingredients Used in Food*, John Wiley & Sons, New York, NY, 1980.

20 Bronchitis and pneumonia

1   Rubenstein, E. and Federman, D., *Scientific American Medicine*, Scientific American, 1984, p. 7:XIX:1.
2   Bicknell, F. and Prescott, F., *The Vitamins in Medicine*, Lee Foundation, Milwaukee, WI, 1953, p. 473.
3   *Op. cit.*, p. 420.
For references pertaining to enhancing immune response see Chapter 6, Immune support.

21 Candidiasis

1   Kroker, G.F., 'Chronic candidiasis and allergy', in Brostoff, J. and Challacombe, S.J. (eds), *Food Allergy and Intolerance*, W.B. Saunders, Philadelphia, PA, 1987, pp. 850–72.
2   Truss, O., *The Missing Diagnosis*, PO Box 26508, Birmingham, AL, 1983.
3   Crook, W.G., *The Yeast Connection*, 2nd ed., Professional Books, Jackson, TN, 1984.
4   Rubinstein, E., Mark, Z., Haspel, J., *et al.*, 'Antibacterial activity of the pancreatic fluid', *Gastroenterol.*, 1985, 88, pp. 927–32.
5   Ransberger, K., 'Enzyme treatment of immune complex diseases', *Arthritis Rheuma.*, 1986, 8, pp. 16–19.
6   Galland, L., 'Nutrition and candidiasis', *J. Orthomol. Psychiatry*, 1985, 15, pp. 50–60.
7   Samaranayake, L.P., 'Nutritional factors and oral candidosis', *J. Oral Pathol.*, 1986, 15, pp. 61–5.
8   Edman, J., Sobel, J.D. and Taylor, M.L., 'Zinc status in women with recurrent vulvovaginal candidiasis', *Am. J. Ob. Gyn.*, 1986, 155, pp. 1,082–5.
9   Boyne, R. and Arthur, J.R., 'The response of selenium-deficient mice to *Candida albicans* infection', *J. Nutr.*, 116, 1986, pp. 816–22.
10   Boero, M., Pera, A., Andruilli, A., *et al.*, 'Candida overgrowth in gastric juice of peptic ulcer subjects on short- and long-term treatment with H_2-receptor antagonists', *Digestion*, 1983, 28, pp. 158–63.
11   Abe, F., Nagata, S. and Hotchi, M., 'Experimental candidiasis in liver injury', *Mycopathologia*, 1987, 100, pp. 37–42.
12   Keeney, E.L., 'Sodium caprylate: a new and effective treatment of moniliasis of the skin and mucous membrane', *Bull. Johns Hopkins Hosp.*, 1946, 78, pp. 333–9.
13   Neuhauser, I. and Gustus, E.L., 'Successful treatment of intestinal moniliasis with fatty acid resin complex', *Arch. Intern. Med.*, 1954, 93, pp. 53–60.
14   Schwabe, A.D., Bennett, L.R. and Bowman, L.P.,'Octanoic acid absorption and oxidation in humans', *J. Applied Physiol.*, 1964, 19, pp. 335–7.
15   Collins, E.B. and Hardt, P., 'Inhibition of *Candida albicans* by *Lactobacillus acidophilus*', *J. Dairy Sci.*, 1980, 63, pp. 830–2.
16   Adetumbi, M.A. and Lau, B.H., 'Allium sativum (garlic) – a natural antibiotic', *Med. Hypothesis*, 1983, 12, pp. 227–37.
17   Amer, M., Taha, M. and Tosson, Z., 'The effect of aqueous garlic extract on the growth of dermatophytes', *Int. J. Dermatol.*, 1980, 19, pp. 285–7.
18   Moore, G.S. and Mycolo   8.
19   Sandhu, D.K., Warraich, M.K. and Singh, S., 'Sensitivity of yeasts isolated from cases of vaginitis to aqueous extracts of garlic', *Mykosen*, 1980, 23, pp. 691–8.
20   Prasad, G. and Sharma, V.D., 'Efficacy of garlic (Allium sativum) treatment against experimental candidiasis in chicks', *Br. Vet. J.*, 1980, 136, pp. 448–51.
21   Duke, J.A., *Handbook of Medicinal Herbs*, CRC Press, Boca Raton, FL, 1985.
22   Leung, A.Y., *Encyclopedia of Common Natural Ingredients Used in Food, Drugs, and Cosmetics*, John Wiley & Sons, New York, NY, 1980.
23   Hahn, F.E. and Ciak, J., 'Berberine', *Antibiotics*, 1976, 3, pp. 577–88.
24   Mahajan, V.M., Sharma, A. and Rattan, A., 'Antimycotic activity of berberine sulphate: an alkaloid from an Indian medicinal herb', *Sabouraudia*, 1982, 20, pp. 79–81.
25   Sharma, R., Joshi, C.K. and Goyal, R.K., 'Berberine tannate in acute diarrhoea', *Indian Pediatr.*, 1970, 7, pp. 496–501.
26   Desai, A.B., Shah, K.M. and Shah, D.M., 'Berberine in treatment of diarrhoea', *Indian Pediatr.*, 1971, 8, pp. 462–5.
27   Sabir, M. and Bhide, N., 'Study of some pharmacologic actions of berberine', *Ind. J. Phys. Pharm.*, 1971, 15, pp. 111–32.
28   Kumazawa, Y., Itagaki, A., Fukumoto, M., *et al.*, 'Activation of peritoneal macrophages by berberine-type alkaloids in terms of induction of cytostatic activity', *Int. J. Immunopharmac.*, 1984, 6, pp. 587–92.
29   Willard, T., 'Tabebuia avellanedae', in Pizzorno, J.E. and Murray, M.T. (eds), *A Textbook of Natural Medicine*, John Bastyr College Publications, Seattle, WA, 1988.

22 Carpal tunnel syndrome

1   Sandez, S.C., 'Carpal tunnel syndrome', *Am. Fam. Phys.*, 1981, 24, pp. 190–204.
2   Phalen, G.S., 'The birth of a syndrome, or carpal tunnel syndrome revisited', *J. Hand Surg.*, 1981, 6, pp. 109–10.
3   Gaby, A., *The Doctor's Guide to Vitamin B6*, Rodale Press, Emmaus, PA, 1984.
4   Ellis, J.M., Folkers, K., Shizukuishi, S., *et al.*, 'Response of vitamin B_6 deficiency and the carpal tunnel syndrome to pyridoxine', *Proc. Natl Acad. Sci.*, 1982, 79, pp. 7,494–8.
5   Ellis, J., Folkers, K., Watabe, T., *et al.*, 'Clinical results of a cross-over treatment with pyridoxine and placebo of the carpal tunnel syndrome', *Am. J. Clin. Nutr.*, 1979, 32, pp. 2,040–6.
6   Ellis, J.M., Azuma, J., Watanabe, T., *et al.*, 'Survey and new data on treatment with pyridoxine of patients having a clinical syndrome including the carpal tunnel and other defects', *Res. Comm. Clin. Path. Pharm.*, 1977, 17, pp. 165–7.
7   Hamfelt, A., 'Carpal tunnel syndrome and vitamin B_6 deficiency', *Clin. Chem.*, 1982, 28, p. 721.
8   Roe, D.A., *Drug-Induced Nutritional deficiencies*, AVI, Westport, CT, 1976, pp. 168–77.

9   Pizzorno, J.E. and Murray, M.T., *A Textbook of Natural Medicine*, John Bastyr College Publications, Seattle, WA, 1985, V:Curcumin.
10 Chandra, D. and Gupta, S., 'Anti-inflammatory and anti-arthritic activity of volatile oil of curcuma longa (Haldi)', *Ind. J. Med. Res.*, 1972, 60, pp. 138–42.
11 Arora, R., Basu, N., Kapoor, V. and Jain, A., 'Anti-inflammatory studies on curcuma longa (turmeric)', *Ind. J. Med. Res.*, 1971, 59, pp. 1,289–95.
12 Srimal, R. and Dhawan, B., 'Pharmacology of diferuloyl methane (curcumin), a non-steroidal anti-inflammatory agent', *J. Pharm. Pharmac.*, 1973, 25, pp. 447–52.
13 Mukhopadhyay, A., Basu, N., Ghatak, N. and Gujral, P., 'Anti-inflammatory and irritant activities of curcumin analogues in rats', *Agents Actions*, 1982, 12, pp. 508–15.
14 Ghatak, N. and Basu, N., 'Sodium curcuminate as an effective anti-inflammatory agent', *Ind. J. Exp. Biol.*, 1972, 10, pp. 235–6.
15 Tassman, G., Zafran, J. and Zayon, G., 'Evaluation of a plant proteolytic enzyme for the control of inflammation and pain', *J. Dent. Med.*, 1964, 19, pp. 73–7.
16 Tassman, G., Zafran, J. and Zayon, G., 'A double-blind crossover study of a plant proteolytic enzyme in oral surgery', *J. Dent. Med.*, 1965, 20, pp. 51–4.
17 Howat, R. and Lewis, G., 'The effect of bromelain therapy on episiotomy wounds – a double blind controlled clinical trial', *J. Ob. Gyn. Br. Commonwealth*, 1972, 79, pp. 951–3.
18 Zatuchni, G. and Colombi, D., 'Bromelains therapy for the prevention of episiotomy pain', *Ob. Gyn.*, 1967, 29, pp. 275–8.

23 Cataracts

1   Straatsma, B., 'Aging-related cataract: laboratory investigation and clinical management', *Annals Int. Med.*, 1985, 102, pp. 82–92.
2   Duarte, A., *Cataract Breakthrough*, International Institute of National Health and Science, Huntingdon Beach, CA, 1982.
3   Varma, S., Kumar, S. and Richards, D., 'Light-induced damage to ocular lens cation pump: prevention by vitamin C', *Proc. Natl Acad. Sci.*, 1979, 76, pp. 3,504–6.
4   Varma, S., Ets, T. and Richards, R., 'Protection against superoxide radicals in rat lens', *Ophthal. Res.*, 1977, 9, pp. 421–31.
5   Bhuyan, K. and Bhuyan, D., 'Superoxide dismutase of the eye: relative functions of superoxide dismutase and catalase in protecting the ocular lens from oxidative damage', *Biochem. Biophys. Acta.*, 1978, 542, pp. 28–38.
6   Rathbun, W. and Hanson, S., 'Glutathione metabolic pathway as a scavenging system in the lens', *Ophthal. Res.*, 1979, 11, pp. 172–6.
7   Garner, W., Garner, M. and Spector, A., 'H_2O_2-induced uncoupling of bovine lens Na+, K+ -ATPase', *Proc. Natl Acad. Sci.*, 1983, 80, pp. 2,044–8.
8   Bellows, J., 'Biochemistry of lens: some studies on vitamin C and lens', *Arch. Ophthal.*, 1936, 16, p. 58.
9   Atkinson, D., 'Malnutrition as an etiological factor in senile cataract', *Eye, Ear, Nose and Throat Monthly*, 1952, 31, pp. 79–83.
10 Bouton, S., 'Vitamin C and the aging eye', *Arch. Int. Med.*, 1939, 63, pp. 930–45.
11 Skalka, H. and Prchal, J., 'Cataracts and riboflavin deficiency', *Am. J. Clin. Nutr.*, 1981, 34, pp. 861–3.
12 Haranaka, R., Okada, N., Kosoto, H., *et al.*, 'Pharmacological action of Hachimijiogan (Ba-wei-wan) on the metabolism of aged subjects', *American Journal of Chinese Medicine*, 1986, 24, pp. 59–67.
13 Fujihira, K., 'Treatment of cataract with Ba-wei-wan', *Journal of Society of Oriental Medicine in Japan*, 1974, 24, pp. 465–79.
14 Whanger, P. and Weswig, P., 'Effects of selenium, chromium and antioxidants on growth, eye cataracts, plasma cholesterol and blood glucose in selenium deficient, vitamin E supplemented rats', *Nutr. Rep. Int.*, 1975, 12, pp. 345–58.
15 Swanson, A. and Truesdale, A., 'Elemental analysis in normal and cataractous human lens tissue', *Biochem. Biophys. Res. Comm.*, 1971, 45, pp. 1,488–96.
16 Bland, J., 'Vitamin E and the accessory lipid antioxidants', in Worthington-Roberts, B. (ed.), *Contemporary Developments in Nutrition*, C.V. Mosby, St Louis, MO, 1981, pp. 135–60.
17 Prchal, J., Conrad, M. and Skalka, H., 'Association of pre-senile cataracts with heterozygosity for galactosemic states and riboflavin deficiency', *Lancet*, 1978, i, pp. 12–13.
18 Hockwin, O., *Drug Treatment of Senile Lens Opacities, Analysis of Possible Ways and Means From the Aging Lens*, Elsevier/North-Holland Biomedical Press, Amsterdam, 1980, p. 281.
19 Burton, G. and Ingold, K., 'Beta-carotene: an unusual type of lipid antioxidant', *Science*, 1984, 224, pp. 569–73.
20 Murata, T., 'The effect of l-hydroxy-5-oxo-5H-pyrido[3,2-a]phenoxazine-3-carboxylic acid (Catalin) on senile cataracts', *Folia Ophthalmol.*, 1980, 31, pp. 1,217–22.
21 Hayashi, H. and Nishida, T., 'The effect of Catalin ophthalmic solution on senile cataracts', *Folia Ophthalmol.*, 1979, 29, pp. 585–98.

24 Cellulite

1   Scherwitz, C. and Braun-Falco, O., 'So-called cellulite', *J. Dermatol. Surg. Oncol.*, 1978, 4, pp. 230–4.
2   Nurnberger, F. and Muller, G., 'So-called cellulite: an invented disease', *J. Dermatol. Surg. Oncol.*, 1978, 4, pp. 221–9.
3   Nurnberger, F., Mende, H. and Roedel, P., 'Behandlungsergebnisse bei der sog. "Cellulitis" mit verteilerenzymen im einfachen blindversuch', *Arch. Dermatol. Forsch.*, 1972, 29, pp. 173–81.
4   Nurnberger, F. and Schroter, B., 'Behandlungsergebnisse bei der sog. Zellulitis mit verteilerenzymen im doppelblindversuch', *Z. Hautkr.*, 1973, 48, pp. 1,009–17.
5   Monograph, *Centella asiatica*, Indena SpA, Milan, 1987.
6   Allegra, C., Pollari, G., Criscuolo, A., *et al.*, 'Centella asiatica extract in venous disorders of the lower limbs. Comparative clinico-instrumental studies with a placebo', *Clin. Terap.*, 1981, 99, pp. 507–13.
7   Marastoni, F., Baldo, A., Redaelli, G. and Ghiringhelli, L., 'Centella asiatica extract in venous pathology of the lower limbs and its evaluation as compared with tribenoside', *Minerva-Cardioangiol.*, 1982, 30, pp. 201–7.

8   Allegra, C., 'Comparative capillaroscopic study of certain bioflavonoids and total triterpenic fractions of Centella asiatica in venous insufficiency', *Clin. Terap.*, 1984, 110, pp. 555–9.

9   Pointel, J.P., Boccalon, H., Cloarec, M., *et al.*, 'Titrated extract of Centella asiatica (TECA) in the treatment of venous insufficiency of the lower limbs', *Angiology*, 1987, 38, pp. 46–50.

10 Monograph, *Escin*. Indena SpA, Milan, Italy, 1987.

11 Aichinger, F., Giss, G. and Vogel, G., 'Neue befunde zur pharmakodynamik von bioflavoiden und des rosskastanien saponins aescin als grundlage ihrer anwendung in der therapie', *Arzniem-Forsch.*, 1964, 14, p. 892.

12 Manca, P. and Passarelli, E., 'Aspetti farmacologici dell'escina, principio attivo dell'aesculus hyppocastanum', *Clin. Terap.*, 1965, 12, pp. 297–328.

13 Annoni, F., Mauri, A., Marincola, F. and Resele, L.F., 'Venotonic activity of escin on the human saphenous vein', *Arzneim-Forsch.*, 1979, 29, 672–5.

14 Lucas, J., 'Erfahrungen mit Aescin in der internen therapie', *Med. Welt.*, 1963, 14, p. 913,.

15 Monograph, *Bladderwrack*, Indena SpA, Milan, Italy, 1987.

25 Cervical dysplasia

1   Robbins, S. and Cotran, R., *Pathologic Basis of Disease*, 3rd ed., W.B. Saunders, Philadelphia, PA, 1984, pp. 1,123–8.

2   Rubin, P., *Clinical Oncology*, 6th ed., American Cancer Society, Washington, DC, 1983, pp. 458–67.

3   Clarke, E., Morgan, R., and Newman, A., 'Smoking as a risk factor in cancer of the cervix: additional evidence from a case-control study', *Am. J. Epid.*, 1982, 115, pp. 59–66.

4   Lyon, J., Gardner, J., West, D., *et al.*, 'Smoking and carcinoma in situ of the uterine cervix', *Am. J. Public Health*, 1983, 73, pp. 558–62.

5   Marshall, J., Graham, S., Byers, T., Swanson, M. and Brasure, J., 'Diet and smoking in the epidemiology of cancer of the cervix', *J. Natl Cancer Instit.*, 1983, 70, pp. 847–51.

6   Clarke, E., Hatcher, J., McKeown-Eyssen, G. and Liekrish, G., 'Cervical dysplasia: association with sexual behavior, smoking, and oral contraceptive use', *Am. J. Ob. Gyn.*, 1985, 151, pp. 612–16.

7   Pelleter, O., 'Vitamin C and tobacco', *Int. J. Vit. Nutr. Res.*, 1977, 16, pp. 147–69.

8   Hoover, R., Bain, C., Cole, P. and Macmahon, B., 'Oral contraceptive use: association with frequency of hospitalization and chronic disease risk indicators', *Am. J. Public Health*, 1978, 68, pp. 335–41.

9   World Health Organization Collaborative Study of Neoplasia and Steroid Contraceptives, 'Invasive cervical cancer and combined oral contraceptives', *Br. Med. J.*, 1983, 290, pp. 961–3.

10 Vessey, M., Lawless, M., McPherson, K. and Yeates, D., 'Neoplasia of the cervix uteri and contraception: a possible adverse effect of the pill', *Lancet*, 1983, ii, pp. 930–4.

11 Krause, M. and Mahan, L., *Food, Nutrition and Diet Therapy*, 7th ed., W.B. Saunders, Philadelphia, PA, 1984.

12 La Vecchia, C., Franceshi, S., Decarlli, A., *et al.*, 'Dietary vitamin A and the risk of invasive cervical cancer', *Int. J. Cancer*, 1984, 34, pp. 319–22.

13 Wassertheil-Smoller, S., Romney, S., Wylie-Rosett, J., *et al.*, 'Dietary vitamin C and uterine cervical dysplasia', *Am. J. Epid.*, 1981, 114, pp. 714–24.

14 Prasad, K. (ed.), *Vitamins, Nutrition and Cancer*, Karger, New York, 1984.

15 Orr, J., Wilson, K., Bodiford, C., *et al.*, 'Nutritional status of patients with untreated cervical cancer, I. Biochemical and immunologic assessment', *Am. J. Ob. Gyn.*, 1985, 151, pp. 625–31.

16 Orr, J., Wilson, K., Bodiford, C., *et al.*, 'Nutritional status of patients with untreated cervical cancer, II. Vitamin assessment', *Am. J. Ob. Gyn.*, 1985, 151, pp. 632–5.

17 Romney, S., Palan, P., Duttagupta, C., *et al.*, 'Retinoids and the prevention of cervical dysplasia', *Am. J. Ob. Gyn.*, 1981, 141, pp. 890–4.

18 Wylie-Rosett, J., Romney, S., Slagel, S., *et al.*, 'Influence of vitamin A on cervical dysplasia and carcinoma in situ', *Nutr. Cancer*, 1984, 6, pp. 49–57.

19 Dawson, E., Nosovitch, J. and Hanigan, E., 'Serum vitamin and selenium changes in cervical dysplasia', *Fed. Proc.*, 1984, 43, p. 612.

20 Romney, S., Duttagupta, C., Basu, J., *et al.*, 'Plasma vitamin C and uterine cervical dysplasia', *Am. J. Ob. Gyn.*, 1985, 151, pp. 978–80.

21 Van Niekerk, W., 'Cervical cytological abnormalities caused by folic acid deficiency', *Acta Cytol.*, 1966, 10, pp.. 67–73.

22 Kitay, D. and Wentz. B., 'Cervical cytology in folic acid deficiency of pregnancy', *Am. J. Ob. Gyn.*, 1969, 104, pp. 931–8.

23 Streiff, R., 'Folate deficiency and oral contraceptives', *J.A.M.A.*, 1970, 214, pp. 105–8.

24 Whitehead, N., Reyner, F. and Lindenbaum, J., 'Megaloblastic changes in the cervical epithelium association with oral contraceptive therapy and reversal with folic acid', *J.A.M.A.*, 1973, 226, pp. 1,421–4.

25 Butterworth, C., Hatch, K., Gore, H., *et al.*, 'Improvement in cervical dysplasia associated with folic acid therapy in users of oral contraceptives', *Am. J. Clin. Nutr.*, 1982, 35, pp. 73–82.

26 Ramaswamy, P. and Natarajan, R., 'Vitamin B6 status in patients with cancer of the uterine cervix', *Nutr. Cancer*, 1984, 6, pp. 176–80.

26 Chronic fatigue syndrome

1   The authors wish to acknowledge Dr Patrick Donovan ND, from whose excellent chapter on the chronic mononucleosis-like syndrome in Pizzorno, J.E. and Murray, M.A., *A Textbook of Natural Medicine* (John Bastyr College Publications, Seattle, WA, 1988) this chapter was derived.

2   Jones, J.F., Ray, G., Minnich, L.L., *et al.*, 'Evidence for active Epstein-Barr virus infection in patients with persistent unexplained illness: elevated anti-early antigen antibioties', *Ann. Intern. Med.*, 1985, 102, pp. 1–7.

3   Straus, S.E., Tosato, F., Armstrong, G., *et al.*, 'Persisting illness and fatigue in adults with evidence of Epstein-Barr virus infection', *Ann. Intern. Med.*, 1985, 102, pp. 7–16.

REFERENCES

4   DuBois, R.E., Seely, J.R., Brus, I., *et al.*, 'Chronic mononucleosis syndrome', *South. Med.*, 1984, 77, pp. 1,376–82.

5   Tobi, M., Morag, A., Ravid, Z., *et al.*, 'Prolonged atypical illness associated with serological evidence of persistent Epstein-Barr virus infection', *Lancet*, 1982, i, pp. 61–4.

6   Jones, J.F., 'Chronic Epstein-Barr virus infection in children', *Pediatr. Infect. Dis.*, 1986, 5, pp. 503–4.

7   Petersdorf, R.G., Adams, R.D., Braunwald, E., *et al.*, *Harrison's Principles of Internal Medicine*, 10th ed., McGraw-Hill, New York, NY, 1983.

8   Paterson, J.K. and Pinninger, J.L., 'Recurrent infectious mononucleosis', *Br. Med. J.*. 1955, 2, p. 476.

9   Issacs, R., 'Chronic infectious mononucleosis', *Blood*, 1948, 3, pp. 858–61.

10   Kaufman, R.E., 'Recurrence in infectious mononucleosis', *Am. Prac.*, 1950, 1, pp. 673–6.

11   Holmes, G.P., Kaplan, J.E., Stewart, J.A., *et al.*, 'A cluster of patients with a chronic mononucleosis-like syndrome. Is Epstein-Barr virus the cause?' *J.A.M.A.*, 1987, 257, pp. 2,297–302.

12   Thorley-Lawson, D.A., Chess, L.M. and Strominger, J.L., 'The suppression of in vitro Epstein-Barr virus infection – a new role for adult human T lymphocytes', *J. Exp. Med.*, 1977, 146, p. 495.

13   Moss, D.J., Rickinson, A.B. and Pope, J.H., 'Long-term T-cell mediated immunity to Epstein-Barr virus in man. III. Activation of cytotoxic T cells in virus-infected leukocyte cultures', *Int. J. Cancer*, 1979, 23, p. 618.

14   Thorley-Lawson, D.A., 'The transformation of adult but not newborn human lymphocytes by Epstein-Barr virus and phytohemagglutinin is inhibited by interferon: the early suppression by T cells of Epstein-Barr infections is mediated by interferon', *J. Immunol.*, 1981, 126, p. 829.

15   Lange, B., Henle, W., Meyers, J.D., *et al.*, 'Epstein-Barr virus related serology in marrow transplant recipients', *Int. J. Cancer*, 1980, 26, pp. 151–7.

16   Henle, W. and Henle, G., 'Epstein-Barr virus-specific serology in immunologically compromised individuals', *Cancer Res.*, 1981, 41, p. 4,222.

17   Henle, G., Henle, W. and Diehl, V., 'Relation of Burkitt's tumor associated herpes-type virus to infectious mononucleosis', *Proc. Natl Acad. Sci.*, 1968, 59, pp. 94–101.

18   Wagh-Mathur, V., Enlow, R.W., Spigland, I., *et al.*, 'Longitudinal study of persistent generalized lymphadenopathy in homosexual men: relation to acquired immunodeficiency syndrome', *Lancet*, 1984, i, p. 1,033.

19   Chang, R.S., Thompson, H. and Pomerantz, S., 'Epstein-Barr virus infection in homosexual men with chronic persistent generalized lymphadenopathy', *J. Infect. Dis.*, 1985, 151, p. 459.

20   Fleisher, G. and Bolognese, R., 'Persistent Epstein-Barr virus infection and pregnancy', *J. Infect. Dis.*, 1983, 147, pp. 982–6.

21   Sumaya, C.V., 'Endogenous reactivation of Epstein-Barr virus infections', *J. Infect. Dis.*, 1977, 135, pp. 374–9.

22   Merlin, T.L., 'Chronic mononucleosis: pitfalls in the laboratory diagnosis', *Hum. Pathol.*, 1986, 17, pp. 1–8.

23   Strauch, B., Andrews, L., Miller, G., *et al.*, 'Oropharyngeal excretion of Epstein-Barr virus by renal transplant recipients and other patients treated with immunosuppression drugs', *Lancet*, 1974, i, p. 234.

24   Henle, W., Ho, C.H., Henle, G. and Kwan, H.C., 'Antibodies to Epstein-Barr virus-related antigens in nasopharyngeal carcinoma: comparison of active cases with long term survivors', *J. Nat. Cancer Inst.*, 1973, 51, pp. 361–9.

25   Pagano, J.S., 'Epstein-Barr virus infection in acquired immunodeficiency syndrome', in *Acquired Immune Deficiency Syndrome*, Alan R. Liss, New York, NY, 1984.

26   Want, T.Y. and Kawaguchi, T.P., *Clinical Laboratory Update: EBV Serologic Profiles*, International Clinical Laboratories, Van Nuys, CA, 1987.

27   Hahnemann, S., *Organon of Medicine*, J.P. Tarcher, Los Angeles, CA, 1982.

28   Lust, B., *Universal Directory of Naturopathy*, Vol. 1, Lust Publications, NJ, 1918.

29   Rubenstein, E. and Federman, D.D. *Scientific American Medicine*, Scientific American, New York, NY, 1988.

30   Montgomery, R., Dryer, R., Conway, T. and Spector, A., *Biochemistry, A Case-oriented Approach*, Mosby, St Louis, MO, 1980.

31   Padova, C., Tritapepe, R., Padova, F., *et al.*, 'S-adenosyl-L-methionine antagonizes oral contraceptive-induced bile cholesterol supersaturation in healthy women: preliminary report of a controlled randomized trial', *Am. J. Gastroenterol.*, 1984, 79, pp. 941–4.

32   Frezza, M., Pozzato, G., Chiesa, L., *et al.*, 'Reversal of intrahepatic cholestasis of pregnancy in women after high dose S-adenosyl-L-methionine (SAMe) administration', *Hepatology*, 1984, 4, pp. 274–8.

33   Bombardieri, G., Milani, A., Bernardi, L. and Rossi, L., 'Effects of S-adenosyl-methionine (SAMe) in the treatment of Gilbert's syndrome', *Curr. Ther. Res.*, 1985, 37, pp. 380–5.

34   Mazzanti, R., Arcangeli, A., Salvadori, G., *et al.*, 'On the antisteatosic effects of S-adenosyl-L-methionine in various chronic liver diseases. A multicenter study', *Curr. Ther. Res.*, 1979, 25, pp. 25–32.

35   Wisniewska-Knypl, J., Sokal, J., Klimczak, J., *et al.*, 'Protective effect of methionine against vinyl chloride-mediated depression of non-protein sulfhydryls and cytochrome P-450', *Toxicology Letters*, 1981, 8, pp. 147–52.

36   Sachan, D.S., Rhew, T.H. and Ruark, R.A., 'Ameliorating effects of carnitine and its precursors on alcohol-induced fatty liver', *Am. J. Clin. Nutr.*, 1984, 39, pp. 738–44.

37   Hosein, E.A. and Bexton, B., 'Protective action of carnitine on liver lipid metabolism after ethanol administration to rats', *Biochem. Pharm.*, 1975, 24, pp. 1,859–63.

38   Sachan, D.A. and Rhew, T.H., 'Lipotropic effect of carnitine on alcohol-induced hepatic stenosis', *Nutr. Rep. Int.*, 1983, 27, pp. 1,221–6.

39   British Herbal Medicine Association, Scientific Committee, *British Herbal Pharmacopoeia*, British Herbal Medicine Association, Cowling, 1983.

40   Kiso, Y., Suzuki, Y., Watanabe, N., *et al.*, 'Antihepatotoxic principles of Curcuma longa rhizomes', *Planta Medica*, 1983, 49, pp. 185–7.

41   Montini, M., Lèvoni, P., Angoro, A. and Pagani, G., 'Controlled trial of cynarin in the treatment of the hyperlipemic syndrome', *Arzneim-Forsch.*, 1975, 25, pp. 1,311–14.

42   Faber, K., 'The dandelion – Taraxacum officinale Weber', *Pharmazie*, 1958, 13, p̦p. 423–35.

43   Hikino, H., Kiso, Y., Wagner, H. and Fiebig, M., 'Antihepatotoxic actions of flavonolignans from Silybum marianum fruits', *Planta Medica*, 1984, 50, pp. 248–50.

44   Vogel, G., Trost, W., Braatz, R., *et al.*, 'Studies on pharmacodynamics, site and mechanism of action of silymarin, the antihepatotoxic principle from Silybum marianum (L.) Gaert', *Arzneim-Forsch.*, 1975, 25, pp. 179–85.

45   Sarre, H., 'Experience in the treatment of chronic hepatopathies with silymarin', *Arzneim-Forsch.*, 1971, 21, pp. 1,209–12.

46   Abonyi, M., Kisfaludy, S. and Szalay, F., 'Therapeutic effect of (+)-cyanidanol-3 in toxic alcoholic liver disease and in chronic active hepatitis', *Acta Physiol. Hung.*, 1984, 64, pp. 455–60.

47   Scevola, D., Magliulo, E., Barbarini, G., *et al.*, 'Possible antiendotoxin activity of (+)-cyanidanol-3 in experimental hepatitis in the rat', *Hepato-gastroenterol.*, 1982, 29, pp. 178–82.

48   Blum, A., Doelle, W., Kortum, K., *et al.*, 'Treatment of acute viral hepatitis with (+)-cyanidanol-3', *Lancet*, 1977, ii, pp. 1,153–5.

49   Piazza, M., Guadagnino, V., Picciotto, L., *et al.*, 'Effect of (+)-cyanidanol-3 in acute HAV, HBV, and non-A, non-B viral hepatitis', *Hepatology*, 1983, 3, pp. 45–9.

50   Kubo, M., Matsuda, H., Tanaka, M., *et al.*, 'Studies on Scutellariae radix. VII. Anti-arthritic and anti-inflammatory actions of methanolic extract and flavonoid components from Scutellaria radix', *Chem. Pharm. Bull.*, 1984, 32, pp. 2,724–9.

51   Kubo, M., Matsuda, H., Tanaka, M., *et al.*, 'Studies on Scutellariae radix. VI. Effects of flavanone compounds on lipid peroxidation in rat liver', *Chem. Pharm. Bull.*, 1982, 30, pp. 1,792–5.

52   Maros, T., Racz, G., Katonaj, B. and Kovacs, V., 'The effects of Cynara scolymus extracts on the regeneration of the rat liver', *Arzneim-Forsch.*, 1966, 16, pp. 127–9 (1st communication); 1968, 18, pp. 884–6.

53   Suzuki, H., Ohta, Y., Takino, T., *et al.*, 'Effects of glycyrrhizin on biochemical tests in patients with chronic hepatitis – double blind trial', *Asian Med. J.*, 1985, 26, pp. 423–38.

54   Nagai, K., 'A study of the excretory mechanism of the liver – effect of liver hydrolysate on BSP excretion', *Jap. J. Gastroenterol.*, 1970, 67, pp. 633–8.

55   Ohbayashi, A., Akioka, T. and Tasaki, H., 'A study of effects of liver hydrolysate on hepatic circulation', *J. Therapy*, 1972, 54, pp. 1,582–5.

56   Fujisawa, K., Suzuki, H., Yamamoto, S., *et al.*, 'Therapeutic effects of liver hydrolysate preparation on chronic hepatitis – a double blind, controlled study', *Asian Med. J.*, 1984, 26, pp. 497–526.

57   Vomel, V.T., 'Influence of a non-specific immune stimulant on phagocytosis of erythrocytes and ink by the reticuloendothelial system of isolated perfused rat livers of different ages', *Arzneim-Forsch.*, 1984, 34, pp. 691–5.

58   Vomel, V.T., 'Influence of a vegetable immune stimulant on phagocytosis of erythrocytes by the reticulohistiocytary system of isolated perfused rat liver', *Arzneim-Forsch.*, 1985, 35, pp. 1,437–9.

59   Sabir, M. and Bhide, N., 'Study of some pharmacologic actions of berberine', *Ind. J. Physiol. Pharm.*, 1971, 15, pp. 111–32.

60   Chandra, R.K., Joshi, P., Au, B., *et al.*, 'Nutrition and immunocompetence of the elderly: effect of short-term nutritional supplementation on cell-mediated immunity and lymphocyte subsets', *Nutr. Res.*, 1982, 2, pp. 223–32.

61   Glaser, R., Strain, E.C., Tarr, K.L., *et al.*, 'Changes in Epstein-Barr virus antibody titers associated with aging', *Proc. Soc. Exp. Biol. Med.*, 1985, 179, pp. 352–5.

62   Burton, G. and Ingold, K., 'B-carotene: an unusual type lipid antioxidant', *Science*, 1984, 224, pp. 569–73.

63   Nomura, A., Stemmermann, G., Heilbrun, L., *et al.*, 'Serum vitamin levels and the risk of cancer of specific sites in men of Japanese ancestry in Hawaii', *Cancer Res.*, 1985, 45, pp. 2,369–72.

64   Byers, T., Vena, J., Mettlin, C., *et al.*, 'Dietary vitamin A and lung cancer risk: an analysis by histologic subtypes', *Amer. J. Epidemiol.*, 1984, 120, pp. 769–76.

65   La Fecchia, C., Ranceschi, S., Decarli, A., *et al.*, 'Dietary vitamin A and the risk of invasive cervical cancer', *Int. J. Cancer*, 1984, 34, pp. 319–22.

66   Peto, R., Doll, R., Buckley, J. and Sporn, M., 'Can dietary beta-carotene materially reduce human cancer rates?', *Nature*, 1981, 290, pp. 201–9.

67   Mathews-Roth, M., 'Antitumor activity of B-carotene, canthaxanthin and phytoene', *Oncology*, 1982, 39, pp. 33–7.

68   Schwartz, J., Suda, D. and Light, G., 'Beta carotene is associated with the regression of hamster buccal pouch carcinoma and the induction of tumor necrosis factor in macrophages', *Biochem. Biophys. Res. Com.*, 1986, 136, pp. 1,130–5.

69   Retura, G., Stratford, F., Levenson, S. and Seifter, E., 'Prophylactic and therapeutic actions of supplemental B-carotene in mice inoculated with C3HBA adenocarcinoma cells: lack of therapeutic action of supplemental ascorbic acid', *J.N.C.I.*, 1982, 69, pp. 73–7.

70   Alam, B. and Alam, S., 'The effect of different levels of dietary B-carotene on DMBA-induced salivary gland tumors', *Nutr. Cancer*, 1987, 9, pp. 93–101.

71   Reinhardt, A., Auperin, D. and Sands, J., 'Mechanism of viricidal activity of retinoids: protein removal from bacteriophage envelope', *Antimicrobial Agents Chemother.*, 1980, 17, pp. 1,034–7.

72   Demetriou, A., Franco, I., Bark, S., *et al.*, 'Effects of vitamin A and beta carotene on intra-abdominal sepsis', *Arch. Surg.*, 1984, 119, pp. 161–5.

73   Rhodes, J., 'Human interferon action: reciprocal regulation by retinoic acid and B-carotene', *J.N.C.I.*, 1983, 70, pp. 833–7.

74   Alexander, M., Newmark, H. and Miller, R., 'Oral beta-carotene can increase the number of OKT4+ cells in human blood', *Immunology Letters*, 1985, 9, pp. 221–4.

75   Anderson, T., Reid, D. and Beaton, G., 'Vitamin C and the common cold: a double blind trial', *Can. Med. Assoc. J.*, 1972, 107, pp. 503–8.

76   Baird, I., Hughes, R., Wilson, H., *et al.*, 'The effect of ascorbic and flavonoids on the occurrence of symptoms normally associated with the common cold', *Am. J. Clin. Nutr.*, 1979, 32, pp. 1,686–90.

77   Scott, J., 'On the biochemical similarities of ascorbic acid and interferon', *J. Theor. Biol.*, 1982, 98, pp. 235–8.

78   Schwerdt, P. and Schwerdt, C., 'Effect of ascorbic acid on rhinovirus replication in WI-38 cells', *Proc. Soc. Exp. Biol. Med.*, 1975, 148, pp. 1,237–43.

79   Leibovitz, B. and Siegal, B., 'Ascorbic acid, neutrophil function, and the immune response', *Int. J. Vit. Nutr. Res.*, 1978, 48, pp. 159–64.

80   Beisel, W., Edelman, R., Nauss, K. and Suskind, R., 'Single-nutrient effects of immunologic functions', *J.A.M.A.*, 1981, 245, pp. 53–8.

81   Chondra, R.K., Heresi, G. and Au, B., 'Serum thymic factor activity in deficiencies of calories, zinc, vitamin A and pyridoxine', *Clin. Exp. Immunol.*, 1980, 42, pp. 332–5.

82   Dardenne, M., Pleau, J., Nabarra, B., *et al.*, 'Contribution of zinc and other metals to the biological activity of the serum thymic factor', *Proc. Natl. Acad. Sci.*, 1982, 79, pp. 5,370–3.

83   Brandon, D.L., 'Interactions of diet and immunity', *Adv. Exp. Med. Biol.*, 1984, 177, pp. 65–90.

84   Bunk, M., Galvin, J., Yung, Y., *et al.*, 'Relationship of cytotoxic activity of natural killer cells to growth rates and serum zinc levels of female RIII mice fed zinc', *Nutr. Cancer*, 1987, 10, pp. 79–87.

85   Cazzola, P., Mazzanti, P. and Bossi, G., 'In vivo modulating effect of a calf thymus acid lysate on human T lymphocyte subsets and CD4+/CD8+ ratio in the course of different diseases', *Curr. Ther. Res.*, 1987, 42, pp. 1,011–17.

86   Genova, R. and Guerra, A., 'Thymomodulin in management of food allergy in children', *Int. J. Tissue Reac.*, 1986, 8, pp. 239–42.

87   Valesini, G., Barnaba, V., Levrero, M., *et al.*, 'Clinical improvement and partial correction of the T-cell defects of acquired immunodeficiency syndrome (AIDS) and lymphadenopathy syndrome (LAS) by a calf thymus lysate', *Eur. J. Clin. Oncol.*, 1986, 22, pp. 531–2.

88   Fiocchi, A., Borella, E., Riva, E., *et al.*, 'A double-blind clinical trial for the evaluation of the therapeutic effectiveness of a calf thymus derivative (Thymomodulin) in children with recurrent respiratory infections', *Thymus*, 1986, 8, pp. 831–9.

89   Minter, M.M., 'Agranulocytic angina: treatment of a case with fetal calf spleen', *Texas State J. Med.*, 1933, 2, pp. 338–43.

90   Kumazawa, Y., Itagaki, A., Fukumoto, M., *et al.*, 'Activation of peritoneal macrophages by berberine alkaloids in terms of induction of cytostatic activity', *Int. J. Immunopharmacol.*, 1984, 6, pp. 587–92.

91   Sabir, M., Akhter, M.H. and Bhide, N.K., 'Further studies on pharmacology of berberine', *Ind. J. Physiol. Pharmacol.*, 1978, 22, pp. 9–23.

92 Wagner, H. and Proksch, A., 'Immunostimulatory drugs of fungi and higher plants', in Wagner, H., Hikino, H., and Farnsworth, N.R., *Economic and Medicinal Plant Research*, vol. 1, Academic Press, London, 1985.
93 Mose, J., 'Effect of echinacin on phagocytosis and natural killer cells', *Med. Welt*, 1983, 34, pp. 1,463–7.
94 Wagner, V.H., Proksch, A., Riess-Maurer, I., *et al.*, 'Immunostimulating polysaccharides (heteroglycans) of higher plants', *Arzneim-Forsch.*, 1985, 35, pp. 1,069–75.
95 Stimple, M., Proksch, A., Wagner, H., *et al.*, 'Macrophage activation and induction of macrophage cytotoxicity in purified polysaccharide fractions from the plant Echinacea purpurea', *Infection Immunity*, 1984, 43, pp. 845–9.
96 Voaden, D. and Jacobsen, M., 'Tumor inhibiters. 3. Identification and synthesis of an oncolytic hydrocarbon from American coneflower roots', *J. Medicinal Chem.*, 1972, 15, pp. 619–23.
97 Ellingwood, F., *American Materia Medica Therapeutics and Pharmacognosy*, Eclectic Medical Publications, Portland, OR, 1983.
98 Culbreth, D., *A Manual of Materia Medica and Pharmacology*, Eclectic Medical Publications, Portland, OR, 1983.
99 Beuscher, N. and Kopanski, L., 'Stimulation der Immunantwort durch Inhaltsstoffe aus Baptisia tinctoria', *Planta Med.*, 1985, 5, pp. 381–4.
100 Lewis W. and Elvin-Lewis, M., *Medical Botany*, John Wiley & Sons, New York, NY, 1977, pp. 98–9.
101 Aron, G. and Irvin, J., 'Inhibition of herpes simplex virus multiplication by the pokeweed antiviral protein', *Antimicrob. Agents Chemother.*, 1980, 17, pp. 1,032–3.
102 Leung, A., *Encyclopedia of Common Natural Ingredients Used in Food, Drugs, and Cosmetics*, John Wiley & Sons, New York, NY, 1980.
103 Pompeii, R., Pani, A., Flora, O., *et al.*, 'Antiviral activity of glycyrrhizic acid', *Experentia*, 1980, 36, pp. 304–5.
104 Abe, N., Ebina, T. and Ishida, N., 'Interferon induction by glycyrrhizin and glycyrrhetinic acid in mice', *Microbial Immunol.*, 1982, 26, pp. 535–9.
105 Yunde, H., Guoliang, M., Shuhua, W., *et al.*, 'Effect of Radix astragalis seuhedysari on the interferon system', *Chin. Med. J.*, 1981, 94, pp. 35–40.
106 Alstat, E.K., 'Lomatium dissectum', *Comp. Med.*, 1987, May/June, pp. 32–4.
107 Chihara, G., Hamuro, J., Maeda, Y., *et al.*, 'Fractionation and purification of the polysaccharides with marked antitumor activity, especially lentinan from Lentinus edodes (Berk.) Sing. (an edible mushroom)', *Cancer Res.*, 1971, 30, pp. 2,776–81.
108 Fukuoka, F., 'Polysaccharide extract active against tumors', *Chem. Abstracts*, 1971, 74, pp. 324–5.
109 Chihara, G., Maeda, Y., Hamuro, J., *et al.*, 'Inhibition of mouse Sarcoma 180 by polysaccharides from Lentinus edodes (Berk.) Sing', *Nature*, 1969, 222, pp. 637–8.
110 Hamuro, J., Rollinghoff, M. and Wagner, H., 'B(1→3) glucan mediated augmentation of alloreactive Murine cytotoxic T-lymphocytes in vivo', *Cancer Res.*, 1978, 38, pp. 3,080–5.
111 Hamuro, J., Rollinghoff, M. and Wagner, H., 'Induction of cytoxic peritoneal exudate cells by T-cell immune adjuvants of the B(1→3) glucan-type lentinan and its analogs', *Immunology*, 1980, 39, pp. 551–9.
112 Fruehauf, J., Bonnard, G. and Herberman, R., 'The effect of lentinan on production of interleukin-1 by human monocytes', *Immunopharm.*, 1982, 5, pp. 65–74.
113 Sipka, S., Abel, G., Scongor, J., *et al.*, 'Effect of lentinan on the chemiluminescence produced by human neutrophils and the murine cell line C4M', *Int. J. Immunopharmacol.*, 1985, 7, pp. 747–51.

27 Coeliac disease

1 Auricchio, S., 'Gluten-sensitive enteropathy and infant nutrition', *J. Ped. Gastroenterol. Nutr.*, 1983, 2 (Suppl. 1), pp. S304–9.
2 Auricchio, S., Follo, D., deRitis, G., *et al.*, 'Does breast feeding protect against the development of clinical symptoms of celiac disease in children?', *J. Ped. Gastroenterol. Nutr.*, 1983, 2, pp. 428–33.
3 Cole, S.G. and Kagnoff, M.F., 'Celiac disease', *Ann. Rev. Nutr.*, 1985, 5, pp. 241–66.
4 Fallstrom, S.P., Winberg, J. and Anderson, H.J., 'Cow's milk malabsorption as a precursor of gluten intolerance', *Acta Paediatrica Scand.* 1965, 54, pp. 101–15.
5 McNicholl, B., Egan-Mitchell, B., Stevens, F.M., *et al.*, 'History, genetics, and natural history of celiac disease – gluten enteropathy', in Walker, D.N. and Kretchmer, N. (eds), *Food, Nutrition and Evolution*, Masson Publications, New York, NY, 1981, pp. 169–78.
6 Simons, F.J., 'Celiac disease as a geographic problem', in Walker, D.N. and Kretchmer, N,. (eds), *Food, Nutrition and Evolution*, Masson Publications, New York, NY, 1981, pp. 179–200.
7 Kasarda, D.D., 'Toxic proteins and peptides in celiac disease: relations to cereal genetics', in Walker, D.N. and Kretchmer, N. (eds), *Food, Nutrition and Evolution*, Masson Publications, New York, NY, 1981, pp. 201–16.
8 Morley, J.E., Levine, A., Yamada, T., *et al.*, 'Effect of exorphins on gastrointestinal function, hormonal release, and appetite', *Gastroenterol.*, 1983, 84, pp. 1,517–23.
9 Morley, J.E., 'Food peptides – a new class of hormones', *J.A.M.A.*, 1982, 247, pp. 2,379–80.
10 Singh, M.M. and Kay, S.R., 'Wheat gluten as a pathogenic factor in schizophrenia', *Science*, 1976, 191, pp. 401–2.
11 Dohan, F.C. and Gasberger, J.C., 'Relapsed schizophrenics: earlier discharge from the hospital after cereal-free, milk-free diet', *Am. J. Psychiatry*, 1973, 130, pp. 685–8.
12 Dohan, F.C., Harper, E.H., Clark, M.H., *et al.*, 'Is schizophrenia rare if grain is rare?' *Biol. Psychiatry*, 1984, 19, pp. 385–99.
13 Robbins, S.L., Cotran, R.S. and Kumar, V., *Pathologic Basis of Disease*, W.B. Saunders, Philadelphia, PA, 1984, pp. 847–8.
14 Ferguson, A., Ziegler, K. and Strobel, S., 'Gluten intolerance (coeliac disease)', *Annals Allergy*, 1984, 53, pp. 637–42.
15 Swinson, C.M., Slavin, G., Coles, E.C. and Booth, C.C., 'Coeliac disease and malignancy', *Lancet*, 1983, i, pp. 111–15.
16 Cooper, B.T., Holmes, K.Y., Ferguson, R., *et al.*, 'Celiac disease and malignancy', *Medicine*, 1980, 59, pp. 249–61.
17 O'Farrelly, C., Whelan, C.A., Feighery, C.P. and Weir, D.G., 'Suppressor-cell activity in coeliac disease induced by alpha-gliadin, a dietary antigen', *Lancet*, 1984, ii, pp. 1,305–6.
18 Stenhammar, L., Kilander, A.F., Nilsson, L.A., *et al.*, 'Serum gliadin antibodies for detection and control of childhood coeliac disease', *Acta Paediatr. Scand.*, 1984, 73, pp. 657–63.
19 Burgin-Wolff, A., Bertele, R.M., Berger, R., *et al.*, 'A reliable screening test for childhood celiac disease: fluorescent immunosorbent test for gliadin antibodies', *J. Pediatr.*, 1983, 102, pp. 655–60.

20   Savilahti, E., Perkkio, M., Kalimo, K., *et al.*, 'IgA antigliadin antibodies: a marker of mucusal damage in childhood coeliac disease', *Lancet*, 1983, i, pp. 320–2.

21   Blazer, S., Naveh, Y., Berant, M., *et al.*, 'Serum IgG antibodies to gliadin in children with celiac disease as measured by an immunofluorescence method', *J. Pediatr. Gastroenterol. Nutr.*, 1984, 3, pp. 205–9.

22   Krause, M.V. and Mahan, K.L., *Food, Nutrition and Diet Therapy*, 7th ed., W.B. Saunders, Philadelphia, PA, 1984, pp. 452–7.

23   Love, A.H.G., Elmes, M., Golden, M., *et al.*, 'Zinc deficiency and celiac disease', in McNicholl, B. McCarthy, C.F. and Fotrell, P.F. (eds), *Perspectives in Celiac Disease*, Baltimore University Press, Baltimore, MD, 1978, pp. 335–42.

24   Messer, M., Anderson, C.M. and Hubbard, L., 'Studies on the mechanism of destruction of the toxic action of wheat gluten in coeliac disease by crude papain', *Gut*, 1964, 5, pp. 295–303.

25   Krainick, H.G. and Mohn, G., 'Weitere Untersuchungen uber den schadlichen Weizenmehleffekt bei del Coliakie. 2. Die Wirkung der enzymatischen Abbauprodukte des Gliadin', *Helv. Paediatr. Acta*, 1959, 14, pp. 124–40.

26   Messer, M. and Baume, P.E., 'Oral papain in gluten intolerance', *Lancet*, 1976, ii, p. 1,022.

27   Baker, P.G., 'Facts about gluten', *Lancet*, 1975, ii, p. 1,307.

28   Corwin, A.H., 'The rotating diet and taxonomy', in Dickey, L.D. (ed.), *Clinical Ecology*, C.C. Thomas, Springfield, IL, 1976, pp. 122–48.

28 Common cold

1   Pizzorno, J.E. and Murray, M.T., *A Textbook of Natural Medicine*, John Bastyr College Publications, Seattle, WA, 1985.

2   Sanchez, A., Reeser, J., Lau, H., *et al.*, 'Role of sugars in human neutrophilic phagocytosis', *Am. J. Clin. Nutr.*, 1973, 26, pp. 1,180–4.

3   Ringsdorf, W., Cheraskin, E. and Ramsay, R., 'Sucrose, neutrophil phagocytosis and resistance to disease', *Dent. Surv.*, 1976, 52, pp. 46–8.

4   Bernstein, J., Alpert, S., Nauss, K. and Suskind, R., 'Depression of lymphocyte transformation following oral glucose ingestion', *Am. J. Clin. Nutr.*, 1977, 30, p. 613.

5   Baird, I., Hughes, R., Wilson, H., *et al.*, 'The effects of ascorbic acid and flavonoids on the occurrence of symptoms normally associated with the common cold', *Am. J. Clin. Nutr.*, 1979, 32, pp. 1,686–90

6   Anderson, T., Reid, D. and Beaton, G., 'Vitamin C and the common cold: a double blind trial', *Can. Med. Assoc. J.*, 1972, 107, pp. 503–8.

7   Anderson, T.W., 'Large scale trials of vitamin C', *Ann. N.Y. Acad. Sci.*, 1975, 258, pp. 494–505.

8   Cheraskin, E., Ringsdorf, W.M. and Sisley, E.L., *The Vitamin C Connection*, Bantam Books, New York, NY, 1983.

9   Prasad, A., 'Clinical, biochemical and nutritional spectrum of zinc deficiency in human subjects; an update', *Nutr. Rev.*, 1983, 41, pp. 197–208.

10   Katz, E. and Margalith, E., 'Inhibition of vaccinia virus maturation by zinc chloride', *Antimicrobial Agents Chemotherapy*, 1981, 19, pp. 213–17.

11   Eby, G.A., Davis, D.R. and Halcomb, W.W., 'Reduction in duration of common colds by zinc gluconate lozenges in a double-blind study', *Antimicrob. Agents Chemother.*, 1984, 25, pp. 20–4.

12   Alexander, M., Newmark, H. and Miller, R., 'Oral beta-carotene can increase the number of OKT4+ cells in human blood', *Immunology Letters*, 1985, 9, pp. 221–4.

13   Reinhardt, A., Auperin, D. and Sands, J., 'Mechanism of viricidal activity of retinoids: protein removal from bacteriophage 6 envelope', *Antimicrob. Agents Chemother.*, 1980, 17, pp. 1,034–7.

14   Chang, H.M. and But, P.P.H., *Pharmacology and Applications of Chinese Materia Medica*, vol. 2, World Scientific Publishing, Teaneck, NJ, 1987, pp. 1,041–6.

15   Wagner, H. and Proksch, A., 'Immunostimulatory drugs of fungi and higher plants', *Economic Medicinal Plant Research*, 1985, 1, pp. 113–53.

16   Wagner, V.H., Proksch, A., Riess-Maurer, I., *et al.*, 'Immunostimulating polysaccharides (heteroglycans) of higher plants', *Arzneim-Forsch.*, 1985, 35, pp. 1,069–75.

17   Abe, N., Ebina, T. and Ishida, N., 'Interferon induction by glycyrrhizin and glycyrrhetinic acid in mice', *Microbial Immunol.*, 1982, 26, pp. 535–9.

29 Constipation

1   Krupp, M.A. and Chatton, M.I., *Current Medical Diagnosis and Treatment*, Lange Medical Publishing, Los Altos, CA, 1984, pp. 350–2.

2   LeRoith, D., Shiloach, J., Roth, J. and Lesniak, M., 'Insulin or a closely related molecule is native to Escherichia coli', *J. Biochem.*, 1981, 256, pp. 6,533–6.

3   Finne, J., Leinonen, M. and Mkel, P.H., 'Antigenic similarities between brain components and bacteria causing meningitis', *Lancet*, 1983, ii, pp. 355–7.

4   Stephansson, K., Dieperink, M.E., Richman, D.P., *et al.*, 'Sharing of antigenic determinants between the nicotinic acetylcholine receptor and proteins in Escherichia coli, Proteus vulgaris, and Klebsiella pneumoniae', *N. Eng. J. Med.*, 1985, 312, pp. 221–5.

5   Weiss, M. and Ingbar, S.H., 'Demonstration of a saturable binding site for thyrotropin in Yersinia enterocolitica', *Science*, 1983, 219, pp. 1,331–5.

6   Ballard, J. and Shiner, M., 'Evidence of cytotoxicity in ulcerative colitis from immunofluorescent staining of the rectal mucosa', *Lancet*, 1974, i, pp. 1,014–17.

7   Donovan, P., 'Bowel toxemia, permeability and disease: new information to support an old concept', in Pizzorno, J.E. and Murray, M.T., *A Textbook of Natural Medicine*, John Bastyr College Publications, Seattle, WA, 1988.

8   Burkitt, D. and Trowell, H., *Western Diseases: Their Emergence and Prevention*, Harvard University Press, Cambridge, MA, 1981.

9   Vahouny, G. and Kritchevsky, D., *Dietary Fiber in Health and Disease*, Plenum Press, New York, NY, 1982.

10   Worthington-Roberts, B., *Contemporary Developments in Nutrition*, C.V. Mosby, St Louis, MO, 1981.

11   Franklin, J.F., 'Treatment of chronic constipation', *J.A.M.A.*, 1986, 256, p. 652.

12   Botez, M.I., *et al.*, 'Neurologic disorders responsive to folic acid therapy', *Can. Med. Assoc. J.*, 1976, 15, p. 217.

13   Roe, D.A., *Drug-Induced Nutritional Deficiencies*, AVI Publications Westport, CT, 1976.

14   Dreisbach, R.H., *Handbook of Poisoning*, Lange Medical Publications, Los Altos, CA, 1983, p. 477.

15   Goth, A., *Medical Pharmacology: Principles and Concepts*, C.V. Mosby, St Louis, MO, 1984, p. 512.

16   Leung, A.Y., *Encyclopedia of Common Natural Ingredients used in Food*, John Wiley & Sons, New York, NY, 1980.

30 Crohn's disease and ulcerative colitis

1   Calkins, B.M., Lilieneld, A.M., Garland, C.F., *et al.*, 'Trends in incidence rates of ulcerative colitis and Crohn's disease', *Dig. Dis. Sci.*, 1984, 29, pp. 913–20.

2   Mayberry, J.F., 'Some aspects on the epidemiology of ulcerative colitis', *Gut*, 1985, 26, pp. 968–74.

3   Robbins, S.L., Cotran, R.S. and Kumar, V., *Pathologic Basis of Disease*, W.B. Sanders, Philadelphia, PA, 1984, pp. 836–41, 859–62.

4   Petersdorf, R., *Harrison's Principles of Internal Medicine*, McGraw-Hill, New York, NY, 1983, pp. 1,738–52.

5   Hentges, D.J. (ed) *Human Intestinal Microflora in Health and Disease*, Academic Press, New York, NY, 1983.

6   Van de Merwe, J.P., 'The human faecal flora and Crohn's disease', *Ant. van Leeuwenhoek*, 1984, 50, pp. 691–700.

7   Chiodini, R.J., Van Kruiningen, H.J., Thayer, W.R., *et al.*, 'Possible role of mycobacteria in inflammatory bowel disease', *Dig. Dis. Sci.*, 1984, 29, pp. 1,073–85.

8   Levi, A.J., 'Diet in the management of Crohn's disease', *Gut*, 1985, 26, pp. 985–8.

9   Jarnerot, J., Jarnmark, I. and Nilsson, K., 'Consumption of refined sugar by patients with Crohn's disease, ulcerative colitis, or irritable bowel syndrome', *Scand. J. Gastroenterol.*, 1983, 18, pp. 999–1,002.

10   Mayberry, J.F., Rhodes, J. and Newcombe, R.G., 'Increased sugar consumption in Crohn's disease', *Digestion*, 1980, 20, pp. 323–6.

11   Grimes, D.S., 'Refined carbohydrate, smooth-muscle spasm and diseases of the colon', *Lancet*, 1976, i, pp. 395–7.

12   Thornton, J.R., Emmett, P.M. and Heaton, K.W., 'Diet and Crohn's disease: characteristics of the pre-illness diet', *Br. Med. J.*, 1979, 279, pp. 762–4.

13   Heaton, K.W., Thornton, J.R. and Emmett, P.M., 'Treatment of Crohn's disease with an unrefined-carbohydrate, fibre-rich diet', *Br. Med. J.*, 1979, 279, pp. 764–6.

14   Morain, C.O., Segal, A.W. and Levi, A.J., 'Elemental diet as primary treatment of acute Crohn's disease: a controlled trial', *Br. Med. J.*, 1984, 288, pp. 1,859–62.

15   Harries, A.D., Danis, V., Heatley, R.V., *et al.*, 'Controlled trial of supplemented oral nutrition in Crohn's disease', *Lancet*, 1983, i, pp. 887–90.

16   Axelsson, C. and Jarnum, S., 'Assessment of the therapeutic value of an elemental diet in chronic inflammatory bowel disease', *Scand. J. Gastroenterol.*, 1977, 12, pp. 89–95.

17   Voitk, A.J., Echave, V., Feller, J.H., *et al.*, 'Experience with elemental diet in the treatment of inflammatory bowel disease', *Arch. Surg.*, 1973, 107, pp. 329–33.

18   Workman, E.M., Jones, A., Wilson, A.J. and Hunter, J.O., 'Diet in the management of Crohn's disease', *Human Nutr: Applied Nutr.*, 1984, 38A, pp. 469–73.

19   Jones, V.A., Workman, E., Freeman, A.H., *et al.*, 'Crohn's disease: maintenance of remission by diet', *Lancet*, 1985, ii, pp. 177–80.

20   Rowe, A. and Uyeyama, K., 'Regional enteritis – its allergic aspects', *Gastroenterol.*, 1953, 23, pp. 554–71.

21   James, A.H., 'Breakfast and Crohn's disease', *Br. Med. J.*, 1977, 276, pp. 943–5.

22   Thornton, J.R., Emmett, P.M. and Heaton, K.W., 'Diet and ulcerative colitis', *Br. Med. J.*, 1980, 280, pp. 293–4.

23   Meyers, S. and Janowitz, H.D., 'Natural history of Crohn's disease; an analytical review of the placebo lesson', *Gastroenterol.*, 1984, 87, pp. 1,189–92.

24   Mekhjian, H.S., Switz, D.M., Melnyk, C.S., *et al.*, 'Clinical features and natural history of Crohn's disease', *Gastroenterol.*, 1979, 77, pp. 898–906.

25   Malchow, H., Ewe, K., Brandes, J.W., Goebell, H., *et al.*, 'European cooperative Crohn's disease study (ECCDS): results of drug treatment', *Gastroenterol.*, 1984, 86, pp. 249–66.

26   Donowitz, M., 'Arachidonic acid metabolites and their role in inflammatory bowel disease', *Gastroenterol.*, 1985, 88, pp. 580–7.

27   Ford-Hutchinson, A.W., 'Leukotrienes: their formation and role as inflammatory mediators', *Fed. Proc.*, 1985, 44, pp. 25–9.

28   Sharon, P. and Stenson, W.F., 'Enhanced synthesis of leukotriene B_4 by colonic mucosa in inflammatory bowel disease', *Gastroenterol.*, 1984, 86, pp. 453–60.

29   Musch, M.W., Miller, R.J., Field, M. and Siegel, M.I., 'Stimulation of colonic secretion by lipoxygenase metabolites of arachidonic acid', *Science*, 1982, 217, pp. 1,255–6.

30   Anonymous, 'Dietary fish oil alters leukotriene generation and neutrophil function', *Nutr. Rev.*, 1986, 44, pp. 137–9.

31   Lee, T.H., Hoover, R.L., Williams, J.D., *et al.*, 'Effect of dietary enrichment with eicosapentaenoic and docosahexanoic acids on in vitro neutrophil and monocyte leukotriene generation and neutrophil function', *N.E.J.M.*, 1985, 312, pp. 1,217–24.

32   Podolsky, D.K. and Isselbacher, K.J., 'Glycoprotein composition of colonic mucosa', *Gastroenterol.*, 1984, 87, pp. 991–8.

33   Kim, Y.S. and Byrd, J.C., 'Ulcerative colitis: a specific mucin defect?', *Gastroenterol.*, 1984, 87, pp. 1,193–5.

34   Boland, C.R., Lance, P., Levin, B., *et al.*, 'Abnormal goblet cell glycoconjugates in rectal biopsies associated with an increased risk of neoplasia in patients with ulcerative colitis: early results of a prospective study', *Gut*, 1984, 25, pp. 1,364–71.

35   Marcus, R. and Watt, J., 'Seaweeds and ulcerative colitis in laboratory animals', *Lancet*, 1969, ii, pp. 489–90.

36   Grasso, P., Sharratt, M., Carpanini, F.M.B. and Ganolli, S.D., 'Studies on carrageenan and large bowel ulceration in mammals', *Food Cosmet. Toxicol.*, 1973, 11, pp. 555–64.

37   Motet, N.K., editorial, 'On animal models for inflammatory bowel disease', *Gastroenterology*, 1972, 62, pp. 1,269–71.

38   Bentiz, K.R., Goldberg, L. and Coulston, F., 'Intestinal effect of carrageenans in the rhesus monkey', *Food Cosmet. Toxicol.*, 1973, 11, pp. 565–75.

39   Bonfils, S., 'Carrageenan and the human gut', *Lancet*, 1970, ii, p. 414.

40   Allan, R.N., 'Extra-intestinal manifestations of inflammatory bowel disease', *Clin. Gastroenterol.*, 1983, 12, pp. 617–32.

41   Pettei, M.J. and Davidson, M., 'Extra gastrointestinal manifestations of inflammatory bowel disease', *J. Ped. Gastroenterol. Nutr.*, 1985, 4, pp. 689–91.

42 Wagner, H., 'Plant constituents with antihepatotoxic activity', in Beal, J.L. and Reinhard, E. (eds), *Natural Products as Medicinal Agents*, Hippocrates-Verlag, Stuttgart, 1981.

43 Hikino, H., Kiso, Y., Wagner, H. and Fiebig, M., 'Antihepatotoxic actions of flavanolignins from Silybum marianum fruits', *Planta Medica*, 1984, 50, pp. 248–50.

44 Kiso, Y., Suzuki, Y., Watanabe, N., *et al.*, 'Antihepatotoxic principles of Curcuma longa rhizomes', *Planta Medica*, 1983, 49, pp. 185–7.

45 Rosenberg, I.H., Bengoa, J.M. and Sitrin, M.D., 'Nutritional aspects of inflammatory bowel disease', *Ann. Rev. Nutr.*, 1985, 5, pp. 463–84.

46 Heatley, H.V., 'Review: nutritional implications of inflammatory bowel disease', *Scand. J. Gastroenterol.*, 1984, 19, pp. 995–8.

47 Motil, K.J. and Grand, R.J., 'Nutritional management of inflammatory bowel disease', *Ped. Clinics North. Amer.*, 1985, 32, pp. 447–69.

48 Best, W.R., Becktel, J.M., Singleton, J.W. and Kern, F., 'Development of a Crohn's disease activity index', *Gastroenterology*, 1976, 70, pp. 439–44.

49 Salyers, A.A., Kurtitza, A.P. and McCarthy, R.E., 'Influence of dietary fibre on the intestinal environment', *Proc. Soc. Exp. Biol. Med.*, 1985, 180, pp. 415–21.

50 Gee, M.I., Grace, M.G.A., Wensel, R.H., *et al.*, 'Nutritional status of gastroenterology outpatients: comparison of inflammatory bowel disease with functional disorders', *J. Am. Diet. Assoc.*, 1985, 85, pp. 1,591–9.

51 Fleming, C.R., Huizenga, K.A., McCall, J.T., *et al.*, 'Zinc nutrition in Crohn's disease', *Dig. Dis. Sci.*, 1981, 26, pp. 865–70.

52 Kruis, W., Rindfleisch, G.E. and Weinzierl, M., 'Zinc deficiency as a problem in patients with Crohn's disease and fistula formation', *Hepato-gastroenterol.*, 1985, 32, pp. 133–4.

53 Schoelmerich, J., Becher, M.S., Hoppe-Seyler, P., *et al.*, 'Zinc and vitamin A deficiency in patients with Crohn's disease is correlated with activity but not with localization or extent of the disease', *Hepato-Gastroenterol.*, 1985, 32, pp. 34–8.

54 Main, A.N.H., Russell, R.I., Fell, G.S., *et al.*, 'Clinical experience of zinc supplementation during intravenous nutrition in Crohn's disease: value of serum and urine zinc measurements', *Gut*, 1982, 23, pp. 984–91.

55 LaSala, M.A., Lifshitz, F., Silverberg, M., *et al.*, 'Magnesium metabolism studies in children with chronic inflammatory disease of the bowel', *J. Ped. Gastroenterol. Nutr.*, 1985, 4, pp. 75–81.

56 Nyhlin, H., Dyckner, T., Ek, B. and Wester, P.O., 'Magnesium in Crohn's disease', *Acta Med. Scand.* (supplement), 1982, 661, pp. 21–5.

57 Ward, C.G., 'Influence of iron on infection', *Am. J. Surg.*, 1986, 151, pp. 291–5.

58 Lehr, L. Schober, O., Hundeshagen, H. and Pichlmayr, R., 'Total-body potassium depletion and the need for preoperative nutritional support in Crohn's disease', *Ann. Surg.*, 1982, 196, pp. 709–14.

59 Skogh, M., Sunquist, T. and Taggeson, C., 'vitamin A in Crohn's disease', *Lancet*, 1980, i, p. 766.

60 Dvorak, A.M., 'Vitamin A in Crohn's disease', *Lancet*, 1980, i, pp. 1,303–4.

61 Wright, J.P., Mee, A.S., Parfitt, A., *et al.*, 'Vitamin A therapy in patients with Crohn's disease', *Gastroenterol.*, 1985, 88, pp. 512–14.

62 Norrby, S., Sjodahl, R. and Taggeson, C., 'Ineffectiveness of vitamin A therapy in severe Crohn's disease', *Acta Chir. Scand.*, 1985, 151, pp. 465–8.

63 Harries, A.D., Brown, R., Heatley, R.V., *et al.*, 'Vitamin D status in Crohn's disease: association with nutrition and disease activity', *Gut*, 1985, 26, pp. 1,197–203.

64 Howard, L., Ovesen, L., Satya-Murti, S. and Chu, R., 'Reversible neurological symptoms caused by vitamin E deficiency in a patient with short bowel syndrome', *Am J. Clin. Nutr.*, 1982, 36, pp. 1,243–9.

65 Lloyd-Still, J. and Green, O.C., 'A clinical scoring system for chronic inflammatory bowel disease in children', *Dig. Dis. Sci.*, 1979, 24, pp. 620–4.

66 Krasinski, S.D., Russell, R.M., Furie, B.C., *et al.*, 'The prevalence of vitamin K deficiency in chronic gastrointestinal disorders', *Am. J. Clin. Nutr.*, 1985, 41, pp. 639–43.

67 Research note, 'Vitamin K deficiency in chronic gastrointestinal disorders', *Nutr. Review*, 1986, 44, pp. 10–12.

68 Elsborg, L. and Larsen, L., 'Folate deficiency in chronic inflammatory bowel diseases', *Scand. J. Gastroenterol.*, 1979, 14, pp. 1,019–24.

69 Hellberg, R., Hulten, L. and Bjorn-Rasmussen, E., 'The nutritional and haematological status before and after primary and subsequent resectional procedures for classical Crohn's disease and Crohn's colitis', *Acta. Chir. Scand.*, 1982, 148, pp. 453–60.

70 Franklin, J.L. and Rosenberg, I.H., 'Impaired folic acid absorption in inflammatory bowel disease: effects of salicylasosulfapyridine (azulfidine)', *Gastroenterol.*, 1973, 64, pp. 517–25.

71 Carruthers, L.B., 'Chronic diarrhoea treated with folic acid', *Lancet*, 1946, i, pp. 849–50.

72 Filipsson, S., Hulten, L. and Lindstedt, G., 'Malabsorption of fat and vitamin B12 before and after intestinal resection for Crohn's disease', *Scand. J. Gastroenterol.*, 1978, 13, pp. 529–36.

73 Hughes, R.G., and Williams, N., 'Leukocyte ascorbic acid in Crohn's disease', *Digestion*, 1978, 17, pp. 272–4.

74 Gerson, C.D. and Fabry, E.M., 'Ascorbic acid deficiency and fistula formation in regional enteritis', *Gastroenterol.*, 1974, 67, pp. 428–33.

75 Middleton, E., 'The flavonoids', *Trends Pharmaceut. Sci.*, 1984, 5, pp. 335–8.

76 Havsteen, B., 'Flavonoids, a class of natural products of high pharmacological potency', *Biochem. Pharmacol.*, 1983, 32, pp. 1,141–8.

77 Petrakis, P.L., Kallianos, A.G., Wender, S.H., *et al.*, 'Metabolic studies of quercetin labeled with C^{14}', *Arch. Biochem. Biophys.*, 1959, 85, pp. 264–71.

78 Mitchell, W., *Naturopathic Applications of the Botanical Remedies*, W. Mitchell, Seattle, WA, 1986,

79 Fleter, H.W. and Lloyd, J.U., *King's Dispensatory*, 1898; republished by Eclectic Medical Publications, Portland, OR, 1983.

80 Leung, A.Y., *Encyclopedia of Common Natural Ingredients Used in Food*, John Wiley & Sons, New York, NY, 1980.

31 Cystitis

1 Branch, W.T., *Office Practice of Medicine*, W.B. Saunders, Philadelphia, PA, 1982, pp. 679–85, 488–504.

2 Krupp, M.A. and Chatton, M.J., *Current Medical Diagnosis and Treatment*, Lange Medical Publishing, Los Altos, CA, 1985, pp. 566–70.

3 Rubenstein, E. and Federman, D.D., *Scientific American Medicine*, Scientific American, New York, NY, 1988, pp. 7:XXIII:1–10.

4 Reilly, B.M., *Practical Strategies in Outpatient Medicine*, W.B. Saunders, Philadelphia, PA, 1984, p. 277.

5 Prodromos, P.N., Brusch, C.A. and Ceresia, G.C., 'Cranberry juice in the treatment of urinary tract infections,' *Southwest Med.*, 1968, 47, p. 17.

6   Sternlieb, P., 'Cranberry juice in renal disease', *New Engl. J. Med.*, 1963, 268, p. 57.

7   Moen, D.V., 'Observations on the effectiveness of cranberry juice in urinary infections', *Wisconsin Med. J.*, 1962, 61, p. 282.

8   Kahn, D.H., Panariello, V.A., Saeli, J., *et al.*, 'Effect of cranberry juice on urine', *J. Am. Diet. Assoc.*, 1967, 51, p. 251.

9   Bodel, P.T., Cotran, R. and Kass, E.H., 'Cranberry juice and the antibacterial action of hippuric acid', *J. Lab. Clin. Med.*, 1959, 54, p. 881.

10 Sobota, A.E., 'Inhibition of bacterial adherence by cranberry juice: potential use for the treatment of urinary tract infections', *J. Urology*, 1984, 131, pp. 1,013–16.

11 Sanchez, A., Reeser, J. Lau, H., *et al.*, 'Role of sugars in human neutrophilic phagocytosis', *Am. J. Clin. Nutr.*, 1973, 26, pp.1,180–4.

12 Ringsdorf, W., Cheraskin, E. and Ramsay, R., 'Sucrose, neutrophil phagocytosis and resistance to disease', *Dent. Surv.*, 1976, 52, pp. 46–8.

13 Bernstein, J., Alpert, S., Nauss, K., and Suskind, R., 'Depression of lymphocyte transformation following oral glucose ingestion', *Am. J. Clin. Nutr.*, 1977, 30, p. 613.

14 *Merck Index*, 10th ed., Merck & Co, Rahway, NJ, 1983, pp. 112–13, 699.

15 Frohne, V., 'Untersuchungen zur frage der harndesifizierenden wirkungen von barentraubenblatt-extracten', *Planta Medica*, 1970, 18, pp. 1–25.

16 Leung, A., *Encyclopedia of Common Natural Ingredients Used in Food, Drugs, and Cosmetics*, John Wiley & Sons, NY, 1980, pp. 292,293 and 316–17.

17 Mitchell, W., *Naturopathic Applications of the Botanical Remedies*, W. Mitchell, Seattle, WA, 1983, p. 8.

18 Adetumbi, M.A. and Lau, B.H., 'Allium sativum (garlic) – a natural antibiotic', *Med. Hypothesis*, 1983, 12, pp. 227–37.

19 Sharma, V.D., Sethi, M.S., Kumar, A., and Rarotra, J.R., 'Antibacterial property of Allium sativum Linn.: in vivo and in vitro studies', *Ind. J. Exp. Biol.*, 1977, 15, pp. 466–80.

20 Elnima, E.I., Ahmed, S.A., Mekkawi, A. and Mossa, J.S., 'The antimicrobial activity of garlic and onion extracts,' *Pharmazie*, 1983, 38, pp. 747–8.

21 Pizzorno, J.E. and Murray, M.T., *A Textbook of Natural Medicine*, John Bastyr College Publications, Seattle, WA, 1988, p.V:Hydras-1-4.

22 Amin, A.H., Subbaiah, T.V. and Abbasi, K.M., 'Berberine sulfate: antimicrobial activity, bioassay, and mode of action', *Can. J. Microbiol.*, 1969, 15, pp. 1,067–76.

23 Johnson, C.C., Johnson, G. and Poe, C.F., 'Toxicity of alkaloids to certain bacteria', *Acta Pharmacol. Toxicol.*, 1952, 8, pp. 71–8.

32 Depression

1   Krupp, M. and Chatton, M., *Current Medical Diagnosis and Treatment*, Chapter 17, Psychiatric disorders, Lange Medical Publications, Los Altos, CA, 1982.

2   Krause, M. and Mahan, L., *Food, Nutrition and Diet Therapy*, W.B. Saunders, Philadelphia, PA, 1984.

3   Sourkes, T., 'Nutrients and the cofactors required for monoamine synthesis in nervous tissue', in Wurtman, R. and Wurtman, J. (eds), *Nutrition and the Brain*, vol. 3, Raven Press, New York, NY, 1979, pp. 265–99.

4   Blair, J., Morar, C., Hamon, C., *et al.*, 'Tetrahydrobiopterin metabolism in depression', *Lancet*, 1984, i, p. 163.

5   Curtius, H., Muldner, H. and Niederwieser, A., 'Tetrahydrobiopterin: efficacy in endogenous depression and Parkinson's disease, *J. Neural Trans.*, 1982, 55, pp. 301–8.

6   Curtius, H., Niederwieser, A., Levine, R., *et al.*, 'Successful treatment of depression with tetrahydrobiopterin', *Lancet*, 1983, i, pp. 657–8.

7   Leeming. R., Harpey, J., Brown, S. and Blair, J., 'Tetrahydrofolate and hydroxycobolamin in the management of dihydropteridine reductase deficiency', *J. Ment Def. Res.*, 1982, 26, pp. 21–5.

8   Lipton, M., Mailman, R. and Nemeroff, C., 'Vitamins, megavitamin therapy and the nervous system', in Wurtman, R. and Wurtman, J. (eds), *Nutrition and the Brain*, Vol. 3, Raven Press, New York, NY, 1979, pp. 183–264.

9   Reynolds, E., Preece, J., Bailey, J. and Coppen, A., 'Folate deficiency in depressive illness', *Br. J. Psychiat.*, 1970, 117, pp. 287–92.

10 Carney, M. and Sheffield, B., 'Associations of subnormal folate and B12 values and effects of replacement therapy', *J. Nerv. Ment. Dis.*, 1970, 150, pp. 404–12.

11 Zucker, D., Livingston, R., Nakra, R. and Clayton, P., 'B12 deficiency and psychiatric disorders: a case report and literature review', *Biol. Psychiatry*, 1981, 16, pp. 197–205.

12 Goggans, F., 'A case of mania secondary to vitamin B12 deficiency', *Am. J. Psychiatry*, 1984, 141, pp. 300–1.

13 Evans, D., Edelsohn, G. and Golden, R., 'Organic psychosis without anaemia or spinal cord symptoms in patients with vitamin B12 deficiency', *Am. J. Psychiatry*, 1983, 140, pp. 218–21.

14 Botez, M., Young, S., Bachevalier, J. and Gauthier, S., 'Effect of folic acid and vitamin B12 deficiencies on 5-hydroxyindoleacetic acid in human cerebrospinal fluid', *Ann. Neurol.*, 1982, 12, pp. 479–84.

15 Reynolds, E., and Stramentinoli, G., 'Folic acid, S-adenosylmethionine and affective disorder', *Psychol. Med.*, 1983, 13, pp. 705–10.

16 Reynolds, E., Carney, M. and Toone, B. 'Methylation and mood', *Lancet*, 1983, ii, p. 196.

17 Bottiglieri, T., Laundry, M., Martin, R., *et al.*, 'S-adenosylmethionine influences monoamine metabolism', *Lancet*, 1984, ii, p. 224.

18 Agnoli, A., Andreoli, V., Casachia, M. and Cerbo, R., 'Effect of S-adenosyl L-methionine (SAMe) upon depressive symptoms', *J. Psychiat. Res.*, 1976, 13, pp. 43–54.

19 Caruso, I., Fumagalli, M., Boccassini, L., *et al.*, 'Antidepressant activity of S-adenosylmethionine', *Lancet*, 1984, i, p. 904.

20 Russ, C., Hendricks, T., Chrisley, B., Kalin, N. and Driskell, J., 'Vitamin B6 status of depressed and obsessive-compulsive patients', *Nutr. Rep. Intl*, 1983, 27, pp. 867–73.

21 Carney, M., Williams, D. and Sheffield, B., 'Thiamin and pyridoxine lack in newly-admitted psychiatric patients', *Br. J. Psychiatr.*, 1979, 135, pp. 249–54.

22 Stewart, J.W., Harrison, W., Quitkin, F. and Baker, H., 'Low level B6 levels in depressed outpatients', *Biolog. Psychiat.*, 1984, 19, pp. 613–16.

23 Nobbs, B., 'Pyridoxal phosphate status in clinical depression', *Lancet*, 1974, i, p. 405.

24 Wynn, V., Adams, P., Folkard, J. and Seed, M., 'Tryptophan, depression and steroidal contraception', *J. Steroid Biochem.*, 1975, 6, pp. 965–70.

25 Bermond, P., 'Therapy of side effects of oral contraceptive agents with vitamin B6', *Acta Vitaminol.-Enzymol.*, 1982, 4, pp. 45–54.

26 Niems, A. and von Borstel, R., 'Caffeine: metabolism and biochemical mechanisms of action', in Wurtman, R. and Wurtman, J. (eds), *Nutrition and the Brain*, vol. 6, Raven Press, New York, NY, 1983, pp. 2–30.

27   Charney, D., Henninger, G. and Jatlow, P., 'Increased anxiogenic effects of caffeine in panic disorders', *Arch. Gen. Psychiatry*, 1984, 42, pp. 233–43.

28   Greden, J., Fontaine, P., Lubetsky, M. and Chamberlain, K., 'Anxiety and depression associated with caffeinism among psychiatric patients', *Am. J. Psychiatry*, 1979, 131, pp. 1,089–94.

29   Bolton, S. and Null, G., 'Caffeine, psychological effects, use and abuse', *J. Orthomol. Psychiatry*, 1981, 10, pp. 202–11.

30   Gilman, A., Goodman, L. and Gilman, A., *The Pharmacological Basis of Therapeutics*, Macmillan, New York, NY, 1980.

31   Brook, M. and Grimshaw, J., 'Vitamin C concentration of plasma and leukocytes as related to smoking habit, age, and sex of humans', *Am. J. Clin. Nutr.*, 1968, 21, pp. 1,254–8.

32   Pelletier, O., 'Smoking and vitamin C levels in humans', *Am. J. Clin. Nutr.*, 1968, 21, pp. 1,259–67.

33   Kinsman, R. and Hood, J., 'Some behavioral effects of ascorbic acid deficiency', *Am. J. Clin. Nutr.*, 1971, 24, pp. 455–64.

34   Kershbaum, A., Pappajohn, D., Bellet, S., Hirabayashi, M. and Shafiiha, H., 'Effect of smoking and nicotine on adrenocortical secretion', *J.A.M.A.*, 1968, 203, pp. 113–16.

35   Bennett, A., Doll, R. and Howell, R., 'Sugar consumption and cigarette smoking', *Lancet*, 1970, i, pp. 1,011–14.

36   Raw, M., Jarvis, M., Feyerbend, C. and Russell, M., 'Comparison of nicotine chewing gum and psychological treatments for dependent smokers', *Br. Med. J.*, 1982, 285, pp. 537–40.

37   West, R., Jarvis, M., Phil, M., *et al.*, 'Effect of nicotine replacement on the cigarette withdrawal syndrome', *Br. J. Addict.*, 1984, 79, pp. 215–19.

38   Ryde, D., 'Hypnotherapy and cigarette smoking', *Practitioner*, 1985, 229, pp. 29–31.

39   Addis, C., 'Effect of avena sativa on cigarette smoking', *Nature*, 1971, 229, p. 496.

40   Petersdorf, R., *Harrison's Principles of Internal Medicine*, McGraw-Hill, New York, NY, 1983.

41   Johnson, D., Dorr, K., Swenson, W. and Service, J., 'Reative hypoglycemia', *J.A.M.A.*, 1980, 243, pp. 1,151–5.

42   Buckley, R., 'Hypoglycemic kindling of limbic system disorder', *J. Orthomol. Psychiatry*, 1978, 7, pp. 118–22.

43   Salzer, H., 'Reactive hypoglycemia as a cause of neuropsychiatric illness', *J. Nat. Med. Assoc.*, 1966, 58, pp. 12–17.

44   Landmann, H. and Sutherland, R., 'Incidence and significance of hypoglycemia in unselected admissions to a psychosomatic service', *Am. J. Dig. Dis.*, 1950, 17, pp. 105–8.

45   Beebe, W. and Wendel, O., 'Preliminary observations of altered carbohydrate metabolism in psychiatric patients', in Pauling, L. and Hawkins, D. (eds), *Orthomolecular Psychiatry Treatment of Schizophrenia*, W.H. Freeman, San Francisco, CA, 1973, pp. 441–54.

46   Gold, M., Pottash, A. and Extein, I. 'Hypothyroidism and depression, evidence from complete thyroid function evaluation', *J.A.M.A.*, 1981, 245, pp. 1,919–22.

47   Joffe, R., Roy-Byrne, P. and Udhe, T., 'Thyroid function and affective illness: a reappraisal', *Biol. Psychiatry*, 1984, 19, pp. 1,685–91.

48   Millen, P., Bishop, M. and Coppen, A., 'Urinary free cortisol and clinical classification of depressive illness', *Psychological Med.*, 1981, 11, pp. 643–5.

49   Altar, C., Bennet, B., Wallace, R. and Yuwiler, A., 'Glucocorticoid induction of tryptophan oxygenase', *Biochem. Pharmacol.*, 1983, 32, pp. 979–84.

50   King, D., 'Can allergic exposure provoke psychological symptoms? A double-blind test', *Biol. Psychiatry*, 1981, 16, pp. 3–19.

51   Bell, I., *Clinical Ecology*, Common Knowledge Press, Bolinas, CA, 1982.

52   Dickey, L. (ed.), *Clinical Ecology*, C.C. Thomas, Springfield, IL, 1976.

53   Lindstrom, K., Riihimaki, H. and Hannininen, K., 'Occupational solvent exposure and neuropsychiatric disorders', *Scan. J. Work. Environ. Health*, 1984, 10, pp. 321–3.

54   Olsen, J. and Sabroe, S., 'A case-referent study of neuropsychiatric disorders among workers exposed to solvents in the Danish wood and furniture industry', *Scand. J. Soc. Med.*, suppl., 1980, 16, pp. 34–43.

55   Schottenfeld, R.S. and Cullen, M.R., 'Organic affective illness associated with lead intoxication', *Am. J. Psychiat.*, 1984, 141, pp. 1,423–6.

56   Crook, W., *The Yeast Connection*, Professional Books, Jackson, TN, 1983.

57   Buist, R., 'The therapeutic predictability of tryptophan and tyrosine in the treatment of depression', *Int. J. Clin. Nutr. Rev.*, 1983, 3, pp. 1–3.

58   Growden, J., 'Neurotransmitter precursors in the diets: their use in the treatment of brain diseases', in Wurtman, R. and Wurtman, J. (eds), *Nutrition and the Brain*, vol 3, Raven Press, New York, NY, 1979, pp. 117–82.

59   Brown, R., 'Tryptophan metabolism in humans', in Hayaishi, O., Ishimura, Y. and Kido, R.(eds), *Biochemical and Medical Aspects of Tryptophan Metabolism*, Elsevier/North Holland Press, Amsterdam, 1980, pp. 227–36.

60   Chouinard, G., *et al.*, 'Tryptophan in the treatment of depression and mania', *Adv. Biol. Psychiat.*, 1983, 10, pp. 47–66.

61   Pardridge, W., 'Regulation of amino acid availability to the brain', in Wurtman, R. and Wurtman, J. (eds), *Nutrition and the Brain*, vol. 1, Raven Press, New York, NY, 1979, pp. 142–204.

62   Gibson, C., 'Control of monoamine synthesis by amino acid precursors', *Adv. Biol. Psychiat.*, 1983, 10, pp. 4–18.

63   Moller, S., Kirk, L., Brandrup, E., *et al.*, 'Tryptophan availability in endogenous depression – relation to efficacy of L-tryptophan treatment', *Adv. Biol. Psychiat.* 1983, 10, pp. 30–46.

64   Beckman, H., 'Phenylalanine in affective disorders', *Adv. Biol. Psychiat.*, 1983, 10, pp. 137–47.

65   Gibson, C. and Gelenberg, A., 'Tyrosine for depression', *Adv. Biol. Psychiat.*, 1983, 10, pp. 148–59.

66   Dishman, R., 'Medical psychology in exercise and sport', *Med. Clin. North Amer.*, 1985, 69, pp. 123–43.

67   Ross, C.E. and Hayes, D., 'Exercise and psychological well-being in the community', *Am. J. Epidemiology*, 1988, 127, pp. 762–71.

33 Diabetes mellitus

1   Burkitt, D. and Trowell, H., *Western Diseases: Their Emergence and Prevention*, Harvard University Press, Cambridge, MA, 1981.

2   Petersdorf, R. (ed.), *Harrison's Principles of Internal Medicine*, 10th ed., McGraw-Hill, New York, NY, 1983.

3   Robbins, S.A. and Cotran, R., *Pathological Basis of Disease*, W.B. Saunders, New York, NY, 1974.

4   Vahouny, G. and Kritchevsky, D., *Dietary Fiber in Health and Disease*, Plenum Press, New York, NY, 1982.

5   Hughs, T., Gwynne, J., Switzer, B., *et al.*, 'Effects of caloric restriction and weight loss on glycemic control, insulin release and resistance and atherosclerotic risk in obese patients with type II diabetes mellitus', *Am. J. Med.*, 1984, 77, pp. 7–17.

6   Goodman, L. and Gilman, A., *The Pharmacological Basis of Therapeutics*, 6th ed., Macmillan, New York, NY, 1980.

REFERENCES

7   Helgason, T. and Johasson, MR., 'Evidence for a food additive as a cause of ketosis-prone diabetes', *Lancet*, 1981, ii, pp. 716–20.

8   Krupp, M. and Chatton, M., *Current Medical Diagnosis and Treatment*, Lange Medical Publications, Los Altos, CA, 1983.

9   Riales, R. and Albrink, M., 'Effect of chromium chloride supplementation on the glucose tolerance and serum lipids, including HDL, of adult men', *Am. J. Clin. Nutr.*, 1981, 34, pp. 2,670–8.

10   Offenbacher, E. and Stunyer, F., 'Beneficial effect of chromium-rich yeast on glucose tolerance and blood lipids in elderly patients', *Diabetes*, 1980, 29, pp. 919–25.

11   Mertz, M., 'Chromium occurrence and function in biological systems', *Physiol. Rev.*, 1969, 49, pp. 163–237.

12   Levine, R., Streeten, D. and Doisy, R., 'Effect of oral chromium supplementation on the glucose tolerance of elderly human subjects', *Metabolism*, 17, pp. 114–25.

13   Schroeder, H., 'The role of chromium in mammalian nutrition', *Am. J. Clin. Nutr.*, 1968, 21, pp. 230–44.

14   Steinberg, M., 'Chromium deficiency and the glucose tolerance factor', *J. John Bastyr Coll. Nat. Med.*, 1979, 1, pp. 32–6.

15   Uusitupa, M., Kumpulainein, J., Voutilainen, E., *et al.*, 'Effect of inorganic chromium supplementation on glucose tolerance, insulin response and serum lipids in noninsulin dependent diabetic', *Am. J. Clin. Nutr.*, 1983, 38, pp. 404–10.

16   Smith, U., 'Insulin resistance in obesity, type II diabetes and stress', *Acta Endocrin.*, supp., 1984, 262, pp. 67–9.

17   Krotkiewski, M., Bjrntorp, P., Sjostrom, L., and Smith, U., 'Impact of obesity on metabolism in men and women', *J. Clin. Invest.*, 1983, 72, pp. 1,150–62.

18   Dolhofer, R. and Wieland, O., 'Increased glycosylation of serum albumin in diabetes mellitus', *Diabetes*, 1980, 24, pp. 417–22.

19   Brownlee, M., Vlassara, H. and Cerami, A., 'Nonenzymatic glycosylation and the pathogenesis of diabetic complications', *Ann. Int. Med.*, 1984, 101, pp. 527–37.

20   Drner, G., Mohnike, A. and Thoelke, H., 'Further evidence for the dependence of diabetes prevalence on nutrition in perinatal life', *Exp. Clin. Endocrinol.*, 1984, 84, pp. 129–33.

21   Schwartz, J.S. and Clancy, C.M., 'Glycosylated hemoglobin assays in the management and diagnosis of diabetes mellitus', *Ann. Int. Med.*, 1984, 101, pp. 710–13.

22   Stickland, M.H., Paton, R.C. and Wales, J.K., 'Haemoglobin Alc concentrations in men and women with diabetes', *Br. Med. J.*, 1984, 289, p. 733.

23   Bolli, G.B., Gottesman, I.S., Campbell, P.J., *et al.*, 'Glucose counterregulation and waning of insulin in the Somogyi Phenomenon (posthypoglycemic hyperglycemia)', *N. Engl. J. Med.*, 1984, 311, pp. 1,214–19.

24   Cogan, D.G., Kinoshita, J.H., Kador, P.F., *et al.*, 'Aldose reductase and complications of diabetes', *Ann. Int. Med.*, 1984, 101, pp. 82–91.

25   Yue, D.K., Hanwell, M.A., Satshell, P.M., *et al.*, 'The effects of aldose reductase inhibition on nerve sorbitol and myoinositol concentrations in diabetic and galactosemic rats', *Metabolism*, 1984, 33, pp. 1,119–22.

26   Chaudhry, P.S., Cambrera, J., Juliani, H.R. and Varma, S.D., 'Inhibition of human lens aldose reductase by flavonoids, sulindac and indomethacin', *Biochem. Pharmacol.*, 1983, 32, pp. 1,995–8.

27   Anderson, J.W. and Ward, K., 'High-carbohydrate, high-fiber diets for insulin-treated men with diabetes mellitus', *Am. J. Clin. Nutr.*, 1979, 32, pp. 2,312–21.

28   Anderson, J.W., 'High polysaccharide diet studies in patients with diabetes and vascular disease', *Cereal Foods World*, 1977, 22, pp. 12–22.

29   Kay, R., Grobin, W. and Trace, N., 'Diets rich in natural fiber improve carbohydrate tolerance in maturity onset, noninsulin dependent diabetics', *Diabetologia*, 1981, 20, pp. 12–23.

30   Simpson, H.C.R., Simpson, R.W., Lousley, S., *et al.*, 'A high carbohydrate leguminous fibre diet improves all aspects of diabetic control', *Lancet*, 1981, i, pp. 1–5.

31   Jenkins, D.J.A., Wolever, T.M.S., Bacon, S., *et al.*, 'Diabetic diets: high carbohydrate combined with high fiber', *Am. J. Clin. Nutr.*, 1980, 33, pp. 1,729–33.

32   Hollenbeck, C.B. Lecklem, J.E., Riddle, M.C. and Conner, W.E., 'The composition and nutritional adequacy of subject-selected high carbohydrate, low fat diets in insulin-dependent diabetes mellitus', *Am. J. Clin. Nutr.*, 1983, 38, pp. 41–51.

33   Anderson, J., *Diabetes. A Practical Approach to Daily Living*, Arco Press, New York, NY, 1981.

34   Pritikin, N. and McGrandy, P., *The Pritikin Program for Diet and Exercise*, Grosset & Dunlap, New York, NY, 1979.

35   Ranic, M. and Berger, M., 'Exercise and diabetes mellitus', *Diabetes*, 1979, 28, pp. 147–63.

36   Koivisto, V.A. and DeFronzo, R.A., 'Exercise in the treatment of type II diabetes', *Acta Endocrin.*, suppl., 1984, 262, pp. 107–11.

37   Vallerand, A.L., Cuerrier, J.P., Shapcott, D., *et al.*, 'Influence of exercise training on tissue chromium concentrations in the rat', *Am. J. Clin. Nutr.*, 1984, 39, pp. 402–9.

38   Pedersen, O., Beck-Nielsen, H. and Heding, L., 'Increased insulin receptors after exercise in patients with insulin-dependent diabetes mellitus', *N. Engl. J. Med.*, 1980, 302, pp. 886–92.

39   Bever, B.O. and Zahnd, G.R., 'Plants with oral hypoglycemic action', *Quart. J. Crude Drug Res.*, 1979, 17, pp. 139–96.

40   Chakravarthy, B.K., Gupa, S., Gambhir, S.S. and Gode, K.D., 'Pancreatic beta-cell regeneration in rats by (-)-epicatechin', *Lancet*, 1981, ii, pp. 759–60.

41   Chakravarthy, B.K., Gupa, S., Gambhir, S.S. and Gode, K.D., '1-Epicatechin – a novel anti-diabetic drug', *Indian Drugs*, 1981, 18, pp. 184–5.

42   Chakravarthy, B.K., Gupa, S. and Gode, K.D., 'Functional beta cell regeneration in the islets of pancreas in alloxan induced diabetic rats by (-)-epicatechin', *Life Sci.*, 1982, 31, pp. 2,693–7.

43   Chakravarthy, B.K., Gupa, S. and Gode, K.D., 'Antidiabetic effect of (-)-epicatechin', *Lancet*, 1982, ii, p. 272.

44   Welihinda, J., Arvidson, G., Gylfe, E., *et al.*, 'The insulin-releasing activity of the tropical plant Momordica charantia', *Acta Biol. Med. Germ.*, 1982, 41, pp. 1,229–40.

45   Keder, P. and Chakrabarti, C.H., 'Effects of bittergourd (Momordica charantia) seed and glibenclamide in streptozotocin induced diabetes mellitus', *Ind. J. Exp. Biol.*, 1982, 20, pp. 232–5.

46   Akhtar, M.S., Athar, M.A. and Yaqub, M., 'Effect of momordica charantia on blood glucose level of normal and alloxan-diabetic rabbits', *Planta Medica*, 1981, 42, pp. 205–12.

47   Sharma, K.K., Gupta, R.K., Gupta, S. and Samuel, K.C., 'Antihyperglycemic effect of onion: effect on fasting blood sugar and induced hyperglycemia in man', *Ind. J. Med. Res.*, 1977, 65, pp. 422–9.

48   Baghurst, K., Raj, M. and Truswell, A., 'Onions and platelet aggregation', *Lancet*, 1977, i, p. 101.

49   Norwell, D. and Tarr, R., 'Garlic, vampires and CHD', *Osteopath. Ann.*, 1984, 12, pp. 276–80.

50   Ribes, G., Sauvaire, Y., Baccou, J.C. *et al.*, 'Effects of fenugreek seeds on endocrine pancreatic secretions in dogs', *Ann. Nutr. Metab.*, 1984, 28, pp. 37–43.

51   Allen, F.M., 'Blueberry leaf extract: physiologic and clinical properties in relation to carbohydrate metabolism', *J.A.M.A.* 1927, 89, pp. 1,577–81.

52   Yudkin, J., 'Dietary factors in arteriosclerosis: sucrose', *Lipids*, 1978, 13, pp. 370–2.

53   Urberg, M. and Zemel, M.B., 'Evidence for synergism between chromium and nicotinic acid in the control of glucose tolerance in elderly humans', *Metabolism*, 1987, 36, pp. 896–9.

54   Mooradian, A.D. and Morley, J.E., 'Micronutrient status in diabetes mellitus', *Am. J. Clin. Nutr.*, 1987, 45, pp. 877–95.

55   McCann, V.J. and Davis, R.E., 'Serum pyridoxal concentrations in patients with diabetic retinopathy', *Aust N.Z. J. Med.*, 1978, 8, pp. 259–61.

56   Jones, C.L. and Gonzales, V., 'Pyridoxine deficiency: a new factor in diabetic retinopathy', *J. Am. Pod. Assoc.*, 1978, 68, pp. 646–53.

57   Lam, S., Harfenist, E., Packham, M., *et al.*, 'Investigation of the possible mechanisms of pyridoxal 5'-phosphate inhibition of platelet reactions', *Thrombosis Res.*, 1980, 20, pp. 633–45.

58   Mann, G.V., 'Hypothesis: the role of vitamin C in diabetic angiopathy', *Perspect. Biol. Med.*, 1974, 17, pp. 210–17.

59   Lubin, B. and Machlin, L., 'Biological aspects of vitamin E', *Ann. N.Y. Acad. Sci.*, 1982, 393, pp. 1–910.

60   Galli, C. and Socin, A., 'Biological actions and possible uses of vitamin E', *Acta Vitaminol. Enzymol.*, 1984, 4, pp. 245–52.

61   Wimhurst, J.M. and Manchester, K.L., 'Comparison of ability of Mg and Mn to activate the key enzymes of glycolysis', *F.E.B.S. Letters*, 1972, 27, pp. 321–6.

62   Editorial, 'Manganese and glucose tolerance', *Nutr. Rev.*, 1968, 26, pp. 207–10.

63   Ceriello, A., Giugliano, D., Russo, P.D. and Passariello, N., 'Hypomagnesemia in relation to diabetic retinopathy', *Diabetes Care*, 1982, 5, pp. 558–9.

64   Davidson, S., 'The use of vitamin B12 in the treatment of diabetic neuropathy', *J. Flor. Med. Assoc.*, 1954, 15, pp. 717–20.

65   Sancetta, S.M., Ayres, P.R. and Scott, R.W., 'The use of vitamin B12 in the management of the neurological manifestations of diabetes mellitus, with notes on the administration of massive doses', *Ann. Int. Med.*, 1951, 35, pp. 1,028–48.

66   Bhatt, H.R., Linnell, J.C. and Matt, D.M., 'Can faulty vitamin B12 (cobalamin) metabolism produce diabetic retinopathy?', *Lancet*, 1983, ii, p. 572.

67   Abdel-Aziz, M.T., Abdou, M.S., Soliman, K., *et al.*, 'Effect of carnitine on blood lipid patterns in diabetic patients', *Nutr. Rep. Int.*, 1984, 29, pp. 1,071–9.

68   Tadros, W.M., Awadallah, R., Doss, H. and Khalifa, K., 'Protective effect of trace elements (Zn, Mn, Cr, Co) on alloxan-induced diabetes', *Ind. J. Exp. Biol.*, 1982, 20, pp. 93–4.

69   Tarui, S., 'Studies of zinc metabolism: III. Effect of the diabetic state on zinc metabolism: a clinical aspect', *Endocrinol. Japan*, 1963, 10, pp. 9–15.

70   Gegersen, G., Harb, H., Helles, A. and Christensen, J., 'Oral supplementation of myoinositol: effects on peripheral nerve function in human diabetics and on the concentration in plasma, erythrocytes, urine and muscle tissue in human diabetics and normals', *Acta Neurol. Scand.*, 1983, 67, pp. 164–71.

71   Norbiato, G., Bevilacqua, M., Merino, R., *et al.*, 'Effects of potassium supplementation on insulin binding and insulin action in human obesity: protein-modified fast and refeeding', *Europ. J. Clin. Invest.*, 1984, pp. 414–19.

72   Strakosch, C.R., Steil, J.N. and Gyry, A.Z., 'Hypokalemia occurring during insulin-induced hypoglycemia', *Aust N.Z. J. Med.*, 1976, 6, pp. 314–16.

73   Reddi, A., DeAngelis, B., Frank, O., *et al.*, 'Biotin supplementation improves glucose and insulin tolerances in genetically diabetic KK mice', *Life Sciences*, 1988, 42, pp. 1,323–30.

74   Roe, D., *Drug Induced Nutritional Deficiencies*, A.V.I. Publishing, Westport, CT, 1976, pp. 168–73.

75   Montgomery, R. *Biochemistry: A Case Oriented Approach*, 3rd ed., Mosby, St Louis, MO, 1980.

76   Coggeshall, J.C., Heggers, J.P., Robson, M.C. and Baker, H., 'Biotin status and plasma glucose in diabetics', *Annals N.Y. Acad. Sci.*, 1985, 447, pp. 389–92.

34 Diarrhoea

1   Rubenstein, E. and Federman, D.D., *Scientific American Medicine*, Scientific American, New York, NY, 1988.

2   Leung, A.Y. *Encyclopedia of Common Natural Ingredients used in Food*, John Wiley & Sons, New York, NY, 1980, pp. 352–4.

3   Wright, J.V., *Healing with Nutrition*, Rodale, Emmaus, PA, 1984.

4   Worthington-Roberts, B.S., *Contemporary Developments in Nutrition*, C.V. Mosby, St Louis, MO., 1981, pp. 29–35.

5   Bhakat, M.P., Nandi, N., Pal, H.K. and Khan, B.S., 'Therapeutic trial of berberine sulphate in non-specific gastroenteritis', *Ind. Med. J.*, 1974, 68, pp. 19–23.

6   Desai, A.B., Shah, K.M. and Shah, D.M., 'Berberine in the treatment of diarrhoea', *Ind. Ped.*, 1971, 8, pp. 462–5.

7   Sharma, R., Joshi, C.K. and Goyal, R.K., 'Berberine tannate in acute diarrhea', *Ind. Ped.*, 1970, 7, pp. 496–501.

8   Choudry, V.P., Sabir, M. and Bhide, V.N., 'Berberine in giardiasis', *Ind. Ped.*, 1972, 9, pp. 143–6.

9   Subbaiah, T.V. and Amin, A.H., 'Effect of berberine sulfate on Entamoeba histolytica', *Nature*, 1967, 215, pp. 527–8.

10   Sack, R.B. and Froehlich, J.L., 'Berberine inhibits intestinal secretory response of vibrio cholerae toxins and Escherichia coli enterotoxins', *Infect. Immun.*, 1982, 35, pp. 471–5.

11   Tai, Y.H., Feser, J.F., Mernane, W.G. and Desjeux, J.F., 'Antisecretory effects of berberine in rat ileum', *Am. J. Physiol.*, 1981, 241, pp. G253–8.

12   Swabb, E.A., Tai, Y.H. and Jordan, L., 'Reversal of cholera toxin-induced secretion in rat ileum by luminal berberine', *Am. J. Physiol.*, 1981, 241, pp. G248–52.

13   Fleter, H.W. and Lloyd, J.U., *King's Dispensatory*, 1898; republished by Eclectic Medical Publications, Portland, OR, 1983.

14   Leung, A.Y., *Encyclopedia of Common Natural Ingredients used in Food*, John Wiley & Sons, New York, NY, 1980.

15   Windholz, M., Budavari, S., Blumetti, R.F. and Otterbein, E.S., *The Merck Index: An Encyclopedia of Chemicals, Drugs, and Biologicals*, Merck, Rahway, NJ, 1983, p. 1,013.

16   Shahani, K.M., Vakil, J.R. and Kilara, A., 'Natural antibiotic activity of Lactobacillus acidophilus and bulgaricus', *Cult. Dairy Prod. J.*, 1977, 12, pp. 8–11.
17   Shahani, K.M. and Friend, B.A., 'Nutritional and therapeutic aspects of lactobacilli', *J. Appl. Nutr.*, 1984, 36, pp. 125–52.
18   Cheney, G., 'Rapid healing of peptic ulcers in patients receiving fresh cabbage juice', *Cal. Med.*, 1949, 70, pp. 10–14.

35 Ear infections

1   Pizzorno, J.E. and Murray, M.T., *A Textbook of Natural Medicine*, John Bastyr College Publications, Seattle, WA, 1985, p.VI:OtitMe-1–4.
2   van Buchen, F.L., Dunk, J.H. and van Hof, M.A., 'Therapy of acute otitis media: myringotomy, antibiotics, or neither?', *Lancet*, 1981, ii, pp. 883–7.
3   Diamant, M. and Diamant, B., 'Abuse and timing of use of antibiotics in acute otitis media', *Arch. Otol.*, 1974, 100, pp. 226–32.
4   Mygind, N., Meistrup-Larsen, K.I., Thomsen, J., *et al.*, 'Penicillin in acute otitis media: a double-blind placebo-controlled trial', *Clin. Otol.*, 1981, 6, pp. 5–13.
5   Saarinen, U.M., 'Prolonged breast feeding as prophylaxis for recurrent otitis media', *Acta Ped. Scand.*, 1982, 71, pp. 567–71.
6   Editorial, 'Breast feeding prevents otitis media', *Nutr. Rev.*, 1983, 41, pp. 241–2.
7   Backon, J. 'Prolonged breast feeding as a prophylaxis for recurrent otitis media: relevance of prostaglandins', *Med. Hypoth.*, 1984, 13, p. 161.
8   McMahan, J.T., Calenoff, E., Croft, D.J., *et al.*, 'Chronic otitis media with effusion and allergy: modified RAST analysis of 119 cases', *Otol. Head Neck Surg.*, 1981, 89, pp. 427–31.
9   Viscomi, G.J., 'Allergic secretory otitis media: an approach to management', *Laryngoscope*, 1975, 85, pp. 751–8.
10   Van Cauwenberge, P.B., 'The role of allergy in otitis media with effusion', *Ther. Umschau.*, 1982, 39, pp. 1,011–16.
11   Bellionin, P., Cantani, A. and Salvinelli, F., 'Allergy: a leading role in otitis media with effusion', *Allergol. Immunol.*, 1987, 15, pp. 205–8.
12   Fiocchi, A., Borella, E., Riva, E., *et al.*, 'A double-blind clinical trial for the evaluation of the therapeutic effectiveness of a calf thymus derivative (Thymomodulin) in children with recurrent respiratory infections', *Thymus*, 1986, 8, pp. 831–9.
13   Genova, R. and Guerra, A., 'Thymomodulin in management of food allergy in children', *Int. J. Tissue Reac.*, 1986, 8, pp. 239–42.
14   Cazzola, P., Mazzanti, P. and Bossi, G., 'In vivo modulating effect of a calf thymus acid lysate on human T lymphocyte subsets and CD4+/CD8+ ratio in the course of different diseases', *Curr. Ther. Res.*, 1987, 42, pp. 1,011–17.

36 Eczema

1   Sampson, H., 'Role of immediate food hypersensitivity in the pathogenesis of atopic dermatitis,' *J. Allergy Clin. Immunol.*, 1983, 71, pp. 473–80.
2   Rubenstein, E. and Federman, D., *Scientific American Medicine*, Scientific American, New York, NY, 1984, p. 2:IV:1.
3   Soter, N. and Baden, H., *Pathophysiology of Dermatologic Disease*, McGraw-Hill, New York, NY, 1984.
4   Siccardi, A., Fortunato, A., Marconi, M., *et al.*, 'Defective bactericidal reaction by the alternative pathway of complement in atopic patients', *Infect. Immun.*, 1981, 33, pp. 710–13.
5   Rawls, W.B. and Ancona, V.C., 'Chronic urticaria associated with hypochlorhydria or achlorhydria', *Rev. Gastroent.*, 1950, Oct., pp. 267–71.
6   Ayres, S., 'Gastric secretion in psoriasis, eczema and dermatitis herpetiformis', *Arch. Derm.*, 1929, Jul. pp. 854–9.
7   Pizzorno, J.E. and Murray, M.T., *A Textbook of Natural Medicine*, John Bastyr College Publications, Seattle, WA, 1985, p. IV:FoodA1.
8   Andres, M.R. and Bingham, J.R., 'Tubeless gastric analysis with a radio-telemetry pill', *C.M.A.*, 1970, 102, pp. 1,087–9.
9   Jordan, J. and Whitlock, F. 'Emotions and the skin: the conditioning of scratch responses in cases of atopic dermatitis', *Br. J. Dermatol.*, 1972, 86, pp. 574–84.
10   Ayres, J., Banks, H., Bixby, F., *et al.*, 'What food is to one', *N.E.J.M.*, 1984, 311, pp. 399–400.
11   Molkhou, P. and Waguet, J., 'Food allergy and atopic dermatitis in children: treatment with oral sodium cromoglycate', *Ann. Allergy*, 1981, 47, pp. 173–5.
12   Jacobs, A., 'Atopic dermatitis: clinical expression and management', *Pediatr. Ann.*, 1976, 5, pp. 763–71.
13   Hansen, A., Knott, E., Wiese, H., *et al.*, 'Eczema and essential fatty acids', *A.J. Dis. Child.*, 1947, 73, pp. 1–18.
14   Manku, M., Horrobin, D., Morse, N., *et al.*, 'Reduced levels of prostaglandin precursors in the blood of atopic patients: defective delta-6-desaturase function as a biochemical basis for atopy', *Prostaglandins, Leukotrienes and Medicine*, 1982, 9, pp. 615–28.
15   Wright, S. and Burton, J., 'Oral evening primrose oil improves eczema', *Lancet*, 1982, ii, p. 1,120.
16   Lee, T., Hoover, R., Williams, J., *et al.*, 'Effect of dietary enrichment with eicosapentaenoic and docosahexaenoic acids on in vitro neutrophil and monocyte leukotriene generation and neutrophil generation', *N.E.J.M.*, 1985, 312, pp. 1,217–24.
17   Strasser, T., Fisher, S. and Weber, P., 'Leukotriene B5 is formed in human neutrophils after dietary supplementation with eicosapentaenoic acid', *Proc. Natl Acad. Sci.*, 1985, 82, pp. 1,540–3.
18   Renaud, S. and Nordoy, A., '"Small is beautiful": alpha-linolenic acid and eicosapentaenoic acid in man', *Lancet*, 1983, i, p. 1,169.
19   Pizzorno, J.E. and Murray, M.T., *A Textbook of Natural Medicine*, John Bastyr College Publications, Seattle, WA, 1985, p. V:Querc.
20   Middleton, E. and Drzewieki, G., 'Flavonoid inhibition of human basophil histamine release stimulated by various agents', *Biochem. Pharmacol.*, 1984, 33, pp. 3,333–8.
21   Middleton, E. and Drzewieki, G., 'Naturally occurring flavonoids and human basophil histamine release', *Int. Arch. Allergy Appl. Immunol.*, 1985, 77, pp. 155–7.
22   Amella, M., Bronner, C., Briancon, F., *et al.*, 'Inhibition of mast cell histamine release by flavonoids and bioflavonoids', *Planta Medica*, 1985, 51, pp. 16–20.
23   Pearce, F., Befus, A.D. and Bienenstock, J., 'Mucosal mast cells. III. Effect of quercetin and other flavonoids on antigen-induced histamine secretion from rat intestinal mast cells', *J. Allergy Clin. Immunol.*, 1984, 73, pp. 819–23.
24   Zile, M.H. and Cullum, M.E., 'The function of vitamin A: current concepts', *Proc. Soc. Exp. Biol. Med.*, 1983, 172, pp. 139–52.

25   Petkov, E., Nikolov, N. and Uzunov, P. 'Inhibitory effects of some flavonoids and flavonoid mixtures on cyclic AMP phosphodiesterase activity of rat heart', *J. Med. Plant Res.*, 1981, 43, pp. 183–6.

26   Beretz, A., Stierle, A., Anton, R. and Cazenavet, J., 'Role of cyclic AMP in the inhibition of human platelet aggregation by quercetin, a flavonoid that potentiates the effect of prostacyclin', *Biochem. Pharm.*, 1981, 31, pp. 3,597–600.

27   Amella, M., Bronner, C., Brincon, F. *et al.*, 'Inhibition of mast cell histamine release by flavonoids and bioflavonoids', *Plant Med.*, 1985, 51, pp. 16–20.

28   Nikaido, T., Ohmoto, T., Noguchi, H., *et al.*, 'Inhibitors of cyclic AMP phosphodiesterase in medicinal plants', *J. Med. Plant. Res.*, 1981, 43, pp. 18–23.

29   Seamon, K., Padgett, W. and Daly, J., 'Forskolin: unique diterpine activator of adenylate cyclase in membranes and intact cells', *Proc. Natl Acad. Sci.*, 1981, 78, pp. 3,363–7.

30   Leung, A.Y., *Encyclopedia of Common Ingredients Used in Food, Drugs and Cosmetics*, J Wiley & Sons, New York, NY, 1980, pp. 80–1.

31   Pizzorno, J.E. and Murray, M.T., *A Textbook of Natural Medicine*, John Bastyr College Publications, Seattle, WA, 1985, p. VI:AtopDe-1.

32   Mann, C. and Staba, E.J., 'The chemistry, pharmacology, and commercial formulation of chamomile', *Herbs, Spices, and Medicinal Plants: Recent Advances in Botany, Horticulture, and Pharmacology*, 1986, 1, pp. 235–80.

33   Evans, F.Q., 'The rationale use of glycyrrhetinic acid in dermatology', *Br. J. Clin. Pract.*, 1958, 12, pp. 269–74.

37 Fibrocystic breast disease

1   Cole, E.N., Sellwood, R.A., England, P.G. and Griffiths, K., 'Serum prolactin concentrations in benign breast disease throughout the menstrual cycle', *J. Cancer*, 1977, 13, pp. 597–603.

2   Peters, F., Schuth, W., Scheurich, B. and Breckwoldt, M., 'Serum prolactin levels in patients with fibrocystic breast disease', *Obstet. Gynecol.*, 1984, 64, pp. 381–5.

3   Boyle, C.A., Berkowitz, G.S., LiVolsi, V.A., *et al.*, 'Caffeine consumption and fibrocystic breast disease: a case-control epidemiologic study', *J.N.C.I.*, 1984, 72, pp. 1,015–19.

4   Minton, J.P., Abou-Issa, H., Reiches, N., Roseman, J.M., 'Clinical and biochemical studies on methylxanthine-related fibrocystic breast disease', *Surgery*, 1981, 90, pp. 299–304.

5   Minton, J.P., Foecking, M.K., Webster, D.J.T. and Matthews, R.H., 'Caffeine, cyclic nucleotides, and breast disease', *Surgery*, 1979, 86, pp. 105–9.

6   Ernster, V.L., Mason, L., Goodson, W.H., *et al.*, 'Effects of caffeine-free diet on benign breast disease: a random trial', *Surgery*, 1982, 91, pp. 263–7.

7   London, R.S., Sundaram, G.S., Schultz, M. *et al.*, 'Endocrine parameters and alpha-tocopherol therapy of patients with mammary dysplasia', *Cancer Res.*, 1981, 41, pp. 3,811–13.

8   London, R.S., Sundaram, G., Manimekalai, S. *et al.*, 'The effect of alpha-tocopherol on premenstrual symptomatology: a double-blind study. II. Endocrine correlates', *J. Am. Col. Nutr.*, 1984, 3, pp. 351–6.

9   Sundaram, G.S., London, R., Margolis, S., *et al.*, 'Serum hormones and lipoproteins in benign breast disease', *Cancer Res.*, 1981, 41, pp. 3,814–16.

10 Band, P.R., Deschamps, M., Falardeau, M., *et al.*, 'Treatment of benign breast disease with vitamin A', *Prev. Med.*, 1984, 13, pp. 549–54.

11 Eskin, B.A., Bartushka, D.G., Dunn, M.R., *et al.*, 'Mammary gland dysplasia in iodine deficiency', *J.A.M.A.*, 1967, 200, pp. 691–5.

12 Estes, N.C., 'Mastodynia due to fibrocystic disease of the breast controlled with thyroid hormone', *A. J. Surg.*, 1981, 142, pp. 764–6.

13 Mielens, Z.E., Rozitis, J. Jr and Sansone, V.J. Jr, 'The effect of oral iodides on inflammation', *Texas Rep. Biol. Med.*, 1968, 26, pp. 117–21.

14 Petrakis, N.L. and King, E.B., 'Cytological abnormalities in nipple aspirates of breast fluid from women with severe constipation', *Lancet*, 1981, ii, pp. 1,203–5.

15 Hentges, D.J., 'Does diet influence human fecal microflora composition?', *Nutr. Rev.*, 1980, 38, pp. 329–36.

16 Goldin, B., Aldercreutz, H., Dwyer, J., *et al.*, 'Effect of diet on excretion of estrogens in pre- and postmenopausal women', *Cancer Res.*, 1981, 41, pp. 3,771–3.

38 Food allergy

1   The authors wish to acknowledge Dr Stephen Barrie, whose chapter Food Allergy in Pizzorno, J.E. and Murray, M.T., *A Textbook of Natural Medicine* (John Bastyr College Publications, Seattle, WA, 1985), formed the basis for this chapter.

2   Adams, F., *The Genuine Works of Hippocrates*, Williams & Williams, Baltimore, MD, 1939.

3   Taken from *Immunology and Clinical Practice*, 1984, 6, p. 123.

4   Gerrard, J.W., Ko, C.G. and Vickers, P., 'The familial incidence of allergic disease', *Ann. All.*, 1976, 36, p. 10.

5   Taub, E.L., *Food Allergy and the Allergic Patient*, C.C. Thomas, Springfield, IL, 1978.

6   Buckley, R., 'Food allergy', *J.A.M.A.*, 1982, 248, p. 2,627.

7   Gell, P.G.H. and Coombs, R.R.A., *Clinical Aspects of Immunology*, Blackwell, Oxford, 1974.

8   Hamburger, R., *Proc. First Intl Symp. on Food Allergy*, Vancouver, BC, 1982.

9   Bryan, W.T.K. and Bryan, M.P., 'The application of the in vitro cytotoxic reactions to clinical diagnosis of food allergy', *Laryngoscope*, 1960, 70, p. 810.

10 Perelmutter, L., 'Non-IgE mediated atopic disease', *Ann. All.*, 1984, 52, p. 640.

11 Paganelli, R., Levinsky, R.J. and Atherton, D.J., 'Detection of specific antigen within circulating immune complexes', *Lancet*, 1979, i, p. 1,270.

12 McGovern, J.J., 'Correlation of clinical food allergy symptoms with serial pharmacological and immunological changes in the patient's plasma', *Ann. Allergy*, 1980, 44, p. 57.

13 Trevino, R.J., 'Immunologic mechanisms in the production of food sensitivities', *Laryngoscope*, 1981, 91, p. 1,913.

REFERENCES

14 Thonnard-Nenmann, E. and Neckers, L.M., 'T-lymphocytes in migraine', *Ann. All.*, 1981, 47, p. 325.

15 Rivlin, J., Kuperman, O., Freier, S., *et al.*, 'Suppressor T-lymphocyte activity in wheezy children', *Clin. Allergy*, 1981, 11, p. 353.

16 Minor, J.D., Tolber, S.G. and Frick, O.L., 'Leukocyte inhibition factor in delayed-onset food sensitivity', *J. Allergy Clin. Immunol.*, 1980, 6, p. 314.

17 Taylor, B., Norman, A.P., Orgel, C.R., *et al.*, 'Transient IgA deficiency and pathogenesis of infantile atopy', *Lancet*, 1973, ii, p. 111.

18 Keller, S.E., Weiss, J.M., Schleifer, S.J., *et al.*, 'Suppression of immunity by stress: effect of graded series of stressors on lymphocyte stimulation in the rat', *Science*, 1981, 213, p. 1,397.

19 Ader, R. (ed.), *Psychoimmunology*, Academic Press, New York, NY, 1981.

20 de Weck, A.L., 'Pathophysiologic mechanisms of allergic and pseudo-allergic reactions to foods, food additives and drugs', *Ann. All.*, 1984, 53, pp. 583–6.

21 Commings, W.A. and Williams, E.W., 'Transport of large breakdown products of dietary protein through the gut wall', *Gut*, 1978, 19, p. 715.

22 Walker, W.A., 'Uptake and transport of macromolecules by the intestine – possible role in clinical disorders', *Gastroenter.*, 1974, 67, p. 531.

23 Lake, A.M., Bloch, K.J., Neutra, M.R. and Waker, W.A., 'Intestinal goblet cell mucous release', *J. Immunol.*, 1979, 122, p. 834.

24 Grusky, F.L., 'Gastrointestinal absorption of unaltered proteins in normal infants', *Pediatrics*, 1955, 16, p. 763.

25 Reinhardt, M.C., 'Macromolecular absorption of food antigens in health and disease', *J. Allergy*, 1984, 53, p. 597.

26 Monroe, J., Carini, C., Brostoff, J. and Zilkha, K., 'Food allergy in migraine', *Lancet*, 1980, ii, p. 1.

27 Atherton, D.J., *et al.*, 'A double-blind controlled crossover trial of an antigen-avoidance diet in atopic eczema', *Lancet*, 1978, i, p. 401.

28 Rea, W.J., 'Recurrent environmentally triggered thrombophlebitis: a five year follow-up', *Ann. Allergy*, 1981, 47, p. 338.

29 Anderson, A.F.R., 'Ulcerative colitis – allergic phenomenon', *Amer. J. Dig. Dis.*, 1942, 9, p. 91.

30 Breneman, J.C., *Basics of Food Allergy*, C.C. Thomas, Springfield, IL, 1977.

31 Egger, J., Graham, P.J., Carter, C.M. and Gumley, D., 'Controlled trial of oligoantigenic treatment in the hyperkinetic syndrome', *Lancet*, 1985, i, p. 540.

32 Rowe, A.H. and Young, E.J., 'Bronchial asthma due to food allergy alone in 95 patients', *J.A.M.A.*, 1959, 169, p. 1,158.

33 Raymond, L.F., 'Allergy and chronic simple glaucoma', *Ann. All.*, 1964, 22, p. 146.

34 Wright, J.V., *Healing with Nutrition*, Rodale, Emmaus, PA, 1984.

35 Dickey, L.D., *Clinical Ecology*, C.C. Thomas, Springfield, IL, 1974.

36 Pizzorno, J.E. and Murray, M.T., *A Textbook of Natural Medicine*, John Bastyr College Publications, Seattle, WA, pp. II:FoodA1–4,5.

37 Dockhorn, R.J. and Smith, T.C., 'Use of a chemically defined hypoallergenic diet in the management of patients with suspected food allergy', *Ann. Allergy*, 1981, 47, pp. 264–6.

38 Rowe, A.H. and Rowe, A., *Food Allergy. Its Manifestations and Control and the Elimination Diets*, C.C. Thomas, Springfield, IL, 1972.

39 Metcalfe, D., 'Food hypersensitivity', *J. All. Clin. Imm.*, 1984, 73, pp. 749–61.

40 Coca, A.F., 'Art of investigating pulse diet record in familial nonreagenic food allergy', *Ann. Allergy*, 1944, 2, p. 1.

41 Rinkel, H.J., Randolph, T. and Zeller, M., *Food Allergy*, C.C. Thomas, Springfield, IL, 1951.

42 Rinkel, H.J., 'Food allergy IV. The function and clinical application of the rotary diversified diet', *J. Pediat.*, 1948, 32, p. 266.

43 Lee, C.H., Williams, R.I. and Binkley, E.L., 'Provocative testing and treatment for foods', *Arch. Otolaryn.*, 1969, 90, p. 113.

44 Rinkel, H.J., Lee, C.H., Brown, D.W., *et al.*, 'The diagnosis of food allergy', *Arch. Otolaryn.*, 1964, 79, p. 71.

45 Miller, J.B., *Food Allergy: Provocative Testing and Injection Therapy*, C.C. Thomas, Springfield, IL, 1972.

46 Levine, S.A., 'Selenium and human chemical hypersensitivities', *Int. J. Biosocial Res.*, 1982, 3, p. 44.

47 Pekarek, R.S., Sandstead, H.H., Jacob, R.A. and Barcome, D.F., 'Abnormal cellular immune responses during acquired zinc deficiency', *Am. J. Clin. Nut.*, 1979, 32, p. 1,466.

48 Pearce, F.L., Befus, A.D. and Bienenstock, J., 'Effect of quercetin and other flavonoids on antigen-induced histamine secretion from rat intestinal mast cells', *J. All. Clin. Immunol.*, 1984, June, p. 822.

49 Horrobin, D.F., *et al.*, 'The nutritional regulation of T lymphocyte function', *Med. Hypothesis*, 1979, 5, p. 969.

39 Gallstones

1 Robbins, S.L., Cotran, R.S. and Kumar, V., *Pathologic Basis of Disease*, W.B. Saunders, Philadelphia, PA, 1984, pp. 942–50.

2 Petersdorf, R., *et al.* (eds), *Harrison's Principles of Internal Medicine*, McGraw-Hill, New York, NY, 1983, pp. 1,821–32.

3 Weisberg, H.F., 'Pathogenesis of gallstones', *Annals Clin. Lab. Sci.*, 1984, 14, pp. 243–51.

4 Trowell, H., Burkitt, D. and Heaton, K., *Dietary Fibre, Fibre-depleted Foods and Disease*, Academic Press, New York, NY, 1985, pp. 289–304.

5 Pixley, F., Wilson, D., McPherson, K., *et al.*, 'Effect of vegetarianism on development of gallstones in women', *Brit. Med. J.*, 1985, 291, pp. 11–12.

6 Kritchevsky, D. and Klurfield, D.M., 'Gallstone formation in hamsters: effect of varying animal and vegetable protein levels', *Amer. J. Clin. Nutr.*, 1983, 37, pp. 802–4.

7 Breneman, J.C., 'Allergy elimination diet as the most effective gallbladder diet', *Annals Allergy*, 1968, 26, pp. 83–7.

8 Necheles, H., Rappaport, B.Z., Green, R., *et al.*, 'Allergy of the gallbladder', *Am. J. Dig. Dis.*, 1949, 7, pp. 238–41.

9 Walzer, M., Gray, I., Harten, M., *et al.*, 'The allergic reaction of the gallbladder: experimental studies in rhesus monkeys', *Gastroenterol.*, 1943, 1, pp. 565–72.

10 De Muro, P. and Ficari, A., 'Experimental studies on allergic cholecystitis', *Gastroenterol.*, 1946, 6, pp. 302–14.

11 Tuzhilin, S.A., Drieling, D.A., Narodetskaja, R.V. and Lukash, L.K., 'The treatment of patients with gallstones by lecithin', *Am. J. Gastroenterol.*, 1976, 65, p. 231.

12 Hanin, I. and Ansell, G.B., *Lecithin. Technological, Biological, and Therapeutic Aspects*, Plenum Press, New York, NY, 1987.

13 Jenkins, S.A., 'Vitamin C and gallstone formation: a preliminary report', *Experentia*, 1977, 33, pp. 1,616–17.

14 Dam, H. and Christensen, F., 'Alimentary production of gallstones in hamsters', *Acta Path. Microbiol. Scand.*, 1952, 30, pp. 236–42.

15 Lee, S.P., Tassmann-Jones, C. and Carlisle, V., 'Oleic acid-induced cholelithiasis in rabbits', *Am. J. Pathol.*, 1986, 124, pp. 18–24.

16 Beynen, A.C., 'Dietary monounsaturated fatty acids and liver cholesterol', *Artery*, 1988, 15, pp. 170–5.

17 Baggio, G., Pagnan, A., Muraca, M., *et al.*, 'Olive-oil-enriched diet: effect on serum lipoprotein levels and biliary cholesterol saturation', *Am. J. Clin. Nutr.*, 1988, 47, pp. 960–4.

18 Hordinsky, B.Z., 'Terpenes in the treatment of gallstones', *Minnesota Medicine*, 1971, 54, pp. 649–51.

19 Bell, G.D. and Doran, J., 'Gallstone dissolution in man using an essential oil preparation', *Brit. Med. J.*, 1979, 278, p. 24.

20 Doran, J., Keighley, R.B. and Bell, G.D., 'Rowachol – a possible treatment for cholesterol gallstones', *Gut*, 1979, 20, pp. 312–17.

21 Ellis, W.R. and Bell, G.D., 'Treatment of biliary duct stones with a terpene preparation', *Brit. Med. J.*, 1981, 282, p. 611.

22 Somerville, K.W., Ellis, W.R., Whitten, B.H., *et al.*, 'Stones in the common bile duct: experience with medical dissolution therapy', *Postgraduate Medical Journal*, 1985, 61, pp. 313–16.

23 Ellis, W.R., Bell, G.D., Middleton, B. and White, D.A., 'Adjunct to bile-acid treatment for gall-stone dissolution: low dose chenodeoxycholic acid combined with a terpene preparation', *Brit. Med. J.*, 1981, 282, pp. 611–12.

24 Bell, G.D., Clegg, R.J., Ellis, W.R., *et al.*, 'How does Rowachol, a mixture of plant monoterpenes, enhance the cholelithic potential of low and medium dose chenodeoxycholic acid?', *British Journal of Pharmacology*, 1982, 13, pp. 278–9.

25 Ellis, W.R., Somerville, K.W., Whitten, B.H. and Bell, G.D., 'Pilot study of combination treatment for gall stones with medium dose chenodeoxycholic acid and a terpene preparation', *Brit. Med. J.*, 1984, 289, pp. 153–6.

40 Glaucoma

1 Krupp, M. and Chatton, M., *Current Medical Diagnosis and Treatment*, Lange Medical Publications, Los Altos, CA, 1982, pp. 77–84.

2 Tengroth, B. and Ammitzboll, T., 'Changes in the content and composition of collagen in the glaucomatous eye – basis for a new hypothesis for the genesis of chronic open-angle glaucoma', *Acta Ophthalmol.*, 1984, 62, pp. 999–1,008.

3 Weiss, J. and Jayson, M., *Collagen in Health and Disease*, Churchill Livingstone, New York, NY, 1982, pp. 388–403.

4 Quigley, H. and Addicks, E., 'Regional differences in the structure of the lamina cribosa and their relation to glaucomatous optic nerve damage', *Arch. Ophthalmol.*, 1983, 99, pp. 137–43.

5 Krakau, T., Bengston, B. and Holmin, C., 'The glaucoma theory updated', *Acta Ophthalmol.*, 1983, 61, pp. 737–41.

6 Rohen, J., 'Why is intraocular pressure elevated in chronic simple glaucoma?', *Ophthalmology*, 1983, 90, pp. 758–65.

7 Bietti, G., 'Further contributions on the value of osmotic substances as means to reduce intraocular pressure', *Trans. Ophthalmol. Soc. UK*, 1966, 86, pp. 247–54.

8 Fishbein, S. and Goodstein, S., 'The pressure lowering effect of ascorbic acid', *Ann. Ophthalmol.*, 1972, 4, pp. 487–91.

9 Linner, E., 'The pressure lowering effect of ascorbic acid in ocular hypertension', *Acta Ophthalmol.*, 1969, 47, pp. 685–9.

10 Shen, T. and Yu, M., 'Clinical evaluation of glycerin-sodium ascorbate solution in lowering intraocular pressure', *Chinese Med. J.*, 1975, 1, pp. 64–8.

11 Virno, M., Bucci, M., Pecori-Giraldi, J. and Missiroli, A., 'Oral treatment of glaucoma with vitamin C', *Eye Ear Nose Throat Monthly*, 1967, 46, pp. 1,502–8.

12 Gabor, M., 'Pharmacologic effects of flavonoids on blood vessels', *Angiologica*, 1972, 9, pp. 355–74.

13 Monboisse, J., Braquet, P. and Borel, J., 'Oxygen-free radicals as mediators of collagen breakage', *Agents Actions*, 1984, 15, pp. 49–50.

14 Hagerman, A. and Butler, L., 'The specificity of proanthocyanidin-protein interactions', *J. Biol. Chem.*, 1981, 250, pp. 4,494–7.

15 Bever, B. and Zahnd, G., 'Plants with oral hypoglycemic action', *Quart. J. Crude Drug Res.*, 1979, 17, pp. 139–96.

16 Stocker, F., 'New ways of influencing the intraocular pressure', *N.Y. St. J. Med.*, 1949, 49, pp. 58–63.

17 Raymond, A.F., 'Allergy and chronic simple glaucoma', *Ann. Allergy*, 1964, 22, pp. 146–50.

41 Gout

1 Robbins, S.L., Cotran, R.S. and Kumar, V., *Pathologic Basis of Disease*, W.B. Saunders, Philadelphia, PA, 1984, pp. 1,356–61.

2 Petersdorf, R., *et al.* (eds), *Harrison's Principles of Internal Medicine*, McGraw-Hill, New York, NY, 1983, pp. 517–24.

3 Rubenstein, E. and Federman, D.D., *Scientific American Medicine*, Scientific American, New York, NY, 1986, pp. 9:IV-1-5, 15:IX-1-11.

4 Krupp, M.A. and Chatton, M.J., *Current Medical Diagnosis and Treatment*, Lange Medical Publications, Los Altos, CA, 1984, pp. 519–22.

5 Wyngaarden, J.B. and Kelly, W.N., 'Gout', in Stanbury, J.B., Wyngaarden, J.B. and Fredrickson, D.S. (eds), *The Metabolic Basis of Inherited Disease*, McGraw-Hill, New York, NY, 1978, pp. 918, 920.

6 Krause, M.V. and Mahan, L.K., *Food, Nutrition, and Diet Therapy*, 7th ed., W.B. Saunders, Philadelphia, PA, 1984, pp. 677–9.

7 Nutrition Foundation, *Present Knowledge in Nutrition*, 5th ed., Nutrition Foundation, Washington DC, 1984, pp. 740–56.

8 Ball, G.V. and Sorensen, L.B., 'Pathogenesis of hyperuricemia in saturnine gout', *N.E.J.M.*, 1969, 280, pp. 1,199–202.

9 Appelboom, T. and Bennett, J.C., 'Gout of the rich and famous', *J. Rheumatol.*, 1986, 13, pp. 618–22.

10 Faller, J. and Fox, I.H., 'Ethanol-induced hyperuricemia', *N.E.J.M.*, 1982, 30, pp. 1,598–602.

11 Scott, J.T., 'Obesity and hyperuricaemia', *Clin. Rheum. Dis.*, 1977, 3, pp. 25–35.

12 Emmerson, B.T., 'Effect of oral fructose on urate production', *Ann. Rheum. Dis.*, 1974, 33, pp. 276–9.

13 Loffler, W., Grobner, W. and Zollner, N., 'Influence of dietary protein on serum and urinary uric acid', *Adv. Exp. Med. Biol.*, 1980, 122A, pp. 209–13.

14 Terano, T., Salmon, J.A., Higgs, G.A. and Moncada, S., 'Eicosapentaenoic acid as a modulator of inflammation, effect on prostaglandin and leukotriene synthesis', *Biochem. Pharmacol.*, 1986, 35, pp. 779–85.

15 Ford-Hutchinson, A.W., 'Leukotrienes: their formation and role as inflammatory mediators', *Fed. Proc.*, 1985, 44, pp. 25–9.

16 Panganamala, R.V. and Cornwell, D.G., 'The effects of vitamin E on arachidonic acid metabolism', *Ann. N.Y. Acad. Sci.*, 1982, 393, pp. 376–91.

17 Lewis, A.S., Murphy, L., McCalla, C., *et al.*, 'Inhibition of mammalian xanthine oxidase by folate compounds and amethopterin', *J. Biol. Chem.*, 1984, 259, pp. 12–15.

18   Spector, T. and Ferone, R., 'Folic acid does not activate xanthine oxidase', *J. Biol. Chem.*, 1984, 259, pp. 10,784–6.
19   Oster, K.A., 'Xanthine oxidase and folic acid', *Ann. Int. Med.*, 1977, 87, p. 252.
20   Taussig, S., Yokoyama, M., Chinen, A., *et al.*, 'Bromelain, a proteolytic enzyme and its clinical application. A review', *Hiroshima J. Med. Sci.*, 1975, 24, pp. 185–93.
21   Bindoli, A., Valente, M. and Cavallini, L., 'Inhibitory action of quercetin on xanthine oxidase and xanthine dehydrogenase activity', *Pharm. Res. Comm.*, 1985, 17, pp. 831–9.
22   Busse, W.W., Kopp, D.E. and Middleton, E., 'Flavonoid modulation of human neutrophil function', *J. Allergy Clin. Immunol.*, 1984, 73, pp. 801–9.
23   Yoshimoto, T., Furukawa, M., Yamamoto, S., *et al.* 'Flavonoids: potent inhibitors of arachidonate 5-lipoxygenase', *Biochem. Biophys. Res. Comm.*, 1983, 116, pp. 612–18.
24   Leuti, M. and Vignali, M., 'Influence of bromelain on penetration of antibiotics in uterus, salpinx and ovary', *Drugs Under Exp. Clin. Res.*, 1978, 4, pp. 45–8.
25   Stein, H.B., Hasan, A. and Fox, I.H., 'Ascorbic acid-induced uricosuria: a consequence of megavitamin therapy', *Ann. Int. Med.*, 1976, 84, pp. 385–8.
26   Gershon, S.L. and Fox, I.H., 'Pharmacological effects of nicotinic acid on human purine metabolism', *J. Lab. Clin. Med.*, 1974, 84, pp. 179–86.
27   Blau, L.W., 'Cherry diet control for gout and arthritis', *Texas Rep. Biol. Med.*, 1950, 8, pp. 309–11.
28   Gabor, M., 'Pharmacologic effects of flavonoids on blood vessels', *Angiologica*, 1972, 9, pp. 355–74.
29   Kuhnau, J., 'The flavonoids. A class of semi-essential food components: their role in human nutrition', *World Rev. Nutr. Diet*, 1976, 24, pp. 117–19.
30   Havsteen, B., 'Flavonoids, a class of natural products of high pharmacological potency', *Biochem. Pharm.*, 1983, 32, pp. 1,141–8.
31   Middleton, E., 'The flavonoids', *Trends Pharm. Sci.*, 1984, 5, pp. 335–8.
32   Brady, L.R., Tyler, V.E. and Robbers, J.E., *Pharmacognosy*, 8th ed., Lea & Febiger, Philadelphia, PA, 1981, p. 480.
33   Duke, J.A., *Handbook of Medicinal Herbs*, CRC Press, Boca Raton, FL, 1985, p. 222.
34   Whitehouse, L.W., Znamirowski, M. and Paul, C.J., 'Devil's claw (Harpagophytum procumbens): no evidence for anti-inflammatory activity in the treatment of arthritic disease', *Can. Med. Assoc. J.*, 1983, 129, pp. 249–51.
35   McLeod, D.W., Revell, P. and Robinson, B.V., 'Investigations of Harpagophytum procumbens (Devil's claw) in the treatment of experimental inflammation and arthritis in the rat', *Br. J. Pharmacol.*, 1979, 66, pp. 140P–141P.

42 Haemorrhoids

1   Robbins, S.L., Cotran, R.S. and Kumar, V., *Pathologic Basis of Disease*, W.B. Saunders, Philadelphia, PA, 1984, pp. 836–41, 859–62.
2   Berkow, R. (ed.), *The Merck Manual of Diagnosis and Therapy*, 14th ed., Merck & Co., Rahway, NJ, 1982, pp. 560–6.
3   Trowell, H., Burkitt, D. and Heaton, K., *Dietary Fibre, Fibre-Depleted Foods and Disease*, Academic Press, London, UK, 1985.
4   Moesgaard, F., Nielsen, M.L., Hansen, J.B. and Knudsen, J.T., 'High-fiber diet reduces bleeding and pain in patients with hemorrhoids', *Dis. Colon Rectum*, 1982, 25, pp. 454–6.
5   Webster, D.J., Gough, D.C. and Craven, J.L., 'The use of bulk evacuation in patients with haemorrhoids', *Br. J. Surg.*, 1978, 65, pp. 291–2.
6   Norman, D.A., Newton, R. and Nicholas, G.V., 'Management of hemorrhoidal disease: an effective, safe and painless outpatient approach utilizing D.C. current', *Am. J. Gastroenterol*, 1989, 84, pp. 482–7.
7   Keesey, W.E., 'Obliteration of hemorrhoids with negative galvanism', *Arch. Phys. Ther., X-ray, and Radium*, 1934, September.

43 Heavy periods

1   Downing, I., Hutchon, D.J.R. and Poyser, N.L., 'Uptake of [3H]-arachidonic acid by human endometrium. Differences between normal and menorrhagic tissue, *Prostaglandins*, 1983, 26, pp. 55–69.
2   Kelly, R.W., Lumsden, M.A., Abel, M.H. and Baird, D.T., 'The relationship between menstrual blood loss and prostaglandin production in the human: evidence for increased availability of arachidonic acid in women suffering from menorrhagia', *Prostaglandins Leukotrienes Med.*, 1984, 16, pp. 69–78.
3   Arvidsson, B., Ekenved, G., Rybo, G. and Solvell, L., 'Iron prophylaxis in menorrhagia', *Acta Ob. Gyn. Scand.*, 1981, 60, pp. 157–60.
4   Taymor, M.L., Sturgis, S.H. and Yahia, C., 'The etiological role of chronic iron deficiency in production of menorrhagia', *J.A.M.A.*, 1964, 187, pp. 323–7.
5   Lithgow, D. and Politzer, W., 'Vitamin A in the treatment of menorrhagia', *S. Afr. Med. J.*, 1977, 51, pp. 191–3.
6   Cohen, J.D. and Rubin, H.W., 'Functional menorrhagia: treatment with bioflavonoids and vitamin C', *Curr. Ther. Res.*, 1960, 2, pp. 539–42.
7   Dasgupta, P.R., Dutta, S., Banerjee, P. and Majumdar, S., 'Vitamin E (alpha tocopherol) in the management of menorrhagia associated with the use of intrauterine contraceptive devices (IUCD)', *Int. J. Fertil.*, 1983, 28, pp. 55–6.
8   Gubner, R. and Ungerleider, H.E., 'Vitamin K therapy in menorrhagia', *South. Med. J.*, 1944, 37, pp. 556–8.
9   Stoffer, C.S., 'Menstrual disorders and mild thyroid insufficiency', *Postgraduate Med.*, 1982, 72, pp. 75–82.
10   Sone, K., Willis, A., Hart, M., *et al.*, 'The metabolism of di-homo-gamma-linolenic acid in man', *Lipids*, 1978, 14, pp. 174–80.
11   Schumann, E., 'Newer concepts of blood coagulation and control of hemorrhage', *Am. J. Ob. Gyn.*, 1939, 38, pp. 1,002–7.
12   Steinberg, A., Segal, H.I. and Parris, H.M., 'Role of oxalic acid and certain related dicarboxylic acids in the control of hemorrhage', *Annals Oto. Rhino. Laryngo.*, 1940, 49, pp. 1,008–21.

44 Hepatitis

1   Krupp, M.A. and Chatton, M.J., *Current Medical Diagnosis and Treatment*, Lange Medical Publishing, Los Altos, CA, 1985, pp. 404–6.

2   Branch, W.T., *Office Practice of Medicine*, W.B. Saunders, Philadelphia, PA, 1982, pp. 679–85.

3   Rubenstein, E. and Federman, D.D., *Scientific American Medicine*, Scientific American, New York, NY, 1988, pp. 4:VII:1–6.

4   Nutrition Review, *Present Knowledge in Nutrition*, The Nutrition Foundation, Washington, DC, 1984, pp. 163–7.

5   Cathcart, R.F., 'The method of determining proper doses of vitamin C for the treatment of disease by titrating to bowel tolerance', *J. Orthomol. Psychiat.*, 1981, 10, pp. 125–32.

6   Klenner, F.R., 'Observations on the dose of administration of ascorbic acid when employed beyond the range of a vitamin in human pathology', *J. Applied Nutr.*, 1971, 23, pp. 61–88.

7   Baetgen, D., 'Results of the treatment of epidemic hepatitis in children with high doses of ascorbic acid for the years 1957–1958', *Medizinische Monatschrift*, 1961, 15, pp. 30–6.

8   Baur, H. and Staub, H., 'Treatment of hepatitis with infusions of ascorbic acid: comparison with other therapies', *J.A.M.A.* 1954, 156, p. 565 (abstract).

9   Knodell, R.G., *et al.*, 'Vitamin C prophylaxis for posttransfusion hepatitis: lack of an effect in a controlled trial', *Am. J. Clin. Nutr.*, 1981, 34, p. 20.

10   Werbach, M.R., *Nutritional Influences on Illness: A Sourcebook of Clinical Research*, Third Line Press, Tarzana, CA, 1987, pp. 211–12.

11   Murata, A., 'Viricidal activity of vitamin C: vitamin C for prevention and treatment of viral diseases', in Hasegawa, T. (ed.), *Proc. First Intersectional Cong. Int. Assoc. Microbiol. Soc.*, vol 3, Tokyo University Press, 1975, pp. 432–42.

12   Cavalieri, S., 'A controlled clinical trial of Legalon in 40 patients', *Gazz, Med. Ital.*, 133, 1974, pp. 628–35.

13   Hirayama, S., Kishikawa, H., Kume, T. and Tada, H., 'Therapeutic effect of liver hydrolysate on experimental liver cirrhosis', *Nisshin Igaku*, 1978, 45, pp. 528–33.

14   Sanbe, K., Murata, T., Fujisawa, K. *et al.*, 'Treatment of liver disease – with particular reference to liver hydrolysates', *Jap. J. Clin. Exp. Med.*, 1973, 50, pp. 2,665–76.

15   Fujisawa, K., Suzuki, H., Yamamoto, S., *et al.*, 'Therapeutic effects of liver hydrolysate preparation on chronic hepatitis – a double blind, controlled study', *Asian Med. J.*, 1984, 26, pp. 497–526.

16   Conn, H. (ed.), *International Workshop on (+)-Cyanidanol-3 in Diseases of the Liver*, Royal Society of Medicine International Symposia Series no. 47, Academic Press, London, 1981.

17   Suzuki, H., *et al.*, 'Cianidanol therapy for HBe-antigen-positive chronic hepatitis: a multicentre, double-blind study', *Liver*, 1986, 6, p. 35.

18   Blum, A., Doelle, W., Kortum, K., *et al.*, 'Treatment of acute viral hepatitis with (+)-cyanidanol-3', *Lancet*, 1977, ii, pp. 1,153–5.

19   Berengo, A. and Esposito, R., 'A double-blind trial of (+)-cyanidanol-3 in viral hepatitis', in *New Trends in the Therapy of Liver Diseases*, Springer-Verlag, Basel, 1975, pp. 177–81.

20   Theodoropoulos, G., Dinos, A., Dimitriou, P. and Archimandritis, A., 'Effect of (+)-cyanidanol-3 in acute viral hepatitis', in Conn, H. (ed.), *Int. Workshop on (+)-Cyanidanol-3 in Diseases of the Liver*, Royal Society of Medicine International Symposia Series, no. 47, Academic Press, London, 1981, pp. 89–91.

21   Demeulenaere, F., Desmet, V., Dupont, E., *et al.*, 'Study of (+)-cyanidanol-3 in chronic active hepatitis. Results of a controlled multicentre study', in Conn, H, (ed.), *Int. Workshop on (+)-Cyanidanol-3 in Diseases of the Liver*, Royal Society of Medicine International Symposia Series no. 47, Academic Press, London 1981, pp. 135–41.

22   Piazza, M., Guadagnino, V., Picciotto, L., *et al.*, 'Effect of (+)-cyanidanol-3 in acute HAV, HBV, and non-A, non-B viral hepatitis', *Hepatology*, 1983, 3, pp. 45–9.

23   Schomerus, H., Wieman, K., Dolle, W., *et al.*, (+)-cyanidanol-3 in the treatment of acute viral hepatitis: a randomized controlled trial', *Hepatology*, 1984, 4, pp. 331–5.

24   Abonyi, M., Kisfaludy, S. and Szalay, F., 'Therapeutic effect of (+)-cyanidanol-3 in toxic alcoholic liver disease and in chronic active hepatitis', *Acta Physiol. Hung.*, 1984, 64, pp. 455–60.

25   Par, A., Horvath, T., Bero, T., *et al.*, 'Inhibition of hepatic drug metabolism by (+)-cyanidanol-3 (catergen) in chronic alcoholic liver disease', *Acta Physiol. Hung.*, 1984, 64, pp. 449–54.

26   Mowrey, D.B., *The Scientific Validation of Herbal Medicine*, Cormorant Books, Lehi, UT, 1986.

27   Faber, K., 'The dandelion – Taraxacum officinale Weber', *Pharmazie*, 1958, 13, pp. 423–35.

28   Wagner, H., 'Plant constituents with antihepatotoxic activity', in Beal, J.L. and Reinhard, E. (eds), *Natural Products as Medicinal Agents*, Hippokrates-Verlag, Stuttgart, 1981.

29   Maros, T., Racz, G., Katonaj, B. and Kovacs, V., 'The effects of Cynara scolymus extracts on the regeneration of the rat liver', *Arzneim-Forsch.*, 1966, 16, pp. 127–9 (1st communication); 1968, 18, pp. 884–6.

30   Schopen, R.D., Lange, O.K., Panne, C. and Kirnberger, E.J., 'Searching for a new therapeutic principle. Experience with hepatic therapeutic agent legalon', *Med. Welt.*, 1969, 20, pp. 888–93.

31   Schopen, R.D. and Lange, O.K., 'Therapy of hepatoses. Therapeutic use of silymarin', *Med. Welt.*, 1970, 21, pp. 691–8.

32   Sarre, H., 'Experience in the treatment of chronic hepatopathies with silymarin', *Arzneim-Forsch.*, 1971, 21, pp. 1,209–12.

33   Canini, F., Bartolucci, A., Cristallini, E., *et al.*, 'Use of silymarin in the treatment of alcoholic hepatic steatosis', *Clin. Ter.*, 1985, 114, pp. 307–14.

34   Salmi, H.A. and Sarna, S., 'Effect of silymarin on chemical, functional, and morphological alteration of the liver. A double-blind controlled study', *Scand. J. Gastroenterol.*, 1982, 17, pp. 417–21.

35   Boari, C., Montanari, M., Galleti, G.P., *et al.*, 'Occupational toxic liver diseases. Therapeutic effects of silymarin', *Min. Med.*, 1981, 72, pp. 2,679–88.

36   Bulfoni, A. and Gobbato, F., 'Evaluation of the therapeutic activity of silymarin in alcoholic hepatology', *Gazz. Med. Ital.*, 1979, 138, pp. 597–608.

37   Saba, P., Galeone, G.F., Salvadorini, F., Guarguaglini, M. and Troyer, C., 'Therapeutic effects of silymarin in chronic liver diseases due to psychodrugs', *Gazz. Med. Ital.*, 1976, 135, pp. 236–51.

38   De Martis, M., Fontana, M., Sebastiani, F. and Parenzi, A., 'La silymaina, farmaco membranotropo: ossevazioni cliniche e sperimentali', *Cl. Terap.*, 1977, 81, pp. 333–62.

39   Suzuki, H., Ohta, Y., Takino, T., Fujisawa, K., *et al.*, 'Effects of glycyrrhizin on biochemical tests in patients with chronic hepatitis – double blind trial', *Asian Med. J.*, 1984, 26, pp. 423–38.

40   Abe, N., Ebina, T. and Ishida, N., 'Interferon induction by glycyrrhizin and glycyrrhetinic acid in mice', *Microbial Immunol.*, 1982, 26, pp. 535–9.

41   Pompeii, R., Pani, A., Flore, O., Marcialis, M. and Loddo, B., 'Antiviral activity of glycyrrhizic acid', *Experientia*, 1980, 36, pp. 304–5.

45 Herpes simplex

1   Rubenstein, E. and Federman, D.D., *Scientific American Medicine*, Scientific American, New York, NY, 1988, pp. 7:XXVI-1-9.

2   Reinhardt, A., Auperin, D. and Sands, J., 'Mechanism of virucidal activity of retinoids: protein removal from bacteriophage envelope', *Antimicrobial Agents Chemother.*, 1980, 17, pp. 1,034–7.

3   Demetriou, A., Franco, I., Bark, S., *et al.*, 'Effects of vitamin A and beta carotene on intra-abdominal sepsis', *Arch. Surg.*, 1984, 119, pp. 161–5.

4   Rhodes, J., 'Human interferon action: reciprocal regulation by retinoic acid and B-carotene', *J.N.C.I.*, 1983, 70, pp. 833–7.

5   Alexander, M., Newmark, H. and Miller, R., 'Oral beta-carotene can increase the number of OKT4+ cells in human blood', *Immunology Letters*, 1985, 9, pp. 221–4.

6   Fitzherbert, J., 'Genital herpes and zinc', *Med. J. Aust.*, 1979, 1, p. 399.

7   Terezhealmy, G., Bottomley, W. and Pellu, G., 'The use of water-soluble bioflavonoid-ascorbic acid complex in the treatment of recurrent herpes labialis', *Oral Surg.*, 1978, 45, pp. 56–62.

8   Brody, I., 'Tropical treatment of recurrent herpes simplex and post-herpetic erythema multiforme with low concentrations of zinc sulphate solution', *Br. J. Dermatol.*, 1981, 104, pp. 191–213.

9   Gibney, M., 'The effect of dietary lysine to arginine ratio on cholesterol kinetics in rabbits', *Athero.*, 1983, 47, pp. 263–70.

10   Nead, D.E., 'Effective vitamin E treatment for ulcerative herpetic lesions', *Dent. Surv.*, 1976, 52, pp. 50–1.

11   Steele, R., Vincent, M., Hensen, S., *et al.*, 'Cellular immune response to herpes simplex type 1 virus in recurrent herpes labialis: in vitro blastogenesis and cytotoxicity to infected cell lines', *J. Inf. Dis.*, 131, 1975, pp. 528–34.

12   Aiuti, F., Sirianni, M., Stella, A., *et al.*, 'A placebo-controlled trial of thymic hormone treatment of recurrent herpes simplex labialis infection in immunodeficient hosts', *Int. J. Clin. Pharm. Ther. Tox.*, 1983, 21, pp. 81–6.

13   Lieb, J., 'Remission of recurrent herpes infection during therapy with lithium' (letter), *N.E.J.M.*, 1979, 301, p. 942.

14   Skinner, G., Hartley, C., Bucham, A., *et al.*, 'The effect of lithium chloride on the replication of Herpes simplex virus', *Med. Microbiol. Immunol.*, 1980, 168, pp. 139–48.

15   Griffith, R., DeLong, D. and Nelson, J., 'Relation of arginine-lysine antagonism to herpes simplex growth in tissue culture', *Chemotherapy*, 1981, 27, pp. 209–13.

16   DiGiovanna, J. and Blank, H., 'Failure of lysine in frequently recurrent herpes simplex infection', *Arch. Dermatol.*, 1984, 120, pp. 48–51.

17   Griffith, R., Norins, A. and Kagan, C., 'A multicentered study of lysine therapy in herpes simplex infection', *Dermatol.*, 1978, 156, pp. 257–67.

18   Leszczynski, D. and Kummerow, F., 'Excess dietary lysine induces hypercholesterolemia in chickens', *Experientia*, 1982, 38, pp. 266–7.

19   Pizzorno, J.E. and Murray, M.T., *A Textbook of Natural Medicine*, John Bastyr College Publications, Seattle, WA, 1985, p. IV:ImmSup-2,3.

20   Pompeii, R., Pani, A., Flore, O., *et al.*, 'Antiviral activity of glycyrrhizic acid', *Experientia*, 1980, 36, p. 304.

46 Hives

1   Czarnetzki, B.M., *Urticaria*, Springer-Verlag, New York, NY, 1986.

2   Mathews, K.P., 'A current view of urticaria', *Med. Clin. North Am.*, 1974, 58, pp. 185–205.

3   Keahey, T.M., 'The pathogenesis of urticaria', *Derm. Clin.*, 1985, 3, pp. 13–28.

4   Winkelmann, R.K., 'Food sensitivity and urticaria or vasculitis', in Brostoff, J. and Challacombe, S.J. (eds), *Food Allergy and Intolerance*, W.B. Saunders, Philadelphia, PA, 1987, pp. 602–17.

5   Ormerod, A.D., Reid, T.M.S. and Main. R.A., 'Penicillin in milk – its importance in urticaria', *Clin. Allergy*, 1987, 17, pp. 229–34.

6   Wicher, K. and Reisman, R.E., 'Anaphylactic reaction to penicillin in a soft drink', *J. Allergy Clin. Immunol.*, 1980, 66, pp. 155–7.

7   Schwartz, H.J. and Sher, T.H., 'Anaphylaxis to penicillin in a frozen dinner', *Ann. Allergy*, 1984, 52, pp. 342–3.

8   Boonk, W.J. and Van Ketel, W.G., 'The role of penicillin in the pathogenesis of chronic urticaria', *Br. J. Derm.*, 1982, 106, pp. 183–90.

9   Lindemayr, H., Knobler, R., Kraft, D. and Baumgartner, G., 'Challenge of penicillin allergic volunteers with penicillin contaminated meat', *Allergy*, 1981, 36, pp. 471–8.

10   Settipane, R.A., Constatine, H.P. and Settipane, G.A., 'Aspirin intolerance and recurrent urticaria in adults', *Allergy*, 1980, 35, pp. 149–54.

11   Genton, C., Frei, P.C. and Pecoud, A., 'Value of oral provocation tests to aspirin and food additives in the routine investigation of asthma and chronic urticaria', *J. Allergy Clin. Immunol.*, 1985, 76, pp. 40–5.

12   Bjarnason, I., Williams, P., Smethurst, P., *et al.*, 'Effect of non-steroidal anti-inflammatory drugs and prostaglandins on the permeability of the human small intestine', *Gut*, 1986, 27, pp. 1,292–7.

13   Asad, S.I., Youlten, L.J.F. and Lessof, M.H., 'Specific desensitisation in aspirin sensitive urticaria', *Clin. Allergy*, 1983, 13, pp. 459–66.

14   Kowalski, M.L., Grzelewski-Ryzmowski, I., Roznieki, J. and Szmidt, M., 'Aspirin-induced tolerance in aspirin sensitive asthmatics', *Allergy*, 1984, 39, pp. 171–8.

15   Atkins, F.M., 'The basis of immediate hypersensitivity reactions to foods', *Nutrition Rev.*, 1983, 41, pp. 229–34.

16   Wraith, D.G., Merrett, J., Roth, A., *et al.*, 'Recognition of food allergic patients and their allergens by the RAST technique and clinical investigation', *Clin. Allergy*, 1975, 9, pp. 25–36.

17   Golbert, T.M., Patterson, R. and Pruzansky, J.J., 'Systemic reactions to ingested antigens', *J. Allergy*, 1969, 44, pp. 96–107.

18   Galant, S.P., Bullock, J. and Frick, O.L., 'An immunological approach to the diagnosis of food sensitivity', *Clin. Allergy*, 1973, 3, pp. 363–72.

19   Pachor, M.L., Andri, L., Nicolis, F., *et al.*, 'Elimination diet and challenge test in diagnosis of food intolerance', *Italian J. Med.*, 1986, 2, pp. 1–6.

20 Rawls, W.B. and Ancona, V.C., 'Chronic urticaria associated with hypochlorhydria or achlorhydria', *Rev. Gastroenterol.*, 1951, 18, pp. 267–71.
21 Baird, P.C., 'Etiology and treatment of urticaria: diagnosis, prevention and treatment of poison-ivy dermatitis', *N.E.J.M.*, 1941, 224, pp. 649–58.
22 Allison, J.R., 'The relation of hydrochloric acid and vitamin B complex deficiency in certain skin diseases', *Southern Med. J.*, 1945, 38, pp. 235–41.
23 Gloor, M., Henkel, K. and Schulz, U., 'Zur pathogenetischen bedeutung von magenfunktionsstoringen bie allergish bedingter chronischer urtikaria', *Derm. Msch.*, 1972, 158, pp. 96–102.
24 Husz, S., Berko, G., Szabo, R. and Simon, N., 'Immunoelectrophoresis in the dermatologic practice. III. Dysproteinemias (chronic urticaria, drug allergy)', *Derm. Msch.*, 1974, 160, pp. 93–100.
25 Lockey, S.D., 'Allergic reactions to F D & C yellow No. 5, tartrazine, an aniline dye used as a coloring and identifying agent in various steroids', *Ann. Allergy*, 1959, 17, pp. 719–21.
26 Collins-Williams, C., 'Clinical spectrum of adverse reactions to tartrazine', *J. Asthma*, 1985, 22, pp. 139–43.
27 Warrington, R.J., Sauder, P.J. and McPhillips, S., 'Cell-mediated immune responses to artificial food additives in chronic urticaria', 1986, 16, pp. 527–33.
28 Natbony, S.F., Phillips, M.E., Elias, J.M., 'Histologic studies of chronic idiopathic urticaria', *J. Allergy Clin. Immunol.* 1983, 71, pp. 177–83.
29 Swain, A.R., Dutton, S.P. and Truswell, A.S., 'Salicylates in foods', *J. Am. Diet. Assoc.*, 1985, 85, pp. 950–60.
30 Kulczycki, A., 'Aspartame-induced urticaria', *Annals Int. Med.*, 1986, 104, pp. 207–8.
31 Thune, P. and Granhold, A., 'Provocation tests with anti-phlogistic and food additives in recurrent urticaria', *Dermatologica*, 1975, 151, pp. 360–72.
32 Juhlin, L., 'Recurrent urticaria: clinical investigation of 330 patients', *Br. J. Derm.*, 1981, 104, pp. 369–81.
33 Simon, R.A., 'Adverse reactions to drug additives', *J. Allergy Clin. Immunol.*, 1984, 74, pp. 623–30.
34 Ziegler, B. and Haustein, U.F., 'Intoleranzreaktionen anf nicht-steroidale antiphogistika und analgetika bei chronisch recidivierendes urtikaria', *Derm. Mschr.*, 1986, 172, pp. 313–17.
35 Moneret-Vautrin, D.A., Faure, G. and Bene, M.C., 'Chewing-gum preservative induced toxidermic vasculitis', *Allergy*, 1986, 41, pp. 546–8.
36 Yang, W.H. and Purchase, E.C.R., 'Adverse reactions to sulfites', *Can. Med. Assoc. J.*, 1985, 133, pp. 865–80.
37 Vaida, G.A., Goldman, M.A. and Bloch, K.J., 'Testing for hepatitis B virus in patients with chronic urticaria and angioedema', *J. Allergy Clin. Immunol.*, 1983, 72, pp. 193–8.
38 Warin, R.P. and Smith, R.J., 'Challenge test battery in chronic urticaria', *Br. J. Derm.*, 1976, 94, pp. 401–10.
39 Schade, C., Kuben, U. and Westphal, H.J., 'Incidence of yeasts and therapeutic results in chronic urticaria', *Derm. Msch.*, 1975, 161, pp. 187–95.
40 Holti, G., 'Management of pruritis and urticaria', *Br. Med. J.*, 1967, I, pp. 155–8.
41 Serrano, H., 'Hypersensitivity to candida albicans and other yeasts in patients with chronic urticaria', *Allergol. Immunopathol.*, 1975, 3, pp. 289–98.
42 James, J. and Warin, R.P., 'An assessment of the role of candida albicans and food yeast in chronic urticaria', *Br. J. Derm.*, 1971, 84, pp. 227–37.
43 Rives, H., Pellerat, J. and Thivolet, J., 'Urticaria chronique et oedeme de quincke', *Dermatologica*, 1972, 144, pp. 193–204.
44 Vivarelli, I. and Mancosu, A., 'Rilievi su due inderizzi terapeutici nella cura dell'orticaria', *Minerva Derm.*, 1967, 42, pp. 441–2.
45 Westphal, H.J., Schade, C. and Kaben, G., 'Spezifische desensibilisierung bei patienten mit sprosspilzbedinger chronischer urtikaria und inestinaler sprosspilzbesiedlung', *Dermatol. Msch.*, 1976, 162, pp. 912–15.
46 Green, G., Koelsche, G. and Kierland, R., 'Etiology and pathogenesis of chronic urticaria', *Ann. Allergy*, 1965, 23, pp. 30–6.
47 Shertzer, C.L. and Lookingbill, D.P., 'Effects of relaxation therapy and hynotizability in chronic urticaria', *Arch. Derm.*, 1987, 123, pp. 913–16.
48 Hannuksela, M. and Kokkonen, E.L., 'Ultraviolet light therapy in chronic urticaria', *Acta Derm. Venereol.*, 1985, 65, pp. 449–50.
49 Olafsson, J.H., Larko, O., Roupe, G., *et al.*, 'Treatment of chronic urticaria with PUVA or UVA plus placebo: a double-blind study', *Arch. Derm. Res.*, 1986, 278, pp. 228–31.
50 Simon, S.W., 'Vitamin B_{12} therapy in allergy and chronic dermatoses', *J. Allergy*, 1951, 22, pp. 183–5.
51 Simon, S.W. and Edmonds, P., 'Cyanocobalamin (B_{12}): comparison of aqueous and repository preparations in urticaria; possible mode of action', *J. Am. Geriatr. Soc.*, 1964, 12, pp. 79–85.

47 Hyperactivity and learning disorders

1 Kaplan, H. and Sadock, B., *Modern Synopsis of Comprehensive Textbook of Psychiatry*, vol. IV, Williams & Wilkins, Baltimore, MD, 1985.
2 Feingold, N., *Why Your Child is Hyperactive*, Random House, New York, NY, 1975.
3 Conners, C., Goyette, C., Southwick, D., Lees, J. and Andrulonis, P., 'Food additives and hyperkinesis: a double-blind experiment', *Pediatrics*, 1976, 58, pp. 154–66.
4 Goyette, C., Conners, C., Petti, T. and Curtis, L., 'Effects of artificial colors on hyperkinetic children: a double-blind challenge study', *Psychopharmacol. Bull.*, 1978, 14, pp. 39–40.
5 Conners, C., *Food Additives and Hyperactive Children*, Plenum Press, New York, NY, 1980.
6 Harley, J., Ray, R., Tomasi, L., *et al.*, 'Hyperkinesis and food additives: testing the Feingold hypothesis', *Pediatrics*, 1978, 61, pp. 811–17.
7 Rowe, K., Hopkins, I. and Lynch, B., 'Artificial food colourings and hyperkinesis', *Aust. Paediatr. J.*, 1979, 15, p. 202.
8 Levy, F., Dumbrell, S., Hobbes, G., *et al.*, 'Hyperkinesis and diet: a double-blind crossover trial with tartrazine challenge', *Med. J. Aust.*, 1978, 1, pp. 61–4.
9 Rowe, K., 'Food additives', *Aust. Paediatr. J.*, 1984, 20, pp. 171–4.
10 Schauss, A., 'Nutrition and behavior: complex interdisciplinary research', *Nutr. Health*, 1984, 3, pp. 9–37.
11 Rippere, V., 'Food additives and hyperactive children: a critique of Conners', *Br. J. Clin. Psych.*, 1983, 22, pp. 19–32.
12 Swanson, J. and Kinsbourne, M., 'Food dyes impair performance of children on a laboratory learning task', *Science*, 1980, 207, pp. 1,485–7.
13 Weiss, B., Williams, J., Margen, S., *et al.*, 'Behavioral responses to artificial food colours', *Science*, 1980, 207, pp. 1,487–9.

14 Weiss, B., 'Food additives and environmental chemicals as sources of childhood behavior disorders', *J. Am. Acad. Child Psychiatry*, 1982, 21, pp. 144–52.

15 Rimland, B., 'The Feingold diet: an assessment of the reviews by Mattes, by Kavale and Forness and others', *J. Learn. Disabil.*, 1983, 16, pp. 331–3.

16 Lipton, M. and Mayo, J., 'Diet and hyperkinesis – an update', *J. Am. Diet. Assoc.*, 1983, 83, pp. 132–4.

17 Anonymous, 'Defined diets and childhood hyperactivity. Consensus conference: Office for Medical Applications of Research, National Institutes of Health', *J.A.M.A.*, 1982, 248, pp. 290–2.

18 Mayron, L., Ott, J., Nations, R. and Mayron, E., 'Light, radiation and academic behavior', *Academic Therapy*, 1974, 10, pp. 33–47.

19 Cook, P. and Woodhill, J., 'The Feingold dietary treatment of the hyperkinetic syndrome', *Med. J. Aust.*, 1976, 2, pp. 85–90.

20 Salzman, L., 'Allergy testing, psychological assessment and dietary treatment of the hyperactive child syndrome', *Med. J. Aust.*, 1976, 2, pp. 248–51.

21 Mattes, J., 'The Feingold diet: a current reappraisal', *J. Learn. Disabil.*, 1983, 16, pp. 319–23.

22 Noonan, J. and Meggos, H., 'Synthetic food colors', in Furia, T. (ed.), *CRC Handbook of Food Additives*, vol. 2, CRC Press, Boca Raton, FL, 1980, pp. 339–83.

23 Prinz, R., Roberts, W. and Hantman, E., 'Dietary correlates of hyperactive behavior in children', *J. Consult. Clin. Psych.*, 1980, 48, pp. 760–9.

24 Langseth, L. and Dowd, J., 'Glucose tolerance and hyperkinesis', *Food Cosmet. Toxicol.*, 1978, 16, pp. 129–33.

25 Sanders, L., Hofeldt, F., Kirk, M. and Levin, J., 'Refined carbohydrate as a contributing factor in reactive hypoglycemia', *Southern Med. J.*, 1982, 75, pp. 1,972–5.

26 Egger, J., Carter, C., Graham, P., Gumley, D. and Soothill, J., 'Controlled trial of oligoantigenic treatment in the hyperkinetic syndrome', *Lancet*, 1985, i, pp. 540–5.

27 O'Shea, J. and Porter, S., 'Double-blind study of children with hyperkinetic syndrome treated with multi-allergen extract sublingually', *J. Learn. Disabil.*, 1981, 14, pp. 189–91.

28 Rapp, D., 'Food allergy treatment for hyperkinesis', *J. Learn. Disabil.*, 1979, 12, pp. 42–50

29 King, D., 'Can allergic exposure provoke psychological symptoms? A double-blind test', *Biol. Psychol.*, 1981, 16, pp. 3–19.

30 David, O., Clark, J. and Voeller, K., 'Lead and hyperactivity', *Lancet*, 1972, ii, pp. 900–3.

31 David, O., Hoffman, S. and Sverd, J., 'Lead and hyperactivity. Behavioral response to chelation: a pilot study', *Am. J. Psychiatry*, 1976, 133, pp. 1,155–88.

32 Reichman, J. and Healey, W., 'Learning disabilities and conductive hearing loss involving otitis media', *J. Learn. Disabil.*, 1983, 16, pp. 272–8.

33 Silva, P., Kirkland, C., Simpson, A., Stewart, I. and Williams, S., 'Some developmental and behavioral problems with bilateral otitis media with effusion', *J. Learn. Disabil.*, 1982, 15, pp. 417–21.

34 Worthington-Roberts, B., 'Suboptimal nutrition and behavior in children', in Worthington-Roberts, B., *Contemporary Developments in Nutrition*, C.V. Mosby, St Louis, MO, 1981, pp. 524–62.

35 Krause, M. and Mahan, L., 'Nutritional care in disease of the nervous system and behavioral disorders', in Krause, M. and Mahan, L., *Food, Nutrition and Diet Therapy*, W.B. Saunders, Philadelphia, PA, 1984, pp. 654–70.

36 Tseng, R., Mellon, J. and Bammer, K., *The Relationship Between Nutrition and Student Achievement, Behavior, and Health – A Review of the Literature*, California State Department of Education, Sacramento, CA, 1980.

37 Pollitt, E. and Leibel, R., 'Iron deficiency and behavior', *J. Pediatrics*, 1976, 88, pp. 372–81.

38 Webb, T. and Oski, F., 'Iron deficiency anemia and scholastic achievement in young adolescents', *J. Pediatrics*, 1973, 82, pp. 827–30.

39 Colgan, M. and Colgan, L., 'Do nutrient supplements and dietary changes affect learning and emotional reactions of children with learning difficulties? A controlled series of 16 cases', *Nutr. Health*, 1984, 3, pp. 69–77.

40 Kerschner, J. and Hawke, W., 'Megavitamins and learning disorders: a controlled double-blind experiment', *J. Nutr.*, 1979, 109, pp. 819–26.

41 Perkins, S., 'Malnutrition: a selected review of its effects on the learning and behavior of children', *Int. J. Early Childhood*, 1977, 5, pp. 173–9.

42 Marlowe, M., Coissairt, A., Welch, K. and Errera, J., 'Hair mineral content as a predictor of learning disabilities', *J. Learn. Disabil.*, 1977, 17, pp. 418–21.

43 Pihl, R. and Parkes, M., 'Hair element content in learning disabled children', *Science*, 1977, 198, pp. 204–6.

44 Benignus, V., Otto, D., Muller, K. and Seipple, K., 'Effects of age and body lead burden on CNS function in young children. EEG spectra', *EEG and Clin. Neurophys.*, 1981, 52, pp. 240–8.

45 Rimland, B. and Larsen, G., 'Hair mineral analysis and behavior: an analysis of 51 studies', *J. Learn. Disabil.*, 1983, 16, pp. 279–85.

48 Hypertension

1 Kaplan, N.M., 'Non-drug treatment of hypertension', *Annals of Internal Medicine*, 1985, 102, pp. 359–73.

2 Miettinen, T.A., 'Multifactorial primary prevention of cardiovascular diseases in middle-aged men. Risk factor changes, incidence, and mortality', *Journal of the American Medical Association*, 1985, 254, pp. 2,097–102.

3 Multiple Risk Factor Intervention Trial Research Group, 'Baseline rest electrocardiographic abnormalities, antihypertensive treatment, and mortality in the Multiple Risk Factor Intervention Trial', *American Journal of Cardiology*, 1985, 55, pp. 1–15.

4 Meneely, G. and Battarbee, H., 'High sodium–low potassium environment and hypertension', *Am. J. Card.*, 1976, 38, pp. 768–81.

5 Freis, E., 'Salt, volume and the prevention of hypertension', *Circ.*, 1976, 53, pp. 589–95.

6 Havlik, R., Hubert, H., Fabsitz, R. and Feinleib, M., 'Weight and hypertension', *Ann. Int. Med.*, 1983, 98, pp. 855–9.

7 Lang, T., Degoulet, P., Aime, F., *et al.*, 'Relationship between coffee drinking and blood pressure: analysis of 6,321 subjects in the Paris region', *Am. J. Card.*, 1983, 52, pp. 1,238–42.

8 Formann, S., Haskell, W., Vranizan, K., *et al.*, 'The association of blood pressure and dietary alcohol: difference by age, sex and estrogen use', *Am. J. Epid.*, 1983, 118, pp. 497–507.

9 Potter, J.F. and Beevers, D.G., 'Pressor effect of alcohol in hypertension', *Lancet*, 1984, i, pp. 119–21.

10 Gruchow, H.W., Sobocinski, M.S. and Barboriak, J.J., 'Alcohol, nutrient intake, and hypertension in US adults', *J.A.M.A.*, 1985, 253, pp. 1,567–70.

11 Schroeder, K.L. and Chen, M.S., 'Smokeless tobacco and blood pressure', *N.E.J.M.*, 1985, 312, p. 919.

12 Hampson, N.B., 'Smokeless is not saltless', *N.E.J.M.*, 1985, 312, pp. 919–20.

13 Bennett, A., Doll, R. and Howell, R., 'Sugar consumption and cigarette smoking', *Lancet*, 1970, i, pp. 1,011–14.

14 Kershbaum, A., Pappajohn, D., Bellet, S., *et al.*, 'Effect of smoking and nicotine on adrenocortical secretion', *J.A.M.A.*, 1968, 203, pp. 113–16.

15 Pelletier, O., 'Smoking and vitamin C levels in humans', *Am. J. Clin. Nutr.*, 1968, 21, pp. 1,254–8.

16 Beattie, A., Campbell, B., Goldberg, A. and Moore, M., 'Blood-lead and hypertension', *Lancet*, 1976, ii, pp. 1–3.

17 Pierkle, J.L., Schwartz, J., Landis, J.R. and Harlan, W.R., 'The relationship between blood lead levels and blood pressure and its cardiovascular risk implications', *Am. J. Epid.*, 1985, 121, pp. 246–58.

18 Glauser, S., Bello, C. and Gauser, E., 'Blood-cadmium levels in normotensive and untreated hypertensive humans', *Lancet*, 1976, i, pp. 717–18.

19 Ford, M., 'Biofeedback treatment for headaches, Raynaud's disease, essential hypertension, and irritable bowel syndrome: a review of the long term follow-up literature', *Biof. Self-Reg.*, 1982, 7, pp. 521–35.

20 Robertson, D., Hollister, A., Kincaid, D., *et al.*, 'Caffeine and hypertension', *A.J. Med.*, 1984, 77, pp. 54–60.

21 Khaw, K.T. and Barrett-Connor, S., 'Dietary potassium and blood pressure in a population', *Am. J. Clin. Nutr.*, 1984, 39, pp. 963–8.

22 Skrabal, F., Aubock, J. and Hortnagl, H., 'Low sodium/high potassium diet for prevention of hypertension: probable mechanisms of action', *Lancet*, 1981, ii, pp. 895–900.

23 Bertino, M., Beauchamp, G. and Engleman, K., 'Long-term reduction in dietary sodium alters the taste of salt', *Am. J. Clin. Nutr.*, 1982, 36, pp. 1,134–44.

24 Kotchen, T., Luke, R., Ott, C., *et al.*, 'Effect of chloride on renin and blood pressure responses to sodium chloride', *Ann. Int. Med.*, 1983, 98, pp. 817–22.

25 Rouse, I.L., Beilin, L.J., Mahoney, D.P., *et al.*, 'Vegetarian diet and blood pressure', *Lancet*, 1983, ii, pp. 742–3.

26 Hodges, R. and Rebello, T., 'Carbohydrates and blood pressure', *Ann. Int. Med.*, 1983, 98, pp. 838–41.

27 Henry, H.J., MacCarron, D.A., Morris, C.D. and Parrott-Garcia, M., 'Increasing calcium intake lowers blood pressure: the literature reviewed', *J. Am. Diet. Assoc.*, 1985, 85, pp. 182–5.

28 Kok, F.J., Vandenfroucke, J.P., Heide-Wessel, C. and Heide, R.M., 'Dietary sodium, calcium, and potassium, and blood pressure', *American Journal of Epidemiology*, 1986, 123, pp. 1,043–8.

29 Resnick, L.M., Sealey, J.E. and Laragh, J.H., 'Short and long-term oral calcium alters blood pressure in essential hypertension', *Federation Proceedings*, 1983, 42, p. 300.

30 Johnson, N.E., Smith, E.L. and Freudenheim, J.L., 'Effects on blood pressure of calcium supplementation of women', *American Journal of Clinical Nutrition*, 1985, 42, pp. 12–17.

31 McCarron, D.A., Henry, H.J. and Morris, C.D., 'Randomised placebo-controlled trial of oral Ca+2 in human hypertension', *Clinical Research*, 1984, 32, p. 37A.

32 Iseri, L. and French, J., 'Magnesium: nature's physiologic calcium blocker', *Am. Heart J.*, 1984, 108, pp. 188–93.

33 Resnick, L.M., Gupta, R.K. and Laragh, J.H., 'Intracellular free magnesium in erythrocytes of essential hypertension: relationship to blood pressure and serum divalent cations', *Proc. Natl Acad. Sci.*, 1984, 81, pp. 6,511–15.

34 Dyckner, T. and Wester, O., 'Effect of magnesium on blood pressure', *Br. Med. J.*, 1983, 286, pp. 1,847–9.

35 Rao, R., Rao, U. and Srikantia, S., 'Effect of polyunsaturated vegetable oils on blood pressure in essential hypertension', *Clin. Exp. Hypertension*, 1981, 3, pp. 27–38.

36 Vergroesen, A., Fleischman, A., Comberg, H., *et al.*, 'The influence of increased dietary linoleate on essential hypertension in man', *Acta Biol. Med. Germ. Band.*, 1978, 37, pp. 879–83.

37 Folkers, K., Watanabe, T. and Kaji, M., 'Critique of coenzyme Q10 in biochemical and biochemical research and in ten years of clinical research on cardiovascular disease', *J. Mol. Med.*, 1977, 2, pp. 431–60.

38 Folkers, K. and Yamamura, Y. (eds) *Biomedical and Clinical Aspects of Coenzyme Q*, vol. 4, Elsevier Science Publishers, Amsterdam, 1984.

39 Yoshioka, M., Matsushita, T. and Chuman, Y., 'Inverse association of serum ascorbic acid level and blood pressure on rate of hypertension in male adults aged 30–39 years', *Int. J. Vit. Nutr. Res.*, 1984, 54, pp. 343–7.

40 Shroeder, H. and Buchman, J., 'Cadmium hypertension', *Arch. Environ. H.*, 1967, 14, pp. 693–7.

41 Grollman, A., Williams, J.R. and Harrison, T.R., 'Reduction of elevated blood pressure by administration of renal extracts', *J.A.M.A.*, 1940, 115, pp. 1,169–76.

42 Petkov, V., 'Plants with hypotensive, antiatheromatous and coronary dilating action', *A.J. Chinese Med.*, 1979, 7, pp. 197–236.

43 Lau, B.H., Adetumbi, M.A. and Sanchez, A., 'Allium sativum (garlic) and atherosclerosis: a review', *Nutrition Research*, 1983, 3, pp. 119–28.

44 Foushee, D., Ruffin, J. and Banerjee, U., 'Garlic as a natural agent for the treatment of hypertension: a preliminary report', *Cytobios*, 1982, 34, pp. 145–52.

45 Ogawa, M., Takahara, A., Ishijima, M. and Tazaki, S., 'Decrease of plasma sulphur amino acids in essential hypertension', *Japanese Circulation Journal*, 1985, 49, pp. 1,217–24.

46 Ammon, H.P.T. and Handel, M., 'Crataegus, toxicology and pharmacology', *Planta Medica*, 1981, 43, pp. 318–22.

49 Hypothyroidism

1 Petersdorf, R., *et al.* (eds), *Harrison's Principles of Internal Medicine*, McGraw-Hill, New York, NY, 1983, pp. 614–23.

2 Mazzaferri, E.L., 'Adult hypothyroidism', *Postgraduate Medicine*, 1986, 79, pp. 64–72.

3 Barnes, B.O. and Galton, L., *Hypothyroidism: The Unsuspected Illness*, Thomas Crowell, New York, NY, 1976.

4 Langer, S.E. and Scheer, J.F., *Solved: The Riddle of Illness*, Keats, New Canaan, CT, 1984.

5 Gold, M., Pottash, A. and Extein, I., 'Hypothyroidism and depression, evidence from complete thyroid function evaluation', *J.A.M.A.*, 1981, 245, pp. 1,919–22.

6 Drinka, P.J. and Nolten, W.E., 'Review: subclinical hypothyroidism in the elderly: to treat or not to treat?', *Am. J. Med. Sci.*, 1988, 295, pp. 125–8.

7 Banovac, K., Zakarija, M. and McKenzie, J.M., 'Experience with routine thyroid function testing: abnormal results in "normal" populations', *J. Florida Med. Assoc.*, 1985, 72, pp. 835–9.

8   Rosenthal, M.J., Hunt, W.C., Garry, P.J. and Goodwin, J.S., 'Thyroid failure in the elderly: microsomal antibodies as discriminate for therapy', *J.A.M.A.*, 1987, 258, pp. 209–13.
9   Althaus, U., Staub, J.J., Ryff-De Leche, A., *et al.*, 'LDL/HDL-changes in subclinical hypothyroidism: possible risk factors for coronary heart disease', *Clinical Endocrinology*, 1988, 28, pp. 157–63.
10   Dean, J.W. and Fowler, P.B.S., 'Exaggerated responsiveness to thyrotrophin releasing hormone: a risk factor in women with artery disease', *Brit. Med. J.*, 1985, 290, pp. 1,555–61.
11   Turnbridge, W.M.G., Evered, D.C. and Hall, R., 'Lipid profiles and cardiovascular disease in the Wickham area with particular reference to thyroid failure', *Clin. Endocrinol.*, 1977, 7, pp. 495–508.
12   Joffe, R, Roy-Byrne, P. and Udhe, T., 'Thyroid function and affective illness: a reappraisal', *Biol. Psychiatry*, 1984, 19, pp. 1,685–91.
13   Krupsky, M., Flatau, E., Yaron, R. and Resnitzky, P., 'Musculoskeletal symptoms as a presenting sign of long-standing hypothyroidism', *Isr. J. Med. Sci.*, 1987, 23, pp. 1,110–13.
14   Hochberg, M.C., Koppes, G.M., Edwards, C.Q., *et al.*, 'Hypothyroidism presenting as a polymyositis-like syndrome', *Arthr. Rheum.*, 1976, 19, pp. 1,363–6.
15   Krause, M.V. and Mahan, L.K., *Food, Nutrition, and Diet Therapy*, 7th edition, W.B. Saunders, Philadelphia, PA, 1984, pp. 170–4.
16   Jennings, I.W., *Vitamins in Endocrine Metabolism*, C.C. Thomas, Springfield, IL, 1970.
17   Prasad, A., 'Clinical, biochemical and nutritional spectrum of zinc deficiency in human subjects: an update', *Ntr. Rev.*, 1983, 41, pp. 197–208.
18   Lennon, D., Nagle, F., Stratman, F., *et al.*, 'Diet and exercise training effects on resting metabolic rate', *Int. J. Obesity*, 1985, 9, pp. 39–47.

50 Insomnia

1   Kaplan, H. and Sadock, B., *Modern Synopsis of Comprehensive Textbook of Psychiatry*, vol. IV, Chapter 24, Williams & Wilkins, Baltimore, MD, 1985, pp. 558–74.
2   Kramer, P. 'Insomnia: importance of the differential diagnosis', *Psychosomatics*, 1982, 23, pp. 129–37.
3   Growdon, J. 'Neurotransmitters in the diet', in Wurtman, R. and Wurtman, J. (eds), *Nutrition and the Brain*, vol. 3, Raven Press, New York, NY, 1979, pp. 117–82.
4   Hartman, E. 'L-trytophan: a rational hypnotic with clinical potential', *Am.J.Psychiatry*, 134, pp. 366–70.
5   Griffiths, W., Lester, B., Coulter, J. and Williams, H., 'Tryptophan and sleep in young adults', *Psychophysiology*, 1972, 9, pp. 345–56.
6   Wyatt, R., Engelman, K., Kupffer, D., *et al.*, 'Effects of L-tryptophan (a natural sedative) on human sleep', *Lancet*, 1970, ii, pp.842–6.
7   Botez, M., Cadotte, M., Beaulieu, R. and Pichette, L., 'Neurologic disorders responsive to folic acid therapy', *Can. Med. Assoc. J.*, 1976, 115, pp. 217–23.
8   Mitchell, W., *Naturopathic Applications of the Botanical Remedies*, Mitchell, Seattle, WA, 1983, pp. 66–7.
9   Leung, A., *Encyclopedia of Common Natural Ingredients Used in Food, Drugs and Cosmetics*, John Wiley & Sons, New York, NY, 1980.
10   Embodden, W., *Narcotic Plants*, Collier Books, New York, NY, 1980.
11   *Merck Index*, 10th ed., Merck & Co., Rahway, NJ, 1983, p. 665.
12   Leathwood, P., Chauffard, F., Heck, E. and Munoz-Box, R., 'Aqueous extract of valerian root (valeriana officinalis L.) improves sleep quality in man', *Pharmacol. Biochem. Behavior.*, 1982, 17, pp. 65–71.
13   Leathwood, P.D. and Chauffard, F., 'Aqueous extract of valerian reduces latency to fall asleep in man', *Planta Medica*, 1985, 54, pp. 144–8.

51 Irritable bowel syndrome

1   Spiro, H., *Clinical Gastroenterology*, 3rd ed., Macmillan, New York, NY, 1983, pp. 713–35.
2   Chin, D., Milhorn, H. and Robbins, J., 'Irritable bowel syndrome', *J. Fam. Pract.*, 1985, 20, pp. 125–38.
3   Fielding, J., 'Detailed history and examination assist positive clinical diagnosis of the irritable bowel syndrome', *J. Clin. Gastroenterol.*, 1983, 5, pp. 495–7.
4   Cann, P., Read, N. and Holdsworth, C., 'What is the benefit of coarse wheat bran in patients with irritable bowel syndrome?', *Gut*, 1984, 25, pp. 168–73.
5   Fielding, J. and Kehoe, M., 'Different dietary fibre formulations and the irritable bowel syndrome', *Irish J. Med. Sci.*, 1984, 153, pp. 178–80.
6   Hollander, E., 'Mucous colitis due to food allergy', *Am. J. Med. Sci.*, 1927, 174, pp. 495–500.
7   Gay, L., 'Mucous colitis, complicated by colonic polyposis, relieved by allergic management', *Am. J. Dig. Dis.*, 1937, 3, pp. 326–9.
8   Jones, V., McLaughlin, P., Shorthouse, M., *et al.*, 'Food intolerance: a major factor in the pathogenesis of irritable bowel syndrome', *Lancet*, 1982, ii, pp. 1,115–18.
9   Petitpierre, M., Gumowski, P. and Girard, J., 'Irritable bowel syndrome and hypersensitivity to food', *Annals Allergy*, 1985, 54, pp. 538–40.
10   Svedlund, J., Sjodin, I., Doteval, G. and Gillberg, R., 'Upper gastrointestinal and mental symptoms in the irritable bowel syndrome', *Scand. J. Gastroenterol.*, 1985, 20, pp. 595–601.
11   Goldsmith, G. and Patterson, M., 'Irritable bowel syndrome: treatment update', *Am. Fam. Phys.*, 1985, 31, pp. 191–5.
12   Ryan, W., Kelly, M. and Fielding, J., 'The normal personality profile of irritable bowel syndrome patients', *Irish J. Med. Sci.*, 1984, 153, pp. 127–9.
13   Narducci, F., Snape, W., Battle, W., Lodon, R. and Cohen, S., 'Increased colonic motility during exposure to a stressful situation', *Dig. Dis. Sci.*, 1985, 30, pp. 40–4.
14   Position paper, Health and Public Policy Committee, American College of Physicians, 'Biofeedback for gastrointestinal disorders', *Annals Int. Med.*, 1985, 103, pp. 291–3.
15   Svedlund, J., Sjodin, I., Ottoson, J. and Doteval, G., 'Controlled study of psychotherapy in irritable bowel syndrome', *Lancet*, 1983, ii, pp. 589–92.
16   Rubenstein, E. and Federman, D.D., *Scientific American Medicine*, Scientific American Inc., New York, NY, 1985, p. 4:III:10.

17   Leicester, R. and Hunt, R., 'Peppermint oil to reduce colonic spasm during endoscopy', *Lancet*, 1982, ii, p. 989.
18   Somerville, K., Richmond, C. and Bell, G., 'Delayed release peppermint oil capsules (Colpermin) for the spastic colon syndrome: a pharmacokinetic study', *Br. J. Clin. Pharmacol.*, 1984, 18, pp. 638–40.
19   Rees, W., Evans, B. and Rhodes, J., 'Treating irritable bowel syndrome with peppermint oil', *Br. Med. J.*, 1979, ii, pp. 835–6.
20   Mowrey, D. and Clayson, D., 'Motion sickness, ginger, and psychophysics', *Lancet*, 1982, i, pp. 655–7.
21   Forster, H.B., Niklas, H. and Lutz, S., 'Antispasmodic effect of some medicinal plants', *Planta Medica*, 1980, 40, pp. 309–19.
22   Hazelhoff, B., Malingre, T.M. and Meijer, D.K., 'Antispasmodic effects of valeriana compounds: an in-vivo and in vitro study on the guinea pig ileum', *Arch. Int. Pharmacodyn.*, 1982, 257, pp. 274–87.

52 Kidney stones

1   Shaw, P., Williams, G. and Green, N., 'Idiopathic hypercalciuria: its control with unprocessed bran', *Br. J. Urol.*, 1980, 52, pp. 426–9.
2   Thom, J., Morris, J., Bishop, A. and Blacklock, N., 'The influence of refined carbohydrate on urinary calcium excretion', *Br. J. Urol.*, 1978, 50, pp. 459–64.
3   Lemann, J., Piering, W. and Lennon, E., 'Possible role of carbohydrate-induced hypercalciuria in calcium oxalate kidney-stone formation', *N.E.J.M.*, 1969, 280, pp. 232–7.
4   Zechner, O., Latal, D., Pfluger, H. and Scheiber, V., 'Nutritional risk factors in urinary stone disease', *J. Urol.*, 1981, 125, pp. 51–5.
5   Robertson, W., Peacock, M. and Marshall, D., 'Prevalence of urinary stone disease in vegetarians', *Eur. Urol.*, 1982, 8, pp. 334–9.
6   Griffith, H., O'Shea, B., Kevany, J. and McCormick, J., 'A control study of dietary factors in renal stone formation', *Br. J. Urol.*, 1981, 53, pp. 416–20.
7   Rose, G. and Westbury, E., 'The influence of calcium content of water, intake of vegetables and fruit and of other food factors upon the incidence of renal calculi', *Urol. Res.*, 1975, 3, pp. 61–6.
8   Ulmann, A., Aubert, J., Bourdeau, A., *et al.*, 'Effects of weight and glucose ingestion on urinary calcium and phosphate excretion: implications for calcium urolithiasis', *J. Clin. Endo. Metab.*, 1982, 54, pp. 1,063–7.
9   Rao, N., Gordon, C., Davis, D. and Blacklock, N. 'Are stone formers maladaptive to refined carbohydrates?', *Br. J. Urol.*, 1982, 54, pp. 575–7.
10   Rushton, H. and Spector, M., 'Effects of magnesium deficiency on intratubular calcium oxalate formation and crystalluria in hyperoxaluric rats', *J. Urol.*, 1982, 127, pp. 598–604.
11   Johansson, G., Backman, U., Danielson, B., *et al.*, 'Biochemical and clinical effects of the prophylactic treatment of renal calcium stones with magnesium hydroxide', *J. Urol.*, 1980, 124, pp. 770–4.
12   Wunderlich, W., 'Aspects of the influence of magnesium ions on the formation of calcium oxalate', *Urol. Res.*, 1981, 9, pp. 157–60.
13   Hallson, P., Rose, G. and Sulaiman, S., 'Magnesium reduces calcium oxalate crystal formation in human whole urine', *Clin. Sci.*, 1982, 62, pp. 17–19.
14   Johansson, G., Backman, U., Danielson, B., *et al.*, 'Magnesium metabolism in renal stone formers. Effects of therapy with magnesium hydroxide', *Scand. J. Urol. Nephrol.*, 1980, 53, pp. 125–30.
15   Prien, E. and Gershoff, S., 'Magnesium oxide-pyridoxine therapy for recurrent calcium oxalate calculi', *J. Urol.*, 1974, 112, pp. 509–12.
16   Gershoff, S. and Prien, E., 'Effect of daily MgO and vitamin B6 administration to patients with recurring calcium oxalate stones', *A.J. Clin. Nutr.*, 1967, 20, pp. 393–9.
17   Will, E. and Bijvoet, L., 'Primary oxalosis: clinical and biochemical response to high-dose pyridoxine therapy', *Metab.*, 1979, 28, pp. 542–8.
18   Lyon, E., Borden, T., Ellis, J. and Vermeulen, C., 'Calcium oxalate lithiasis produced by pyridoxine deficiency and inhibition with high magnesium diets', *Invest. Urol.*, 1966, 4, pp.133–42.
19   Murthy, M., Farooqui, S., Talwar, H., *et al.*, 'Effect of pyridoxine supplementation on recurrent stone formers', *Int. J. Clin. Pharm. Ther. Tox.*, 1982, 20, pp. 434–7.
20   Azoury, L., Garti, N., Perlberg, S. and Sarig, S., 'May enzyme activity in urine play a role in kidney stone formation?', *Urol. Res.*, 1982, 10, pp. 185–9.
21   Sarig, S., Azoury, R. and Garti, N., 'Biological control to diminish dangers of urolithiasis', *Urol. Int.*, 1985, 40, pp. 274–6.
22   Nakagawa, Y., Margolis, H., Yokoyama, S., *et al.*, 'Purification and characterization of a calcium oxalate monohydrate crystal growth inhibitor from human kidney tissue culture medium', *J. Biol. Chem.*, 1981, 256, pp. 3,936–44.
23   Dharmsathaphorn, K., Freeman, D., Binder, H. and Dobbins, J., 'Increased risk of nephrolithiasis in patients with steatorrhea', *Dig. Dis. Sci.*, 1982, 27, pp. 401–5.
24   Editorial, 'Citrate for calcium nephrolithiasis', *Lancet*, 1986, i, p. 955.
25   Pak, C.Y.C. and Fuller, C., 'Idiopathic hypocitraturic calcium-oxalate nephrolithiasis successfully treated with potassium citrate', *Annals Int. Med.*, 1986, 104, pp. 33–7.
26   Recker, R., 'Calcium absorption and achlorhydria', *N.E.J.M.*, 1985, 313, pp. 70–3.
27   Nicar, M.J. and Pak, C.Y.C., 'Calcium bioavailability from calcium carbonate and calcium citrate', *J. Clin. Endocrinol. Metab.*, 1985, 61, pp. 391–3.
28   Seelig, M.S., 'Magnesium deficiency with phosphate and vitamin D excess: role in pediatric cardiovascular disease', *Card. Med.*, 1978, 3, pp. 637–50.
29   Scott, R., Cunningham, C., McLelland, A., *et al.*, 'The importance of cadmium as a factor in calcified upper urinary tract stone disease – a prospective 7-year study', *Br. J. Urol.*, 1982, 54, pp. 584–9.
30   Anton, R. and Haag-Berrurier, M., 'Therapeutic use of natural anthraquinone for other than laxative actions', *Pharmacology*, 1980, 20, pp. 104–12.
31   Berg, W., Hesse, A., Hensel, K., *et al.*, 'Influence of anthraquinones on the formation of urinary calculi in experimental animals', *Urologe A.*, 1976, 15, pp. 188–91.
32   Riley, K., 'The biological efficacy of aloes', *J. John Bastyr Coll. Nat. Med.*, 1981, 2, pp. 18–27.
33   Trease, G. and Evans, W., *Pharmacognosy*, Baillière, Tindall, London, 1978, pp. 373–401.
34   Samaan, K., 'The pharmacological basis of drug treatment of spasm of the ureter or bladder and of ureteral stone', *Br. J. Urol.*, 1933, 5, pp. 213–24.
35   Mitchell, W., *Naturopathic Application of the Botanical Remedies*, W. Mitchell, Seattle, WA, 1983.

53 Macular degeneration of the eye

1   Scharrer, A. and Ober, M., 'Anthocyanosides in the treatment of retinopathies', *Klin. Monatsbl. Augenheilkd.*, 1981, 178, pp. 386–9.
2   Caselli, L., 'Clinical and electroretinographic study on the activity of anthocyanosides', *Arch. Med. Int.*, 1985, 37, pp. 29–35.
3   Lebuisson, D.A., Leroy, L. and Rigal, G., 'Treatment of senile macular degeneration with Ginkgo biloba extract. A preliminary double-blind, drug versus placebo study', *Presse Med.*, 1986, 15, pp. 1,556–8.
4   Newsome, D.A., Swartz, M., Leone, N.C., *et al.*, 'Oral zinc in macular degeneration', *Arch. Ophthalmol.*, 1988, 106, pp. 192–8.

54 Migraine

1   Rubenstein, E. and Federman, D.D., *Scientific American Medicine*, Scientific American, New York, NY, 1987, pp. 11:XI:1-3, CTM:II:10.
2   Branch, W.T., *Office Practice of Medicine*, W.B. Saunders, Philadelphia, PA, 1982; pp. 389–93.
3   Blacklow, R.S., *Signs and Symptoms: Applied Pathologic Physiology and Clinical Interpretation*, J.B. Lippincott, Philadelphia, PA, 1983, pp. 54–72.
4   Rose, F.C. 'The pathogenesis of a migraine attack', *T.I.N.S.*, 1983, 6, p. 247.
5   Shinhoj, E., 'Hemodynamic studies within the brain during migraine', *Arch. Neurol.*, 1979, 29, pp. 257–66.
6   Blacklow, R.S., *MacBrydes Signs and Symptoms*, 6th ed., J.B. Lippincott, New York, NY, 1983, pp. 64–8.
7   Olesen, J., 'The ischemic hypothesis of migraine', *Arch. Neurol.*, 1987, 44, pp. 321–2.
8   Hanington, E., 'The platelet and migraine', *Headache*, 1986, 26, pp. 411–15.
9   Spence, J.D., Wong, D.G., Melendez, L.J., *et al.*, 'Increased incidence of mitral valve prolapse in patients with migraine', *Can. Med. Assoc. J.*, 1984, 131, pp. 1,457–60.
10 Gamberini, G., D'Alessandro, R., Labriola, E., *et al.*, 'Further evidence on the association of mitral valve prolapse and migraine', *Headache*, 1984, 24, pp. 39–40.
11 Lanzi, G., Grandi, A.M., Gamba, G., *et al.*, 'Migraine, mitral valve prolapse and platelet function in the pediatric age group', *Headache*, 1986, 26, pp. 142–5.
12 Welch, K.M.A., 'Migraine: a biobehavioral disorder', *Arch. Neurol.*, 1987, 44, pp. 323–7.
13 Mansfield, L.E., Vaughan, T.R., Waller, S.T., *et al.*, 'Food allergy and adult migraine: double-blind and mediator confirmation of an allergic etiology', *Ann. Allergy*, 1985, 55, pp. 126–9.
14 Carter, C.M. Egger, J. and Soothill, J.F., 'A dietary management of severe childhood migraine', *Hum. Nutr: Appl. Nutr.*, 1985, 39A, pp. 294–303.
15 Hughes, E.C., Gott, P.S. Weinstein, R.C. and Binggeli, R., 'Migraine: a diagnostic test for etiology of food sensitivity by a nutritionally supported fast and confirmed by long-term report', *Ann. Allergy*, 1985, 55, pp. 28–32.
16 Egger, J., Carter, C.M., Wilson, J., *et al.*, 'Is migraine food allergy?', *Lancet*, 1983, ii, pp. 865–9.
17 Monro, J., Brostoff, J., Carini, C. and Zilkhan, K., 'Food allergy in migraine', *Lancet*, 1980, ii, pp. 1–4.
18 Grant, E.C.G., 'Food allergies and migraine', *Lancet*, 1979, i, pp. 966–9.
19 Little, C.H., Stewart, A.G. and Fennessy, M.R., 'Platelet serotonin release in rheumatoid arthritis as studied in food intolerant patients', *Lancet*, 1983, ii, pp. 297–9.
20 Littlewood, J., Glover, V., Petty, R., *et al.*, 'Platelet phenolsulphotransferase deficiency in dietary migraine', *Lancet*, 1982, i, pp. 983–6.
21 Littlewood, J.T., Glover, V. and Sandler, M. 'Red wine contains a potent inhibitor of phenolsulphotransferase', *Br. J. Clin. Pharm.*, 1985, 19, pp. 275–8.
22 Gerrard, J.M., White, J.G. and Krivit, W., 'Labile aggregation stimulating substance, free fatty acids and platelet aggregation', *J. Lab. Clin. Med.*, 1976, 87, pp. 73–82.
23 Sanders, T.A.B. and Roshanai, F., 'The influence of different types of omega-3 polyunsaturated fatty acids on blood lipids and platelet function in healthy volunteers', *Clin. Sci.*, 1981, 64, pp. 91–9.
24 Woodcock, B.E., Smith, E., Lambert, W.H., *et al.*, 'Beneficial effect of fish oil on blood viscosity in peripheral vascular disease', *Br. Med. J.*, 1984, 288, pp. 592–4.
25 Parker, G.B., Tupling, H. and Pryor, D.S., 'A controlled trial of cervical manipulation for migraine', *Aust. N.Z. J. Med.*, 1978, 8, pp. 589–93.
26 Pinkham, I.D., 'British dental migraine study group', *Dent. Pract.* 1982, 13, p. 1.
27 Watts, P.G., Peet, K.M.S. and Juniper, R.P., 'Migraine and the temporomandibular joint: the final answer?', *Br. Dent. J.*, 1986, 161, pp. 170–3.
28 Fischer-Williams, M., Nigl, A.L. and Sovine, D.L., *A Textbook of Biological Feedback*, Human Sciences Press, New York, NY, 1986, pp. 215–16.
29 Solomon, S. and Guglielmo, K.M., 'Treatment of headache by transcutaneous electrical stimulation', *Headache*, 1985, 25, pp. 12–15.
30 Doeer-Proske, H. and Wittchen, H.U., 'A muscle and vascular oriented program for the treatment of chronic migraine patients. A randomized clinical comparative study', *Z. Psychosom. Med. Psychoanal.*, 1985, 31, pp. 247–66.
31 Vesnina, V.A., 'Current methods of migraine reflexotherapy (acupuncture, electropuncture, and electroacupuncture)', *Zh. Nevropatol. Psikhiatr.*, 1980, 80, pp. 703–9.
32 Kurkland, H.D., 'Treatment of headache pain with auto-acupressure', *Dis. Nerv. Sys.*, 1976, 37, pp. 127–9.
33 Lenhard, L. and Waite, P.M., 'Acupuncture in the prophylactic treatment of migraine headache: pilot study', *N.Z. Med. J.*, 1983, 96, pp. 663–6.
34 Facchinetti, F., Nappi, G., Savoldi, F. and Genazzani, A.R., 'Primary headaches: reduced circulating beta-lipotropin and beta-endorphin levels with impaired reactivity to acupuncture', *Cephalgia*, 1981, 1, pp. 195–201.
35 Markelova, V.F., Vesnina, V.A., Malygina, S.I. and Dubovskaia, L.A., 'Changes in blood serotonin levels in patients with migraine headaches before and after a course of reflexotherapy', *Zh. Nevropatol. Psikhiatr.*, 1984, 84, pp. 1,313–16.
36 Laiten, J., 'Acupuncture for migraine prophylaxis: a prospective clinical study with six months' follow-up', *Am. J. Chin. Med.*, 1975, 3, pp. 271–4.
37 Leung, A.Y. *Encyclopedia of Common Natural Ingredients Used in Food*, John Wiley & Sons, New York, NY, 1980.
38 Dreisbach, R.H., *Handbook of Poisoning: Prevention, Diagnosis and Treatment*, Lange Medical Publishing, Los Altos, CA, 1983, pp. 392–4.

39 Johnson, E.S., Kadam, N.P., Hylands, D.M. and Hylands, P.J. 'Efficacy of feverfew as prophylactic treatment of migraine', *Br. Med. J.*, 1985, 291, pp. 569–73.

40 Makheja, A.M. and Bailey, J.M., 'The active principle in feverfew', *Lancet*, 1981, ii, p. 1,054.

41 Makheja, A.M. and Bailey, J.M., 'A platelet phospholipase inhibitor from the medicinal herb feverfew (Tanacetum parthenium)', *Prostagland. Leukotri. Med.*, 1982, 8, pp. 653–60.

42 Heptinstall, S., White, A., Williamson, L. and Mitchell, J.R.A., 'Extracts of feverfew inhibit granule secretion in blood platelets and polymorphonuclear leukocytes', *Lancet*, 1985, i, pp. 1,071–4.

43 Editors, 'Hot peppers and substance P', *Lancet*, 1983, i, p. 1,198.

44 Wang, J.P., Hsu, M.F. and Teng, C.M., 'Antiplatelet effect of capsaicin', *Thrombosis Research*, 1984, 36, pp. 497–507.

45 Buck, S.H. and Burks, T.F., 'The neuropharmacology of capsaicin: review of some recent observations', *Pharm. Rev.*, 1986, 38, pp. 179–226.

46 Duke, J.A., *Handbook of Medicinal Herbs*, CRC Press, Boca Raton, FL, 1985, pp. 317–18.

47 Atkinson, M., 'Migraine headache', *Ann. Int. Med.*, 1944, 21, p. 990.

48 Grenfill, R.F., 'Treatment of migraine with nicotinic acid', *Am. Pract.*, 1949, 3, p. 542.

49 Friedman, A.P. and Brenner, C., 'The use of sodium nicotinate in the treatment of headache', *N.Y. J. Med.*, 1948, 48, p.78.

50 Galland, L.D., Baker, S.M. and McLellan, R.K., 'Magnesium deficiency in the pathogenesis of mitral valve prolapse', *Magnesium*, 1986, 5, pp. 165–74.

51 Fernandes, J.S., Pereira, T., Carvalho, J., *et al.*, 'Therapeutic effect of a magnesium salt in patients suffering from mitral valvular prolapse and latent tetany', *Magnesium*, 1985, 4, p. 283.

52 Melnykowycz, J. and Johansson, K.R., 'Formation of amines by intestinal microorganisms and the influence of chlortetracycline', *J. Exp. Med.*, 1955, 101, pp. 507–17.

53 Watanabe, A., Obata, T. and Nagashima, H., 'Berberine therapy of hypertyraminemia in patients with liver cirrhosis', *Acta Med. Okayama*, 1982, 36, pp. 277–81.

55 Morning sickness

1 Jarnfelt-Samsioe, A., Ericksson, B., *et al.*, 'Serum bile acids, gamma-glutamyltransferase and routine liver function tests in emetic and nonemetic pregnancies', *Gyn. Obs. Invest.*, 1986, 21, pp. 169–76.

2 Gaby, A., *The Doctor's Guide to B6*, Rodale Press, Emmaus, PA, 1984, Ch. 3.

3 Weinstein, B., Wohl, Z., Mitchell, M., *et al.*, 'Oral administration of pyridoxine hydrochloride in the treatment of nausea and vomiting of pregnancy', *Am. J. Ob. Gyn.*, 1944, 47, pp. 389–94.

4 Merkel, R., 'The use of menadione bisulfite and ascorbic acid in the treatment of nausea and vomiting of pregnancy', *Am. J. Ob. Gyn.*, 1952, 64, pp. 416–18.

5 Mowrey, D. and Clayson, D., 'Motion sickness, ginger, and psychophysics', *Lancet*, 1982, i, pp. 655–7.

6 Grontved, A. and Hentzer, E., 'Vertigo-reducing effect of ginger root', *O.R.L.*, 1986, 48, pp. 282–6.

7 Grontved, A., Brask, T., Kambskard, J. and Hentzer, E., 'Ginger root against seasickness. A controlled trial on the open sea', *Acta Otolaryngol.*, 1988, 105, pp. 45–9.

8 Wolkind, S. and Zajicek, E., 'Psycho-social correlates of nausea and vomiting in pregnancy', *H. Psychosom. Res.*, 1978, 22, pp. 1–5.

9 Fitzgerald, C.M., 'Nausea and vomiting in pregnancy', *Br. J. Med. Psycho.*, 1984, 57, pp. 159–65.

56 Mouth ulcers

1 Little, J.W., 'Food allergens and basophil histamine release in recurrent aphthous stomatitis', *Oral Surgery*, 1982, 54, pp. 388–95.

2 Ship, I.I., Merritt, A.D., and Stanley, H.R., 'Recurrent aphthous ulcers', *Am. J. Med.*, 1962, 32, pp. 32–43.

3 Wray, D., Ferguson, M.M., Mason, D.K.,*et al.*, 'Recurrent aphthae: treatment with vitamin B12, folic acid, and iron', *Br. Med. J.*, 1975, 2, pp. 490–3.

4 Wray, D.W., Ferguson, M.M., Hutcheon, A.W. and Dagg, J.H., 'Nutritional deficiencies in recurrent aphthae', *J. Oral. Path.*, 1978, 7, pp. 418–23.

5 Thomas, H.C., Ferguson, A., McLennan, J.G. and Mason, D.K., 'Food antibodies in oral disease: a study of serum antibodies to food proteins in aphthous ulceration and other oral diseases', *J. Clin. Path.*, 1973, 26, pp. 371–4.

6 Wilson, C.W.M., 'Food sensitivities, taste changes, aphthous ulcers and atopic symptoms in allergic disease', *Ann. Allergy*, 1980, 44, pp. 302–7.

7 Rays, R.A., Hamerlinck, F. and Cormane, R.H., 'Immunoglobulin-bearing lymphocytes and polymorphonuclear leukocytes in recurrent aphthous ulcers in man', *Arch. Oral Biol.*, 1977, 22, pp. 147–53.

8 Lehner, T., 'Pathology of recurrent oral ulceraton and oral ulceration in Behcet's syndrome: light, electron and fluorescence microscopy', *J. Path.*, 1969, 97, pp. 481–3.

9 Hay, K.D. and Reade, P.C., 'The use of an elimination diet in the treatment of recurrent aphthous ulceration of the oral cavity', *Oral Surg.*, 1984, 57, pp. 504–7.

10 Ferguson, R., Bashu, M.K., Asquith, P. and Cooke, W.T., 'Jejunal mucosal abnormalities in patients with recurrent aphthous ulceration', *Br. Med. J.*, 1975, 1, pp. 11–13.

11 Ferguson, M.M., Wray, D., Carmichael, H.A., *et al.*, 'Coeliac disease associated with recurrent aphthae', *Gut*, 1980, 21, pp. 223–6.

12 Wray, D., 'Gluten-sensitive recurrent aphthous stomatitis', *Dig. Dis. Sci.*, 1981, 26, pp. 737–40.

13 Walker, D.M., Rhodes, J., Llewelyn, J., *et al.*, 'Gluten hypersensitivity in recurrent aphthous ulceration', *J. Dent. Res.*, 1979, 58 (Special Issue C), p. 1,271.

14 Pearce, F.L., Befus, A.D., and Bienenstock, J., 'Mucosal mast cells III: effect of quercetin and other flavonoids on antigen-induced histamine secretion from rat intestinal mast cells', *J. Allergy Clin. Immunol.*, 1984, 73, pp. 819–23.

15   Busse, W.W., Kopp, D.E., and Middleton, E., 'Flavonoid modulation of human neutrophil function', *J. Allergy Clin. Immunol.*, 1984, 73, pp. 801–9.
16   Kowolik, M.J., Muir, K.F. and MacPhee, I.T., 'Di-sodium cromoglycate in the treatment of recurrent aphthous ulceration', *Br. Dent. J.*, 1978, 144, pp. 384–9.

57 Multiple sclerosis

1   Ellison, G.W., Visscher, B.R., Graves, M.C. and Fahey, J.L., 'Multiple sclerosis', *Annals Int. Med.*, 1984, 101, pp. 514–26.
2   Robbins, S.L., Cotran, R.S. and Kumar, V., *Pathologic Basis of Disease*, 3rd ed., W.B. Saunders, Philadelphia, PA, 1984, pp. 1,410–12.
3   Petersdorf, R.G., *Harrison's Principles of Internal Medicine*, McGraw-Hill, New York, NY, 1983, pp. 2,098–103.
4   Huddlestone, J.R. and Oldstone, M.B.A., 'T suppressor (Tg) lymphocytes fluctuate in parallel with changes in the clinical course of patients with multiple sclerosis', *J. Immunol.* 1979, 123, pp. 1,615–18.
5   Hewson, D.C., 'Is there a role for gluten-free diets in multiple sclerosis', *Human Nutr. Appl. Nutr.*, 1984, 38A, pp. 417–20.
6   Butcher, P.J., 'Milk consumption and multiple sclerosis – an etiological hypothesis', *Medical Hypothesis*, 1986, 19, pp. 169–78.
7   Agranoff, B.A. and Goldberg, D., 'Diet and the geographical distribution of multiple sclerosis', *Lancet*, 1974, ii, pp. 1,061–6.
8   Swank, R.L., 'Multiple sclerosis: a correlation of its incidence with dietary fat', *Am. J. Med. Sci.*, 1950, 220, pp. 421–30.
9   Alter, M., Yamoor, M. and Harshe, M., 'Multiple sclerosis and nutrition', *Arch. Neurol.*, 1974, 31, pp. 267–72.
10   Swank, R.L., 'Multiple sclerosis: twenty years on low fat diet', *Arch. Neurol.*, 1970, 23, pp. 460–74.
11   Swank, R.L., Lerstad, O., Strom, A. *et al.*, 'Multiple sclerosis in rural Norway: its geographic distribution and occupational incidence in relation to nutrition', *N.E.J.M.*, 1952, 246, pp. 721–8.
12   Bernsohn, J. and Stephanides, L.M., 'Aetiology of multiple sclerosis', *Nature*, 1963, 10, pp. 523–30.
13   Shukla, V.K.S., Jensen, G.E. and Clausen, J., 'Erythrocyte glutathione peroxidase deficiency in multiple sclerosis', *Acta Neurol. Scand.*, 1977, 56, pp. 542–50.
14   Szeinberg, A., Golan, R., Ezzer, B., *et al.*, 'Decreased erythrocyte glutathione peroxidase activity in multiple sclerosis', *Acta Neurol. Scand.*, 1979, 60, pp. 265–71.
15   Jensen, G.E., Gissel-Nielsen, G. and Clausen, J., 'Leukocyte glutathione peroxidase activity and selenium level in multiple sclerosis', *J. Neurol. Sci.* 1980, 48, pp. 61–7.
16   Mazzella, G.L., Sinfoiani, E., Savoldi, F., *et al.*, 'Blood cells glutathione peroxidase activity and selenium in multiple sclerosis', *Eur. Neurol.*, 1983, 22, pp. 442–6.
17   Wikstrom, J., Westermarck, T. and Palo, J., 'Selenium, vitamin E and copper in multiple sclerosis', *Acta Neurol. Scand.* 1976, 54, pp. 287–90.
18   Swank, R.L. and Pullen, M.H., *The Multiple Sclerosis Diet Book*, Doubleday, Garden City, NY, 1977.
19   Neu, I.S., 'Essential fatty acids in the serum and cerebrospinal fluid of multiple sclerosis patients', in Gonsette, R.E. and Delmotte, P. (eds), *Immunological and Clinical Aspects of Multiple Sclerosis*, MTP Press, Boston, MA, 1984, Chapter 35.
20   Homa, S.T., Belin, J., Smith, A.D., *et al.*, 'Levels of linolenate and arachidonate in red blood cells of healthy individuals and patients with multiple sclerosis', *J. Neurol. Neurosurg. Psychiat.*, 1980, 43, pp. 106–10.
21   Wright, H.P., Thompson, R.H.S. and Zilkha, K.J., 'Platelet adhesiveness in multiple sclerosis', *Lancet*, 1965, ii, pp. 1, 109–10.
22   Cullen, C.F. and Swank, R.L., 'Intravascular aggregation and adhesiveness of the blood elements associated with alimentary lipemia and injection of large molecular substances: effect on blood-brain barrier', *Circulation*, 1954, 9, pp. 335–46.
23   Haeren, A.F., Tourtellotte, W.W., Richard, K.A., *et al.*, 'A study of the blood cerebrospinal fluid-brain barrier in multiple sclerosis', *Neurology*, 1964, 14, pp. 345–51.
24   Swank, R.L. and Nakamura, H., 'Oxygen availability in brain tissues after lipid meals', *Am. J. Physiol.*, 1960, 198, pp. 217–20.
25   Millar, J.H.D., Zilkha, K.J., Langman, M.J.S., *et al.*, 'Double-blind trial of linolate supplementation of the diet in multiple sclerosis', *Br. Med. J.*, 1973, i, pp. 765–8.
26   Bates, D., Fawcett, P.R.W., Shaw, D.A. and Weightman, D., 'Polyunsaturated fatty acids in treatment of acute remitting multiple sclerosis', *Br. Med. J.*, 1978, ii, pp. 1,390–1.
27   Paty, D.W., Cousin, H.K., Read, S. and Adlakkha, K., 'Linoleic acid in multiple sclerosis: failure to show any therapeutic benefit', *Acta Neurol. Scand.*, 1978, 58, pp. 53–8.
28   Dworkin, R.H., Bates, D., Millar, J.H.D. and Paty, D.W., 'Linoleic acid and multiple sclerosis: a reanalysis of three double-blind trials', *Neurology*, 1984, 34, pp. 1,441–5.
29   Dworkin, R.H., Bates, D., Millar, J.H.D., Shaw, D.A. and Paty, D. W., 'Dietary supplementation with polyunsaturated fatty acids in acute remitting multiple sclerosis', in Gonsette, R.E. and Delmotte, P. (eds), *Immunological and Clinical Aspects of Multiple Sclerosis*, MTP Press, Boston, MA, 1984, Chapter 34.
30   Field, E.J. and Joyce, G., 'Multiple sclerosis: effect of gamma linolenate administration upon membranes and the need for extended clinical trials of unsaturated fatty acids', *Eur. Neurol.* 1983, 22, pp. 78–83.
31   Meade, C.J., Mertin, J., Sheena, J. and Hunt, R., 'Reduction by linoleic acid of the severity of experimental allergic encephalomyelitis in the guinea pig', *J. Neurol. Sci.*, 1978, 35, pp. 291–308.
32   Hughes, D., Kieth, A.B., Mertin, J. and Caspary, E.A., 'Linoleic acid therapy in severe experimental allergic encephalomyelitis in the guinea pig: suppression by continuous treatment', *Clin. Exp. Immunol.*, 1980, 41, pp. 523–31.
33   Johnston, D.V. and Mashall, L.A., 'Dietary fat, prostaglandins and the immune response', *Progress Food Nutr. Sci.*, 1984, 8, pp. 3–25.
34   Meade, G.J. and Mertin, J., 'Fatty acids and immunity', *Adv. Lipid Res.*, 1978, 16, pp. 127–65.
35   Mertin, J. and Stackpoole, A., 'The spleen is required for suppression of experimental allergic encephalomyelitis by prostaglandin precursors', *Clin. Exp. Immunol.*, 1979. 36, pp. 449–55.
36   Mertin, J. and Stackpoole, A., 'Suppression by essential fatty acids of experimental allergic encephalomyelitis is abolished by indomethacin', *Prostaglandins Med.*, 1978, 1, pp. 283–91.
37   Renaud, S. and Norday, A., '"Small is beautiful": alpha-linolenic acid and eicosapentaenoic acid in man', *Lancet*, 1983, i, pp. 1,169.
38   Holman, R.T., Johnson, S.B. and Hatch, T.F., 'A case of human linolenic acid deficiency involving neurological abnormalities', *Am. J. Clin. Nutr.*, 1982, 65, pp. 617–23.

39   Horrobin, D.F., 'Multiple sclerosis: the rational basis for treatment with colchicine and evening primrose oil', *Med. Hypothesis*, 1979, 5, pp. 365–78.
40   Dyerberg, J., 'Linolenate-derived polyunsaturated fatty acids and prevention of atherosclerosis', *Nutr. Rev.*, 1986, 44, pp. 125–34.
41   Nutrition Foundation, *Present Knowledge in Nutrition*, 5th ed., Nutrition Foundation, Washington DC, 1984.
42   Gupta, J.K., Ingegno, A.P., Cook, A.W. and Pertschuk, L.P. 'Multiple sclerosis and malabsorption', *Am. J. Gastroenterol.*, 1977, 68, pp. 560–6.
43   Lange, L.S. and Shiner, M., 'Small-bowel abnormalities in multiple sclerosis', *Lancet*, 1976, ii, pp. 1,319–22.
44   Soll, R.W. and Grenoble, P.B., *MS Something Can Be Done and You Can Do It*, Contemporary Books, Chicago, IL, 1984.
45   Liversedge, L.A., 'Treatment and management of MS', *Br. Med. Bull.*, 1976, 33, pp. 78–83.
46   Hunter, L.A., Rees, B.W.G. and Jones, L.T., 'Gluten antibodies in patients with multiple sclerosis', *Hum. Nutr. Clin. Nutr.*, 1984, 38A, pp. 142–83.
47   Boschetty, V. and Cernoch, J. 'Aplikace kysliku za pretlaku u nekterych neurologickych onemocneni', *Bratisl. Lek. Listy*, 1970, 53, pp. 298–302.
48   Baixe, J.H., 'Bilan de onze années d'activité en medicine hyperbaré', *Med. Aer. Spatiale Med. Subaquatique Hyperbare*, 1978, 17, pp. 90–2.
49   Neubauer, R.A., 'Treatment of multiple sclerosis with monoplace hyperbaric oxygenation', *J. Fl. Med. Assoc.*, 1978, 65, p. 101.
50   Fischler, B.H., Marks, M. and Reich, T., 'Hyperbaric-oxygen treatment of multiple sclerosis', *N.E.J.M.*, 1983, 308, pp. 181–6.
51   Barnes, M.P., Bates, D., Cartlidge, N.E.F., *et al.*, 'Hyperbaric oxygen and multiple sclerosis: short term results of a placebo-controlled, double blind trial', *Lancet*, 1985, i, pp. 297–300.
52   Wiles, C.M., Clarke, C.R.A., Irwin, H.P., *et al.*, 'Hyperbaric oxygen in multiple sclerosis: a double blind trial, *Br. Med. J.*, 1986, 292, pp. 367–71.

58 Obesity

1   Krause, M.V. and Mahan, L.K., *Food, Nutrition, and Diet Therapy*, 7th ed., W.B. Saunders, Philadelphia, PA, 1984.
2   Bray, G.A., 'Obesity: definition, diagnosis and disadvantages', *Med. J. Australia*, 1985, 142, pp. 52–8.
3   Raymond, C.A., 'Biology, culture, dietary changes conspire to increase incidence of obesity', *J.A.M.A.*, 1986, 256, pp. 2,157–8.
4   Kolata, G., 'Obese children: a growing problem', *Science*, 1986, 232, pp. 20–1.
5   Bjorntorp, P., 'Classification of obese patients and complications related to the distribution of surplus fat', *Am. J. Clin. Nutr.*, 1987, 45, pp. 1,120–5.
6   Ashwell, M., Cole, T.J. and Dixon, A.K., 'Obesity: new insight into the anthropometric classification of fat distribution shown by computed tomography', *Br. Med. J.*, 1985, 290, pp. 1,692–4.
7   Gillum, R.F., 'The association of body fat distribution with hypertension, hypertensive heart disease, coronary heart disease, diabetes and cardiovascular risk factors in men and women aged 18–79 years', *J. Chron. Dis.*, 1987, 40, pp. 421–8.
8   Contaldo, F., di Biase, G., Panico, S., *et al.*, 'Body fat distribution and cardiovascular risk in middle-aged people in southern Italy', *Atherosclerosis*, 1986, 61, pp. 169–72.
9   Williams, P.T., Fortmann, S.P., Terry, R.B., *et al.*, 'Associations of dietary fat, regional adiposity, and blood pressure in men', *J.A.M.A.*, 1987, 257, pp. 3,251–6.
10   Haffner, S.M., Stern, M.P., Hazuda, H.P., *et al.*, 'Role of obesity and fat distribution in non-insulin-dependent diabetes mellitus in Mexican Americans and non-Hispanic whites', *Diabetes Care*, 1986, 9, pp. 153–61.
11   Dietz, W.H. and Gortmaker, S.L., 'Do we fatten our children at the television set?', *Pediatrics*, 1985, 75, pp. 807–12.
12   Foreyt, J.P., Mitchell, R.E., Garner, D.T., *et al.*, 'Behavioral treatment of obesity: results and limitations', *Behavioral Therapy*, 1982, 13, pp. 153–61.
13   Kolata, G., 'Why do people get fat?', *Science*, 1985, 227, pp. 1,327–8.
14   Bennett, W. and Gurin, J., *The Dieter's Dilemma*, Basic Books, New York, NY, 1982.
15   Trowell, H., Burkitt, D. and Heaton, K., *Dietary Fibre, Fibre-depleted Foods and Disease*, Academic Press, New York, NY, 1985.
16   Anderson, J.W. and Bryant, C.A., 'Dietary fiber: diabetes and obesity', *Am. J. Gastroenterol.*, 1986, 81, pp. 898–906.
17   Palgi, A., Read, J.L., Greenberg, I., *et al.*, 'Multidisciplinary treatment of obesity with a protein-sparing modified fast: results in 668 outpatients', *Am. J. Public Health*, 1985, 75, pp. 1,190–4.
18   Valenta, L. and Elias, A.N., 'Modified fasting in treatment of obesity', *Postgraduate Medicine*, 1986, 79, pp. 263–7.
19   Wadden, T.A., Stunkard, A.J., Day, S.C., *et al.*, 'Less food, less hunger: reports of appetite and symptoms in a controlled study of a protein-sparing modified fast', *Int. J. Obesity*, 1987, 11, pp. 239–49.
20   Kirchner, M.A., Schneider, G., Ertel, N.H. and Gorman, J., 'An eight-year experience with a very-low-calorie formula diet for control of major obesity', *Int. J. Obesity*, 1988, 12, pp. 69–80.
21   Thompson, J.K., Jarvie, G.J., Lahey, B.B. and Cureton, K.J., 'Exercise and obesity: etiology, physiology, and intervention', *Psychol. Bull.*, 1982, 91, pp. 55–79.
22   Rossner, S., Zweigbergk, D.V., Ohlin, A. and Ryttig, K., 'Weight reduction with dietary fibre supplements. Results of two double-blind studies', *Acta Med. Scand.*, 1987, 222, pp. 83–8.
23   Shearer, R.S., 'Effect of bulk producing tablets on hunger intensity and dieting pattern', *Curr. Ther. Res.*, 1976, 19, pp. 433–41.
24   Hylander, B., and Rossner, S., 'Effects of dietary fibre intake before meals on weight loss and hunger in a weight-reducing club', *Acta Med. Scand.*, 1983, 213, pp. 217–20.
25   Walsh, D.E., Yaghoubian, V. and Behforooz, A., 'Effect of glucomannan on obese patients: a clinical study', *Int. J. Obesity*, 1984, 8, pp. 289–93.
26   Dean, D.H. and Hiramoto, R.N. 'Weight loss during pancreatin feeding of rats', *Nutrition Reports International*, 1984, 29, pp. 167–72.
27   Bailey, C.J., Thornburn, C.C. and Flatt, P.R., 'Effects of ephedrine and atenol on the development of obesity and diabetes in ob/ob mice', *Gen. Pharmac.*, 1986, 17, pp. 243–6.
28   Dulloo, A.G. and Miller, D.S., 'The thermogenic properties of ephedrine/methylxanthine mixtures: animal studies', *Am. J. Clin. Nutr.*, 1986, 43, pp. 388–94.
29   Dulloo, A.G. and Miller, D.S., 'The thermogenic properties of ephedrine/methylxanthine mixtures: human studies', *Int. J. Obesity*, 1986, 10, pp. 467–81.
30   Pozniak, P.C., 'The carcinogenicity of caffeine and coffee: a review', *J. of the American Dietetic Association*, 1985, 85, pp. 1,127–33.

31   Nomura, F., Ohnishi, K., Satomura, Y., *et al.*, 'Liver function in moderate obesity – study in 534 moderately obese subjects among 4,613 male company employees', *Int. J. Obesity*, 1986, 10, pp. 349–54.

32   Racz-Kotilla, E., Racz, G. and Solomon, A., 'The action of Taraxacum officinale extracts on the body weight and diuresis of laboratory animals', *Planta Medica*, 1974, 26, pp. 212–17.

59 Osteoarthritis

1   Robbins, S.L., Cotran, R.S. and Kumar, V., *Pathologic Basis of Disease*, W.B. Saunders, Philadelphia, PA, 1984, pp. 1,356–61.

2   Petersdorf, R., *et al.* (eds), *Harrison's Principles of Internal Medicine*, McGraw-Hill, New York, NY, 1983, pp. 517–24.

3   Bland, J.H. and Cooper, S.M., 'Osteoarthritis: a review of the cell biology involved and evidence for reversibility. Management rationally related to known genesis and pathophysiology', *Sem. Arthr. Rheum.*, 1984, 14, pp. 106–33.

4   Sokoloff, L. (ed.), *Osteoarthritis*, Clinics in Rheumatic Diseases, 1985, 11, no. 2.

5   Perry, G.H., Smith, M.J.G. and Whiteside, C.G., 'Spontaneous recovery of the hip joint space in degenerative hip disease', *Ann. Rheum. Dis.*, 1972, 31, pp. 440–8.

6   Brooks, P.M., Potter, S.R. and Buchanan, W.W., 'NSAID and osteoarthritis – help or hindrance', *J. Rheumatol.*, 1982, 9, pp. 3–5.

7   Newman, N.M. and Ling, R.S.M., 'Acetabular bond destruction related to non-steroidal anti-inflammatory drugs', *Lancet*, 1985, ii, pp. 11–13.

8   Solomon, L., 'Drug induced arthropathy and necrosis of the femoral head', *J. Bone Joint. Surg.*, 1973, 55B, pp. 246–51.

9   Ronningen, H. and Langeland, N., 'Indomethacin treatment in osteoarthritis of the hip joint', *Acta Orthop. Scand.*, 1979, 50, pp. 169–74.

10   Dequeker, J., Burssens, A. and Bouillon, R., 'Dynamics of growth hormone secretion in patients with osteoporosis and in patients with osteoarthrosis', *Hormone Res.*, 1982, 16, pp. 353–6.

11   Krause, M.V. and Mahan, L.K., *Food, Nutrition and Diet Therapy*, 7th edition, W.B. Saunders, Philadelphia, PA, 1984, pp. 677–9.

12   Hartz, A.J., Fischer, M.E., Bril, G., *et al.*, 'The association of obesity with joint pain and osteoarthritis in the Hanes data', *J. Chron. Dis.*, 1986, 39, pp. 311–19.

13   Childers, N.F. and Russo, G.M., *The Nightshades and Health*, Horticulture Publications, Somerville, NJ, 1973.

14   Kaufman, W., *The Common Form of Joint Dysfunction: Its Incidence and Treatment*, E.L. Hildreth Company, Brattleboro, VT, 1949.

15   Hoffer, A., 'Treatment of arthritis by nicotinic acid and nicotinamide', *Canadian Medical Association Journal*, 1959, 81, pp. 235–9.

16   Marcolongo, R., Giordano, N., Colombo, B., *et al.*, 'Double-blind multicentre study of the activity of S-adenosyl-methionine in hip osteoarthritis', *Current Therapeutic Research*, 1985, 37, pp. 82–94.

17   Di Padova, C., 'S-adenosylmethionine in the treatment of osteoarthritis. Review of clinical studies', *Am. J. Med.*, 1987, 83, Supplement 5A, pp. 60–5.

18   Verbuggen, G. and Veys, M., 'Glycosaminoglycan polysulphate, the first ways to counteract biochemical abnormalities in osteoarthritic joints', *Acta Rheumatologica*, 1980, 4, pp. 171–7.

19   Vacha, J., Pesakova, V., Krajickova, J. and Adam, M., 'Effect of glycoaminoglycan polysulphate on the metabolism of cartilage ribonucliec acid', *Arzneim-Forsch.*, 1984, 34, pp. 607–9.

20   Annefeld, M., 'Ultrastructural and morphometrical studies on the articular cartilage of rats: the destructive effects of dexamethasone and the chondroprotective effect of Rumalon', *Agents Action*, 1985, 17, pp. 319–21.

21   Anderman, G. and Dietz, M., 'The influence of the route of administration on the bio-availability of an endogenous macromolecule: chondroitin sulphate (CSA)', *Eur. J. Drug Metabol. Pharmakokin.*, 1982, 7, pp. 11–16.

22   Turazza, G., Spreafico, P.L. and Frandoli, G., 'Comparative investigation on the effects of nicotinic acid alone and in association with a synthetic, heparin-like sulfated polyanion on fibrinolysis, platelet aggregation and lipidic fractions', *Arzneim-Forsch.*, 1973, 23, pp. 654–7.

23   Lund-Olesen, K. and Menander, K.B., 'Orgotein: a new anti-inflammatory metalloprotein drug: preliminary evaluation of clinical efficacy and safety in degenerative joint disease', *Curr. Ther. Res.*, 1974, 16, pp. 706–17.

24   Huskisson, E.C. and Scott, J., 'Orgotein in osteoarthritis of the knee joint', *Eur. J. Rheumatol. Inflam.*, 1981, 4, p. 212.

25   Zidenberg-Cherr, S., Keen, C.L., Lonnerdal, B. and Hurley, L.S., 'Dietary superoxide dismutase does not affect tissue levels', *Am. J. Clin. Nutr.*, 1983, 37, pp. 5–7.

26   Machtey, I. and Ouaknine, L., 'Tocopherol in osteoarthritis: a controlled pilot study', *Journal of the American Geriatrics Society*, 1978, 26, pp. 328–30.

27   Schwartz, E.R., 'The modulation of osteoarthritic development by vitamins C and E', *Int. J. Vit. Nutr. Res.*, supplement, 1984, 26, pp. 141–6.

28   Bates, C.J., 'Proline and hydroxyproline excretion and vitamin C status in elderly human subjects', *Clinical Sci. Molecular Med.*, 1977, 52, pp. 535–43.

29   Prins, A.P., Lipman, J.M., McDevitt, C.A. and Sokoloff, L., 'Effect of purified growth factors on rabbit articular chondrocytes in monolayer culture', *Arthr. Rheum.*, 1982, 25, pp. 1,228–32.

30   Krystal, G., Morris, G.M. and Sokoloff, L., 'Stimulation of DNA synthesis by ascorbate in cultures of articular chondrocytes', *Arth. Rheum.*, 1982, 25, pp. 318–25.

31   Anand, J.C., 'Osteoarthritis and pantothenic acid', *J. Coll. Gen. Pract.*, 1963, 5, pp. 136–7.

32   Anand, J.C., 'Osteoarthritis and pantothenic acid', *Lancet*, 1963, ii, p. 1,168.

33   'Calcium pantothenate in arthritis conditions. A report from the General Practitioner Research Group', *Practitioner*, 1980, 224, pp. 208–11.

34   Wright, V., 'Treatment of osteo-arthritis of the knees', *Ann. Rheum. Dis.*, 1964, 23, pp. 389–91.

35   Clarke, G.R., Willis, L.A., Stenner, L. and Nichols, P.J.R., 'Evaluation of physiotherapy in the treatment of osteoarthrosis of the knee', *Rheumatol. Rehabilitation*, 1974, 13, pp. 190–7.

36   Vanharantha, H., 'Effect of short-wave diathermy on mobility and radiological stage of the knee in the development of experimental osteoarthritis', *Am. J. Phys. Med.*, 1982, 61, pp. 59–65.

37   Bingham, R., Bellew, B.A. and Bellew, J.G., 'Yucca plant saponin in the management of arthritis', *J. Applied Nutr.*, 1975, 27, pp. 45–50.

38   Morales, T.I., Wahl, L.M. and Hascall, V.C., 'The effect of lipopolysaccharides on the biosynthesis and release of proteoglycans from calf articular cartilage cultures', *J. Biol. Chem.*, 1984, 259, pp. 6,720–9.

39   Brady, L.R., Tyler, V.E. and Robbers, J.E., *Pharmacognosy*, 8th ed., Lea & Febiger, Philadelphia, PA, 1981, p. 480.

40   Whitehouse, L.W., Znamirowski, M. and Paul, C.J., 'Devil's claw (Harpagophytum procumbens): no evidence for anti-inflammatory activity

in the treatment of arthritic disease', *Canadian Medical Association Journal*, 1983, 129, pp. 249–51.

41 McLeod, D.W., Revell, P. and Robinson, B.V., 'Investigations of Harpagophytum procumbens (Devil's claw) in the treatment of experimental inflammation and arthritis in the rat', *British Journal of Pharmacology*, 1979, 66, pp. 140P–141P.

42 Gabor, M., 'Pharmacologic effects of flavonoids on blood vessels', *Angiologica*, 1972, 9, pp. 355–74.

43 Kuhnau, J., 'The flavonoids. A class of semi-essential food components: their role in human nutrition', *World Review Nutrition and Dietetics*, 1976, 24, pp. 117–91.

44 Havsteen, B., 'Flavonoids, a class of natural products of high pharmacological potency', *Biochemical Pharmacology*, 1983, 32, pp. 1,141–8.

45 Middleton, E., 'The flavonoids', *Trends in Pharmaceutical Science*, 1984, 5, pp. 335–8.

60 Osteoporosis

1 Pizzorno, J.E. and Murray, I r., *A Textbook of Natural Medicine*, John Bastyr College Publications, Seattle, WA, 1985.

2 Grossman, M., Kirsner, J. a..u Gillespie, I., 'Basal and histalog-stimulated gastric secretion in control subjects and in patients with peptic ulcer or gastric cancer', *Gastroenterology*, 1963, 45, pp. 15–26.

3 Recker, R., 'Calcium absorption and achlorhydria', *New England Journal of Medicine*, 1985, 313, pp. 70–3.

4 Nicar, M.J., and Pak, C.Y.C., 'Calcium bioavailability from calcium carbonate and calcium citrate', *Journal of Clinical Endocrinology and Metabolism*, 1985, 61, pp. 391–3.

5 Lore, F., Nuti, R., Vattimo, A. and Caniggia, A., 'Vitamin D metabolites in postmenopausal osteoporosis', *Horm. Metabol. Res.*, 1984, 16, p. 58.

6 Gallagher, J., Riggs, L., Eisman, J., *et al.*, 'Intestinal calcium absorption and serum vitamin D metabolites in normal subjects and osteoporotic patients: effect of age and dietary calcium', *J. Clin. Invest.*, 1979, 64, pp. 729–36.

7 Heaney, R., 'Nutritional factors and estrogen in age-related bone loss', *Clin. Invest. Med.*, 1981, 5, pp. 147–55.

8 Ellis, F., Holesh, S. and Ellis, J., 'Incidence of osteoporosis in vegetarians and omnivores', *Am. J. Clin. Nutr.*, 1972, 25, pp. 55–8.

9 Marsh, A., Sanchez, T., Chaffe, F., *et al.*, 'Bone mineral mass in adult lacto-ovo-vegetarian and omnivorous adults', *Am. J. Clin. Nutr.*, 1983, 37, pp. 453–6.

10 Licata, A., Bou, E., Bartter, F. and West, F., 'Acute effects of dietary protein on calcium metabolism in patients with osteoporosis', *J. Geron.*, 1981, 36, pp. 14–19.

11 Thom, J., Morris, J., Bishop, A. and Blacklock, N.J., 'The influence of refined carbohydrate on urinary calcium excretion', *Br. J. Urol.*, 1978, 50, pp. 459–64.

12 Marcus, R., 'The relationship of dietary calcium to the maintenance of skeletal integrity in man – an interface of endocrinology and nutrition', *Metabol.*, 1982, 31, pp. 93–102.

13 Lee, C.J., Lawler, G.S. and Johnson, G.H., 'Effects of supplementation of the diets with calcium and calcium-rich foods on bone density of elderly females with osteoporosis', *Am. J. Clin. Nutr.*, 1981, 34, pp. 819–23.

14 Editorial, 'Citrate for calcium nephrolithiasis', *Lancet*, 1986, i, p. 955.

15 Pak, C.Y.C. and Fuller, C., 'Idiopathic hypocitraturic calcium-oxalate nephrolithiasis successfully treated with potassium citrate', *Ann. Int. Med.*, 1986, 104, pp. 33–7.

16 Johansson, G., Backman, U., Danielson, B., *et al.*, 'Biochemical and clinical effects of the prophylactic treatment of renal calcium stones with magnesium hydroxide', *J. Urol.*, 1980, 124, pp. 770–4.

17 Cohen, L. and Kitzes, R., 'Infrared spectroscopy and magnesium content of bone mineral in osteoporotic women', *Isr. J. Med. Sci.*, 1981, 17, pp. 1,123–5.

18 Rude, R.K., Adams, J.S., Ryzen, E., *et al.*, 'Low serum concentration of 1,25-dihydroxyvitamin D in human magnesium deficiency', *J. Clin. Endo. Metabol.*, 1985, 61, pp. 933–40.

19 Seelig, M.S., 'Magnesium deficiency with phosphate and vitamin D excess: role in pediatric cardiovascular nutrition', *Cardio. Med.*, 1978, 3, pp. 637–50.

20 Newcomer, A., Hodgson, S., McGill, D. and Thomas, P., 'Lactase deficiency: prevalence in osteoporosis', *Ann. Int. Med.*, 1978, 89, pp. 218–20.

21 Barker, H., Frank, O., Thind, I.C., *et al.*, 'Vitamin profiles in elderly persons living at home or in nursing homes versus profile in healthy young subjects', *J. Am. Geriatrics Society*, 1979, 10, pp. 444–50.

22 Infante-Rivard, C., Krieger M., Gascon-Barre, M. and Rivard, G.E., 'Folate deficiency among institutionalized elderly, public health impact', *J. Am. Geriatrics Society*, 1986, 34, pp. 211–14.

23 Brattstrom, L.E., Hultberg, B.L. and Hardebo, J.E., 'Folic acid responsive postmenopausal homocysteinemia', *Metabolism*, 1985, 34, pp. 1,073–7.

24 Editorial, 'The function of the vitamin K-dependent proteins, bone GLA protein (BGP) and kidney GLA proteins (KGP)', *Nutr. Rev.*, 1984, 42, pp. 230–3.

25 Krasinski, S.D., Russell, R.M., Furie, B.C., *et al.*, 'The prevalence of vitamin K deficiency in chronic gastrointestinal disorders', *Am. J. Clin. Nutr.*, 1985, 41, pp. 639–43.

26 Nielsen, F.H., 'Boron – an overlooked element of potential nutrition importance', *Nutrition Today*, 1988, Jan/Feb, pp. 4–7.

27 McCaslin, F.E. Jr and Janes, J.M., 'The effect of strontium lactate in the treatment of osteoporosis', *Proc. Staff Meetings Mayo Clin.*, 1959, 34, p. 329.

28 Rao, C., Rao, V. and Steinman, B., 'Influence of bioflavonoids on the metabolism and crosslinking of collagen', *Ital. J. Biochem.*, 1981, 30, pp. 259–70.

29 Duke, J.A., *Handbook of Medicinal Herbs*, CRC Press, Boca Raton, FL, 1985.

30 Leung, A.Y., *Encyclopedia of Common Natural Ingredients Used in Food, Drugs, and Cosmetics*, John Wiley & Sons, New York, NY, 1980.

31 *British Herbal Pharmacopoeia*, British Herbal Medicine Association, West Yorks, 1983.

32 Elghamry, M.I. and Shihata, I.M., 'Biological activity of phytoestrogens', *Planta Medica*, 1965, 13, pp. 352–7.

33 Albert-Puleo, M., 'Fennel and anise as estrogenic agents', *J. Ethnopharmacology*, 1980, 2, pp. 337–44.

34 Costello, C.H. and Lynn, E.V., 'Estrogenic substances from plants: I. Glycyrrhiza', *J. Am. Pharm. Soc.*, 1950, 39, pp. 177–80.

35 Baron, J., 'Smoking and oestrogen-related disease', *A.J. Epid.*, 1984, 119, pp. 9–22.

36   Aloia, J.F., Cohn, S.H., Vaswani, A., *et al.*, 'Risk factors for postmenopausal osteoporosis', *Am. J. Med.*, 1985, 78, pp. 95–100.

37   Krolner, B., Toft, B., Nielsen, S. and Tondevold, E., 'Physical exercise as prophylaxis against involutional vertebral bone loss: a controlled trial', *Clin. Sci.*, 1983, 64, pp. 541–6.

38   Yeater, R. and Martin, R., 'Senile osteoporosis: the effects of exercise', *Postg. Med.*, 1984, 75, pp. 147–9.

39   Donaldson, C., Hulley, S., Vogel, J., *et al.*, 'Effect of prolonged bed rest on bone mineral', *Metabolism*, 1970, 19, pp. 1,071–84.

61 Periodontal disease

1   Carranza, F., *Glickman's Clinical Periodontology*, W.B. Saunders, Philadelphia, PA, 1984.

2   Robbins, S. and Cotran, R., *Pathologic Basis of Disease*, W.B. Saunders, Philadelphia, PA, 1979, pp. 893–5.

3   Page, R. and Schroeder, H., 'Current status of the host response in chronic marginal peridontitis', *J. Periodontal*, 1981, 52, pp. 477–91.

4   James, K., 'Complement: activation, consequences, and control', *Am. J. Med. Tech.*, 1982, 48, pp. 735–43.

5   Hyyppa, T., 'Gingival IgE and histamine concentrations in patients with periodontitis', *J. Clin. Periodontal*, 1984, 11, pp. 132–7.

6   Addya, S., Chakravarti, K., Basu, A., *et al.*, 'Effects of mercuric chloride on several scavenging enzymes in rat kidney and influence of vitamin E supplementation', *Acta Vitaminol. Enzymol.*, 1984, 6, pp. 103–7.

7   Bartold, P., Wiebkin, O. and Thonard, J., 'The effect of oxygen-derived free radicals on gingival proteoglycans and hyaluronic acid', *J. Periodontal Res.*, 1984, 19, pp. 390–400.

8   Christen, A., 'The clinical effects of tobacco on oral tissue', *J.A.D.A.*, 1970, 81, pp. 1,378–82.

9   Bastaan, R. and Reade, P., 'The effects of tobacco on oral and dental tissues', *Aust. Dent. J.*, 1976, 21, pp. 308–15.

10   Pelletier, O., 'Smoking and vitamin C levels in humans', *Am. J. Clin. Nutr.*, 1968, 21, pp. 1,259–67.

11   Junqueira, L. and Carneiro, J., *Basic Histology*, Lange Med Publishing, Los Altos, CA, 1980, p. 312.

12   Bartold, P., Wiebkin, O. and Thonard, J., 'The active role of gingival proteoglycans in periodontal disease', *Med. Hypothesis*, 1983, 12, pp. 377–87.

13   Bartold, P., Wiebkin, O. and Thonard, J., 'Proteoglycans of human gingival epithelium and connective tissue', *Biochem. J.*, 1983, 11, pp. 119–27.

14   Alvares, O., 'Nutrition, diet and oral health', Chapter 14 in Worthington-Roberts, B. (ed.), *Contemporary Developments in Nutrition*, C.V. Mosby, St Louis, MO, 1981.

15   Alvares, O., Altman, L., Springmeyer, S., *et al.*, 'The effect of subclinical ascorbate deficiency on periodontal disease in nonhuman primates', *J. Periodontal Res.*, 1984, 16, pp. 628–36.

16   Woolfe, S., Hume, W. and Kenney, E., 'Ascorbic acid and periodontal disease: a review of the literature', *J. Western Soc. Periodontal.*, 1980, 28, pp. 44–60.

17   Alfano, M., Miller, S. and Drummond, J., 'Effect of ascorbic acid deficiency on the permeability and collagen biosynthesis of oral mucosal epithelium', *Ann. N.Y. Acad. Sci.*, 1975, 258, pp. 253–63.

18   Alvares, O. and Siegel, I., 'Permeability of gingival sulcular epithelium in the development of scorbutic gingivitis', *J. Oral Path.*, 1981, 10, pp. 40–8.

19   Stephens, C. and Snyderman, R., 'Cyclic nucleotides regulate the morphologic alterations required for chemotaxis in monocytes', *J. Immunol.*, 1982, 128, pp. 1,192–7.

20   Krause, M. and Mahan, L., *Food, Nutrition and Diet Therapy*, W.B. Saunders, Philadelphia, PA, 1984.

21   Burton, G. and Ingold, K., 'Beta-carotene: an unusual type of lipid antioxidant', *Science*, 1984, 224, pp. 569–73.

22   Prasad, A., 'Clinical, biochemical and nutritional spectrum of zinc deficiency in human subjects: an update', *Nutr. Rev.*, 1983, 41, pp. 197–208.

23   Freeland, J., Cousins, R. and Schwartz, R., 'Relationship of mineral status and intake to periodontal disease', *Am. J. Clin. Nutr.*, 1976, 29, pp. 745–9.

24   Nordstrom, J., 'Trace mineral nutrition in the elderly', *Am. J. Clin. Nutr.*, 1982, 36, pp. 788–95.

25   Harrap, G., Saxton, C. and Best, J., 'Inhibition of plaque growth by zinc salts', *J. Periodontal Res.*, 1983, 18, pp. 634–42.

26   Hsieh, S., Hayali, A. and Navia, J., 'Zinc', in Curzon, M. and Cutress, T. (eds), *Trace Elements in Dental Disease*, John Wright PSG Inc., Boston, MA, 1983, Chapter 9, pp. 99–220.

27   Aleo, J., Padh, H. and Subramoniam, A., 'Possible role of calcium in periodontal disease', *J. Periodontal*, 1984, 55, pp. 642–7.

28   Hazan, S. and Cowan, E., *Diet, Nutrition and Periodontal Disease*, American Society of Preventative Dentistry, Chicago, IL, 1975.

29   Kim, J. and Shklar, G., 'The effect of vitamin E on the healing of gingival wounds in rats', *J. Periodontal*, 1983, 54, pp. 305–8.

30   Monboisse, J., Braquet, P. and Borel, J., 'Oxygen-free radicals as mediators of collagen breakage', *Agents Actions*, 1984, 15, pp. 49–50.

31   Rao, C., Rao, V. and Steinman, B., 'Influence of bioflavonoids on the metabolism and cross linking of collagen', *Ital. J. Biochem.*, 1981, 30, pp. 259–70.

32   Ronziere, M., Herbage, D., Garrone, R. and Frey, G., 'Influence of some flavonoids on reticulation of collagen fibrils in vitro', *Biochem. Pharm.*, 1981, 30, pp. 1,771–6.

33   Jones, C., Cummings, C., Ball, J. and Beighton, P., 'A clinical and ultrastructural study of osteogenesis imperfecta after flavonoid (Catergen) therapy', *S. Afr. Med. J.*, 1984, 66, pp. 907–10.

34   Pearce, F., Befus, A. and Bienenstock, J., 'Effect of quercetin and other flavonoids on antigen-induced histamine secretion from rat intestinal mast cells', *J. Allerg. Clin. Immunol.*, 1984, 73, pp. 819–23.

35   Busse, W., Kopp, D. and Middleton, E., 'Flavonoid modulation of human neutrophil function', *J. Allerg. Clin. Immunol.*, 1984, 73, pp. 801–9.

36   Vogel, R., Fink, R., Schneider, L., *et al.*, 'The effect of folic acid on gingival health', *J. Periodontal*, 1976, 47, pp. 667–8.

37   Vogel, R., Fink, R., Schneider, L., *et al.*, 'The effect of topical application of folic acid on gingival health', *J. Oral. Med.*, 1978, 33, pp. 20–2.

38   Pack, A. and Thomson, M., 'Effects of topical and systemic folic acid supplementation on gingivitis in pregnancy', *J. Clin. Periodontal*, 1980, 7, pp. 402–4.

39   Pack, A. and Thomson, M., 'Effects of extended systemic and topical folate supplementation on gingivitis of pregnancy', *J. Clin. Periodontal*, 1982, 9, pp. 275–80.

40   Pack, A., 'Folate mouthwash: effects on established gingivitis in periodontal patients', *J. Clin. Periodontal.*, 1984, 11, pp. 619–28.

41   Whitehead, N., Reyner, F. and Lindenbaum, J., 'Megaloblastic changes in the cervical epithelium associated with oral contraceptive therapy and reversal with folic acid', *J.A.M.A.*, 1973, 226, pp. 1,421–4.

42   da Costa, M. and Rothenberg, S., 'Appearance of folate binder in leukocytes and serum of women who are pregnant or taking oral contraceptives', *J. Lab. Clin. Med.*, 1974, 83, pp. 207–14.
43   Ringsdorf, W., Cheraskin, E. and Ramsay, R., 'Sucrose, neutrophil phagocytosis and resistance to disease', *Dent. Surv.*, 1976, 52, pp. 46–8.
44   Sanchez, A., Reeser, J., Lau, H. *et al.*, 'Role of sugars in human neutrophilic phagocytosis', *Am. J. Clin. Nutr.*, 1973, 26, pp. 1,180–4.
45   Gineste, M., de Grousaz, P., Duffort, J.F. *et al.*, 'Influence of 3-methoxy 5,7,3′4′-tetrahydroxyflavan (ME) on experimental periodontitis in the golden hamster', *J. Biol. Buccale*, 1984, 12, pp. 259–65.
46   Abbas, F., van der Velden, U. and Hart, A., 'Relation between wound healing after surgery and susceptibility to periodontal disease', *J. Clin. Periodontal.*, 1984, 11, pp. 221–9.

62 Premenstrual syndrome

1   Abraham, G.E., 'Nutritional factors in the etiology of the premenstrual tension syndromes', *J. Repro. Med.*, 1983, 28, pp. 446–64.
2   Piesse, J.W., 'Nutritional factors in the premenstrual syndrome', *Int. Clin. Nutr. Rev.*, 1984, 4, pp. 54–81.
3   Halbreich, U., Assael, M., Ben-David, M. and Bornstein, R., 'Serum-prolactin in women with premenstrual syndrome', *Lancet*, 1976, 2, pp. 654–6.
4   Griggs, M. and Briggs, M., 'Relationship between monoamine oxidase activity and sex hormone concentration in human blood plasma', *J. Repro. Fert.*, 1972, 28, pp. 447–50.
5   Schildkraut, J.J. and Kety, S.S., 'Biogenic amines and emotion', *Science*, 1967, 156, pp. 21–30.
6   Krause, M. and Mahan, C., *Food, Nutrition and Diet Therapy*, W.B. Saunders, Philadelphia, PA, 1984.
7   Lipton, M., Mailman, R. and Nemeroff, C., 'Vitamins, megavitamin therapy and the nervous system', in Wurtman, R. and Wurtman, J. (eds), *Nutrition and the Brain*, Raven Press, New York, NY, 1979, pp. 183–264.
8   O'Brien, P.M. and Symonds, E.M., 'Prolactin levels in the premenstrual syndrome', *Br. J. Obst. Gyn.*, 1982, 89, pp. 306–8.
9   Facchinetti, F., Nappi, G., Petraglia, A., *et al.*, 'Oestradiol/progesterone imbalance and the premenstrual syndrome', *Lancet*, 1983, ii, p. 1,302.
10   Walsh, C.H. and O'Sullivan, D.J., 'Studies of glucose tolerance, insulin and growth hormone secretion during the menstrual cycle in healthy women', *Irish J. Med. Sci.*, 1975, 144, pp. 18–24.
11   Horrobin, D.F., 'The role of essential fatty acids and prostaglandins in the premenstrual syndrome', *J. Repro. Med.*, 1983, 28, pp. 465–8.
12   Goei, G.S. and Abraham, G.E., 'Effect of nutritional supplement, Optivite, on symptoms of premenstrual tension', *J. Repro. Med.*, 1983, 28, pp. 527–31.
13   Biskind, M.S., 'Nutritional deficiency in the etiology of menorrhagia, metrorrhagia, cystic mastitis and premenstrual tension; treatment with vitamin B complex', *J. Clin. Endo. Met.*, 1943, 3, pp. 227–34.
14   Barr, W., 'Pyridoxine supplements in the premenstrual syndrome', *Practitioner*, 1984, 228, pp. 425–7.
15   Stokes, J. and Mendels, J., 'Pyridoxine and premenstrual tension', *Lancet*, 1972, i, p. 1,177.
16   Editor, 'Metabolism of beta-carotene by the bovine corpus luteum', *Nutr. Rev.*, 1983, 41, pp. 357–8.
17   London, R.S., Sundaram, G.S., Murphy, L. and Goldstein, P.J., 'Evaluation and treatment of breast symptoms in patients with the premenstrual syndrome', *J. Repro. Med.*, 1983, 28, pp. 503–8.
18   Goldin, B. and Gorsbach, S., 'The effect of milk and lactobacillus feeding on human intestinal bacterial enzyme activity', *Am. J. Clin. Nutr.*, 1984, 39, pp. 756–61.
19   Abraham, G.E. and Lubran, M.M., 'Serum and red cell magnesium levels in patients with premenstrual tension', *Am. J. Clin. Nutr.*, 1981, 34, pp. 2,364–6.
20   Abraham, G.E. and Hargrove, J.T., 'Effect of vitamin B_6 on premenstrual symptomatology in women with premenstrual tension syndromes: a double-blind crossover study', *Infert.*, 1980, 3, pp. 155–65.
21   Judd, A.M., Macleod, R.M. and Login, I.S., 'Zinc acutely, selectively and reversibly inhibits pituitary prolactin secretion', *Brain Res.*, 1984, 294, pp. 190–2.
22   Kappas, A., Anderson, K., Conney, A., *et al.*, 'Nutrition-endocrine interactions: induction of reciprocal changes in the delta-4-5-alpha-reduction of testosterone and the cytochrome p-450-dependent oxidation of estradiol by dietary macro-nutrients in man', *Proc. Natl. Acad. Sci.*, 1983, 80, pp. 7,646–9.
23   Pizzorno, J.E. and Murray, M.T., *A Textbook of Natural Medicine*, John Bastyr College Publications, Seattle, WA, 1985, p. VI:PreMns-1-5.
24   Leung, A., *Encyclopedia of Common Natural Ingredients Used in Food, Drugs and Cosmetics*, John Wiley & Sons, New York, NY, 1980, pp. 14,15.
25   Mitchell, M., *Naturopathic Applications of the Botanical Remedies*, John Bastyr College Publications, Seattle, WA, 1983, p. 77.
26   Hunter, R.G., Henry, G.W. and Henicke, R.M., 'The action of papain and bromelain on the uterus', *Am. J. Ob. Gyn.*, 1957, 73, pp. 867–80.
27   Felton, G., 'Does kinin released by pineapple stem bromelain stimulate production of prostaglandin E1-like compounds?', *Hawaii Med. J.*, 1977, 36, pp. 39–47.
28   Wagner, H., 'Plant constituents with antihepatotoxic activity', in Beal, J.L. and Reinhard, E. (eds), *Natural Products as Medicinal Agents*, Hippokrates-Verlag, Stuttgart, 1981.
29   Sarre, H., 'Experience in the treatment of chronic hepatopathies with silymarin', *Arzneim-Forsch.*, 1971, 21, pp. 1,209–12.
30   Reynolds, J.E. (ed.), *Martindale: The Extra Pharmacopoeia*, Pharmaceutical Press, London, 1982.

63 Prostate enlargement

1   Hinman, F., *Benign Prostatic Hyperplasia*, Springer-Verlag, New York, NY, 1983.
2   Horton, R., 'Benign prostatic hyperplasia: a disorder of androgen metabolism in the male', *J. Am. Geri. Soc.*, 1984, 32, pp. 380–5.
3   Judd, A.M., MacLeod, R.M. and Login, I.S., 'Zinc acutely, selectively and reversibly inhibits pituitary prolactin secretion', *Brain Res.*, 1984, 294, pp. 190–2.

4   Vescovi, P.P., Gerra, G., Rastelli, G., et al., 'Pyridoxine (vit. B$_6$) decreases opioids-induced hyperprolactinemia', Horm. Metabol. Res., 1985, 17, pp. 46–7.
5   Bush, I.M., et al., 'Zinc and the prostate', presented at the annual meeting of the A.M.A., 1974.
6   Fahim, M., Fahim, Z., Der, R. and Harman, J., 'Zinc treatment for the reduction of hyperplasia of the prostate', Fed. Proc., 1976, 35, p. 361.
7   Leake, A., Chisholm, G.D. and Habib, F.K., 'The effect of zinc on the 5-alpha-reduction of testosterone by the hyperplastic human prostate gland', J. Steroid Biochem., 1984, 20, pp. 651–5.
8   Wallace, A.M. and Grant, J.E., 'Effect of zinc on androgen metabolism in the human hyperplastic prostate', Biochem. Soc. Trans., 1975, 3, pp. 540–2.
9   Lahtonen, R., 'Zinc and cadmium concentrations in whole tissue and in separated epithelium and stroma from human benign prostatic hypertrophic glands', Prostate, 1985, 6, pp. 177–83.
10   Sinquin, G., Morfin, R.F., Charles, J.F. and Floch, H.H., 'Testosterone metabolism by homogenates of human prostates with benign hyperplasia: effects of zinc, cadmium, and other bivalent cations', J. Steroid Biochem., 1984, 20, pp. 733–80.
11   Leake, A., Chrisholm, G.D., Busuttil, A. and Habib, F.K., 'Subcellular distribution of zinc in the benign and malignant human prostate: evidence for a direct zinc androgen interaction', Acta Endocrinol., 1984, 105, pp. 281–8.
12   Login, I.S., Thorner, M.O. and MacLeod, R.M., 'Zinc may have a physiological role in regulating pituitary prolactin secretion', Neuroendocrinology, 1983, 37, pp. 317–20.
13   Evans, G.W., 'Normal and abnormal zinc absorption in man and animals: the tryptophan connection', Nutrition Reviews, 1980, 38, pp. 137–41.
14   Evans, G.W. and Johnson, E.C., 'Effect of iron, vitamin B-6 and picolinic acid on zinc absorption in the rat', Journal of Nutrition, 1981, 111, pp. 68–75.
15   Krieger, I., Cash, R. and Evans, G.W., 'Picolinic acid in acrodermatitis enteropathica: evidence for a disorder of tryptophan metabolism', Journal of Pediatric Gastroenterology and Nutrition, 1984, 3, pp. 62–8.
16   Boosalis, M.G., Evans, G.W. and McClain, C.J., 'Impaired handling of orally administered zinc in pancreatic insufficiency', American Journal of Clinical Nutrition, 1983, 37, pp. 268–71.
17   Hart, J.P. and Cooper, W.L., Vitamin F in the Treatment of Prostatic Hyperplasia, Report number 1, Lee Foundation for Nutritional Research, Milwaukee, WI, 1941.
18   Scott, W.W., 'The lipids of the prostatic fluid, seminal plasma and enlarged prostate gland of man', J. Urol., 1945, 53, pp. 712–18.
19   Boyd, E.M. and Berry, N.E., 'Prostatic hypertrophy as part of a generalized metabolic disease. Evidence of the presence of a lipopenia', J. Urol., 1939, 41, pp. 406–11.
20   Dumrau, F., 'Benign prostatic hyperplasia: amino acid therapy for symptomatic relief', Am. J. Ger., 1962, 10, pp. 426–30.
21   Feinblatt, H.M. and Gant, J.C., 'Palliative treatment of benign prostatic hypertrophy: value of glycine, alanine, glutamic acid combination', J. Maine Med. Assoc., 1958, 49, pp. 99–102.
22   Ask-Upmark, E., 'Prostatitis and its treatment', Acta Med. Scand., 1967, 181, pp. 355–7.
23   Carilla, E., Briley, M., Fauran, F., et al., 'Binding of Permixon, a new treatment for prostatic benign hyperplasia, to the cytosolic androgen receptor in the rat prostate', J. Steroid Biochem., 1984, 20, pp. 521–3.
24   Champlault, G., Patel, J.C. and Bonnard, A.M., 'A double-blind trial of an extract of the plant Serenoa repens in benign prostatic hyperplasia', Br. J. Clin. Pharmacol., 1984, 18, pp. 461–2.
25   Tasca, A., Barulli, M., Cavazzana, A., et al., 'Treatment of obstructive symptomatology caused by prostatic adenoma with an extract of Serenoa repens. Double-blind clinical study vs. placebo', Minerva Urol. Nefrol., 1985, 37, pp. 87–91.
26   Boccafoschi, C. and Annoscia, S., 'Comparison of Serenoa repens extract with placebo by controlled clinical trial in patients with prostatic adenomatosis', Urologia, 1983, 50, pp. 1,257–9.
27   Fahim, W.S., Harman, J.M., Clevenger, T.E., et al., 'Effect of Panax ginseng on testosterone level and prostate in male rats', Arch. Androl., 1982, 8, pp. 261–3.
28   Ohkoshi, M., Kawamura, N. and Nagakubo, I., 'Clinical evaluation of Cernilton in chronic prostatitis', Jap. J. Clin. Urol., 1967, 21, pp. 73–85.
29   Saito, Y., Diagnosis and treatment of chronic prostatitis with special reference to experience with Cernilton', Clin. Exp. Med., 1967, 44, pp. 387–93.

64 Psoriasis

1   Voorhees, J. and Duell, E., 'Imbalanced cyclic AMP–cyclic GMP levels in psoriasis', Advances in Cyclic Nucleotide Research, 1975, 5, pp. 755–7.
2   Robbins, S. and Cotran, R., Pathological Basis of Disease, W.B. Saunders & Co., Philadelphia, PA, 1979, p. 1,449.
3   Proctor, M., Wilkenson, D., Orenberg, E., et al., 'Lowered cutaneous and urinary levels of polyamines with clinical improvement in treated psoriasis', Arch. Dermatol., 1979, 115, pp. 945–9.
4   Editorial, 'Polyamines and psoriasis', Arch. Dermatol., 1979, 115, p. 943–4.
5   Editorial, 'Polyamines in psoriasis', J. Invest. Dermatol., 1983, 81, pp. 385–7.
6   Haddox, M., Frassir, K. and Russel, D., 'Retinol inhibition of ornithine decarboxylase induction and G1 progression in CHD cells', Cancer Research, 1979, 39, pp. 4,930–8.
7   Kuwano, S. and Yamauchi, K., 'Effect of berberine on tyrosine decarboxylase activity of Streptococcus faecalis', Chem. Pharm. Bull., 1960, 8, pp. 491–6.
8   Rosenberg, E. and Belew, P., 'Microbial factors in psoriasis', Arch. Dermatol., 1982, 118, pp. 1,434–44.
9   Rao, M. and Field, M., 'Enterotoxins and anti-oxidants', Biochem. Soc. Trans., 1984, 12, pp. 177–80.
10   Thurmon, F.M., 'The treatment of psoriasis with sarsaparilla compound', N.E.J.M., 1942, 227, pp. 128–33.
11   Weber, G. and Galle, K., 'The liver, a therapeutic target in dermatoses', Med. Welt, 1983, 34, pp. 108–11.
12   Monk, B.E. and Neill, S.M., 'Alcohol consumption and psoriasis', Dermatologica, 1986, 173, pp. 57–60.
13   Hikino, H., Kiso, Y., Wagner, H. and Fiebig, M., 'Antihepatotoxic actions of flavanolignans from Silybum marianum fruits', Planta Medica, 1984, 50, pp. 248–50.
14   Adzet, T., 'Polyphenolic compounds with biological and pharmacological activity', Herbs Spices Medicinal Plants, 1986, 1, pp. 167–84.
15   Chafin, A., Vesley D., Hudson, J., et al., 'Inhibition of growth and guanylate cyclase activity of undifferentiated prostate adenocarcinoma by

an extract of balsam pear (Momardica charantia abbreviata)', *Proc. Natl. Acad. Sci.*, 1978, 75, pp. 989–93

16 Haddox, M. Stephenson, J., Moser, M., *et al.*, 'Ascorbic acid modulation of splenic cell cyclic GMP metabolism', *Life Sciences*, 1979, 24, pp. 1,555–6.

17 Rainsford, K.D., Brune, K. and Whitehouse, M.W., 'Trace elements in the pathogenesis of inflammation', *Agents and Actions*, Suppl. 8, 1981, pp. 164–72.

18 Donadini, A., Dazzaglia, A. and Desirello, G., 'Plasma levels of Zn, Cu and Ni in healthy controls and in psoriatic patients', *Acta Vitamin Enzymol.*, 1980, 1, pp. 9–16.

19 Fratino, P., Pelfini, C., Jucci, A. and Bellazi, R., 'Glucose and insulin in psoriasis: the role of obesity and genetic history', *Panminerva Medica*, 1979, 21, p. 167.

20 Juhlin, L., Bedquist, L., Echman, G., *et al.*, 'Blood glutathione-peroxide levels in skin diseases: effect of selenium and vitamin E treatment', *Acta Dermat. Vener.*, 1982, 62, pp. 211–14.

21 Lithell, H., Bruce, A., Gustafsson, B., *et al.*, 'A fasting and vegetarian diet treatment trial on chronic inflammatory disorders', *Acta Derm. Vener.*, 1983, 63, pp. 397–403.

22 Bazex, A., 'Diet without gluten and psoriasis', *Ann. Derm. Symp.*, 1976, 103, p. 648.

23 Bittiner, S.B., Tucker, W.F.G., Cartwright, I. and Bleehen, S.S., 'A double-blind, randomized, placebo-controlled trial of fish oil in psoriasis', *Lancet*, 1988, i, pp. 378–80.

24 Ziboh, V.A., Cohen, K.A., Ellis, C.N., *et al.*, 'Effects of dietary supplementation of fish oil on neutrophil and epidermal fatty acids', *Arch. Dermatol.*, 1986, 122, pp. 1,277–82.

25 Maurice, P.D.L., Allen, B.R., Barkley, A.S.J., *et al.*, 'The effects of dietary supplementation with fish oil in patients with psoriasis', *Brit. J. Dermatol.*, 1987, 117, pp. 599–606.

26 Seville, R.H., 'Psoriasis and stress', *Br. J. Dermatol.*, 1977, 97, p. 297.

27 Winchell, S.A. and Watts, R.A., 'Relaxation therapies in the treatment of psoriasis and possible pathophysiologic mechanisms', *J. Am. Acad. Dermatol.*, 1988, 18, pp. 101–4.

28 Parrish, J. 'Phototherapy and photochemotherapy of skin diseases', *J. Invest. Dermatol.*, 1981, 77, pp. 167–71.

29 Larko, O. and Swanbeck, G., 'Is UVB treatment of psoriasis safe?', *Acta Dermat. Vener.*, 1982, 62, pp. 507–12.

30 Boer, J., Hermans, J., Schothorst, A. and Suurmond, D., 'Comparison of phototherapy (UV-B) and photochemotherapy (PUVA) for clearing and maintenance therapy of psoriasis', *Arch. Dermatol.*, 1984, 120, pp. 52–7.

31 Katayama, H. and Hori, H., 'The influence of UVB irradiation on the excretion of the main urinary metabolite of prostaglandin F1a and F2a in psoriatic and normal subjects', *Acta Dermatol. Vener.*, 1984, 64, pp. 1–4.

32 Urabe, H., Nishitani, K. and Kohda, H., 'Hyperthermia in the treatment of psoriasis', *Arch. Dermatol.*, 1981, 117, pp. 770–4.

33 Orenberg, E., Deneau, D. and Farber, E., 'Response of chronic psoriatic plaques to localised heating induced by ultrasound', *Arch. Dermatol.*, 1980, 116, pp. 893–70.

65 Rheumatoid arthritis

1 Petersdorf, R., *et al.* (eds), *Harrison's Principles of Internal Medicine*, McGraw-Hill, New York, NY, 1983, pp. 1,977–86.

2 Krupp, M.A. and Chatton, M.J. (eds), *Current Medical Treatment and Diagnosis*, Lange Medical Publications, Los Altos, CA, 1982, pp. 487–91.

3 Smith, M.D., Gibson, R.A. and Brooks, P.M., 'Abnormal bowel permeability in ankylosing spondylitis and rheumatoid arthritis', *Journal of Rheumatology*, 1985, 12, pp. 299–305.

4 Zaphiropoulos, G.C., 'Rheumatoid arthritis and the gut', *British Journal of Rheumatology*, 1986, 25, pp. 138–40.

5 Segal, A.W., Isenberg, D.A., Hajirousou, V., *et al.*, 'Preliminary evidence for gut involvement in the pathogenesis of rheumatoid arthritis', *British Journal of Rheumatology*, 1986, 25, pp. 162–6.

6 McCrae, F., Veerapen, K. and Dieppe, P., 'Diet and arthritis', *Practitioner*, 1986, 230, pp. 359–61.

7 Darlington, L.G., Ramsey, N.W. and Mansfield, J.R., 'Placebo-controlled, blind study of dietary manipulation therapy in rheumatoid arthritis', *Lancet*, 1986, i, pp. 236–8.

8 Hicklin, J.A., McEwen, L.M. and Morgan, J.E., 'The effect of diet in rheumatoid arthritis', *Clinical Allergy*, 1980, 10, pp. 463–7.

9 Panush, R.S., 'Delayed reactions to foods. Food allergy and rheumatic disease', *Annals of Allergy*, 1986, 56, pp. 500–3.

10 Lucas, P. and Power, L., 'Dietary fat aggravates active rheumatoid arthritis', *Clinical Research*, 1981, 29, p. 754A.

11 Ziff, M., 'Diet in the treatment of rheumatoid arthritis', *Arthritis Rheumatism*, 1983, 26, pp. 457–61.

12 Lindahl, O., Lindwall, L., Spangberg, A., *et al.*, 'Vegan diet regimen with reduced medication in the treatment of bronchial asthma', *Journal of Asthma*, 1985, 22, pp. 45–55.

13 Kremer, J., Michaelek, A.V., Lininger, L., *et al.*, 'Effects of manipulation of dietary fatty acids on clinical manifestation of rheumatoid arthritis', *Lancet*, 1985, i, pp. 184–7.

14 Lee, T.H. and Arm, J.P., 'Prospects for modifying the allergic response by fish oil diets', *Clinical Allergy*, 1986, 16, pp. 89–100.

15 Terano, T., Salmon, J.A., Higgs, G.A. and Moncada, S., 'Eicosapentaenoic acid as a modulator of inflammation, effect on prostaglandin and leukotriene synthesis', *Biochemical Pharmacology*, 1986, 35, pp. 779–85.

16 Bruch, C.A. and Johnson, E.T., 'A new dietary regimen for arthritis, value of cod liver oil on a fasting stomach', *Journal of the National Medical Association*, 1959, 51, pp. 266–70.

17 Skoldstam, L., Larsson, L. and Lindstrom, F.D., 'Effects of fasting and lactovegetarian diet on rheumatoid arthritis', *Scandinavian Journal of Rheumatology*, 1979, 8, pp. 249–55.

18 Kroker, G.P., Stroud, R.M., Marshall, R.T., *et al.*, 'Fasting and rheumatoid arthritis: a multicenter study', *Clinical Ecology*, 1984, 2, pp. 137–44.

19 Tarp, U., Overvad, K., Hansen, J.C. and Thorling, E.B., 'Low selenium level in severe rheumatoid arthritis', *Scandinavian Journal of Rheumatology*, 1985, 14, pp. 97–101.

20 Tarp, U., Overvad, K., Thorling, E.B., Hansen, J.C. and Graudal, H., 'Selenium treatment in rheumatoid arthritis', *Scandinavian Journal of Rheumatology*, 1985, 14, pp. 364–8.

21 Munthe, E. and Aseth, J., 'Treatment of rheumatoid arthritis with selenium and vitamin E', *Scandinavian Journal of Rheumatology*, 1984, 53 (suppl.), p. 103.

REFERENCES

22 Panganamala, R.V. and Cornwell, D.G., 'The effects of vitamin E on arachidonic acid metabolism', *Annals of the New York Academy of Sciences*, 1982, 393, pp. 376–91.

23 Pandley, S.P., Bhattacharya, S.K. and Sundar, S., 'Zinc in rheumatoid arthritis', *Indian Journal of Medical Research*, 1985, 81, pp. 618–20.

24 Simkin, P.A., 'Treatment of rheumatoid arthritis with oral zinc sulfate', *Agents and Actions* (supplement), 1981, 8, pp. 587–95.

25 Mattingly, P.C. and Mowat, A.G., 'Zinc sulphate in rheumatoid arthritis', *Annals of the Rheumatic Diseases*, 1982, 41, pp. 456–7.

26 Pasquier, C., Mach, P.S., Raichvarg, D., *et al.*, 'Manganese-containing superoxide-dismutase deficiency in polymorphonuclear leukocytes of adults with rheumatoid arthritis', *Inflammation*, 1984, 8, pp. 27–32.

27 Rosa, G.D., Keen, C.L., Leach, R.M. and Hurley, L.S., 'Regulation of superoxide dismutase activity by dietary manganese', *Journal of Nutrition*, 1980, 110, pp. 795–804.

28 Subramanian, N., 'Histamine degradation potential of ascorbic acid', *Agents and Actions*, 1978, 8, pp. 484–7.

29 Levine, M., 'New concepts in the biology and biochemistry of ascorbic acid', *New England Journal of Medicine*, 1986, 314, pp. 892–902.

30 De Witte, T.J., Geerdink, P.J., Lamers, C.B., *et al.*, 'Hypochlorhydria and hypergastrinemia in rheumatoid arthritis', *Annals of the Rheumatic Diseases*, 1979, 38, pp. 14–17.

31 Henriksson, K., Uvnas-Moberg, K., Nord, C.E., *et al.*, 'Gastrin, gastric acid secretion, and gastric microflora in patients with rheumatoid arthritis', *Annals of the Rheumatic Diseases*, 1986, 45, pp. 475–83.

32 Cohen, A. and Goldman, J., 'Bromelains therapy in rheumatoid arthritis', *Pennsylvania Medical Journal*, 1964, 67, pp. 27–30.

33 Taussig, S., 'The mechanism of the physiological action of bromelain', *Medical Hypothesis*, 1980, 6, pp. 99–104.

34 Ransberger, K., 'Enzyme treatment of immune complex diseases', *Arthritis Rheuma*. 1986, 8, pp. 16–19.

35 Amella, M., Bronner, C., Briancon, F., *et al.*, 'Inhibition of mast cell histamine release by flavonoids and bioflavonoids', *Planta Medica*, 1985, 51, pp. 16–20.

36 Middleton, E., 'The flavonoids', *Trends in Pharmaceutical Science*, 1984, 5, pp. 335–8.

37 Tarayre, J.P. and Lauressergues, H., 'Advantages of a combination of proteolytic enzymes, flavonoids and ascorbic acid in comparison with non-steroidal anti-inflammatory agents', *Arzneim-Forsch.*, 1977, 27, pp. 1,144–9.

38 Bonica, J., Lindblom, U. and Iggo, A. (eds), *Advances in Pain Research and Therapy*, vol. 5, Raven Press, New York, NY, 1983.

39 Kaufman, W., *The Common Form of Joint Dysfunction: Its Incidence and Treatment*, E.L. Hildreth, Brattleboro, VT, 1949.

40 Hoffer, A. 'Treatment of arthritis by nicotinic acid and nicotinamide', *Canadian Medical Association Journal*, 1959, 81, pp. 235–9.

41 Seltzer, S., Dewart, D., Pollack, R. and Jackson, E., 'The effects of dietary tryptophan on chronic maxillofacial pain and experimental pain tolerance', *Journal of Psychiatric Research*, 1982, 17, pp. 181–6.

42 Seltzer, S., 'Pain relief by dietary manipulation and tryptophan supplements', *Journal of Endodontics*, 1985, 11, pp. 449–53.

43 Sorenson, J.R.J. and Hangarter, W., 'Treatment of rheumatoid and degenerative disease with copper complexes: a review with emphasis on copper salicylate', *Inflammation*, 1977, 2, pp. 217–38.

44 Lewis, A.J., 'The role of copper in inflammatory disorders', *Agents and Actions*, 1984, 15, pp. 513–19.

45 Walker, R.W., and Keats, D.M., 'An investigation of the therapeutic value of the "copper bracelet" – dermal assimilation of copper in arthritic/rheumatoid conditions', *Agents and Actions*, 1976, 6, pp. 454–8.

46 Chung, M.H., Kessner, L. and Chan, P.C., 'Degradation of articular cartilage by copper and hydrogen peroxide', *Agents and Actions*, 1984, 15, pp. 328–35.

47 Menander-Huber, K.B., 'Orgotein in the treatment of rheumatoid arthritis', *European Journal of Rheumatology and Inflammation*, 1981, 4, pp. 201–11.

48 Zidenberg-Cherr, S., Keen, C.L., Lonnerdal, B. and Hurley, L.S., 'Dietary superoxide dismutase does not affect tissue levels', *American Journal of Clinical Nutrition*, 1983, 37, pp. 5–7.

49 Capasso, F., 'The effect of an aqueous extract of Tanacetum parthenium L. on arachidonic acid metabolism by rat peritoneal leucocytes', *Journal of Pharmacy and Pharmacology*, 1986, 38, pp. 71–2.

60 Makheja, A.M. and Bailey, J.M., 'A platelet phospholipase inhibitor from the medicinal herb feverfew (Tanacetum parthenum)', *Prostaglandins, Leukotrienes and Medicine*, 1982, 8, pp. 653–60.

51 Heptinstall, S., White, A., Williamson, L. and Mitchell, J.R.A., 'Extracts of feverfew inhibit granule secretion in blood platelets and plymorphonuclear leucocytes', *Lancet*, 1985, i, pp. 1,071–4.

52 Duke, J.A., *Handbook of Medicinal Herbs*, C.R.C. Press, Boca Raton, FL, 1985.

53 Leung, A.Y., *Encyclopedia of Common Natural Ingredients Used in Food, Drugs, and Cosmetics*, John Wiley & Sons, New York, NY, 1980.

54 Whitehouse, L.W., Znamirowski, M. and Paul, C.J., 'Devil's claw (Harpagophytum procumbens): no evidence for anti-inflammatory activity in the treatment of arthritic disease', *Canadian Medical Association Journal*, 1983, 129, pp. 249–51.

55 McLeod, D.W., Revell, P. and Robinson, B.V., 'Investigations of Harpagophytum procumbens (Devil's claw) in the treatment of experimental inflammation and arthritis in the rat', *British Journal of Pharmacology*, 1979, 66, pp. 140P–141P.

56 Gabor, M., 'Pharmacologic effects of flavonoids on blood vessels', *Angiologica*, 1972, 9, pp. 355–74.

57 Kuhnau, J., 'The flavonoids. A class of semi-essential food components: their role in human nutrition', *World Review Nutrition and Dietetics*, 1976, 24, pp. 117–91.

58 Havsteen, B., 'Flavonoids, a class of natural products of high pharmacological potency', *Biochemical Pharmacology*, 1983, 32, pp. 1,141–8.

59 Shimizu, K., Amagaya, S. and Ogihara, Y., 'Combination of shosaikoto (Chinese traditional medicine) and prednisolone on the anti-inflammatory action', *J. of Pharmaco. Dyn.*, 1984, 7, pp. 891–9.

60 Yamamoto, M., Kumagai, A. and Yokoyama, Y., 'Structure and actions of saikosaponins isolated from Bupleurum falcatum L.', *Arzniem-Forsch.*, 1975, 25, pp. 1,021–40.

61 Hiai, S., Yokoyama, H., Nagasawa, T. and Oura, H., 'Stimulation of the pituitary-adrenocortical axis by saikosaponin of Bupleuri radix', *Chem. Pharm. Bull.*, 1981, 29, pp. 495–9.

62 Cyong, J., 'A pharmacological study of the anti-inflammatory activity of Chinese herbs. A review', *Acupunct. Electro-Ther.*, 1982, 7, pp. 173–202.

63 Hikino, H., 'Recent research on Oriental medicinal plants', *Economic and Medicinal Plant Research*, 1985, 1, pp. 53–85.

64 Kumagai, A., Nanaboshi, M., Asanuma, Y., *et al.*, 'Effects of glycyrrhizin on thymolytic and immunosuppressive action of cortisone', *Endocrinol. Japan*, 1967, 14, pp. 39–42.

65 Srimal, R. and Dhawan, B., 'Pharmacology of diferuloyl methane (curcumin), a nonsteroidal anti-inflammatory agent', *J. Pharm. Pharmac.*, 1973, 25, pp. 447–52.

66 Mukhopadhyay, A., Basu, N., Ghatak, N. and Gujral, P., 'Anti-inflammatory and irritant activities of curcumin analogues in rats', *Agents Actions*, 1982, 12, pp. 508–15.

67   Ghatak, N. and Basu, N., 'Sodium curcuminate as an effective anti-inflammatory agent', *Ind. J. Exp. Biol.*, 1972, 10, pp. 235–6.
68   Shibata, S., Tanaka, O., Shoji, J. and Saito, H., 'Chemistry and pharmacology of Panax', *Economic and Medicinal Plant Research*, 1985, 1, pp. 217–84.
69   Baranov, A.I., 'Medicinal uses of ginseng and related plants in the Soviet Union: recent trends in the Soviet literature', *J. Ethnopharmacology*, 1982, 6, pp. 339–53.
70   Farnsworth, N.R., Kinghorn, A.D., Soejarto, D.D. and Waller, D.P., 'Siberian ginseng (Eleutherococcus senticosus): current status as an adaptogen', *Economic and Medicinal Plant Research*, 1985, 1, pp. 156–215.
71   Lewis, W.H. and Elvin-Lewis, M.P., *Medical Botany*, John Wiley & Sons, New York, NY, 1977.
72   Kubo, M., Matsuda, H., Tanaka, M., *et al.*, 'Studies on Scutellariae radix. VII. Anti-arthritic and anti-inflammatory actions of methanolic extract and flavonoid components from Scutellaria radix', *Chem. Pharm. Bull.*, 1984, 32, pp. 2,724–9.
73   Kimura, Y., Okuda, H. and Arichi, S., 'Studies on Scutellariae radix. VIII. Effects of various flavonoids on arachidonate metabolism in leukocytes', *Planta Medica*, 1985, 54, pp. 132–6.

66 Rosacea

1   Ryle, J. and Barber, H., 'Gastric analysis in acne rosacea', *Lancet*, 1920, ii, pp. 1,195–6.
2   Poole, W., 'Effect of vitamin B complex and S-factor on acne rosacea', *S. Med. J.*, 1957, 50, pp. 207–10.
3   Barba, A., Rosa, B., Angelini, G., *et al.*, 'Pancreatic exocrine function in rosacea', *Dermatologica*, 1982, 165, pp. 601–6.
4   Tulipan, L., 'Acne rosacea: a vitamin B complex deficiency', *N.Y. State J. Med.*, 1929, 29, pp. 1,063–4.
5   Johnson, L. and Eckardt, R., 'Rosacea keratitis and conditions with vascularization of the cornea treated with riboflavin', *Arch. Ophth.*, 1940, 23, p. 899.

67 Seborrhoeic dermatitis

1   Eppic, J., 'Seborrhea capitis in infants: a clinical experience in allergy therapy', *Ann. Allergy*, 1971, 29, pp. 323–4.
2   Nisenson, A., 'Seborrheic dermatitis of infants and Leiner's disease: a biotin deficiency', *J. Ped.*, 1957, 51, pp. 537–49.
3   Nisenson, A., 'Treatment of seborrheic dermatitis with biotin and vitamin B complex', *J. Ped.*, 1972, 81, pp. 630–1.
4   Schreiner, A., Slinger, W., Hawkins, V., *et al.*, 'Seborrheic dermatitis: a local metabolic defect involving pyridoxine', *J. Lab. Clin. Med.*, 1952, 40, pp. 121–30.
5   Effersoe, H., 'The effect of topical application of pyridoxine ointment on the rate of sebaceous secretion in patients with seborrheic dermatitis', *Acta Dermatol.*, 1954, 3, pp. 272–7.
6   Callaghan, T., 'The effect of folic acid on seborrheic dermatitis', *Cutis*, 1967, 3, pp. 584–8.
7   Andrews, G., Post, C. and Domonkos, A., 'Seborrheic dermatitis: supplemental treatment with vitamin B12', *N.Y. State J.M.*, 1950, 50, pp. 1,921–5.
8   Bicknell, F. and Prescott, F., *The Vitamins in Medicine*, Lee Foundation for Nutritional Research, WI, 1962, p. 309.

68 Sinus infection

1   Yerushalmi, A., Karman, S. and Lwoff, A., 'Treatment of perennial allergic rhinitis by local hyperthermia', *Proc. Natl Acad. Sci.*, 1982, 79, pp. 4,766–9.
For references on botanical and nutritional recommendations, see Chapter 6, Immune support.

69 Sore throat

1   Editorial, 'Study links bacterial cause to 40 per cent of pharyngitis cases', *Am. Fam. Phy.*, 1983, 29, pp. 336–8.
2   Braude, A., *Medical Microbiology and Infectious Diseases*, W.B. Saunders, Philadelphia, PA, 1981, p. 816.
3   Bridges-Webb, C., Darvas, G. and Miller, L., 'Sore throat', *Aust. Fam. Phys.*, 1981, 10, pp. 510–15.
4   Rubenstein, E. and Federman, D.D., *Scientific American Medicine*, Scientific American, New York, NY, 1984, p. 7:I:9.
5   McKowen, T., *The Role of Medicine: Dream, Mirage, or Nemesis?*, Nuffield Provincial Hospitals Trust, London, 1975.
6   Brook, I., 'Treatment of group A streptococcal pharyngotonsillitis', *J.A.M.A.*, 1982, 247, p. 2,496.
7   Rinehart, J.F., 'Studies relating vitamin C deficiency to rheumatic fever and rheumatoid arthritis. Experimental, clinical, and general considerations. I. Rheumatic fever', *Ann. Int. Med.*, 1935, 9, pp. 586–99.
8   Rinehart, J.F., 'Studies relating vitamin C deficiency to rheumatic fever and rheumatoid arthritis: experimental, clinical, and general considerations. II. Rheumatoid (atrophic) arthritis', *Ann. Int. Med.*, 1935, 9, pp. 671–89.
9   Reichenberg, J., 'A scientific basis for the active principle of garlic (allium sativum) and its use as a hypocholesterolemic and antibacterial/ antifungal agent', *J. John Bastyr Col. Nat. Med.*, 1980, 2, pp. 28–32.
10   Lau, B. and Adetumbi, M., 'Allium sativum (garlic) – a natural antibiotic', *Med. Hypoth.*, 1983, 12, pp. 227–37.
11   Hahn, F. and Ciak, J., 'Berberine', *Antibiotics*, 1976, 3, pp. 577–84.

70 Tendinitis and bursitis

1   Southmayd, W. and Hoffman, M., *Sports Health: The Complete Book of Athletic Injuries*, Putman, New York, NY, 1981.
2   Carranza, F., *Glickman's Clinical Periodontology*, W.B. Saunders, Philadelphia, PA, 1984.
3   Krause, M. and Mahan, L., *Food, Nutrition and Diet Therapy*, W.B. Saunders, Philadelphia, PA, 1984.
4   Burton. G. and Ingold. K., 'Beta-carotene: an unusual type of lipid antioxidant', *Science*, 1984, 224, pp. 569–73.
5   Prasad, A., 'Clinical, biochemical and nutritional spectrum of zinc deficiency in human subjects: an update', *Nutr. Rev.*, 1983, 41, pp. 197–208.
6   Kim, J. and Shklar, G., 'The effect of vitamin E on the healing of gingival wounds in rats', *J. Periodontal.*, 1983, 54, pp. 305–8.
7   Havsteen, B., 'Flavonoids, a class of natural products of high pharmacological potency', *Biochem. Pharmacol.*, 1983, 32, pp. 1,141–8.
8   Yoshimoto, T., Furukawa, M., Yamamoto, S., *et al.*, 'Flavonoids: potent inhibitors of arachidonate 5-lipoxygenase', *Biochem. Biophys. Res. Commun.*, 1983, 116, pp. 612–18.
9   Amella, M., Bronner, C., Briancon, F., *et al.*, 'Inhibition of mast cell histamine release by flavonoids and bioflavonoids', *Planta Medica*, 1985, 51, pp. 16–20.
10 Middleton, E., 'The flavonoids', *Trends Pharmaceut. Sci.*, 1984, 5, pp. 335–8.
11 Miller, M.J., 'Injuries to athletes', *Med. Times*, 1960, 88, pp. 313–14.
12 Cragin, R.B., 'The use of bioflavonoids in the prevention and treatment of athletic injuries', *Med. Times*, 1962, 90, pp. 529–30.
13 Klemes, I.S., 'Vitamin B12 in acute subdeltoid bursitis', *Indust. Med. Surg.*, 1957, 26, pp. 290–2.
14 Pizzorno, J.E. and Murray, M.T., *A Textbook of Natural Medicine*, John Bastyr College Publications, Seattle, WA, 1985, V:Curcumin.
15 Chandra, D. and Gupta, S., 'Anti-inflammatory and anti-arthritic activity of volatile oil of curcuma longa (Haldi)', *Ind. J. Med. Res.*, 1972, 60, pp. 138–42.
16 Arora, R., Basu, N. Kapoor, V. and Jain, A., 'Anti-inflammatory studies on curcuma longa (turmeric)', *Ind. J. Med. Res.*, 1971, 59, pp. 1,289–95.
17 Srimal, R. and Dhawan, B., 'Pharmacology of diferuloyl methane (curcumin), a non-steroidal anti-inflammatory agent', *J. Pharm. Pharmac.*, 1973, 25, pp. 447–52.
18 Mukhopadhyay, VA., Basu, N., Ghatak, N. and Gujral, P., 'Anti-inflammatory and irritant activities of curcumin analogues in rats', *Agents Actions*, 1982, 12, pp. 508–15.
19 Ghatak, N. and Basu, N., 'Sodium curcuminate as an effective anti-inflammatory agent', *Ind. J. Exp. Biol.*, 1972, 10, pp. 235–6.
20 Tassman, G., Zafran, J. and Zayon, G., 'Evaluation of a plant proteolytic enzyme for the control of inflammation and pain', *J. Dent. Med.*, 1964, 19, pp. 73–7.
21 Tassman, G., Zafran, J. and Zayon, G., 'A double-blind crossover study of a plant proteolytic enzyme in oral surgery', *J. Dent. Med.*, 1965, 20, pp. 51–4.
22 Howat, R. and Lewis, G., 'The effect of bromelain therapy on episiotomy wounds – a double blind controlled clinical trial', *J. Ob. Gyn. Br. Commonwealth*, 1972, 79, pp. 951–3.
23 Zatuchni, G. and Colombi, D., 'Bromelains therapy for the prevention of episiotomy pain', *Ob. Gyn.*, 1967, 29, pp. 275–8.
24 Krusen, F.H., Kottke, F.J. and Ellwood, P.M., *Handbook of Physical Medicine and Rehabilitation*, W.B. Saunders, Philadelphia, PA, 1971, pp. 297–321.

71 Ulcers

1   Guslandi, M., 'Importance of defensive factors in the prevention of peptic ulcer recurrence', *Acta Gastro-Enterologica Belgica*, 1983, 46, pp. 411–18.
2   Petersdorf, R., *Harrison's Principles of Internal Medicine*, 10th ed., McGraw-Hill, New York, NY, 1983.
3   Siegel, J., 'Gastrointestinal ulcer – Arthus reaction!', *Ann. Allergy*, 1974, 32, pp. 127–30.
4   Andre, C., Moulinier, B., Andre, F. and Daniere, S., 'Evidence for anaphylactic reactions in peptic ulcer and varioliform gastritis', *Ann. Allergy*, 1983, 51, pp. 325–8.
5   Siegel, J., 'Immunologic approach to the treatment and prevention of gastrointestinal ulcers', *Ann. Allergy*, 1977, 38, pp. 27–9.
6   Rebhun, J., 'Duodenal ulceration in allergic children', *Ann. Allergy*, 1975, 34, pp. 145–9.
7   Rydning, A., Berstad, A., Aadland, E. and Odegaard, B., 'Prophylactic effects of dietary fibre in duodenal ulcer disease', *Lancet*, 1982, ii, pp. 736–9.
8   Rubenstein, E. and Federman, D.D., *Scientific American Medicine*, Scientific American, New York, NY, 1985, p. 4:II:3.
9   Schumpelik, V.V. and Farthmann, E., 'Untersuchung zur protektiven wirkung von vitamin A beim stressulkus der ratte', *Arz.-For. (Drug Res.)*, 1976, 20, p. 386.
10 Harris P.L., Hove, E.L., Mellott, M. and Hickman, K., 'Dietary production of gastric ulcers in rats and prevention by tocopherol administration', *Proc. Soc. Exp. Biol. Med.*, 1947, 4, pp. 273–7.
11 Muller-Lissner, S.A., 'Bile reflux is increased in cigarette smokers', *Gastroenterol.*, 1986, 90, pp. 1,205–9.
12 Formmer, D.J., 'The healing of gastric ulcers by zinc sulphate', *Med. J. Austr.*, 1975, 2, p. 793.
13 Feldman, E.J. and Sabovich, K.A., 'Stress and peptic ulcer disease', *Gastroenterol.*, 1980, 78, pp. 1,087–9.
14 Doll, R., Hill, I., Hutton, C. and Underwood, D., 'Clinical trial of a triterpenoid liquorice compound in gastric and duodenal ulcer', *Lancet*, 1962, ii, pp. 793–6.
15 Reed, P., Vincent-Brown, A., Cook, P., *et al.*, 'Comparative study on carbenoxolone and cimetidine in the management of duodenal ulcer', *Acta Gastro-Enterologica*, 1983, 46, pp. 459–68.
16 Johnson, B. and McIsaac, R., 'Effect of some anti-ulcer agents on mucosal blood flow', *Br. J. Pharmacol.*, 1981, i, p. 308.
17 Rees, W.D.W., Rhodes, J., Wright, J.E., *et al.*, 'Effect of deglycyrrhizinated liquorice on gastric mucosal damage by aspirin', *Scand. J. Gastroent.*, 1979, 14, pp. 605–7.
18 Turpie, A.G., Runcie, J. and Thomson, T.J., 'Clinical trial of deglycyrrhizinate liquorice in gastric ulcer', *Gut*, 1969, 10, pp. 299–303.
19 Montgomery, R.D. and Cookson, J.B., 'The treatment of gastric ulcer. A comparative trial of carbenoxolone and a deglycyrrhizinated liquorice preparation (Caved-S)', *Clinical Trials Journal*, 1972, 1, pp. 33–8.

20 Morgan, A.G., McAdam, W.A.F., Pacsoo, C. and Darnborough, A., 'Comparison between cimetidine and Caved-S in the treatment of gastric ulceration, and subsequent maintenance therapy', *Gut*, 1982, 23, pp. 545–51.

21 Glick, L., 'Deglycrrhizinated liquorice in peptic ulcer', *Lancet*, 1982, ii, p. 817.

22 Tewari, S.N. and Wilson, A.K., 'Deglycyrrhizinated liquorice in duodenal ulcer', *Practitioner*, 1972, 210, pp. 820–5.

23 Kassir, Z.A., 'Endoscopic controlled trial of four drug regimens in the treatment of chronic duodenal ulceration', *Irish Med. J.*, 1985, 78, pp. 153–6.

24 Cheney, G., 'Rapid healing of peptic ulcers in patients receiving fresh cabbage juice', *Cal. Med.*, 1949, 70, pp. 10–14.

25 Cheney, G., 'Anti-peptic ulcer dietary factor', *J. Am. Diet. Assoc.*, 1950, 26, pp. 668–72.

26 Shive, W., Snider, R.N., DuBiler, B., *et al.*, 'Glutamine in treatment of peptic ulcer', *Tex. J. Med.*, 1957, 53, pp. 840–3.

72 Vaginitis

1 The authors wish to acknowledge Dr Paul Reilly ND, from whose excellent chapter on vaginitis in Pizzorno, J.E. and Murray, M.A., *A Textbook of Natural Medicine* (John Bastyr College Publications, Seattle, WA, 1988) this chapter was derived.

2 Eschenbach, D., 'Vaginal infection', *Clin. Ob. Gyn.*, 1983, 26, pp. 186–202.

3 Woo, B. and Branch, W.T., 'Vaginitis', in Branch, W.T., *Office Practice of Medicine*, W.B. Saunders, Philadelphia, PA, 1982, pp. 461–70.

4 McCue, J., Kamanoff, A., Pass, T. and Friedland, G., 'Strategies for diagnosing vaginitis', *J. Fam. Prac.*, 1979, 9, pp. 395–402.

5 Stamey, T., 'The role of introital enterobacteria in recurrent urinary infections', *J. Urol.*, 1973, 109, pp. 467–72.

6 Netto, N.R., Rangel, P., Da Silva, R., *et al.*, 'The importance of vaginal infection on recurrent cystitis in women', *Int. Surg.*, 1979, 64, pp. 79–82.

7 Larsen, B. and Galask, R., 'Vaginal microbial flora: practical and theoretic relevance', *Ob. Gyn.*, 1980, 55 (supplement), pp. 100S–113S.

8 Meeker, C.I., 'Candidiasis – an obstinate problem', *Med. Times*, 1978, 106, pp. 26–32.

9 Gardner, H., 'Vulvovaginitis: prevalence and diagnosis', *Med. Times*, 1978, 106, pp. 21–5.

10 Hildebrandt, R.J., 'Trichomoniasis: always with us – but controllable', *Med. Times*, 1978, 106, pp. 44–8.

11 Holmes, K. and Handsfield, H., 'Sexually transmitted diseases', in Petersdorf, R. (ed.), *Harrison's Principles of Internal Medicine*, 10th ed., McGraw-Hill, New York, NY, 1983, pp. 889–902.

12 Miles, M.R., Olsen, L., Rogers, A., *et al.*, 'Recurrent vaginal candidiasis – importance of an intestinal reservoir', *J.A.M.A.*, 1977, 238, pp. 1,836–7.

13 Heidrich, F., Berg, A., Gergman, F., *et al.*, 'Clothing factors and vaginitis', *J. Fam. Prac.*, 1984, 19, pp. 491–4.

14 Kudelco, N., 'Allergy in chronic monilial vaginitis', *Ann. Allergy*, 1971, 29, pp. 266–7.

15 Fleury, F.J., 'Is there a "non-specific" vaginitis?', *Med. Times*, 1978, 106, pp. 37–43.

16 Vontver, L. and Eschenbach, D., 'The role of Gardnerella vaginalis in nonspecific vaginitis', *Clin. Ob. Gyn.*, 1981, 24, pp. 439–60.

17 Balsdon, M., Pead, L., Taylor, G. and Maskell, R., 'Corynebacterium vaginale and vaginitis: a controlled trial of treatment', *Lancet*, 1980, i, pp. 501–3.

18 Spiegel, C., Amsel, R., Exhenbach, D., *et al.*, 'Anaerobic bacteria in nonspecific vaginitis', *N.E.J.M.*, 1980, 303, pp. 601–7.

19 Holmes, K.K., 'The chlamydia epidemic', *J.A.M.A.*, 1981, 245, pp. 1,718–23.

20 Khatamee, M., 'Chlamydia mycoplasma: what are the hidden risks of these STDs?', *Mod. Med.*, 1984, 52, pp. 156–74.

21 Sirisnha, S., Daziy, M., Moongkarndi, P., *et al.*, 'Impaired local immune response in vitamin A deficient rats', *Clin. Exp. Immunol.*, 1980, 40, pp. 127–35.

22 Alexander, M.M., Newmark, H. and Miller, R., 'Oral betacarotene can increase the number of OKT4+ cells in human blood', *Immunol. Letters*, 1985, 9, pp. 221–4.

23 Sharaf, A. and Gomaa, N., 'Interrelationship between vitamins of the B-complex group and oestradiol', *J. Endo.*, 1974, 62, pp. 241–4.

24 Beisel, W.R., Edelman, R., Nauss, K., and Suskind, R., 'Single-nutrient effects on immunologic functions', *J.A.M.A.*, 1981, 245, pp. 53–8.

25 Stankova, L., Gerhardt, N., Nagel, L. and Bigley, R., 'Ascorbate and phagocyte function', *Inf. Immun.*, 1975, 12, pp. 252–6.

26 Havsteen, B., 'Flavonoids, a class of natural products of high pharmacological potency', *Biochem. Pharm.*, 1983, 32, pp. ,1,141–8.

27 Holden, M. and Resnick, R., 'The in-vitro action of synthetic crystalline vitamin C (ascorbic acid) on herpes virus', *J. Immunol.*, 1936, 31, pp. 455–62.

28 Terezhalmy, G., Bottomley, W. and Pelley, G., 'The use of water soluble bioflavonoid-ascorbic acid complex in the treatment of recurrent herpes labialis', *Oral Surg.*, 1978, 45, pp. 60–2.

29 Stephens, L., McChesney, A. and Nockels, C., 'Improved recovery of vitamin E treated lambs that have been experimentally infected with intertracheal chlamydia', *Br. Vet. J.*, 1979, 135, pp. 291–3.

30 Kavinoky, N.R., 'Vitamin E and the control of climacteric symptoms', *Ann. West. Med. Surg.*, 1950, 4, pp. 27–33.

31 Hain, A.M. and Sym, J.C.B., 'The control of menopausal flushes by vitamin E', *Br. Med. J.*, 1943, ii, pp. 8–9.

32 Christy, C.J., 'Vitamin E in menopause', *Am. J. Ob. Gyn.*, 1945, 50, pp. 84–7.

33 McLaren, H.C., 'Vitamin E in the menopause', *Br. Med. J.*, 1949, ii, pp. 1,378–81.

34 Watteville, H.D., Borth, R. and Gsell, M., 'Effect of dl-alpha-tocopherol acetate on progesterone metabolism', *J. Clin. Endo.*, 1948, 89, pp. 982–91.

35 Ant, M., 'Diabetic vulvovaginitis treated with vitamin E suppositories', *Am. J. Ob. Gyn.*, 1954, 67, pp. 407–10.

36 Finkler, R.S., 'The effect of vitamin E in the menopause', *J. Clin. Endo.*, 1949, 9, pp. 89–94.

37 Whitacre, F. and Barrera, B., 'War amenorrhea', *J.A.M.A.*, 1944, 124, pp. 399–403.

38 Pories, W., Henzel, J., Rob, C., and Strain, W., 'Acceleration of wound healing in man with zinc sulphate given by mouth', *Lancet*, 1967, i, pp. 121–4.

39 Sandstead, H., Lanier, V. Jr., Shepard, G., and Gillespie, D., 'Zinc and wound healing', *Am. J. Clin. Nut.*, 1970, 23, pp. 514–19.

40 Liszewski, R., 'The effect of zinc on wound healing: a collective review', *J. Am. Osteop. Assoc.*, 1981, 81, pp. 104–6.

41 Greenberg, S., Harris, D., Giles, P., *et al.*, 'Inhibition of Chlamydia trachomatis growth by zinc', *Antimicrob. Agents Chemo.*, 1985, 27, pp. 953–7.

42 Krieger, J. and Rein, M., 'Zinc sensitivity of Trichomonas vaginalis: in vitro studies and clinical implications', *J. Inf. Dis.*, 1982, 146, pp. 341–5.

43 Willmott, F., Say, J., Downey, D. and Hookham, A., 'Zinc and recalcitrant trichomoniasis' (letter), *Lancet*, 1983, i, p. 1,053.

44 Tennican, P., Carl, G., Frey, J., *et al.*, 'Topical zinc in the treatment of mice infected intravaginally with Herpes genitalis virus', *Proc. Soc. Exp. Bio. Med.*, 1980, 164, pp. 593–7.

45 Gordon, Y., Asher, Y. and Becker, Y., 'Irreversible inhibition of Herpes simplex virus replication in BSC-cells by zinc ions', *Antimicrob. Agents Chemo.*, 1975, 8, pp. 377–80.

46 Griffith, R., Norins, A.L. and Kagan, C., 'A multicentered study of lysine therapy in Herpes simplex infection', *Dermatologia*, 1978, 156, pp. 257–67.

47 McCune, M., Perry, H., Muller, S. and O'Fallon, W.M., 'Treatment of recurrent Herpes simplex infections with L-lysine monohydrochloride', *Cutis*, 1984, 34, pp. 366–73.

48 Lieb, J., 'Remission of recurrent herpes infection during therapy with lithium' (letter), *N.E.J.M.*, 1979, 301, p. 942.

49 Skinner, G., Hartley, C., Bucham, A., *et al.*, 'The effect of lithium chloride on the replication of Herpes simplex virus', *Med. Microbiol. Immunol.*, 1980, 168, pp. 139–48.

50 Mitchell, W., *Naturopathic Applications of the Botanical Remedies*, John Bastyr College Publications, Seattle, WA, 1983.

51 Madison, E., *Class Lectures in Botanical Medicines*, John Bastyr College of Naturopathic Medicine, Seattle, WA, 1984.

52 Mowbray, W., 'The antibacterial activity of chlorophyll', *Br. Med. J.*, 1957, i, pp. 268–70.

53 Goldberg, S., 'The use of water soluble chlorophyll in oral sepsis', *Am. J. Surg.*, 1943, 62, pp. 117–22.

54 Smith, L. and Livingston, A., 'Chlorophyll: an experimental study of its water soluble derivatives in wound healing', *Am. J. Surg.*, 1943, 62, pp. 358–69.

55 Sharma, V., Sethi, M.S., Kumar, A. and Rarotra, J.R., 'Antibacterial property of Allium sativum Linn: in vivo and in vitro studies', *Ind. J. Exp. Bio.*, 1977, 15, pp. 466–8.

56 Moore, G. and Atkins, R., 'The fungicidal and fungistatic effects of an aqueous garlic extract on medically important yeast-like fungi', *Mycologia*, 1977, 69, pp. 341–8.

57 Cavallito, C. and Bailey, J., 'Allicin, the antibacterial principle of Allium sativum. I. Isolation, physical properties and antibacterial action', *J. Am. Chem. Soc.*, 1944, 66, pp. 1,950–1.

58 Barone, F. and Tansey, M., 'Isolation, purification, identification, synthesis, and kinetics of activity of the anticandidal component of Allium sativum, and a hypothesis for its mode of action', *Mycologia*, 1977, 69, pp. 793–825.

59 Prat, M., 'Algunas consideraciones sobre la accion antibiotica del Allium sativum y sus preparados' (trans.), *Biol. Abstr.*, 1950, 24, p. 24,264.

60 Hahn, F. and Ciak, J., 'Berberine', *Antibiotics*, 1976, 3, pp. 577–88.

61 Sabir, M. and Bhide, N., 'Study of some pharmacological actions of berberine', *Ind. J. Phys. Pharm.*, 1971, 15, pp. 111–32.

62 Sabir, M., Mahajan, V., Mohaptra, L. and Bhide, N. 'Experimental study of the antitrachoma action of berberine', *Ind. J. Med. Res.*, 1976, 64, pp. 1,160–7.

63 Dutta, N. and Panse, M., 'Usefulness of berberine (an alkaloid from Berberis aristata) in the treatment of cholera (experimental)', *Ind. J. Med. Res.*, 1962, 50, pp. 732–5.

64 Punnonen, R. and Lukola, A., 'Oestrogen-like effect of ginseng', *Br. Med. J.*, 1980, 281, p. 1,110.

65 Dodds, E.C. and Lawson, W., 'A simple aromatic oestrogenic agent with an activity of the same order as that of oestrone', *Nature*, 1937, 139, pp. 627–8.

66 Zondeck, B. and Bergmann, E., 'Phenol methyl ethers as oestrogenic agents', *Biochem. J.*, 1938, 32, pp. 641–5.

67 Albert-Puleo, M., 'Fennel and anise as oestrogenic agents', *J. Ethnopharm.*, 1980, 2, pp. 337–44.

68 Kulshrestha, W.K., Singh, N., Saxena, R. and Kohli, R., 'A study of central pharmacological activity of alkaloid fraction of Apium graveolens Linn', *Ind. J. Med. Res.*, 1970, 58, pp. 99–102.

69 Pena, E.F., 'Maleluca alternafolia oil: its use for trichomonal vaginitis and other vaginal infections', *Ob. Gyn.*, 1962, 19, pp. 793–5.

70 Vincent, J., Veomett, R. and Riley, R., 'Antibacterial activity associated with Lactobacillus acidophilus', *J. Bact.*, 1959, 78, pp. 477–84.

71 Shook, D., 'A clinical study of a povidone iodine regimen for resistant vaginitis', *Curr. Ther. Res.*, 1963, 5, pp. 256–63.

72 Maneksha, S., 'Comparison of povidone iodine (Betadine) vaginal pessaries and lactic acid pessaries in the treatment of vaginitis', *J. Int. Med. Res.*, 1974, 2, pp. 236–9.

73 Reeve, P., 'The inactivation of Chlamydia trachomatis by povidone iodine', *J. Antimicrob. Chemo.*, 1976, 2, pp. 77–80.

74 Ratzen, J., 'Monilial and trichomonal vaginitis – topical treatment with povidone iodine treatments', *Cal. Med.*, 1969, 110, pp. 24–7.

75 Mayhew, S., 'Vaginitis: a study of the efficacy of povidone iodine in unselected cases', *J. Int. Med. Res.*, 1981, 9, pp. 157–9.

76 Gershenfeld, L., 'Povidone iodine as a trichomoniacide', *Am. J. Pharm.*, 1962, 134, pp. 324–31.

77 Gershenfeld, L., 'Povidone iodine as a vaginal microbicide', *Am. J. Pharm.*, 1962, 134, pp. 278–9.

78 Singha, H., 'The use of a vaginal cleansing kit in non-specific vaginitis', *Practitioner*, 1979, 223, pp. 403–4.

79 Swate, T. and Weed, J., 'Boric acid treatment of vulvovaginal candidiasis', *Ob. Gyn.*, 1974, 43, pp. 894–5.

80 Keller Van Slyke, K., 'Treatment of vulvovaginal candidiasis with boric acid powder', *Am. J. Ob. Gyn.*, 1981, 141, pp. 145–8.

73 Varicose veins

1 Rose, S., 'What causes varicose veins?' *Lancet*, 1986, i, pp. 320–1.

2 Berkow, R. (ed.), *The Merck Manual of Diagnosis and Therapy*, 14th ed., Merck & Co., Rahway, NJ, 1982, pp. 560–6.

3 Trowell, H., Burkitt, D., and Heaton, K., *Dietary Fibre, Fibre-Depleted Foods and Disease*, Academic Press, London, UK, 1985.

4 Vahouny, G. and Kritchevsky, D., *Dietary Fibre in Health and Disease*, Plenum Press, New York, NY, 1982.

5 Latto, C., Wilkinson, R.W. and Gilmore, O.J.A., 'Diverticular disease and varicose veins', *Lancet*, 1973, i, pp. 1,089–90.

6 Allegra, C., Pollari, G., Criscuolo, A., *et al.*, 'Centella asiatica extract in venous disorders of the lower limbs. Comparative clinico-instrumental studies with a placebo', *Clin. Terap.*, 1981, 99, pp. 507–13.

7 Monograph, *Centella asiatica*, Indena SpA, Milan, Italy, 1987.

8 Allegra, C., 'Comparative capillaroscopic study of certain bioflavonoids and total triterpenic fractions of Centella asiatica in venous insufficiency', *Clin. Terap.*, 1984, 110, p. 550.

9 Pointel, J.P., Boccalon, H., Cloarec, M., *et al.*, 'Titrated extract of Centella asiatica (TECA) in the treatment of venous insufficiency of the lower limbs', *Angiology*, 1987, 38, pp. 46–50.

10 Marastoni, F., Baldo, A., Redaelli, G. and Ghiringhelli, L., 'Centella asiatica extract in venous pathology of the lower limbs and its evaluation as compared with tribenoside', *Minerva-Cardioangiol.*, 1982, 30, pp. 201–7.

11 Felter, H.W. and Lloyd, J.U., *King's American Dispensatory*, 18th ed., 1898; reprinted by Eclectic Medical Publications, Portland, OR, 1983, pp. 990–2.

12 Aichinger, F., Giss, G. and Vogel, G., 'Neue befunde zur pharmakodynamik von bioflavoiden und des rosskastanien saponins aescin als grundlage ihrer anwendung in der therapie', *Arzneim-Forsch.*, 1964, 14, p. 892.

13 Manca, P. and Passarelli, E., 'Aspetti farmacologici dell'escina, principio attivo dell'aesculus hyppocastanum', *Clin. Terap.*, 1965, 32, pp. 297–328.

14 Annoni, F., Mauri, A., Marincola, F. and Resele, L.F., 'Venotonic activity of escin on the human saphenous vein', *Arzneim-Forsch.*, 1979, 29, pp. 672–5.

15 Lucas, J., 'Erfahrungen mit Aescin in der internen therapie', *Med. Wel.*, 1963, 14, p. 913.

16 Monograph, *Butcher's Broom*, Indena SpA, Milan, Italy, 1987.

17 Capra, C., 'Studio farmacologico e tossicologico di componenti del Ruscus aculeatus', *Fitoterapia*, 1972, 43, p. 99.

18 Marcelon, G., Verbeuren, T.J., Lauressergues, H. and Vanhoutte, P.M., 'Effect of Ruscus aculeatus on isolated canine cutaneous veins', *Gen. Pharmacol.*, 1983, 14, p. 103.

19 Gabor, M. 'Pharmacologic effects of flavonoids on blood vessels', *Angiologica*, 1972, 9, pp. 355–74.

20 Kuhnau, J., 'The flavonoids. A class of semi-essential food components: their role in human nutrition', *World Review Nutrition and Dietetics*, 1976, 24, pp. 117–91.

21 Pourrat, H., 'Anthocyanidin drugs in vascular disease', *Plant Med. Phytothera.*, 1977, 11, pp. 143–51.

22 Kreysel, H.W., Nissen, H.P. and Enghoffer, E., 'A possible role of lysosomal enzymes in the pathogenesis of varicosis and the reduction in their serum activity by venostasin', *V.A.S.A.*, 1983, 12, pp. 377–82.

23 Visudhiphan, S., Poolsuppasit, S., Piboonnakarintr, O. and Tumliang, S., 'The relationship between high fibrinolytic activity and daily capsicum ingestion in Thais', *Am. J. Clin. Nutr.*, 1982, 35, pp. 1,452–8.

24 Bordia, A.K., Josh, H.K. and Sanadhya, Y.K., 'Effect of garlic oil on fibrinolytic activity in patient with CHD', *Atherosclerosis*, 1977, 28, pp. 155–9.

25 Baghurst, K.I., Raj, M.J. and Truswell, A.S., 'Onions and platelet aggregation', *Lancet*, 1977, i, p. 101.

26 Srivastava, K., 'Effects of aqueous extracts of onion, garlic and ginger on the platelet aggregation and metabolism of arachidonic acid in the blood vascular system: in vitro study, *Prost. Leukotri. Med.*, 1984, 13, pp. 227–35.

27 Ako, H., Cheung, A. and Matsura, P., 'Isolation of a fibrinolysis enzyme activator from commercial bromelain', *Arch. Int. Pharmacodyn.*, 1981, 254, pp. 157–67.

Useful Addresses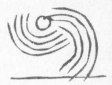

Physician Referral Sources

British Naturopathic and Osteopathic Association
Frazer House
6 Netherhall Gardens
London NW3 5RR
United Kingdom

Institute for Complementary Medicine
21 Portland Place
London W1N 3AF
United Kingdom

American Association of Naturopathic Physicians
P.O. Box 20386
Seattle, WA 98112
USA

Naturopathic Medical Schools

British College of Naturopathy and Osteopathy
Frazer House
6 Netherhall Gardens
London NW3 5RR
United Kingdom

National College of Naturopathic Medicine
11231 S.E. Market Street
Portland, OR 97216
USA

Bastyr College
144 N.E. 54th Street
Seattle, WA 98105
USA

Comprehensive information on suppliers and resources may be found in *Green Pages* (Macdonald Optima).

Index

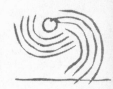

☐ Pears Medical Encyclopaedia	Dr Bennett/Dr Brown	£9.99
☐ RCN Manual of Family Health	Royal College of Nursing	£12.50
☐ Woman's Book of Yoga	Louise Taylor	£9.99
☐ The Body Shop Book	The Body Shop Team	£12.99
☐ Complete Handbook of Pregnancy	Wendy Rose-Neil	£14.99
☐ The Personal Touch	Dr Glen Wilson	£14.99
☐ The Intimate Touch	Dr Glen Wilson	£14.99

Little, Brown and Company now offers an exciting range of quality titles by both established and new authors. All of the books in this series are available from:

Little, Brown & Company (UK),
P.O. Box 11,
Falmouth,
Cornwall TR10 9EN.

Alternatively you may fax your order to the above address. Fax No. 01326 317444.

Payments can be made as follows: cheque, postal order (payable to Little, Brown and Company) or by credit cards, Visa/Access. Do not send cash or currency. UK customers and B.F.P.O. please allow £1.00 for postage and packing for the first book, plus 50p for the second book, plus 30p for each additional book up to a maximum charge of £3.00 (7 books plus). Overseas customers including Ireland, please allow £2.00 for the first book plus £1.00 for the second book, plus 50p for each additional book.

NAME (Block Letters) _____

ADDRESS _____

_____

_____

☐ I enclose my remittance for £ _____
☐ I wish to pay by Access/Visa Card

Number ☐☐☐☐☐☐☐☐☐☐☐☐☐☐☐☐

Card Expiry Date _____